INDUSTRIAL THERAPY

INDUSTRIAL THERAPY

Edited by

Glenda L. Key, P.T.

President and Founder
KEY Method
Minneapolis, Minnesota

with 354 illustrations

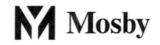 Mosby

A Harcourt Health Sciences Company

St. Louis   London   Philadelphia   Sydney   Toronto

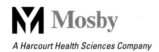

A Harcourt Health Sciences Company

Executive Editor: Martha Sasser
Associate Developmental Editor: Kellie F. White
Editorial Assistant: Amy Dubin
Production and Editing: Diane B. Oehler, Publishers Services, Inc.
Manufacturing Supervisor: Karen Lewis
Design: Julie Anderson, Publishers Services, Inc.

To my Mother—for her quiet bravery.

First Edition
Copyright © 1995 by Mosby, Inc.

Printed in the United States of America

Mosby, Inc.
11830 Westline Industrial Drive
St. Louis, Missouri 63146

ISBN 0-8151-5046-6
00010203 98765432

CONTRIBUTORS' LIST

Mark L. Anderle, MS, CRC, CIRS
National Rehabilitation Consultants
Roseville, Minnesota

Mark A. Anderson, MA, PT
The Saunders Group
Chaska, Minnesota

D'Arcy Bain, BPT, CAT(c)
D'Arcy Bain Physiotherapy
Winnipeg, Manitoba
Canada

Ronald E. Bates
Executive Vice President
KEY Method
Minneapolis, Minnesota

Susan M. Brookins, PT, OTR/L, MS
St. Joseph Medical Center
Industrial Rehabilitation
Joliet, Illinois

Peter M. Budnick
Dept. of Mechanical Engineering
University of Utah
Salt Lake City, Utah

Oliver Corbeel, PT
Holmes Regional Medical Center
Melbourne, Florida

Linda M. Demers, PT
Saco, Maine

Ed Dobrzykowski, MHS, PT, ATC
Formations in Health Care, Inc.
Chicago, Illinois

Douglas H. Frey, MS, PT
Elmira, New York

James A. Gould, MS, PT
Options Physical Therapy
LaCrosse, Wisconsin

Stephanie Hatlestad, PT, ATC, MBA
Minnetonka, Minnesota

John Hilson, Jr., PT
Alden Industrial Rehabilitation Center
Meadville, Pennsylvania

Robert L. Karol, PhD, LP
Karol Neuropsychological Services & Consulting
Eden Prairie, Minnesota

Glenda L. Key, PT
KEY Method
Minneapolis, Minnesota

Robert B. King, PT
HealthFocus
Lakewood, Colorado

Tom G. Mayer, MD
PRIDE
Dallas, Texas

Michael S. Melnik, MS, OTR
Prevention Plus
Minneapolis, Minnesota

Denise M. Miller, OT
KEY Method
Minneapolis, Minnesota

Philip C. Moe, PT
Midwest Back Center
Sioux Falls, South Dakota

Cherilyn G. Murer, JD, CRA
Murer Consultants
Joliet, Illinois

Richard W. Nelson, MA, CRC, CIRS
Director
National Rehabilitation Consultants
Roseville, Minnesota

Jane O'Callaghan, BS, MED, PT, OT
TOC Consulting
Toronto, Ontario
Canada

H. Duane Saunders, MS, PT
The Saunders Group
Chaska, Minnesota

Robin Saunders, MS, PT
Saunders Therapy Centers
St. Paul, Minnesota

Gary J. Smith, EdD, PT
Eastern Washington University
Department of Physical Therapy
Cheney, Washington

Mark R. Stultz, MSIE, PT
The Saunders Group
Chaska, Minnesota

Sharon Switzer-McIntyre, BSci, PT
TOC Consulting
Toronto, Ontario
Canada

Anne K. Tramposh, MS, PT, CIRS
Advantage Health
Kansas City, Missouri

Robert L. Volski, PT, ATC, CES
Fort Myers, Florida

David R. Worth, BAS, MAS, PhD
Rankin Occupational Safety and Health
North Adelaide
Australia

PREFACE

The medical community has been tossed upside down in recent years. As a result, opportunities have opened up for therapists to have an impact on industry like never before.

With that in mind, this textbook was compiled to give direction on how to deliver and implement high quality, successful programs that yield measurable results in industry. This medical-industrial relationship has blossomed into a spectrum of worker care opportunities. Safe job placement upon hire, injury prevention, functional capacity assessment for safe return to work, job analysis, job modification, Work Hardening, and Work Conditioning are but a few services now being sought after by industry.

Whether the reader is a student just beginning their professional journey, a practicing therapist ex-ploring the opportunities and challenges of Industrial Therapy, or an experienced Industrial Therapist, this book will be a valuable resource to guide you in the concept, the philosophy, and the how-to's of each category.

The thirty-one experts who have contributed their knowledge and experience in these pages represent active practitioners in private practice clinics, hospitals, and industrial settings across the United States, and in Canada and Australia. They bring the reader an orientation toward real-world applications and real-world consequences.

It is intended, therefore, for readers to be able to apply this expertise in their own practices and meet these opportunities with confidence and success.

Glenda L. Key

ACKNOWLEDGMENTS

An edited textbook such as this is not possible without the commitment, generosity, and hard work of many people. I first wish to acknowledge and thank all of the contributors for the time and energy they took out of their already busy schedules. Their efforts and willingness to share their expertise and experience contributes to the growth of others in Industrial Therapy and to the profession as a whole. The Providers of KEY Method deserve recognition for this text, in that they provide a constant source of professional encouragement and motivation. It is their sharing of experiences along with their dedication and trust that help us advance in this specialized field. I also want to acknowledge and thank my superb staff who, with their dedication to quality, backed me up and cheered me on throughout this process.

I thank the numerous academicians who encouraged the writing of this book for their use in the education of our future therapists. And, I thank those who have been inspirational or encouraging in these efforts including Marilyn Moffat, Mary Lou Barnes, Rosemary Skully, Jim Gould, George Davies, Gary Soderberg, Jan Richardson, Annette Iglarsh, Trish Montgomery, and David Worth. At Mosby, I am grateful to Martha Sasser for her acumen, and to Kellie White for her patience and persistence. Lance Nelson deserves a great deal of credit and I thank him for working tirelessly with me on this project, keeping the process moving with humor and tenacity.

I want to acknowledge and thank my family for their unwavering support in all that I do. A special thank you to Ron Bates, my husband, partner and dear friend for his vision, encouragement, and belief in me.

To all of you who read this, I thank you for contributing to the efforts of *Industrial Therapy*. It is truly through your interest, actions, and interactions that this distinct body of study will continue to develop further within our profession.

Glenda Key

"Think you can or think you can't
Either way you'll be right"
Anonymous

INTRODUCTION

Industrial Therapy (IT) is a term chosen to refer to the full range of worker-oriented endeavors designed to keep them healthy and productive, and if injured, to restore them to maximum job function as quickly and as cost-effectively as possible.

Readers may have seen or used terms such as "industrial medicine" or "industrial rehabilitation" in reference to Physicians or Therapists restoring function to injured body parts. What is now being done for the worker, however, goes beyond treating injuries. Therapists are implementing an increasing variety of measures that focus on education, capability strengthening, job matching, ergonomics, attitude and behavioral change, and a host of other approaches to enhance wellness and prevent injuries. The term "Industrial Therapy" is used to encompass this expanded spectrum of modalities that has evolved.

What began as a basic focus on alleviating pain and healing the injured body part has been transformed and enlarged to include a comprehensive body of disciplines. Industrial Therapy is a rapidly emerging field which links the medical and industrial communities. It draws together the expertise and resources of medicine, engineering, and industry. The field includes Physical Therapists, Occupational Therapists, Physicians, Rehabilitation Counselors, Exercise Physiologists, hospital and insurance administrators, and other managers and health care workers. Virtually every aspect of working life is given attention, where the attention proves to expedite goals, reduce costs, or enhance the bottom line.

The purpose of this book is to examine and illustrate the role that Therapists play in each aspect of the Industrial Therapy continuum, and how the multiplicity of disciplines are applied toward the emerging concept of industrial "wellness." Therapists' role in worker wellness is ever-expanding, and their interactions with the other professionals are continuously changing.

The evolution of a field is often driven by changes in thinking and philosophy. One way to trace the evolution of Industrial Therapy is to follow the change in mind-set regarding what should happen when a worker becomes injured.

The Medical Model

In the beginning, the prevailing wisdom could be described as follows:

> *When a worker is injured, steps must be taken to alleviate the pain and heal the injured body part, after which the worker is ready to go back to work.*

In this "medical model," the physician was the principal, and in many cases, the only provider treating the patient throughout the acute care, rehabilitation, and return-to-work phases. Therapists, if involved, received the referral from the physician and were a subordinate appendage in the process.

The major deficiency in this approach was that the release criteria for returning to work—alleviated pain and healed body parts—were not necessarily related to the worker's ability to resume specific job functions. As a result, workers often returned to the job deconditioned or unable to perform the job, without changing improper workstyles that may have originally caused the injury. High rates of reinjury were the consequence.

Conditioning Orientation

Gradually, Physicians, Therapists, employers, and other stakeholders realized that deconditioned workers represented a risk, and that a modification in thinking was required:

> *The worker is not ready to resume work until the healed body part and other musculoskeletal functions have been restrengthened to levels required by job demands.*

To effectuate this approach, practitioners placed workers in a reconditioning phase following pain alleviation and healing. This was typically accomplished by by strengthening programs using conventional weight training equipment and methods. Although these programs represented an advance over no program, some deficiences remained. The postures, motions, and number of repetitions on weight training equipment did not necessarily replicate those required by the job. For this reason, certain workers were still being returned to the job at risk.

Functional Orientation

Over time, through observation, trial and error, practitioners' thinking evolved further. They began to assess and plan in terms of an injured worker's ability to execute the real-world job in terms of specific postures, motions, and resistances, not just once or ten times, but as many times and for as long as the work day required. As these considerations took hold, the focus shifted from healing and general conditioning to restoring real-world job functions.

A new mind-set thus emerged:

> *More is needed than alleviating pain, healing and conditioning the injured body part. The worker must be able to perform the specific job tasks under the requisite conditions and time frame.*

Under this evolved thinking, the rehabilitation process began to incorporate job function–oriented assessment, planning and rehabilitation. A Functional Capacity Assessment (FCA) was performed to determine the worker's static and dynamic capabilities and limits. Job Analysis (JA) was included to methodically identify the specific job demands, risk points, and functional requirements. Work Conditioning evolved from traditional weight training to include simulating specific job postures and motions.

This functional orientation achieved more complete restoration of job function, faster return to work, and reduced reinjury rates. But a new set of problems soon became apparent.

Psychosocial Factors

An injury that interrupts a person's working life dramatically impacts the worker's self-esteem, peer group acceptance, family life, and social life. These psychosocial impediments can often present a greater hurdle than the physiological needs. Therapists discovered that restoring function is more than a matter of musculoskeletal exercise and strengthening for this category of injured worker. Often, psychosocial factors have to be addressed along with the musculoskeletal rehabilitation.

Industrial Therapy thinking evolved further:

> *Restoring job function is often inhibited by dramatic changes in the injured worker's self-esteem, peer group acceptance, employer relationship, family life, social life, and fear of reinjury. Rehabilitation must therefore focus on the "whole person."*

With this additional enlightenment, the rehabilitation process began to include intervention by psychologists and counselors, the development of classes for insight and coping strategies, and the inclusion of workers, peers, and family at appropriate stages in the rehabilitation process. The addition of psychosocial components to Work Conditioning is now referred to as Work Hardening.

Prevention Education

Rehabilitating the "whole person" through functional orientation and psychosocial intervention has yielded desired outcomes faster and more cost-efficiently, but the total costs of injuries have continued to rise. As a result, employers, payors, and enlightened providers have been progressively more receptive to the concept of preventing injuries in the first place, giving rise to yet another advance in thinking:

> *Injuries can be averted in the first place if workers can be taught safer workstyles and accident prevention strategies.*

The prevention concept began with a focus on the back—safe postures, lifting, and materials handling techniques—because back injuries have always been the most common and costly category of industrial disability. Typically, education took the form of classes to heighten awareness and demonstrate proper techniques. In many cases noticeable improvements in workstyles and injury rates would occur following such programs, but within a few months, old habits and injury rates would often return.

Prevention Process

Gradually, employers and providers realized that a prevention program must be more than a short-term event. It must be a process that is companywide, continuous, and an integral part of the organization's culture. This thinking can be represented as follows:

> *Changes in behavior, in the form of safer workstyles, do not endure unless they are accompanied by a change in attitude on the part of top management, supervisors, and workers.*

Accordingly, successful approaches to prevention begin by gaining the commitment and support of top management. Input is obtained from department managers, supervisors, and employees, so the program can be tailored to fit the organization's unique needs, and everyone has a sense of ownership in the final design. Top management is encouraged to provide the authority and resources to empower managers and supervisors to implement and maintain the program.

Changes in prevention behavior and attitudes have significantly reduced the incidence of injury, but another opportunity for improvement has been gaining recognition.

Preventative Job Placement

Some workers are at risk in a job, even if their attitude and workstyles are as healthy as possible. Certain musculoskeletal attributes may not be compatible with the specific demands of a particular job. Thinking along these lines can be expressed as follows:

Changing attitude, behavior, and workstyles are insufficient if the worker is poorly matched to the demands of the job.

Physicians began using x-ray information to make job matching decisions, while Therapists attempted to relate flexibility and mobility information to job capabilities. Some practitioners began to think in terms of using Functional Capacity Assessments to ensure safer, healthier job placement. But since FCAs are more extensive than is required for this specialized purpose, a scaled-down job matching tool called Job Placement Assessment (JPA) evolved. At the same time, job requirements were being more thoroughly identified and analyzed in what was becoming known as Job Analysis (JA). Eventually, JPA and JA were used in combination to complete the job matching equation. However, the scope of Job Analysis used preventatively in placement decisions is an abbreviated version of the complete JA used for post injury rehabilitation planning.

Safer job placement has reduced injury rates, but there remained instances in which certain jobs still represented risk given the worker's particular musculoskeletal attributes. In some cases, this has been addressed with Work Conditioning, but therapists are increasingly adding a focus on job modification and redesign.

Ergonomics

At some point during the course of selecting workers to fit the job, it was inevitable that therapists would begin thinking in terms of modifying jobs to fit the worker. What has become known as ergonomics is based on this point of view:

Matching the worker's capabilities to the job is insufficient if the job environment or work station is unsafe. It is often better to modify the job to fit the worker.

Ergonomic assessment has become a component in a growing number of Job Analyses, with the information used to correct environmental risks, redesign workstations, and even redesign the tools used on the job.

Beyond Injury Orientation

The foregoing discussion covered the enhancements that have evolved beyond the traditional medical model: conditioning, functional orientation, psychosocial intervention, prevention education and processes, job placement, job modification, and ergonomics. Injury prevention and rehabilitation have been significantly advanced in the process.

Taking a step back, however, it can be seen that most of these strategies are driven from a negative orientation toward reacting to injury or preventing injury. It is generally recognized that avoiding a negative is an inferior strategy to striving for a positive. Playing to win is better than playing to avoid losing. The best defense is a good offense. Accordingly, even with a growing awareness of the many successful ways to reduce injuries, and the benefits of doing so, "prevention" is still a hard sell. When an employer or employee must be convinced to adopt a new attitude or new behavior, they are more effectively persuaded if they see the outcome in positive terms.

For this reason, people in the field of Industrial Therapy have sought ways to position activities with a more positive orientation. The answer for many has been the concept of wellness:

"Avoiding injury" is a negative mind-set that gives rise to defensive thinking and reduced motivation. "Employees who live healthy, feel good, and do their best" is a more positive orientation from which to drive innovation and gain employer and employee acceptance.

The positive prospect of a healthier, happier, more productive workforce is a more positive call to action than an injury avoidance mind-set. A more emotionally engaging image has a better chance of persuading employers to inaugurate a number of programs they might otherwise postpone or forego under an avoidance mentality.

Many companies are introducing on-the-job stretching and exercise sessions, formal and informal educational programs, and home study and exercise. Therapists are finding that under the banner of industrial "wellness," these programs are gaining greater acceptance and popularity.

Beyond Wellness Orientation

To many employers operating under a bottom line orthodoxy, "wellness" can be dismissed as simply a "feel good" term that might be desirable, but not practical or affordable in today's global competitive arena. For this reason, a further orientation is evolving:

> *What we're really talking about here is productivity. Injuries hamper productivity. Expeditious return to work restores it. Improved functional capacities increase it. Prevention protects it. Ergonomics facilitates it. Wellness supports productivity.*

Economists and business leaders understand that the major advantage American industry holds in the global economy is productivity per worker. The American worker still produces more value than anyone else, and this translates to a higher standard of living.

As other countries acquire the technology, capital, economic systems, and infrastructure to challenge this position, American industry must seek innovative advantages in other aspects of the equation—new ways to increase productivity and lower the cost of doing business. When rates of injury are reduced; when injured workers are returned to productivity faster; when jobs are redesigned to fit the worker; when wellness becomes part of a company's culture; with each new advance in Industrial Therapy, employers, payors, and therapists have seen that the benefits outweigh the costs. Productivity increases and costs decrease. In this light, Industrial Therapy can be seen as a major component of a strategy to ensure that American productivity remains on the cutting edge of global economic activity.

CONTENTS

I

Industrial Therapy in the Contemporary Workplace

James A. Gould

Susan M. Brookins

Glenda L. Key

Ed Dobrzykowski

Denise M. Miller

Linda M. Demers

1

What Is Industrial Therapy?

James A. Gould

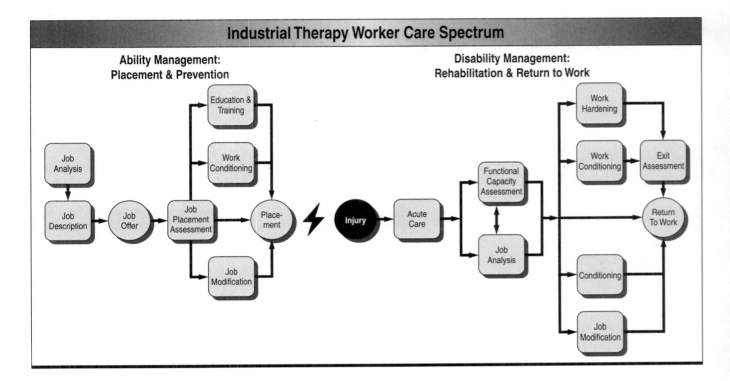

Industrial Therapy is a system which encompasses a wide spectrum of treatment based upon the principle that a person working in industry, as anywhere else, has physical, emotional, vocational, educational, psychological, and sociological needs which must be met to gain successful employment, or in the case of injury, rehabilitated, and reemployed.[19]

Industrial Therapy evolved from the realization that musculoskeletal problems rank second only to acute respiratory conditions such as the flu or common cold as a cause of work loss days. The spine is identified as the most commonly affected area of the musculoskeletal system, followed by lower and upper extremities.[9,10,16,17,18,31]

Formerly, the traditional medical model was the customary solution for treating injured workers. Presently, to deal with rising costs of Workers' Compensa-

tion claims, insurance premiums, medical care, litigation, lost productivity, and the advent of regulations such as the Americans with Disabilities Act (ADA), additional components of treatment and therapy are utilized to accelerate return-to-work, enhance worker capabilities, reduce injury and reinjury rates, lower costs, and lessen exposure to legal and regulatory problems. Utilizing both new and traditional aspects of the medical model comprise the worker care continuum known as Industrial Therapy.

This chapter describes and discusses each aspect of Industrial Therapy, from its role in hiring and job placement, to injury prevention, and injured worker rehabilitation. A review of the traditional medical model of treatment will provide insight into why many new treatment approaches in Industrial Therapy have emerged.

TRADITIONAL MEDICAL MODEL

The medical model has evolved and helped a multitude of people. Traditional medicine continues to be instrumental in rehabilitation, especially in acute care phases. Other conditions and procedures have been introduced into the rehabilitation process, in an attempt to yield the best outcome for the worker at an affordable cost to the employer.

It is important to note that we are not examining shortcomings in medical people, but only certain medical *processes* that have not fully met the more specialized requirements of Industrial Therapy.

Intervention vs Prevention

Despite genuine concern for prevention, the traditional model has been treatment orientated. In most cases, it is reverted to when the "pound of cure" is invariably more expensive than a more proactive, preventive approach, thus creating problems.

Recognizing the benefits of proactive prevention, Industrial Therapy has incorporated many elements of assessment, risk identification, education, and preventive activities to intercept problems before they occur, or become more costly.

Real World Context

Originally a doctor cared for most patients in their own homes. Home visits provided some input to the physician as to what would be expected of the patient during recovery. Rehabilitation could be directed to functional outcomes, using home activities and household effects which would be an integral part of the patient's daily routine.

As physicians cut back on home care, they became one more step removed from their patients and the environment within which they live and work. Therefore, the traditional model tends to separate the worker both physically and mentally from the work place. The medical clinic and rehabilitation site are apt to be located away from the work place, and exercise programs are often accomplished without relating them to functions required therein.

The examination procedure begins with the patient relating the history of onset through verbal description, without audio or visual aids. The medical practitioner then does not effectively envision the work place, the tasks required, the type of movements and number of repetitions leading up to the incident, the parameters of the physical environment, or the psychodynamics of the worker-supervisor or worker-worker interaction. With all input coming from the patient, the quality of the analysis is directly related to the patient's ability to accurately provide verbal description. There is rarely on-site analysis (Figures 1.1, *A*, *B*).

Further, the physical examination is conducted using the planar movements of flexion-extension, lateral flexion, and rotation to each side. In some situations, combined movements are utilized in the examination, but seldom is there actual loading of the patient with the size and weight of the object which caused the injury. There is no assessment of the patient's ability to function with the load at the particular heights or directions of the work situation or injurious movement.

After the examination and subsequent tests, conducted in the clinic, a diagnosis is made and a plan of remediation is adopted. This plan may include further examination and evaluation which is again conducted at the office of the specialist with the only link between the incident, the work place, and the injury being the patient's ability to accurately describe details to the practitioner.

In its quest for outcomes that work in the real world, Industrial Therapy has integrated the real world context into several points in the care continuum. Simulating not just physical, but also psychological and interpersonal job aspects during assessment and treatment results in a more efficient, more successful return to work.

Patient Involvement and Empowerment

Traditional medicine's evolution has been characterized by shifting progressively more power and control from the patient to the provider. The patient's role is essentially passive.

Today, in most instances, the sick or injured travel to the physician's office. This transfer from "their" environment to the doctor's environment should be understood, as it constitutes a shift in power and control from the patient to the physician.[28]

Characteristic long waits at the physicians office can also create anxiety and increases the person's concentration on the injury. A well known aspect of pain modulation is that pain perception increases when a person concentrates on it. Long waits for treatment can undermine the development of a positive attitude.

Finally, involvement is reduced by having a subordinate employee (nurse, receptionist) instruct the patient to disrobe for examination and diagnosis. In addition to further depersonalizing the treatment, this practice also precludes the medical practitioner from observing at least some functional movement; the act of undressing and the biomechanical movements allowed or impaired by the injury.

FIGURE 1.1   **A,** In a traditional physical examination, the worker is separated physically and mentally from the work place. **B,** With Industrial Therapy, injured workers capabilities and limitations are examined within job and functional contexts.

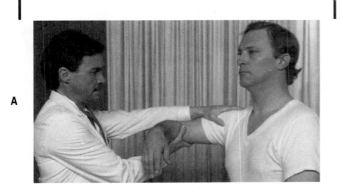

A

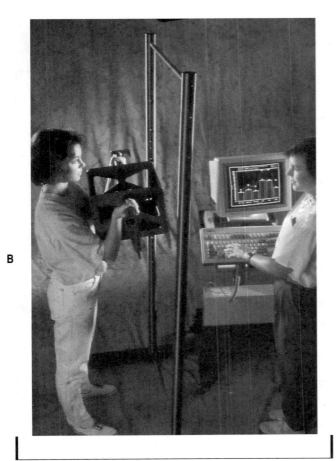

B

In summary, to seek medical help in the traditional model, the patient is often treated impersonally in a foreign setting which is sterile and devoid of most familiar and comforting aspects.

Recognizing the benefits of gaining the injured worker's commitment and maximum effort, Industrial Therapy has sought to increase the worker's involvement in their rehabilitation, and to provide more support and empowerment to achieve success.

Psychological Factors

The medical practitioner in the traditional model has been conditioned to approach a work related injury with suspicion—that injured workers are "malingerers until proven innocent." This image of the malingering patient is fueled by a minority of injured workers who try to exaggerate their symptoms in order to increase benefits or prolong the term of disability. But the stereotype rubs off on all injured workers. As a result, in the traditional medical model, the patient with a work related injury is surrounded by doubts as to the validity of the injury and its effects upon the body.

To preclude negative attitudes and to foster positive ones, Industrial Therapy has integrated a "presumption of innocence" into the process, which facilitates unprejudiced decisions and creates a more supportive environment.

Resource Coordination

In the traditional medical model, once all tests and examinations have been completed, a diagnosis is made and a rehabilitation program is established. In many situations, a patient is only treated by one specialist at a time.

On completion of an introductory course of treatment with a Physical Therapist, a patient may be passed on to another practitioner, like an Occupational Therapist, with nothing more than a written document to bridge the transfer. Any psychological intervention being conducted with the patient is not available to these specialists, as this remains confidential. If psychological intervention is mentioned in the record, however, it automatically prejudices the candidate in a negative manner for all who read the chart.

Recognizing the benefits of interdisciplinary coordination and communication, Industrial Therapy has instituted a teamwork approach to rehabilitation. In addition, psychosocial considerations are integrated into the care continuum at several points to instill confidence and a positive mind set (Figures 1.2, A, B).

The Rehabilitation Center

In the traditional medical model, the patient is sent for rehabilitation with clinically-based programs which utilize planar movements, often without the effects of gravity, and with stabilization which is not present in their normal functional movement patterns in the real world. Repetitions of activities are kept within easily monitored numbers, such as ten repetitions repeated from one to five times per day. The number of repetitions required of the worker and the forces produced are often not correlated to the demands of the job.

For example, Williams flexion exercises, frequently utilized for back rehabilitation, are completed in a supine position, non-weight bearing, and require repetitions of five to fifteen. It is easy to see that this does not translate to an eight hour day in which a person is expected to lift boxes weighing 15 pounds once every minute with a ten minute break after two hours and a half hour lunch.

Another example is the use of cuff weights, or an NK table for knee rehabilitation in which a person is required to lift a percentage of his or her maximum capacity ten times at a self-selected velocity. These exercises under-replicate the person's normal walking speed. Studies show that the average self-selected velocity of a person on an NK table lifting a manageable weight is 60 degrees per second and slows as the weight is increased.[6] Other studies show that the knee's average velocity during normal walking is 240 degrees per second. This means that a person successfully completing an NK table program is capable of walking only one fourth normal speed. In addition, it has been shown that although training at faster speeds develops strength at slower speeds, training at slower speeds does not similarly translate upward.[6] As a consequence, the patient is released back to work and leisure with inadequate capabilities and vulnerability to future risks.

FIGURE 1.2 Comparative resource coordination. **A,** The traditional medical model sequential approach; and, **B,** The Industrial Therapy model team approach.

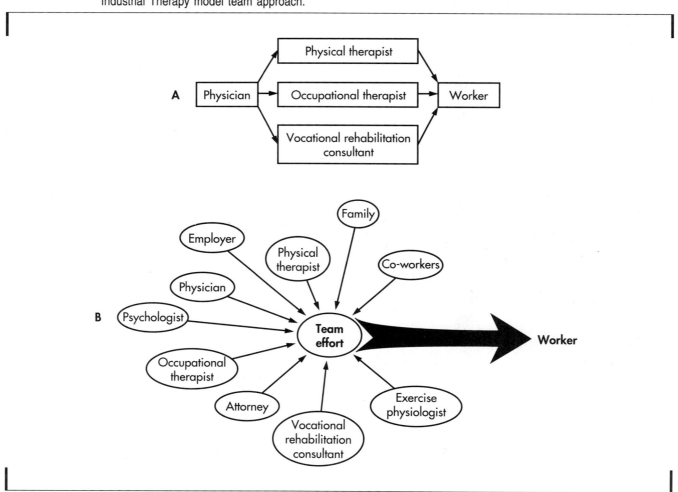

To ensure that restored capabilities hold up in the real world, Industrial Therapy has integrated a great deal of precise simulation into its strengthening, Work Conditioning, and Work Hardening programs (Figures 1.3, A, B).

Return to Work

In the traditional model, a person returns to work only when discharged from all medical services, and cannot seek follow-up treatment without jeopardizing job status. The person often returns to work without guidance or support to an eight hour work day, on a job which initially created the injury, and an appointment to see the physician in charge after four weeks.

In some situations, a "light work" detail is arranged at the work place to ease the person back into the job (Figure 1.4, page 8). This sounds good, but in reality the light work is typically not related to their normal work assignment. In addition, management looks on the worker in this position in a negative manner, and their coworkers may ridicule the worker. This negative atmosphere undermines the worker's assimilation back into the work environment.

Industrial Therapy goes to great lengths to analyze actual job demands so treatment is focused on rebuilding and strengthening the capabilities necessary to return to that job, or a modified version of the job. In addition, psychosocial aspects are incorporated in the rehabilitation process to further facilitate readjustments required at work, home, and in the community.

Summary

The medical model has followed processes that although workable in many contexts, requires the incorporation of new components and approaches to provide the best outcome for the injured worker at an affordable cost to the employer.

The evolution of Industrial Therapy has been driven by the need for more successful and cost effec-

FIGURE 1.3 Injured workers are strengthened in simulated environments **(A)** so that progress translates to real-world job capabilities **(B).**

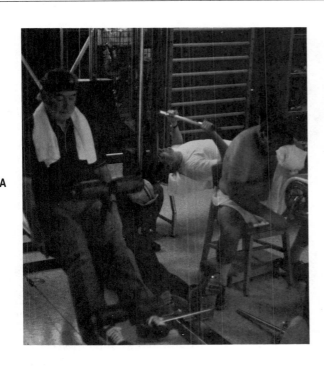
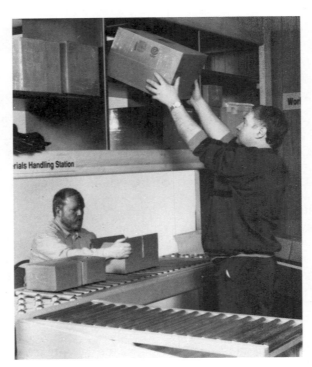

(1.3, **A,** From Cardiopulmonary Physical Therapy, 2nd Edition, Irwin & Tecklin)

FIGURE 1.4 Interim "light work" can sometimes be demeaning or demoralizing to the worker on the mend.

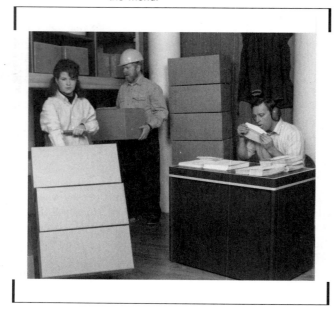

tive approaches to worker wellness and rehabilitation. Advancements have been accomplished by:

1. Increasing the focus on prevention
2. Bringing more real world context into rehabilitation procedures
3. Increasing worker involvement and empowerment in the process
4. Developing a teamwork orientation
5. Fostering more positive perceptions and attitudes
6. Providing more comprehensive preparation and support to facilitate reintegration into the working world

THE WORKER CARE SPECTRUM

Industrial Therapy today is multifaceted to mirror the many aspects of the worker/work-site interaction. Proper intervention is not only physical but educational and emotional as well, both pre and post injury.[14]

The Worker Care Spectrum schematic developed by KEY Method in Minneapolis (see page 3) provides an excellent visualization of the areas comprising the Industrial Therapy continuum of care. Industrial Therapy involves a variety of persons and specialties working with optimal interaction to move the patient rapidly toward the goal of good health. It is important to note that Industrial Therapy focuses on both treating disability and enhancing ability.

Each aspect of the Worker Care Spectrum will be covered in detail in later chapters in this book, but a brief introductory description of the components and processes follows.

Job Placement Assessments

Job Placement Assessments (JPA) or preplacement assessments objectively measure the worker's capabilities in a variety of tasks related to the jobs available. They are essential mechanisms for properly interfacing the worker with the machines at the job site. Job applicants do not generally undergo employment testing, but this particular assessment procedure is in reality a worker's best friend for two reasons. The first, is that the worker is placed in a job that he or she can perform safely.[11] The second is that an unknown weakness or range of motion deficit can be detected and remedied to better prepare the worker for safely performing the assigned job, as well as expanding job opportunities in the future.[3]

Job Placement Assessment incorporates consideration of physiological factors, but it places greater emphasis on functional capabilities to perform job-related movements. Physiological range of motion or strength, either alone or in cardinal patterns, or isolated activities do not translate well to the work place where movements are coupled and repetitions numerous.

There are a number of functional assessment tools available which may be called Functional Capacity Assessments, physical capacity evaluations, work assessments, or worker Functional Capacity Assessments. For purposes of clarity in this chapter and throughout this book, all such functional assessment tools will be referred to under the term "Functional Capacity Assessments" (FCA).

Job Analysis

Job Analysis can be divided into two components—1) the tasks involved and 2) the person's interactions within the job site.

Task Analysis. Every job consists of a series of tasks done over a period of time. An Industrial Therapist works closely with the company to develop a job description which details physical demands of the job.[12] This includes measuring the components of the job such as lifts, bends, push/pull resistance, materials handling requirements, repetitions, heights, distances, and the length of the time involved in each activity.

With the advent of the Americans with Disabilities Act (Box 1.1), those tasks which are "essential func-

FIGURE 1.5   A, Traditional hiring sequence before ADA; **B,** New hiring sequence required by ADA.

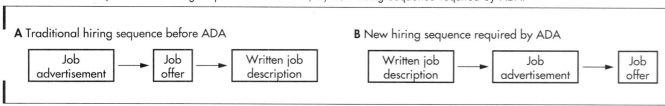

tions" of the job must now be defined in an objective manner to avoid suits under this Act regarding denial of a job to an applicant (Figure 1.5, *A, B*).[4]

Job-Site Analysis.   The job site is another aspect which needs to be carefully analyzed to prevent injury.[4,20] Machinery developed to enhance the manufac-

---

BOX 1.1

Americans with Disabilities Act

The Americans with Disabilities Act (ADA) which went into full effect in July of 1992 is certain to transform Industrial Therapy in a number of ways. ADA requires employers to work with individuals to develop harmonious relationships between the work site, job demands, and worker abilities.

Employers must have written job descriptions which are objective, thorough, and complete. Job descriptions must delineate the requirements of the job and be on file before the position is advertised. Figure 1.5 summarizes the key differences between the job hiring process before and after ADA.

The potential employee cannot be denied a job unless, through established physical manipulative skill testing, it can be demonstrated that the applicant cannot fulfill the job demands and that the work place cannot be adapted without undue cost to the employer as measured by the size and revenues of the company. The cost to adapt a work site may be deemed prohibitive for a small company but not for a large company.

The ramifications of the ADA will evolve over time as employees and employers test the limits of the guidelines through litigation. Industrial Therapy's components and procedures must provide the kind of objective measurement and evaluation that will enable employers to comply with these new regulations.

---

ture of a product may not be "employee friendly." Having been designed by a mechanical engineer to effectively build, box, or fasten a particular product, the human factor may not have been a consideration or a priority in development. Therefore, working heights of counters, shelves, or doors should be analyzed to best match the worker to the work site. The power needed to pull a lever or push a dolly, or the height of a lift may need to be altered to suit an employee who must interface with the machine.[13]

An Industrial Therapist should be an integral part of the design team of any product to assess compatibility of employee to machine. A change in the design phase can preempt a tremendous cost of redesign or injury in the production line phase.

Acute Care and Rehabilitation

The Industrial Therapist also deals with the worker post-injury to maximize function and minimize time away from the job.[30] Early intervention is paramount in the acute phase to insure rest from function while at the same time maintaining mobility for the worker's health.

Injury assessment is accomplished with full knowledge of the work setting and tasks involved. When the medical practitioner is familiar with the site, machines, hours, and tasks, analysis is not dependent on the worker's ability to adequately describe the work place. This facilitates the examination and enhances problem identification.

Entry into the rehabilitation phase is also facilitated by familiarity with job demands of the worker, coupled with assessment information from the examination and Functional Capacity Assessment. Rehabilitation is conducted using simulation of motions, resistances, repetitions, and often the actual machines to which the worker must return.

Functional Capacity Assessment

Static testing on an individual or single axis testing does not translate well to the work place where tri-planer movements are routine. Therefore, testing the patient for their ability to perform a full body task in light of the specific area of injury is important.[22] Knee flexion of 110 degrees may be a goal for the clinic, but stepping up into a bus is the functional goal for the patient.

Rehabilitation and medicine have become specialized to the point of sometimes losing sight of the total picture. A clinician can focus on the knee and ignore the total gait or the knee's input to complete the task of lifting. To this end, Functional Capacity Assessment analyzes the total performance with acknowledgment of the single joint's contribution to overall performance (Figure 1.6).

Task requirements dictate what part of the body is the focus of FCA. If a person lifts and carries, then the focus of the assessment is the whole body. Alternatively, the assessment may be focused more specifically on the upper extremity in the case of a receptionist, or on the lower extremity, in the case of a heavy machine operator who must apply force to pedals from a sitting position. The focus could also be on both upper and lower extremities if the job entails moving levers with the hands and pushing pedals with the feet, as many heavy equipment operators do on a daily basis.[8]

A Functional Capacity Assessment performed at the beginning of a rehabilitation program enables assessment of the worker's beginning capabilities so that improvement can be measured.[7] The FCA also provides baseline information that drives the planning, implementing, and monitoring of other Worker Care Spectrum components.

If a Job Placement Assessment had been done prior to injury, this information would help clarify the worker's normal pre-injury capacity. A Job Analysis, either before or after the injury, in combination with the FCA would help determine when return to work is possible.

Functional Capacity Assessment also yields defensible data to support decisions regarding worker's compensation payments, disability classification, in-

FIGURE 1.6 The injured knee is rehabilitated best when assessed and strengthened in ways that simulate the ultimate job functionality.

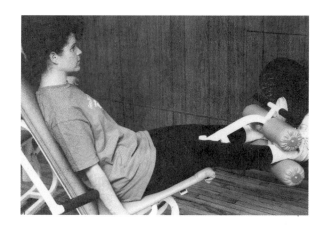

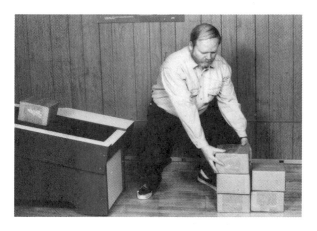

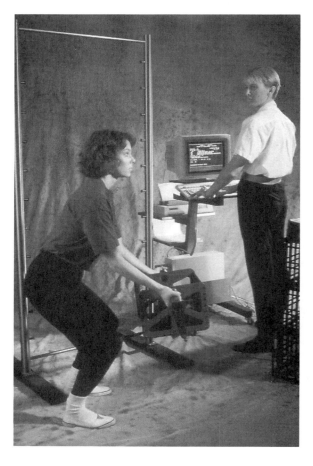

surance settlements, litigation "awards," job abilities, and rehabilitation goals.

In summary, FCA is good for the worker vocationally, financially, and emotionally.

Job Analysis

A Job Analysis connected to rehabilitation is essential to compare and contrast the Functional Capacity Assessment when setting rehabilitative goals. At this point in the spectrum, Job Analysis is more corrective than preventive, and it is performed in a way that it will not mitigate against the rehabilitation program underway.

Ergonomics—the study of fitting the work place to the worker—is involved at this point. Again, a review of the heights, weights, lifts, pulls, and pushes is imperative. Worker height, arm span, weight, range of motion, and functional strength and endurance need to be analyzed against information from the work place, to see if alterations to the work site can be accomplished in an economically feasible manner.

Ergonomics applied to the worker post-injury involves analyzing the cause, in order to avoid perpetuation rather than prevention (at this point).

Industrial Therapy allows for an assessment of the whole person in perspective to the job site. Besides physical assessment, there may be a psychosocial aspect to the problem. The psychosocial component may be addressed simply by counseling at the work place, or it may require more complex intervention by a psychologist or psychiatrist. In many cases, intervention can be in the form of lower cost preventive counseling and assertiveness training or stress management.

Work Hardening

Industrial Therapy focuses on physical rehabilitation at the work place with exercises using models or actual machinery to which the person will return. The sessions are set up to simulate actual work conditions during a four to eight hour Work Hardening program.

Work Hardening is designed to gradually strengthen and condition the worker to maximum possible function. This measured approach is intended to minimize the risk of reinjury that would be present when the worker returns to work. The traditional medical model has involved a more abrupt change for the worker—from no work and three sets of ten exercise repetitions on their back, to eight hours of 2,300 repetitions in a weight-bearing position—a transition few are able to make safely.

A Work Hardening program is individualized for each worker based on the results of their Functional Capacity Assessment in relationship to the requirements identified in Job Analysis. The program is designed to restore essential functionality in areas affected by the injury.

Work Hardening as a rehabilitation method is not new, but the multidimensional aspect with team medical involvement is a new format which has proven beneficial. Work Hardening differs from basic conditioning, in that it is a multifaceted physical program which incorporates psychosocial intervention. Studies have shown that Work Hardening yields higher return-to-work percentages.[23] KEY Method in Minneapolis has established a summary (Figure 1.7, page 12) that illustrates Work Hardening and its many aspects.[21]

Work Conditioning

Work Conditioning is a term which has been developed to delineate the physical conditioning aspect of the Work Hardening program. Both Figure 1.7 and Table 1.1 on page 12 summarize the differences between conditioning, Work Conditioning, and Work Hardening.[21]

Work Conditioning is a departure from, or an enhancement of, the medical model's conditioning programs to include the aspect of time and job task simulation.[21]

The traditional medical model conditioning program involves multiple repetitions of a particular exercise or activity, with a compressed time element. A circumscribed number of repetitions are done in rapid succession until completion, exhaustion, or fatigue.

The traditional model's determination of muscle fatigue is when force produced by an exercising muscle falls below half of the force produced in the first maximal contraction.[6] The number of repetitions to reach this half force is dependent upon the physical condition of the worker.

Another traditional form of determining when an exercise should cease, is when a person is unable to complete a full arc of movement with the maximum weight of a single repetition, or percentage of the maximum weight, as determined by an exercise specialist. The exercise repetitions are completed with little or no rest between arc swings, so fatigue comes quickly. Although these forms of exercise are excellent ways to build strength and endurance, the factor of time is not attended to in a proper manner.

In most cases, a worker lifting a 20 lb box at work will lift the box in spurts and starts over an eight hour day. Although the worker may not reach fatigue in any given bout of work, as measured by the preceding method, the effect of the load accumulates over the period of time the worker is on the job. As a result, although bout fatigue may not be apparent in a physical conditioning exercise session, it can cumulate to general fatigue four to six hours into the day.

TABLE 1.1   Comparison of Work Hardening or Work Conditioning with Conditioning

**Work Hardening or
Work Conditioning**

1. Extensive treatment program lasting 4-8 weeks
2. Frequency of treatment; 5 days per week, 4 hours per day
3. Movements required in the work place are used for establishing the treatment plan
4. Initiated and supervised by professional therapist
5. Work simulation included
6. Structured body mechanics
7. Preceded by Functional Capacity Assessment
8. Uses job requirements as objectives
9. Uses incremental task achieved as progress measure
10. Capability level of worker based on safe performance of job tasks and job site ergonomics
11. Considered to be a complete program. Could be part of a multi-discipline organization

Conditioning

1. Extensive exercise program lasting 2-4 weeks
2. Frequency of treatment; 3-5 days per week, 2-4 hours per day
3. Movements required in the work place are used for establishing the treatment plan
4. Initiated and supervised by professional therapist
5. Work simulation is not included
6. Structured body mechanics
7. Preceded by traditional clinical evaluation
8. Uses fitness levels as objectives
9. Uses fitness goal attainment as progress measure
10. Capability level of worker based on physical fitness
11. Preparation for, or one facet of, a Work Hardening or Work Conditioning program

(Adapted with permission from Key GL, Work Hardening or Work Conditioning, *PT Today,* Summer 1991.)

FIGURE 1.7   Comparisons of Work Hardening, Work Conditioning, and Functional exercise programs.

Work hardening

Work conditioning

Functional exercise programs
1. Clinical evaluation
2. Flexibility, mobility, aerobic conditioning

3. Functional capacity assessment
4. Program management (internal)
5. Body mechanics education
6. Job simulation (based on job requirements)
7. Job modification
8. Exit functional assessment

9. Case management
10. Nutrition education
11. Psychosocial
12. Vocational rehabilitation
13. Job matching/placement
14. Vocational retraining

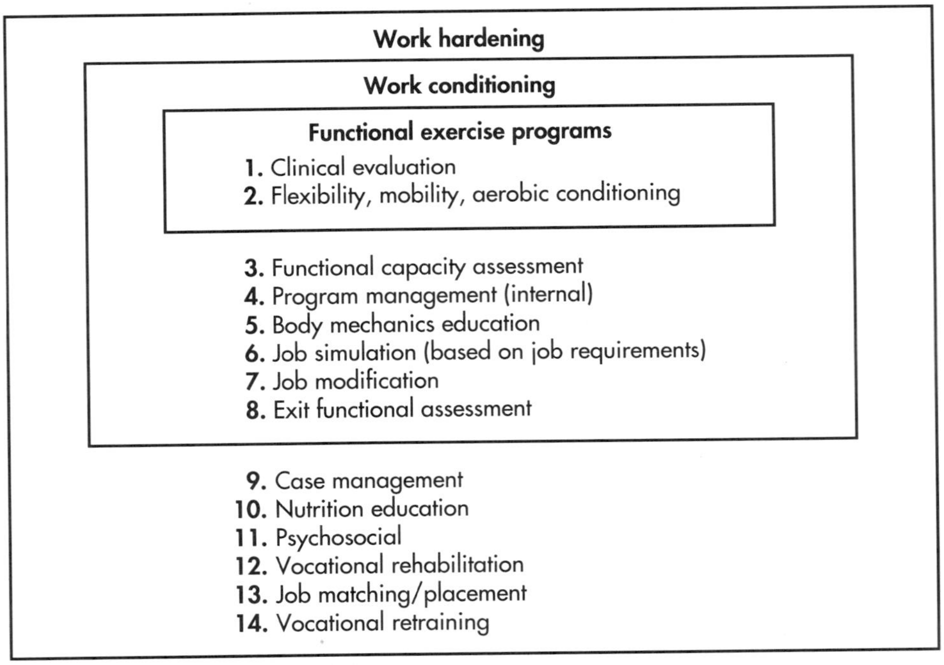

(Reprinted with permission from Key GL.)

Work Conditioning, therefore, expands the task demands of weight and heights, typically in a four hour session in which multiple tasks are accomplished. These activities involve or simulate job requirements, but in a controlled environment which can be observed, modified, corrected, and reinforced. A staff member in the Work Conditioning program can observe and monitor the workers' responses, and consult with the worker throughout the time-task work period to assure that activities are done properly. Work Conditioning enables a worker to build up the number of repetitions and weights imposed, to eventually match those required on the job.

The Work Conditioning program advances toward restored function, an end point that simulates the size of the load, the positions in which the load is required to be moved, and the pace at which the tasks are expected to be accomplished. These parameters are determined by a job site and task analysis.

In addition, Work Conditioning incorporates some psychosocial factors, in that it is usually conducted individually in the presence of other participants. In working alongside others who are also recovering, the worker can obtain visual and auditory encouragement to continue with the activity. Discussion sessions with health providers during the "work day" in the Work Conditioning environment allows workers to reveal anxiety and pain as they occur, with instantaneous feedback regarding the relevance to their continued progression toward a healthy return to work and leisure activities.

Work Conditioning may often include manipulative and dexterity exercises to provide load simulation for workers whose job involves movement such as threading bolts, soldering wires to panels, pulling levers, or pressing buttons in a coordinated manner.[5]

The worker may simulate the manufacture or fabrication of a product in the Work Conditioning period by lifting the "finished product" to a cart or table at the completion of the project. This is done at a graduated rate to a point that replicates the work environment and, in many cases, encompasses the same components which the worker will use on the job. These components are often supplied by the company to the Work Conditioning site for use by the injured worker in the rehabilitation process.

The scope of tasks simulated is limited only by the job description supplied by the companies working with the conditioning center. A close cooperation between the Work Conditioning center and the company is essential for maximum efficiency and minimum time loss. Work Hardening and Work Conditioning programs are excellent methods of returning injured workers to the work environment sooner and with less recidivism.

Prevention

An Industrial Therapist must work with a company to develop a "healthy environment" for workers.[24] Surveys and analyses of needs should be conducted and prevention programs developed for all employees.[26] Educational programs can be general, such as the mechanisms of safe lifting, "back school," upper extremity, cumulative trauma prevention, or proper use of protective measures. Prevention may also address a specific problem recurring in an identified target group, such as carpal tunnel syndrome prevention in computer operators,[13,27] or impingement syndrome in the shoulders of workers doing overhead work, like an auto mechanic who works on cars raised on hoists.

Prevention can involve activity programs such as group exercise at the work site, group calisthenics, as is done in China, development of fitness centers and specific programs for cardiopulmonary fitness, muscular fitness, or coordination activities done as a group or individually.[26]

Prevention can also come in the form of stress management programs, family counseling, coping skills, or assertiveness training. Such programs can help avoid psychosomatic manifestations of inner-conflict. They can also help to prevent injury that stems from mental distraction associated with preoccupation with family problems or worker interaction conflict.

Prevention pays for itself in decreased medical care claims, reduced injury rates, and reduced insurance premiums to the company.[1] Prevention programs are also responsible for increased production in some industries.[2]

INDUSTRIAL THERAPY PARTICIPANTS

In the traditional medical model, main participants were the injured worker, the employer, and the physician. Industrial Therapy has incorporated a number of additional participants which can have a dramatic effect on enhancing outcomes. A brief description of who they are and their role in the process follows.

Worker. The worker endeavors to do productive work which creates a sense of accomplishment and pride, as well as earn an income which provides support for self and any dependants.

Employer. The employer aims to supply a product, or provide a service which is of marketable quality with the least interruptions of the process. This includes providing a safe, worker-friendly environment which is supportive to all on the job site.

Physician. The physician serves as a team player to determine physical or emotional problems while working with and supporting team members who assume the responsibility of intervention at many points in the process.

Physical Therapist. The Physical Therapist works to enhance the physical abilities of the worker, to attain and maintain their physical health, to meet the task demands in the work environment, in a preventative, as well as rehabilitative manner.

Occupational Therapist. The Occupational Therapist works to enhance the worker's ability to perform physical and manipulative tasks, as well as conduct occupational testing for returning to work, or alternate job selection.

Vocational Rehabilitation Consultant. Vocational Rehabilitation Consultants work to match the skills of the worker with those that the job requires. They also act as team coordinators helping all participants to reach consensus on the patient's goals and objectives.

Psychologist-Counselor. The psychologist-counselor can play a contributing role in many phases of the Worker Care Spectrum, but their participation is vital in Work Hardening programs. Prevention in the form of stress management and assertiveness training, family counseling, worker interaction counseling, and total environmental dynamics are essential components of an effective Work Hardening program. Intervention may also include overcoming fear of failure, re-injury, and education.

Attorney. Although the author does not feel that the attorney should be included, in this age of litigation, the attorney is involved in case management from the standpoint of worker and employer rights, as well as fair and equitable compensation to either party. These professionals need to be knowledgeable and efficient in their actions to ensure proper settlement and management of their cases.

Case Manager. Case management is becoming a method of monitoring and controlling health care costs. The most effective case managers are intimately knowledgeable of the situation, the persons involved, and the services available. Sometimes case managers operate from distant locations, and are required to make decisions without complete knowledge of either the workplace or the worker. When this happens, they are at the same disadvantage as the traditional medical practitioner in trying to make fair decisions outside the full context of the job environment and the worker's functional interactions.

SUMMARY

The evolution of Industrial Therapy has been driven by the need for more successful and cost effective approaches to worker wellness and rehabilitation. A multi-faceted variety of components and processes have been integrated along with traditional medical services to encompass the Industrial Therapy spectrum. Industrial Therapy has introduced an increasing focus on prevention; brought more real world context into rehabilitation procedures; increased worker involvement and empowerment in the process; developed a teamwork orientation; fostered more positive perceptions and attitudes; and provided more comprehensive preparation and support to facilitate reintegration into the working world.

Industrial Therapy involves a wide diversity of input and challenge. The Industrial Therapist must endeavor to maintain knowledge of all aspects of the care spectrum in order to effectively benefit those for whom he or she provides a service.

From wellness to injury rehabilitation, the Industrial Therapist must maintain a responsive, positive interaction with the patient and other involved parties; provide informed diagnosis and problem (case) management; maintain a firm understanding of the job demands and work place into which the worker is desiring to return; and finally, be aware of the psychosocial aspects of any individual who interacts with others at home or in the work place.

REFERENCES

1. Allers V: Workplace preventive programs cut costs of illness and injuries, *Occupational Health and Safety* 58:26-29, 1989.
2. Burrous N: An industrial response to low-back injuries and their prevention, *Topics in Acute Care and Trauma Rehabilitation* 2:78-82, 1988.
3. Button R, Pater R: Pretraining is essential tool for fall and back injuries, *Occupational Health and Safety* 57:23-25, 1988.
4. Chaffin D, Andersson GBJ: *Occupational Biomechanics*, New York, 1991, John Wiley and Sons.
5. Cobb K: RSI: the new computer age health assault. *Prevention* 43:58-64, 1991.
6. Davies GJ: *Isokinetics in Clinical Usage*, La Crosse, Wisc., 1990, S & S Publishers.
7. Davis LM: Use whole brain learning methods to control repetitive motion injuries, *Occupational Health and Safety* 59:26, 1990.
8. Donkin SW: *Sitting on the Job*, Boston, Mass., 1989, Houghton Mifflin.
9. Feffer H: Low-back pain: view in 1988, *Topics in Acute Care and Trauma Rehabilitation* 1:7, 1988.
10. Gabor A: On-the-job straining, *U.S. News and World Report* 108:51-53, 1990.

11. Gates SJ: Muscle weakness is leading cause for nurses' lower back injuries, pain, *Occupational Health and Safety* 57:57, 1988.
12. Glad I, Kirschenbaum A: Study shows work environments, job tasks may cause back pain, *Occupational Health and Safety* 58:44-46, 1989.
13. Goldoftas B: Hands that hurt: repetitive motion injuries on the job, *Technology Review* 94:42-50, 1991.
14. Harvey DA: Health and safety first, *BYTE* 16:119-128, 1991.
15. Isernhagen SJ: *Work Injury*, Rockville, Md., 1988, Aspen Publishing.
16. Jensen R: Epidemiology of work-related back pain, *Topics in Acute Care and Trauma Rehabilitation* 2:1-15, 1988.
17. Joyce M: Ergonomics offers solutions to numerous health complaints, *Occupational Health and Safety* 57:58-66, 1988.
18. Kelsey JL: *Epidemiology of Musculoskeletal Disorders*, New York, 1982, Oxford University Press.
19. Key G: Industrial Physical Therapy: An Introduction. Chapter by Gould, J, *Orthopedic and Sports Physical Therapy*, St Louis, 1990, Mosby.
20. Key G: The Worker Care Spectrum, *Newswork*, 1991.
21. Key, G: Work Hardening or Work Conditioning; Semantics or Reality, *PT Today*, Summer 1991.
22. Kreighbaum E, Barthels K: *Biomechanics—A Qualitative Approach for Studying Human Movement*, New York, 1985, Macmillan.
23. Mayer TG, et al: A Prospective Two-Year Study of Functional Restoration in Industrial Low Back Injury, *JAMA*, vol 258, October, 1987.
24. Morgan D: Concepts in functional training and postural stabilization for the low-back injured, *Topics in Acute Care and Trauma Rehabilitation* 2:8-17, 1988.
25. Nelson R, Nestor D: Standardized assessment of industrial low-back injuries, *Topics in Acute Care and Trauma Rehabilitation* 2:16-30, 1988.
26. Niemeyer LO: Components of a good report, *Industrial Rehabilitation Quarterly* 1:9, 1988.
27. Saal J: Diagnostic studies of low-back injuries, *Topics in Acute Care and Trauma Rehabilitation* 2:31-49, 1988.
28. Smith RB: Workplace stretching programs reduce costly accidents, injuries, *Occupational Health and Safety* 59:24-25, 1990.
29. Stix G: Handful of Pain, *Scientific American* 264:118-120, 1991.
30. Toffler A: *Power Shift*, New York, 1990 Bantam Books,.
31. Tramposh A: Musculoskeletal injuries demand new treatment model, *Occupational Health and Safety* 58:21-24, 1989.
32. Tramposh AK: Work-related therapy for the injured reduces return-to-work barriers, *Occupational Health and Safety* 57:55-56, 1988.
33. White A: Treatment of the upper back, part 1: the epidemiology and diagnostics, perspectives of the physician, *Topics in Acute Care and Trauma Rehabilitation* 2:50-66, 1988.

2

The Industrial Therapy Team

Susan M. Brookins

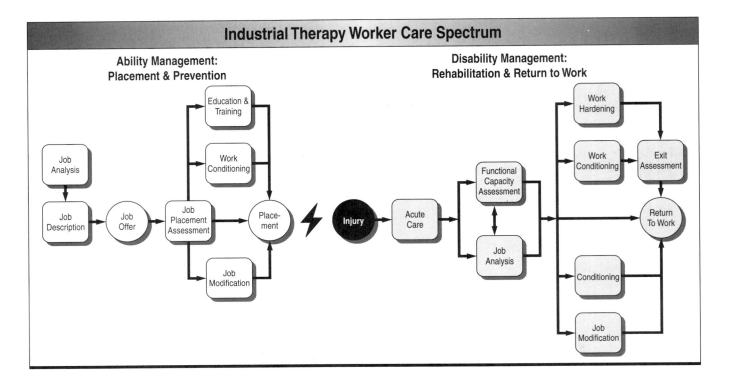

Industrial Therapy Worker Care Spectrum

Ability Management: Placement & Prevention

Disability Management: Rehabilitation & Return to Work

The National Council on Rehabilitation in August of 1943 defined rehabilitation as "the restoration of the handicapped (person with a disability) to the fullest physical, mental, social, vocational, and economic usefulness of which they are capable."[15]

This definition focuses beyond the injured body part, to encompass the whole person and their life activities. Accordingly, rehabilitation is viewed as a holistic process, and basic to it, is the value of the human being. The view is that every human being is deserving of respect,[7] and is entitled to an inherent right to earn a living in a democratic society.[13]

The provision of treatment specific to the industrially injured person has improved rapidly over the last two decades. One could safely say the birth of Work Hardening began when treatment goals included work related outcomes. These grass roots work-related programs wore many masks, and the treatment protocols

varied. Services were also provided by any combination of specialty professions, from one discipline approach to the multidisciplinary service providers.

Presently, all of these models continue to provide programs called Work Hardening, but the one factor which constantly remains threaded through all such processes is a focus on the injured worker and his or her identifiable needs. In the arena of industrial rehabilitation the term "functional" has taken on a new priority in the realm of treatment goals.

This chapter will focus on people and their roles in the rehabilitation process which follows acute care. It will describe the role of each player, and interaction as a team in Functional Capacity Assessment, Work Conditioning, and Work Hardening, and the Return-To-Work-Transition. Although Job Analysis, Education, and Prevention come into play during hiring and as independent programs, they will be discussed primarily to the extent within which they are included in post-injury rehabilitation programs.

THE TEAM CONCEPT

Origins

It has become apparent that injured workers are returned to maximum function more quickly and cost-effectively, with minimized risk of reinjury, if providers take a holistic approach to the treatment process. Service providers have become more specialized in addressing the full range and complexity of the individual's needs by increasingly utilizing the holistic process.

As a result, rehabilitation has become progressively more interdisciplinary in nature, integrating a myriad of specialties and resources into a comprehensive approach for serving the needs of the whole individual.

The complexity of the workers' needs dictates a team approach, as delineated in the models developed by such founders in the field as Blankenship,[5] Isernhagen,[10] Key,[11] Matheson,[12] and Tramposh.[16] The team approach has also been endorsed by the Commission on Accreditation of Rehabilitation Facilities (CARF).[6]

Participants

The team that applies its specialized skills is composed of people with varied academic and experiential backgrounds. The interdisciplinary team collaborates as a group, shares common goals, is cohesive, mutually supportive, respects individual differences, values, personalities, and skills, does problem solving, and has decision-making responsibilities. Although the team is multidirectional, the interaction of each member contributes to the goals of the whole.

Table 2.1 on page 18 indicates the involvement of each team member in the components of the Worker Care Spectrum. Current staffing patterns in industrial rehabilitation programs continue to vary from the Physical Therapist or Occupational Therapist in the private practice setting or hospital-based program to the multidisciplinary team approach. Even in the multidisciplinary team model, the membership varies from program to program. Experience indicates that there is a lot of cross over services being provided by the various disciplines.

Primary and Auxiliary Teams

If one looks critically at the goal of increasing function in light of work related goals, one has to acknowledge that there are primary and secondary influencing fac-

tors. This concept can then be expanded to include both a primary and auxiliary team approach. The members of the auxiliary team have enough influence to affect the progress of the worker's participation in the programs provided by the primary team. Their role and influence cannot be ignored.

The focus of this chapter is to identify the players involved in the primary team—the industrial therapy team—and to describe their individual roles in the treatment process. In addition, the roles of the auxiliary team members will be addressed as well, since their influence is having an increasing impact on successful rehabilitation.

THE WORKER

First and foremost, the role of the worker will be discussed, since the worker is a member of both primary and auxiliary teams.

Experience tells us that the workers admitted into our programs do not always fit into an ideal or standardized profile. They come to us with any combination of incidental baggage and influences. Those of us working in the field can well recognize these characteristics which manifest themselves in various combinations and degrees of severity.

The injured worker undergoes a dramatic change in roles. At one time this person was gainfully employed, productive in the employed community, and fulfilling expectations of the employer and fellow employees. In addition, he or she was meeting familial and social expectations in their life away from work. Then an incident or series of incidents has prevented this person from continuing the role of a worker.

In the past, this injured worker has been viewed as a ''patient'' who passively receives medical management. Today, the injured worker is being seen as an active participant in a team rehabilitation process. How the care givers view the individual can affect the individual's attitude and behavior. These ramifications are summarized in Table 2.2 on page 19 and discussed below.

The Patient Model

In this model, as the recipient of traditional medical management, the patient may assume certain new personality characteristics. The injury may become all-consuming, with the worker focusing blame on others, specifically the employer. Some view the injury as the employer's fault, and the employer's responsibility to cure. In many cases the search is for a cure that is ''100% pain free.''

Often the anticipation of a settlement is perceived as the Big Score that is expected to solve all the ensuing

TABLE 2.1 Industrial Rehabilitation Team: Typical involvement in the rehabilitation process (A = Typically always involved; S = Typically sometimes involved)

	Job placement assessment	Job analysis	Education and prevention	Acute care	Whole body assessment	Work conditioning	Work hardening	Special purpose assessment	RTW transition
Primary team									
Physical therapist or Occupational therapist	A	A	A	A	A	A	A	A	A
Psychologist			S	S			A	S	A
Vocational rehab consultant		S	S		S	S	A	S	
Exercise physiologist		S	S		S	S	S	S	
Work simulator technician		S				S	A		
Social worker			S	S			S		
Rehabilitation nurse						S	S		
Auxiliary team									
Physician				A	A	S	S	A	S
Employer	A	A	S		A	A	A		A
Family				S		S	S		A
Attorney	S			S	S		S		S
External service providers									
Insurance representative			S	A	A	A	A		A
Case manager	S	S	S	S	S	S	S	S	S
Ergonomist	S	S	S			S	S		S
Industrial engineer	S	S	S				S		S
Dietitian			S				S		
Orthotist/prosthetist				S			S		
Educators			S			S	S		
Financial counselor			S				S		
Special prog. consultants			S	S		S	S		S

T A B L E 2 . 2 How injury affects workers' perceptions and roles.

The "Worker" Usually . . .	The "Patient" Sometimes . . .
Accepts supervision	Considers supervision as criticism
Has rapport with coworkers	Is suspicious of coworkers
Sets realistic goals	Looks to others to set goals
Accepts responsibility	Transfers responsibility to others
Manages financial resources	Expects a settlement to solve financial status
Manages personal time	Loses sense of time
Manages outside influences	Waits for outside influences to take control
Follows corrective instructions	Is resistant to change
Adheres to safety factors	Ignores safety
Has emotional balance	Under or over reacts
Has the ability to avoid alcohol and drug dependency	Becomes alcohol and drug dependent

(From ERGOS: Work Simulator User's Training Manual, Work Recovery, 1991.)

problems. Some patients wait for outside influences to change and ameliorate their situation. Particular patients may wander aimlessly through the day, often becoming drug or alcohol dependent, and over or under reacting emotionally.[8] When certain patients are asked to describe their daily activities they frequently cannot account for how they fill their waking hours.

When asked what their return to work goals are, many patients do not know. They may not have received proper counseling, or they've waited for "someone else" to solve their problem. They may give answers such as "the doctor hasn't said anything" or "when I'm pain free."

The Team Member Model

In the milieu of industrial therapy, the worker becomes empowered with the responsibility to be an active participant on the treatment team, bringing to the team concept a personal ownership in the treatment process and outcome. The worker should help to identify treatment goals, then take the responsibility to actuate those goals by participating in the treatment process.

Becoming a team member in an industrial therapy program requires the injured worker to reject the passive recipient mind set and adopt a team member orientation. There has to be a cultivation of the ability to place the injury and related problems in perspective. The worker has to focus on abilities, including accepting responsibilities for outcomes, managing time, and resisting distracting influences. In other words, the worker becomes a doer, not the recipient of services. The worker is expected to set goals and through participation in the rehabilitation process actuate outcomes. The worker once again has to take control of life

and accept the responsibility for his or her own actions.[8]

Typically this orientation takes the form of participating in an industrial therapy program where the worker has the primary responsibility, with the assistance of the industrial rehab team, to identify treatment goals that are focused on return to work. Then on a daily basis the team works toward reaching these goals, documenting achievement and progress. The worker keeps the other team members apprised of their progress in relationship to the established treatment plan, work attitudes and habits, and safety issues, which are revitalized during this process. The worker may also assist the team in developing the work station and work simulation track.

The Team

The Industrial Therapy Team is comprised of many players who have various degrees of influence on the outcome: Return to Work. These team members can be divided into categories by virtue of their relationship to the worker—the focal point—in the rehabilitation process.

The primary treatment team consists of members responsible for implementing the rehabilitation procedures, or the disability management as identified in the Worker Care Spectrum (refer to page 16)[11].

The auxiliary team, by virtue of the influence their roles in the process play an essential role on the expected outcome. Finally there are the external service providers, who essentially address return to work barriers. The organization chart in Figure 2.1 on page 20 includes a complete listing of primary and auxiliary team members, as well as additional external service providers and consultants.

FIGURE 2.1   Organization of the Industrial Rehabilitation Team

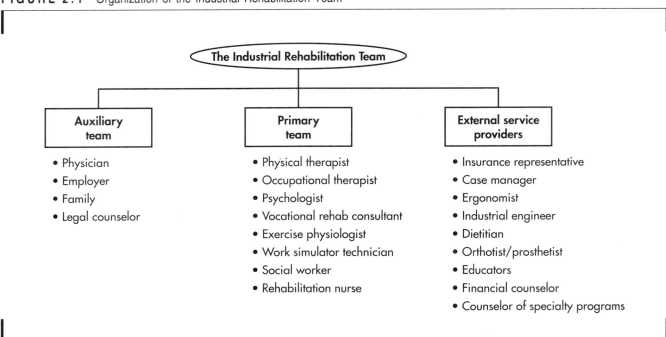

THE PRIMARY REHABILITATION TEAM

The primary rehabilitation team members are those most directly involved in the rehabilitation process itself. For CARF accredited facilities, the primary team is identified as including a Physical Therapist, Occupational Therapist, Psychologist, and a Vocational Specialist.[6]

When reviewing the job descriptions of these team members, one will note many overlaps in functions provided. This is due to the philosophical approaches an organization may take when identifying the specific roles of these team members in their respective organizations. By way of example, the intake process may be delegated to the Vocational Rehabilitation Consultant in one organization and to the PT or OT in another.

The following role descriptions are based on the author's experience in the field as well as the responses received from a questionnaire sent to practitioners in the field.

Physical Therapist

In 1991 The American Physical Therapy Association (APTA) assembled an Industrial Rehabilitation Advisory Committee to develop guidelines identifying the role of Physical Therapist, distinguishing between the contemporary practices of Work Conditioning and Work Hardening, as well as standardizing terminology.

The guidelines were approved by APTA in November of 1992.[2]

In essence, Work Conditioning is defined as programs focusing on physical issues of flexibility, strength, endurance, coordination, and work-related functions for the goal of returning to work. Whereas Work Hardening is identified as being interdisciplinary in nature focusing on the physical, functional, behavioral, and vocational needs of the injured worker with the goal being returning to work.

APTA identifies the role of Physical Therapy as providing the physical and functional components of both of these programs. APTA guidelines parallel CARF's requirements for the "core" team members.

The following job descriptions for these defined "core" team members are presented as a prototype for developing job descriptions specific to the needs of a given organization. When developing these job descriptions the information here can be rearranged into the organization's own format.

Occupational Therapist

In 1986 the American Occupational Therapy Association (AOTA) published guidelines for Work Hardening[1] and in 1989 published the book *Work in Progress— Occupational Therapy in Work Programs*.[9] In the Preface of the document *Work Hardening Guidelines*, the role of Occupational Therapy personnel is defined as providing "an individualized, work-oriented activity process

BOX 2.1

Job Description

Title: Physical Therapist   **Date:**_____
Service: Industrial Therapy
Qualifications: Graduate of an APTA approved curriculum and licensure in the state practicing. Experience in work related treatment programs, Job Analysis, and ergonomics is desirable.

Reports to:_____

Job Responsibilities
Evaluation:

1. The PT participates in the screening process to determine the appropriateness of the referral for services. This includes reviewing medical and work histories.
2. The PT may conduct an intake interview with the prospective client gleaning medical and work histories from the client's viewpoint. A job description/analysis provided by the employer may be reviewed at this time with the client.
3. The PT may conduct an on-site Job Analysis including acquiring information from the employer regarding return to work expectations, the advisability and practicality of job site modification or alternative placement.
4. The PT may test muscle strength, range of motion or neuromuscular function.
5. The PT may administer a Functional Capacity Assessment (FCA) in preparation for a Work Conditioning or Work Hardening program.

Treatment:

1. The PT will develop and implement an individualized treatment plan for Work Conditioning or Work Hardening based on the client's current capabilities and known physical demand work requirements.
2. Program goals should be established with input from the person served.
3. Implementing a Work Hardening program includes techniques to improve strength, endurance, movement, flexibility, motor control, and cardiopulmonary capacity as related to the performance of work tasks. Work Conditioning includes practice, modification, and instruction in work related activities. In Work Hardening, the treatment plan includes developing a work station and job simulation approach to improve the client's functional ability to perform simulated or real work activities. The program should foster appropriate work behavior traits and attitudes such as punctuality, response to supervision, working with peers, pacing, competitiveness, and safety. The program should also include increasing physical and psychological tolerances including endurance, stress management, and pain management. Promotion of client responsibility and self management is emphasized in both Work Conditioning and Work Hardening.

Program Management

The PT may assume the responsibility for being the client's program manager, coordinating all the services the client receives in the program and providing communication and feedback to the client. The PT needs to collaborate with all team members including the Physician, Employer, Rehabilitation Case Manager, Insurance Company, and Attorney. The PT in this role represents the client at staffings and case conferences discussing progress, revision of goals and discharge planning. The APTA guidelines include assisting the client to obtain additional services of alcohol and other drug dependency counseling, engineering and ergonomic services, medical services, nutrition and weight control services, orthotic and prosthetic services, and smoking cessation counseling as appropriate for clients in Work Hardening.[2]

Documentation

The PT is responsible for documenting evaluation findings, progress, discharge status and plans, attainment of goals, staffing and case conferences as well as various forms of communication with other team members. The PT reviews the client's documentation of daily activity log sheets and time cards, recording attendance, and daily charges.

Discharge Planning

The PT as client program manager is responsible for discharge planning, formulating recommendations for return to work which may include a collaboration with the employer regarding modification of work stations or tools, light duty assignment, or alternative placement. The PT can assist the employer with issues regarding accessibility and reasonable accommodations in compliance with the American's with Disabilities Act (ADA). Follow-up recommendations may be made.

Continued

BOX 2.1 *cont'd*

Education

The PT can participate in the educational component of the program. Often times topics covered include safe job performance and injury prevention, pain management, body mechanics, and lifting techniques. The PT may also do presentations to referral sources and more specifically for the employer on site. The PT should participate in research, attend conferences, and in-services.

Consultation

In a consultative role the PT may participate in quality assessment, peer review, follow-up programs, program evaluation and outcome assessments. In addition, the PT may consult with referral sources and employers regarding program feasibility for industrial injury prevention, risk analysis, conduct trainer programs, and ADA issues. The PT may be required to supervise PT students. The PT may be required to serve as an expert witness in legal cases. The PT may also consult with other team members in their areas of expertise.

Developed by

_____

Approved by

_____

_____ **Date**

_____

_____ **Date**

_____ **Review date(s)**

---

that involves a client in simulated or actual work tasks. These tasks are structured and graded progressively to increase psychological, physical, and emotional tolerance and improve endurance, general productivity and work feasibility. The eventual goal of Work Hardening services is to improve the client's occupational performance skills to allow effective functioning in homebound, sheltered, modified or competitive work."[1]

One of the unique skills OT's bring to Work Hardening by virtue of their training, is their complex task analysis. This is specifically helpful in performing Job Analysis and developing work stations and job simulation tracks for the clients. The OT also brings skills in assessing and implementing treatment techniques addressing the psychological aspects of treatment planning and implementation. This aspect is steeped in the history of providing OT services in the psychiatric milieu where the value of work as a therapeutic approach had already established precedence.

BOX 2.2

Job Description

Title: Occupational Therapist   **Date:**_____
Service: Industrial Therapy
Qualifications: Graduate of an AOTA approved curriculum and licensure in the state where required. Experience in work related treatment programs, Job Analysis, and ergonomics is desired.

Reports to:_____

Job Responsibilities
Evaluation:

1. The OT participates in the screening process to determine the appropriateness of the referral for services. This includes reviewing medical and work histories.
2. The OT may conduct an intake interview with the prospective client gleaning medical and work

Continued

BOX 2.2 *cont'd*

history from the client's viewpoint. A job description/analysis provided by the employer may be reviewed at this time with the client.

3. The OT may conduct an on site Job Analysis including acquiring information from the employer regarding return to work expectations, the advisability and practicality of job site modifications or alternative placement.

4. The OT may test muscle strength, range of motion, sensation, or fine or gross motor coordination.

5. The OT may administer a Functional Capacity Assessment (FCA) in preparation for a Work Conditioning or Work Hardening program.

Treatment:

1. The OT will develop and implement an individualized treatment plan based on the client's current capabilities and known physical demand work requirements.

2. Program goals should be established with input from the person served.

3. Implementation of Work Hardening services includes developing a work station and job simulation approach to improve the client's functional ability to perform specific work related tasks. The program should foster appropriate work behavior traits and attitudes such as punctuality, response to supervision, working with peers, pacing, competitiveness, and safety. The program should also include increasing physical and psychological tolerances including endurance, stress management, and pain management.

Program Management

The OT may assume the responsibility for being the client's program manager, coordinating all the services the client receives in the program and providing communication and feedback to the client. The OT needs to collaborate with all team members including the Physician, Employer, Rehabilitation Case Manager, Insurance Company, and Attorney. The OT in this role represents the client at staffings and case conferences discussing progress review, revision of goals and discharge planning.

Documentation

The OT is responsible for documenting evaluation findings, progress, discharge status and plans, attainment of goals, staffing and case conferences as well as various forms of communication with other team members. The OT reviews the client's documentation on the daily activity log

sheets and time cards, documenting attendance, and daily charges.

Discharge Planning

The OT as client program manager is responsible for discharge planning, formulating recommendations for return to work which may include a collaboration with the employer regarding modifications of the work station or tools, light duty assignments or alternative placement. The OT can assist the employer with issues regarding accessibility and reasonable accommodations in compliance with the American's with Disabilities Act (ADA). Follow-up recommendations may be made.

Education

The OT can participate in the educational components of the program. Often times topics covered are joint protection, stress management, pain management, body mechanics, and lifting techniques. The OT may also do presentations to referral sources and more specifically for the employer on site. The OT should participate in research, attend conferences, and in-services.

Consultation

In a consultative role the OT may participate in quality assessment, peer review, follow-up programs, and program evaluation. In addition, the OT may consult with referral sources and employers regarding risk analysis and ADA issues, or conduct trainer programs. The OT may be required to supervise OT students, and serve as an expert witness in legal cases. The OT may consult with other team members in their areas of expertise.

Developed by

_____

Approved by

_____

_____ **Date**

_____

_____ **Date**

_____ **Review date(s)**

The Vocational Rehabilitation Consultant

Vocational Rehabilitation as a process is goal-oriented, is comprised of an individualized sequence of services designated to assist the injured worker to achieve vocational adjustment, culminating in gainful activity and rendering that worker a productive wage earning, tax paying member of society. The goal therefore is employability.[4]

Historically, there has been rehabilitation legislation supporting the need for vocational oriented services. Initially, early legislation was geared toward the military and veterans (the National Defense Act 1916, Smith-Hughes Act 1917, and Soldier Act 1918) followed by the Vocational Rehabilitation Act of 1920 which marked the beginning of the public rehabilitation program.

The history of vocational rehabilitation programs in the U.S. has been characterized by steady growth.[4] Most recently, the ADA has been added to the legislative series aimed at employability of persons with disabilities.

The role of the Vocational Rehabilitation Consultant is to help the client achieve vocational adjustment by providing comprehensive evaluation, and the development of a treatment plan upon which the delivery of services is subsequently determined. In Vocational Rehabilitation, workability is the focus of the therapeutic goal, as well as the treatment process itself. In Industrial Therapy the goal of returning to work is a complex issue. It supersedes the injured worker's capabilities to just meet the physical demand characteristics of the job.[10]

Creation of a positive milieu for return-to-work necessitates a comprehensive approach that may include such factors as the worker's interests, aptitudes, and transferability of skills. Job availability, job seeking skills, job placement, work motivation, job site modifications and vocational training are also important. The Vocational Specialist offers the injured worker reinforcement in dealing with the adjustment process of returning to work. This includes the reestablishment of relationships with the employer and co-workers, as well as reduction of the anticipated non-medical concerns that interfere with the return-to-work process.

These individuals may participate in the intake interviews, and offer counseling in group or individually in areas such as stress management, self esteem, personal adjustment, relaxation training, communication skills development, goal setting, and job seeking skills.

BOX 2.3

Job Description

Title: Vocational Rehabilitation
Consultant   **Date:**_____
Service: Industrial Therapy
Qualifications: "An individual with a Master's degree in vocational rehabilitation or a vocationally related field, or who is eligible for, or is a professional member of the National Rehabilitation Counseling Association or the American Rehabilitation Counseling Association or who is certified by the Commission on Rehabilitation Counselor Certification or by the Commission on Certification of Work Adjustment and Vocational Evaluation Specialists."[6] Experience in industrial rehabilitation programs is desirable.

Reports to:_____

Job Responsibilities
Evaluation:
1. The Vocational Rehabilitation Consultant participates in the screening process to determine the appropriateness of the referral for services. This includes reviewing medical, work and educational histories.
2. The Vocational Rehabilitation Consultant may conduct an intake interview with the prospective client gleaning educational, social, and work history from the client's viewpoint. A job description or analysis provided by the employer may be reviewed at this time with the client.
3. The Vocational Rehabilitation Consultant may conduct an on site Job Analysis including acquiring information from the employer regarding return-to-work expectations, the advisability and practicality of job site modifications or alternative placement.
4. The Vocational Rehabilitation Consultant may recommend that a Functional Capacity Assessment be performed for additional information.
5. The Vocational Rehabilitation Consultant may evaluate occupational interest, intelligence, work aptitude, personality, achievement, and general educational development skills to determine transferability of skills or criteria for enrollment in vocational training.

Continued

BOX 2.3 *cont'd*

Treatment

The Vocational Rehabilitation Consultant provides counseling and guidance specific to vocational issues and influencing factors for return to work. The Vocational Rehabilitation Consultant provides job coaching, placement services, post employment, and follow-up services.

Program Management

The Vocational Rehabilitation Consultant may assume the responsibility for case management. In this capacity, the Vocational Rehabilitation Consultant assumes the responsibilities for coordinating the medical and vocational return to work plan, including family and employer involvement and the cost-benefit of treatment options.[17]

Documentation

The Vocational Rehabilitation Consultant is responsible for documenting evaluation findings, case management reports, rehabilitation plans, status reports, and ongoing consultative reports. A case closure report is required.

Discharge Planning

The Vocational Rehabilitation Consultant participates in discharge planning, formulating recommendations for return to work. Discharge planning, in collaboration with the employer, is essential and includes modification of work station or tools and job placement. The Vocational Rehabilitation Consultant can assist the employer in meeting ADA requirements.

Education

The Vocational Rehabilitation Consultant can participate in the educational component of the program. Topics covered include legal issues, client's rights, reestablishing relationships with employers and coworkers, motivation and appropriate work behaviors, or how to apply for a job. The Vocational Rehabilitation Consultant may also do presentations to referral sources and employers.

Consultation

In a consultative role, the Vocational Rehabilitation Consultant may participate in quality assessment, peer review, program evaluation, and follow-up programs. In addition, the Vocational Rehabilitation Consultant may consult with referral sources and employers regarding case management issues. The Vocational Rehabilitation Consultant may be required to serve as an expert witness. The Vocational Rehabilitation Consultant, on an ongoing basis consults with other team members in their areas of expertise.

Developed by

_____

Approved by

_____

_____   Date

_____

_____   Date

_____   Review date(s)

The Psychologist

The multidisciplinary approach to the industrial rehabilitation process is by nature a holistic approach. The injured worker enters into the rehabilitation process not only with physical injury, but also the psychological complexities associated with this interruption in life routines. These psychological overlays may delay or alter the injured worker's progress in the rehabilitation process and return to work.

Manifestations of decreased motivation, frustration, anger, fear and anxiety, or depression, often cause resistance to participation in the rehabilitation process. This may take the form of non-compliance, magnification of symptoms, behavioral changes, or in the extreme, dependence on drugs or alcohol. These psychological overlays also may affect their familial and social relationships, roles, and responsibilities. Dependency or aggressive behavior patterns may emerge. In effect, the injured worker may lose control, as well as the ability to be goal oriented.

As a team member in an industrial therapy program, it is the role of the psychologist to help the injured worker establish a stable, emotional status that is conducive to reinstatement as a team member with a positive goal-oriented focus. The goal of treatment is to decrease the injured worker's psychological distress and increase their taking control, also to provide the other team members a framework within which they are to respond to the injured worker's behavioral patterns.

The psychologist may provide support for the injured worker's family, facilitating insight regarding the behavioral changes they may be dealing with, as well as how to reinforce progress in the rehabilitative process. The psychologist's treatment plan may include using group dynamics or individual counseling sessions. Biofeedback, relaxation techniques, pain management, stress management, and even hypnosis may be integral parts of the treatment plan.

BOX 2.4

Job Description

Title: Psychologist   **Date:**_____
Service: Industrial Therapy
Qualifications: Completion of a professional educational track in the field of psychology. Licensure or certification by respective state law governing the practice of psychology. Experience or specialization in industrial psychology is desirable.

Reports to:_____

Job Responsibilities
Evaluation:
1. The Psychologist participates in the screening process to determine the appropriateness of the referral for services. This includes reviewing medical and psychological case histories.
2. The Psychologist may conduct an intake interview with the perspective client.
3. The Psychologist may administer such test batteries as the MMPI, personality inventories, behavior assessments, and pain profiles.

Treatment
The Psychologist provides individual counseling, biofeedback, hypnosis, visual imagery exercises, support group sessions. Topics addressed include pain management techniques, stress management techniques, and goal setting. When necessary, family counseling may be appropriate.

Documentation
The Psychologist is responsible for documenting evaluation findings, counseling sessions, group support sessions, progress reports, and discharge summaries.

Discharge Planning
The Psychologist participates in the discharge plan, providing input for formulating recommendations for work readiness and return to work.

Education
The Psychologist participates in the educational component of the program. Sessions include topics like stress management, pain management, and return to work issues. Educational sessions may include family members. The Psychologist may also give presentations to referral sources and employers as well as the treatment team.

Consultation
The Psychologist attends staffings and case conferences, representing the psychological perspective in reviewing progress, revising goals, and changing program plans. In a consultative role, the Psychologist may participate in quality assessment, peer review, program evaluation, and follow-up programs. In addition, the Psychologist may consult with referral sources and the medical treatment providers regarding the injured worker's psychological status and recommended management. The Psychologist may be required to serve as an expert witness.

Developed by

_____

Approved by

_____

_____   **Date**

_____   **Date**

_____   **Review date(s)**

OTHER REHABILITATION DISCIPLINES

Depending on the philosophy of staffing industrial therapy programs, organizations may include other disciplines on their treatment teams. These other disciplines will now be described.

Certified Occupational Therapy Assistant (COTA) and Physical Therapist Assistant (PTA)

The COTA and PTA must be graduates of an approved curriculum of AOTA and APTA respectively. In some states, certification or licensure is required. Both must work under the direct supervision of a PT or OT. In Work Hardening, their responsibilities include supervising the worker performing their exercises and work simulation tracks (floor supervision). They may participate in the evaluation process if appropriately trained, provide general supervision of the worker's daily activities, assist in the development of work circuits, upgrade daily work task assignments, monitor body mechanics, and participate in providing group activities and educational components.

These assistants are responsible for documenting observations of the worker's performance in the case record and contribute input during team conferences. Some, after having additional training, may also administer a FCA or perform a job analysis.

Exercise Physiologist

The Exercise Physiologist must be a graduate of an accredited program; having a Masters Degree is preferable, as well as having experience in providing services in the medical arena with knowledge of orthopedics or cardiac rehabilitation programs.

Responsibilities include fitness and exercise testing with the development of an exercise prescription. Assessments may include strength, flexibility, body composition, and submaximal or maximal exercycle or treadmill testing.

The Exercise Physiologist may be responsible for developing the conditioning exercise program, and monitoring its content, frequency, duration, intensity, and progression. Warm-up, stretching and cool down programs should also be under the Exercise Physiologist.

The Exercise Physiologist also contributes to the educational components, especially in the areas of fitness, body mechanics, and nutrition. In some programs the Exercise Physiologist participates in case management and supervision of work circuits.

The Exercise Physiologist documents observations in case records and contributes to team conferences. In some instances, after having additional training, the Exercise Physiologist may also conduct FCA's and perform Job Analyses. It should be noted that some organizations also employ the services of certified athletic trainers (ATC's) and corporate fitness specialists in these capacities.

Work Simulator Technician

Another provider of services in industrial rehabilitation has multiple job titles. Some are known as Work Simulators, Industrial Rehabilitation Technicians, Work Trainers, or Work-Floor Foremen. These individuals usually bring their experience and expertise from a variety of industrial trades and occupations, and typically have supervisory experience. They function under the direct supervision of a core team member.

Responsibilities include designing and constructing work stations to simulate the injured worker's job tasks, then monitoring the worker's performance with special attention to safety, pacing, work habits, and progress toward job goals. They often are the "foreman" in the simulated work setting. This technician may participate in job site evaluations and work station modifications. They document observations in the case record and participate in team conferences.

Social Worker

In some programs a Social Worker is identified as part of the service team. These individuals may also participate in the intake interview process and then counsel the client pertaining to social or vocational problems arising from the worker's injury. They arrange for services not provided within the program and make appropriate referrals to community resources. These individuals participate in team conferences and document observations and responses to services in the case record, including follow-up services.

Rehabilitation Nurse

Some programs incorporate the clinical services of a Rehabilitation Nurse who can monitor the client's medical status and medications, and can provide education in health related behaviors and their relationship to the work place. Topics may include nutrition, monitoring vital signs, blood pressure, use of medications, substance abuse and other medical conditions as indicated. As a team member, the nurse participates in team conferences and makes entries in the case record.

THE AUXILIARY TEAM

The auxiliary team members in industrial therapy, by virtue of influence, play an essential role on the expected outcome: return to work. Coordinating the agendas and goals of these team members is often the ultimate challenge. Members of this team can vary. The author will address only the physician, employer, family, and legal consult in this chapter.

The Physician

Physicians providing services to the injured worker have various specialties, including the specialization in industrial or occupational medicine. Typically more than one physician is involved in the case. Each contributes to the care of the injured worker in individual areas of expertise depending on the nature of the injury. Their services may be sought by the injured worker, the insurance provider, lawyer, case manager, or employer.

The Physician's role, often in frequent interaction with the Vocational Rehabilitation Consultant, is to complete a diagnostic work-up, provide or prescribe appropriate medical tests or treatments, and monitor the progression of the healing process.

In the case of industrial injury, it is imperative that the physician has a clear understanding of the injured worker's work place and job duties, since the final release for return to work is the decision of the physician. The physician may also be required to make disability determinations and provide expert witness if legal action is taken.

The Employer

The employer's role in industrial rehabilitation is indeed powerful. The relationship maintained with the worker prior to and during the rehabilitation process ultimately determines the achievement of the primary goal: return to work. When the employer hires the worker, each party has certain expectations. The employer expects the worker to produce a desired product or service, and the employee expects certain benefits, not the least of which is a salary. Other customary benefits include health benefits, Workers' Compensation, disability benefits, and unemployment compensation.

This relationship constitutes an employment agreement, whether expressed or implied, that governs how the mutual needs of each party will be met. Both have the responsibility for a safe work environment, safe working protocols and practices. Ideally these conditions need to be in writing, acknowledged, accepted, and practiced in a spirit of equal mutual responsibility by employer and employee.

When a worker becomes injured, the employment agreement is not severed. The employer has the responsibility to assure that the employee receives the appropriate medical services as identified in the insurance policy endorsed by the employer. The employee is also entitled to Workers' Compensation benefits as determined by the respective state laws.

Unfortunately, many employers feel their responsibilities end here, expecting the primary industrial rehabilitation team to rehabilitate the worker for return to work. Current trends are showing that employer's continued involvement in the rehabilitation process does indeed shorten the lost time and accelerate a successful return to work.

The employer may work with the industrial rehabilitation team in providing preventative programs and delegate a representative to maintain contact with the injured worker. The employer might also participate in case management, Job Analysis, work station modification, and return to work policies, including part-time and light-duty.

An example of an employer involvement in preventative measures is the Boeing study, which indicated that work perception and psychosocial factors affect the reporting of back injuries.[3] Through this study, the employer recognized that there were factors other than physical that contributed to lost time due to reported back injury. The management of perception and psychosocial factors can affect the overall cost of work injuries.

The Americans with Disabilities Act (ADA), which became effective July 1, 1992 for employers with 25 or more employees, (as of July 1, 1994, 15 or more employees) will continue to drive a movement toward creative practices in dealing with return to work issues in the future.

The Family

Traditionally the relationship of the family to the worker has been one of financial dependency. The disruption of the financial relationship, superimposed on the disruption in the family's established daily routine, play a significant influence in the rehabilitation process. The major issue is to maintain financial stability during the healing process. Secondary to that, is the extent to which the family provides emotional support for the injured worker.

It is important that the family understands the nature of the injury, the possible limitations it might impose, the elements of the rehabilitation process, and the psychosocial impact on the injured worker.

The family first of all must address the financial responsibilities it has incurred. This often means a budgeting process, formal or informal, to manage cash flow. If the employer has an Employee Assistance

Program which offers financial counseling and assistance, the family's financial problems might be partially alleviated. This would reinforce the positive influence of the auxiliary team approach.

In some instances, the spouse assumes additional responsibility of contributing to the financial security of the family by either entering the work force or taking on a second job. This may necessitate degrees of role reversal in relationship to child care or household responsibilities.

Financial security is an obvious need, but the not so obvious need of emotional support is vital. As mentioned earlier in this chapter, the injured worker may adopt different personality characteristics. Most often these changes evolve progressively and family members do not understand why their loved one seems to be a different person. The worker's emotional make-up and stability have been altered, and family members need to be aware of these changes in order to respond appropriately.

Another factor to consider is that the pain experienced by the injured worker cannot be readily seen by the bystander. The injured worker has less tolerance for family activities that cause pain. The injured worker may refrain from participation in these activities and appear distant, disinterested, or withdrawn. Open communication between the worker and family members is crucial for understanding and coping.

The family has to exert a great deal of patience and understanding in response to emotional dips, while at the same time provide stability. If possible, the family should accompany the injured worker to the intake interview, group presentations on stress management, nutrition classes, back-schools, and case conferences. This increases the family's coping skills and supportive influence on the injured worker's efforts at pain management.

Family members need to encourage the worker to assume responsibility for the rehabilitation process and ultimate return to work. They should encourage and reinforce the injured worker's diligence in performing home programs, especially over the weekends when therapy is not available. At the very least, the family should encourage participation in family and social activities.

The Attorney

If the injured worker becomes dissatisfied with the process, or benefit payments are interrupted for any reason, a new team member may be added. The attorney has the responsibility to represent the client's best interests in a timely manner, particularly if the rights of the injured worker are in jeopardy.

Experience has indicated, however, that Workers' Compensation cases become immensely more complicated and more costly when litigation is involved. This financial impact is aptly characterized by James Courtney, III, "The legal community is essentially a financial physician."[10]

It is the attorney's responsibility to see that all the necessary documents pertaining to the job and medical history are obtained and that a good case history is completed. The attorney often also fulfills the role of case manager, and is therefore responsible for assuring that the client receives the appropriate rehabilitation services required. When return to work issues are clouded, it is the attorney's responsibility to see that return to work requirements are made possible, or that alternative services are provided that will afford the client the opportunity to return to the working community.

There are other members of the auxiliary team including but not limited to the Workers' Compensation Commission and the unions. Since their roles are dictated mostly by law or contractual agreements, it is outside the bounds of this chapter to cover all the possible changes of their roles and relationships.

EXTERNAL SERVICE PROVIDERS

Finally there are external service providers. Included in this group are insurance representatives, case managers, ergonomists, industrial engineers, dietitians, orthotists, prosthetists, educators, financial counselors, and counselors of specialty programs, such as smoking cessation and substance abuse. The services of these individuals in their respective fields is aimed at overcoming return to work barriers.

Case Manager

The case manager is typically a rehabilitation professional, often a Vocational Rehabilitation Consultant, who either works directly for an insurance company or a private rehabilitation service provider. The case manager assumes the responsibility of triaging appropriate services for the injured worker in a cost effective manner.

The case manager coordinates the services provided and facilitates the communication between all team members and service providers. This ensures that consolidated goals and realistic time frames are established. The case manager chooses the providers of service and schedules these services. Although the case manager is usually accountable to the financial provider, responsibilities include being an advocate of the injured worker in the quest to regain the status of worker.

Office Support Services

Most industrial therapy programs require the support services of a marketing representative and clerical staff. The role of these team members is not to be underestimated. The individual responsible for marketing the industrial rehabilitation program needs to develop a marketing plan, including designing marketing materials. This individual needs to do a marketing analysis and develop marketing strategies. Time is spent calling on referral sources, conducting tours of the facility, and possibly arranging for programs to be presented at the facility or referral source office.

The marketing representative does frequent mailings and telephone contacts. Follow-up and service calls are very important. The marketer attends or exhibits at relevant meetings and seminars and is active in community organizations.

The program secretary or office manager is also a marketer of sorts. Often this person is the first contact someone has with the organization. The secretary therefore needs to fully understand the services provided in order to field questions and give appropriate information. The primary responsibilities of the secretary includes receptionist's tasks, managing the office, and processing the correspondence of the organization.

Often it is the responsibility of the office coordinator to verify insurance coverage, schedule appointments, complete the billing process, maintain program statistics, and manage the storage of case records.

SUMMARY

The evolution of Industrial Therapy has taught us that the injured worker's needs extend far beyond healing the injured body part. Professionals have discovered that addressing the full range of needs holistically yields better rehabilitation outcomes. The most beneficial results have been more complete restoration of function, faster return to work, and lower overall costs.

As this multifaceted orientation has evolved, Industrial Therapy has been characterized by increased specialization in each area of need, and a growing recognition that when these specialists work together as a team, commensurate benefits ensue.

Over time, the injured worker's role has evolved from a "passive recipient" of care to an active team member and participant in the rehabilitation process. Concurrently, the team has been enhanced by including everyone who has a stake in the outcome, or who can contribute important benefits to the process.

The evolution of this team concept in Industrial Therapy is sure to continue, characterized by increasing levels of expertise and specialization, continuing innovation, and growing progress toward the excellent management of not only disability, but of ability as well.

REFERENCES

1. AJOT: Guidelines for Work Hardening, 40(12):841–843, 1986.
2. APTA: Guidelines for Programs in Industrial Rehabilitation, November, 1992.
3. Bigos S, Battel M, Spengler D, Fisher L, Fordyce W, Hanson T, Nachemson A, Wortley M: A Prospective Study of Work Perceptions and Psychosocial Factors Affecting the Report of Back Injury, *Spine* 16:1, 1991.
4. Bitter J: *Introduction to Rehabilitation*, St Louis, 1979, Mosby.
5. Blankenship KL: Work Capacity Evaluation and Industrial Consultation (seminar manual), American Therapeutics, 1985.
6. CARF: 1992 Standards Manual for Organizations Serving People with Disabilities, The Commission of Accreditation of Rehabilitation Facilities.
7. DiMichael SG: The Current Scene, In Miliken D, Rusdem H editors: Vocational Rehabilitation of the Disabled; an overview, New York, 1969, New York University Press.
8. ERGOS Work Simulator User's Training Manual, Work Recovery Inc., 1991.
9. Hertfelder S, Givin C, editor: Work in Progress, Occupational Therapy in Work Programs, *AOTA*, 1989.
10. Isernhagen SI: Work Injury Management and Prevention, Aspen Series In Lewis CB series editor, 1988, Aspen Publications.
11. Key, GL: Work Hardening or Work Conditioning—Semantics or Reality?, *Phys Ther Today* vol 14, 1991.
12. Matheson LN (with contributions by Ogden-Niemeyer L): Industrial Rehabilitation Resource book 1990 including the 1988 edition of the Work Capacities Evaluation Training Manual.
13. McGowan JF, Porter TL: An Introduction to the Vocational Rehabilitation Process, Washington, DC, Government Printing Office, 1967.
14. Ogden-Niemeyer L, Jacobs K: Work Hardening State of the Art, New Jersey, 1989, Slack.
15. Townsend MR: Sheltered Workshops—a Handbook, National Association of Sheltered Workshops, ed 2, Home-bound Programs, Washington, DC, 1966.
16. Tramposh A, Lett CF, et al: The Successful Approach manual for the Functionally Fit for Work Process seminar Wx: Work Capacities, 1989.
17. Williams JD: Insuring the Success of Work Hardening; the Role of the Rehabilitation Counselor in Return to Work (an abstract) CAIRE Conference; Work Injury Management, Advances in Prevention, Evaluation and Treatment of Work Injuries, Denver, 1989.

CHAPTER

3

The Impact and Outcomes of Industrial Therapy

Glenda L. Key

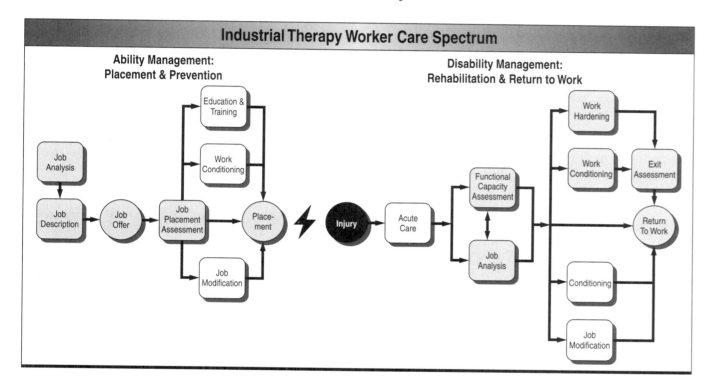

The post World War II dominance American industry enjoyed in technology, capital, and market penetration has been gradually chipped away as foreign economies have grown. Profit margins and total profits have been under continuing pressure. America's productivity and living standard are still number one, but holding that position has become a formidable challenge. With differences in technology, capital, and marketing narrowed, American industry must seek competitive advantages in new areas.

Industrial Therapy, through injury prevention and expeditious return to work, represents one such area. Lowering medical and disability costs, reducing work loss days, and enhancing wellness and productivity represent significant opportunities for competitive advantages in the global arena.

Under increasing scrutiny from financial executives, payors, and litigants, all parties to the rehabilitation process need strong support for the recommendations and treatment procedures they bring to the process. Everyone is being made progressively more accountable for the outcome of their efforts.

Recent Trends

Injuries have always been a factor in the production of goods and services, but there are a number of developments that are accelerating the costs of injuries, and driving the demand for more financially favorable outcomes.

One significant influence is the emergence of a more highly skilled work force. In an earlier era when most production jobs were lower skilled or unskilled, replacements for injured workers could be quickly recruited and trained. Today, with a preponderance of skilled jobs, it takes significantly more time and money to recruit replacements and progress them to the previous job-holder's level of productivity. Because of this, industry has learned that the best way to minimize costs and restore productivity is to return the injured worker to the job quickly, safely, and as cost-effectively as possible.

With today's workforce more skilled than ever before, the most financially favorable outcomes are to prevent injuries from happening in the first place, and to find ways to restore the injured worker to safe productivity levels as quickly as possible. In this light, the preferred outcome has become synonymous with what is in the best interest of the worker.

Another trend is the increasing incidence of litigation. The United States has 5% of the world's population, and 33% of the world's attorneys.[4] These attorneys have to generate revenue. Lawyers do not benefit when the worker and employer implement an amicable rehabilitation and return-to-work program. They only make money if the employer-employee relationship falters. As attorneys become increasingly involved, case closure entails higher legal fees and higher settlements.

Chapter Focus

This chapter will focus on outcomes management, defined as the process of monitoring, compiling, and analyzing the results of client care for the purpose of discovering the most effective programs and procedures, improving quality, and reducing cost (Figure 3.1).

The discussion will include the kinds of outcomes being sought by parties involved in Industrial Therapy, the nature and uses of outcome studies, and how the Industrial Therapy practice can implement an outcome orientation in the provision of their services.

SOURCES OF DEMAND FOR OUTCOMES

In the environment described above, the demand for statistically verifiable and reproducible outcomes is growing rapidly. If an employer or payor can be shown in hard numbers how to significantly reduce the incidence of injuries, or restore an injured worker to maximum productivity faster or less expensively, they are ready to listen. In addition, the parties involved in Industrial Therapy have emerging needs that are bolstering the demand for outcome studies.

Employees need to return to work quickly, to the

FIGURE 3.1 Outcomes Management Process

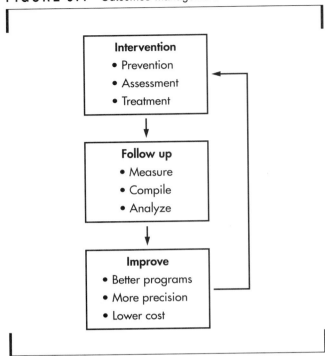

same job status, with confidence that the risk of reinjury is minimized or eliminated.

Physicians need strong support for their recommendations and treatment procedures in legal and reimbursement disputes. They also need confidence in the capabilities of the Industrial Therapists in referring their patients, particularly since they are barred from owning or controlling the Therapy practice to whom they refer.

Employers need reliable outcome data to guide prevention strategies, streamline return to work time frames and costs, direct wellness efforts, deter or defend against legal challenges, and minimize insurance rates, particularly when self-insured.

Vocational Rehabilitation Consultants need to develop new ways to achieve case progression and closure more efficiently and effectively.

Attorneys need statistically reliable, supporting information to strengthen their case in court and maximize the amount of settlement.

Insurance Companies are under pressure from both competitors and regulators to keep premiums down by shortening the return to work cycle, streamlining rehabilitation steps, restoring a higher percentage of pre-injury function, lowering the rate of reinjury, reducing the incidence of fraudulent claims, implementing effective case management practices, and keeping the process out of litigation.

Industrial Therapists, as ammunition in recruiting new prospects or justifying recommendations and reimbursements, need quantitative support that their treatment outcomes have derived from effective methods and not by chance or random occurrence.

Legislators need accurate outcome information in order to identify areas requiring legislative action, and to establish standards for treatment and reimbursement.

TYPES OF OUTCOMES BEING SOUGHT

Employers, employees, insurers, and providers are focusing primarily on the following goals:

Reduced rates of injury

Reduced rates of reinjury post rehabilitation

Reduced total costs of injuries

Higher return to work rates

Shorter, more predictive return to work time frames

Maximized restored function - same employer/same job

Minimized legal exposure

Minimized incidence of litigation

Legally defensible assessment and treatment procedures

Financially justifiable Industrial Therapy programs

Improved worker morale

Improved employer-employee relationships

Reduced Rates of Injury and Reinjury

In a classic brain teaser, a room is flooding because someone has left the water running with the sink drain plugged. There is a floor drain, a bucket, and a mop. The question posed is what should be done to prevent further damage? The answer is to shut off the water. In Industrial Therapy, the first priority should be to shut off the injuries.

There are a number of measures directed toward this outcome: safer job placement through Job Placement Assessment and Job Analysis; safer working conditions through ergonomic analysis, job modification and job rotation; safer workstyles through education and training; better return to work decisions through Functional Capacity Assessment; and strengthened capabilities through Work Hardening, Work Conditioning, and ongoing fitness programs. By monitoring outcomes and statistically relating them to these prevention measures, continuing progress against injury rates can be accomplished.

Outcome Study A

A study of 220 Michigan establishments (with more than 100 employees) correlated differences in em-

ployer-reported levels of achievement in prevention policies and activities with disability outcome measures. The study indicated the benefits of performance on the following prevention policies and activities.[4]

A 10% increase in performance level of this activity . . .	. . . Yields this% reduction in lost workdays/100 workers
Proactive RTW programs	13.6%
Safety diligence	13.0%
Safety training	6.5%

Employers are also discovering ways to detect propensities toward injuries before they happen.

Outcome Study B

A state transportation authority has found that Functional Capacity Assessments enable them to predict whether an employee is at risk of injury. Among 36 employees injured from 1985 to 1992, 75% had been categorized as "at risk" by FCA's performed when these employees were hired.[9]

Therapists can use outcome information like this to show employers existing tools that have reduced the incidence of injuries and their attendant problems and costs, and that they do not have to accept their current injury rates as unavoidable "givens."

Reduced Costs of Injuries

The costs of Workers' Compensation claims and ratings, litigation, health care, and lost productivity have been skyrocketing in recent years.[7] Concurrently, intensifying competition has been bringing all costs under closer scrutiny than ever before.

While implementing measures to prevent injuries and reinjuries, employers are also seeking ways to streamline rehabilitation and return to work time frames and costs without compromising other objectives. There is a growing demand for outcome statistics to support every component of the rehabilitation plan, from assessment methodologies to goal setting, program design, treatment components, duration, and fees.

Whether in Functional Capacity Assessment, Job Analysis, Work Conditioning, or Work Hardening, there is an increasing preference for objectivity over opinion, proof over speculation, reliability over happenstance, accuracy over guesswork, and science over art. Whenever outcome statistics support a new approach to reducing rehabilitation time or expense, employers and payors are ready to listen.

Outcome Study C

The Potlach Corporation instituted Job Placement Assessment (JPA) in September of 1988 to help stem the costs of lost work days and Workers' Compensation claims. Two years later the experiences of 70 employees hired before the use of JPA's were compared to 70 hired after the use of JPA's. The results showed that JPA's reduced lost work days and Workers' Compensation costs:[6]

	70 Hirees — no JPA's	70 Hirees — with JPA's
Lost work days	520	26
Workers' Comp. costs	$3,000,000	$880,000

Outcome information expressed in terms of productivity and pocketbook concerns can be used by therapists to get the employer's attention, and begin to propose proven methods of impacting these important bottom line issues.

Higher Return to Work Rates

Employers and payors have realized that in most cases, rehabilitating injured workers is preferable to paying long term disability costs or hiring, training, and progressing replacement workers to comparable productivity levels. A key objective, therefore, is to return progressively higher percentages of injured workers to their pre-injury employment status.

Using outcome statistics to evaluate treatment effectiveness has been instrumental in fine tuning the components of the Worker Care Spectrum toward higher return to work rates. In addition, rehabilitation has adopted a team approach to planning and implementation, and new disciplines and treatment components were brought into the process. For example, when it was found that psychosocial factors tended to stifle motivation and progress, psychological professionals were added to the team, and the client's family and peer group were involved in appropriate components of the care continuum.

Outcome Study D

A research team at the University of Texas Health Science Center at Dallas used Functional Capacity Assessments to monitor and guide a treatment program for 116 chronic low back pain patients. This group's results were compared with a group of 72 patients who did not receive the treatment program. The outcome study indicated higher return to work rates as follows:[8]

	Treatment group	Comparison group
RTW after 1 year	85%	39%
Add'l surgery in 1st year	4%	12%
Medical visits 1st year:		
Percent visiting	33%	75%
Visits per person	2.3	21.0

Often, procedures like Functional Capacity Assessments are seen as "extra costs" over and above the way people are accustomed to accomplish successful outcomes. Outcome studies enable therapists to change the perceptions from "costs" to "bottom line contributors."

Faster Return to Work

The length of time off work directly affects costs, productivity, and the prospects for maximum recovery. Outcome studies have shown that return to work is accelerated by the earliest possible intervention post injury, by accurate and reliable Functional Capacity Assessment for rehabilitation goal-setting and implementation, and by individualized planning for each client.

Outcome Study E

A 1987 study comparing early intervention with return–to–work rates indicated that cases referred to a Vocational Rehabilitation Consultant within one month after injury were returned to work at a remarkable 86% success rate. Cases referred beyond two years post-injury experienced only a 37% return–to–work rate.[1]

Referral delay vs reemployment

Delay: injury to referral (mos.)	No. cases	% Reemployed
0–1	190	86%
2–3	278	75%
4–6	118	68%
7–12	86	65%
13–18	54	54%
19–24	38	47%
25+	107	37%

There is a tendency to look only at treatment options for opportunities to shorten the return to work time frame, but some providers are finding opportunities in the assessment phase.

Outcome Study F

Waite studied the impact of FCAs on shortening the amount of time required for vocational evaluation of injured workers. The analysis indicated that clients undergoing a KEY Method FCA required a median of 18 fewer days of vocational evaluation.[11]

Employers are undoubtedly inundated with proposals to accelerate the return to work time frame safely and cost effectively. Outcome studies are one way to stand out from the crowd of competing appeals, and to explain approaches in monetary terms employers understand.

Maximized Restored Function

As mentioned, restoring the injured worker to full pre-injury productivity is the ideal outcome. Work Conditioning and Work Hardening have been instrumental in addressing the physical and psychological needs for successful recovery of function. In addition, Functional Capacity Assessment in conjunction with Job Analysis have enabled workstyle and job modifications that further enhance the workers' productivity levels. Finally, ongoing employee fitness programs have been shown to bolster morale and productivity.

Outcome Study G

At Saatchi & Saatchi Advertising, morale was shown to improve in 75% of the fitness participants and productivity increased among 63%.[6]

Employers with low worker enthusiasm, substandard productivity, and high absenteeism understand the competitive disadvantages that result. Through outcome studies that measure such factors, there is an opportunity to demonstrate the positive role of Industrial Therapy.

Everything the employer does to accelerate return to work, maximize restored function, and promote an on-going healthy work culture sends the kind of positive signals that restore enthusiasm and commitment to mutual goals.

Minimized Legal Exposure

Legal exposure stems from two main sources: government encroachment and injury liability.

Under increasing government encroachment, primarily regarding OSHA and the Americans with Disabilities Act, employers are seeking more reliable support. They want confirmation that their work environments, work stations, and tools are safe. They want assurance that their hiring and placement policies and procedures are defensible. Outcome studies that can back up the employer's approach to Job Placement Assessments, Ergonomics, and prevention programs can be invaluable in substantiating that compliance actions are appropriate and sound.

Regarding injuries, reducing injury rates and increasing return to work rates directly lessens the amount of legal exposure. A lower than average rate of injury not only reduces sheer numbers of potential legal cases, it also provides support that the company's working conditions are safer than most.

Similarly, a higher than average return to work rate does more than reduce the number of frustrated workers who might resort to litigation. It provides support that the company is doing more to help its injured workers regain their jobs.

Minimized Incidence of Litigation

Where exposure remains, litigation looms as a possibility but is mitigated by some relevant factors. First, it helps to organize rehabilitation around the team concept with the client taking an active role. By sharing in the responsibility for rehabilitation, a more positive attitude develops, and a less likely "them-us" view of the process results.

Further, if mistakes are made, the team concept causes more of a problem-solving response rather than a blaming response that can lead to litigation. Finally, as employers more actively and visibly stand behind their workers with prevention and rehabilitation programs, they present a more attractive win-win alternative to the win-lose litigation process.

Legally Defensible Treatment Procedures

When litigation is involved, the worker's attorney will try to prove that whatever has gone wrong is the fault of improper working conditions or improper therapeutic judgments, recommendations, or procedures. As assessment and treatment approaches become more objective, reliable, predictive, and supportable with outcome statistics, it becomes increasingly difficult to successfully challenge therapeutic components in a court of law.

In addition, regulators and the courts tend to judge more favorably, those companies that have objective and systematic procedures. When companies objectively predetermine an employees' safe capabilities and risk points, take measured steps to make the workplace safer, or proactively accelerate rehabilitation and return to work, such good faith efforts can go a long way in ameliorating court judgments and settlement amounts.

Financially Justifiable Programs and Procedures

Employers and payors are increasingly challenging the proposed length, scope, and complexity of Industrial Therapy components. Outcome studies not only help support the recommended prevention or treatment program before the fact, they also help demonstrate that positive outcomes after the fact correlate closely with the quality of treatment provided.

Outcome Study H

The Association of Quality Health Clubs analyzed the return six corporations obtained on dollars invested in employee fitness programs.

Fitness program returns on invested dollars

Company	Dollars returned per dollar invested
Coors	$ 6.15
Kennecott	$ 5.78
Equitable Life	$ 5.52
General Mills	$ 3.90
Motorola	$ 3.15
Pepsi	$ 3.00

With permission from IRSA, 1992.[6]

Sometimes it is difficult to convince financial people as to the cause and effect of alleged financial benefits. However, at a very minimum, dollar and cents payout measures get a discussion started that, without these numbers, might never have occurred.

Improved Worker Morale

As Industrial Therapy becomes a more structured and effective system of prevention and rehabilitation, it sends a positive, morale-building signal to the workforce that the company stands behind its employees. In addition, outcome studies have shown that employee fitness programs enhance morale. Further, they have also shown that high morale is associated with lower levels of reported injuries.

Outcome Study I

A study by Boeing indicated that workers with positive work perceptions and psychosocial responses on psychological tests (MMPI) showed the lowest incidence of back injury reporting. Those indicating that they "hardly ever" enjoy their job report 2.5 times the back injury claims of those indicating that they "almost always" enjoy their job.[2]

As mentioned earlier, there are a number of ways in which Industrial Therapy programs can positively impact morale. However when problems arise, employers are more likely to think of motivational seminars, retreats, and other responses that attend to the mind. Outcome studies enable Therapists to gain consideration for approaches that attend to the body.

Improved Employer-Employee Relationships

A good working relationship between the employer and employee is another component of minimizing costly turnover and enhancing worker morale. This relationship impacts costs and productivity in a number of ways.

Outcome Study J

British Columbia Hydroelectric employees who participated in fitness programs revealed a turnover rate of 3.5% versus the company's average rate of 10.4%.[3]

USES OF OUTCOME INFORMATION

It is evident from the foregoing that outcome studies dramatize to industry, ways to protect profits and maintain productivity and competitiveness. Industrial Therapists can bring such studies to the attention of industry, and provide proven solutions. In doing so, they will attract more referrals and solidify their customer base.

One readily accessible source of outcome information is a growing presence of published studies in industry journals such as:

- *American Journal of Physical Medicine*
- *Journal of the American Association of Occupational Health Nurses*
- *Journal of American Medical Association*
- *Journal of Applied Physiology*
- *Journal of Hand Therapy*
- *Journal of Occupational Medicine*
- *Journal of Occupational Therapy*
- *Journal of Orthopaedic and Sports Physical Therapy*
- *Journal of Public Health*
- *Journal of Rehabilitation*
- *Physical Therapy*
- *Risk and Benefits Journal*
- *Spine*
- *WORK: A Journal of Prevention, Assessment, & Rehabilitation*

Published studies are certainly better than relying on judgment, opinion, or guesswork, but a growing number of Industrial Therapists are discovering the advantages of generating their own outcome studies.

Citing first hand knowledge enhances the Therapist's credibility, whether for purposes of justifying reimbursement, testifying in legal proceedings, or marketing services to new prospects. Moreover, augmenting published information with first-hand experiences enables the practice to more precisely tailor programs and procedures to their own customer base and internal operating culture.

The major ways in which outcome information can be used by Industrial Therapists is as follows:

- To influence legislative endeavors
- To improve assessment and treatment procedures

- To support treatment and reimbursement
- To deter or win litigation
- To educate customers and clients
- To market industrial therapy services to new prospects

Influence Legislative Endeavors

With the skyrocketing costs of health care, Federal and State legislatures are developing plans and legislation to regulate and control medical practices and costs. Unfortunately, legislators are not always knowledgeable about professions outside of traditional medicine, and may therefore design solutions that assume physicians are the only players.

Therapist organizations are educating lawmakers as to their important role. Outcome studies are instrumental in gaining the attention and credibility required to ensure the Therapist's role is acknowledged and incorporated in new legislation.

Improve Assessment and Treatment Procedures

By diligently following-up with clients in their work place, post-assessment or post-treatment results can be tracked to evaluate whether attempted improvements in assessment protocols or treatment procedures have yielded the prevention, return-to-work, or productivity outcomes that were sought. An effective process keeps therapists in touch with what is working as intended, and what is not. As the volume of data and case histories increases, outcomes of various programs and treatments become more predictable, and a clearer understanding of variability in results emerges.

In some instances, outcome studies indicate shortcomings in programs or procedures that the Therapist may have been using for years. In such instances, paradigms may have to be broken. Indeed, a commitment to use outcome studies to guide experimentation and implementation requires a commitment from principals on down, and a culture of monitoring and adjusting every aspect of Industrial Therapy.

Support Treatment and Reimbursement

Although the financial pressures to cut costs and streamline procedures are growing steadily, the pressure to play it safe from the standpoint of risk exposure often inhibits experimentation and adoption of new approaches. With the presence of reimbursement caps, there is growing pressure to reduce treatment procedures to their lowest common denominator at the expense of quality.

Outcome studies can be used to relieve these sources of pressure—to defend against further cuts in cost or quality, or to support that reductions can be achieved without adverse consequences. In short, outcome studies help to reduce the amount of haggling over procedures and costs, and free up the Therapist to spend more time serving their clients.

Deter or Win Litigation

In courtroom proceedings regarding injury cases, there is a growing demand for objective, reliable, and valid data to support or discredit allegations regarding the nature of the injury and the appropriateness of assessment and treatment. When opinions or judgments are pitted against statistically sound outcome studies, the numbers prevail. In defending an assessment or treatment process, the Therapist who follows outcome-verified protocols or procedures has much less exposure than the Therapist who improvises. In many instances, the mere presence of strong outcome study validations can deter an attorney from litigation. For more information on using Functional Capacity Assessment in this regard, see Chapter 13.

Educate Customers and Clients

Many companies are keenly aware of certain problems that they have, but are unaware of others. It is quite common to accept problems as an inevitable consequence of doing business, or to believe that everything is as good as it can be. Many companies are not aware that Job Placement Assessments can significantly reduce the incidence of injuries below what may be perceived as an unavoidable "given."

Many companies are not aware that absenteeism and turnover can be reduced by a companywide commitment to employee fitness programs. Many companies do not realize there are a multitude of proven approaches to returning injured workers to their jobs more successfully and efficiently. It is difficult, however, to convince a company to address unperceived problems, or to fix what they do not see as broken. That is where outcome studies can play an important role.

Statistically verified benefits that impact productivity and the bottom line can quickly get management's attention and interest—the necessary first step in any process of education. When the time comes to convince employees to embrace prevention and wellness strategies, hard numbers can provide the convincing evidence that a new program or policy will yield real benefits.

Market IT Services to New Prospects

As mentioned, it is difficult to propose solutions when management is unaware of the problems, or views them as unavoidable "givens." In addition, the complexity of Industrial Therapy components such as Job Placement Assessment, Ergonomics, Functional Capacity Assessments and Work Hardening further complicate the communication and decision process. Outcome studies that indicate bottom line results are one way to cut through to what is really important to prospects.

OUTCOME MANAGEMENT STRATEGIES

In light of the expanding role outcome studies are playing, and how they further the professional interests of therapists, it behooves the Industrial Therapy practice to develop an outcome oriented culture, and to make tracking, collecting, and analyzing information an automatic, everyday occurrence.

Establishing The Culture

Therapists are typically quite familiar with the clinical measures necessary for the delivery and progression of patient care. They must become equally well versed in outcome measures that are useful to employers, payors, attorneys, and other entities.

It is important to establish a measurement orientation on the part of therapists and everyone else in the practice or clinic. Measurement and record keeping for outcomes must become a reflex, a habit, an everyday part of assessment and treatment procedures. Follow up with clients after return to work should also be instituted as a formal procedure.

A sound outcomes management system necessitates standardized measurement and information processing procedures. Some therapists may view these functions as diverting their time from patient care. Others may see it as the overintrusion of science into the art of their profession. These paradigms must be addressed, and everyone in the practice must realize that outcome management is an inevitable development. It will further the mission of the practice, and Industrial Therapy as a whole.

Cost and Time Considerations

At the outset, however, it is also important to weigh the costs and time associated with the benefits derived. Measurement for the sake of measurement; analysis for the sake of analysis can overburden the staff and interfere with the provision of quality care. The Therapist and practice must therefore devote careful time making hard choices as to what should or should not be measured.

What Outcomes to Measure

Certainly, outcomes can be effective in marketing services to new prospects. Since the primary objectives of Industrial Therapy are to safely place employees, keep them healthy and productive, and to return injured employees to maximum safe function as quickly as possible, the most important outcomes to track should be those that relate to these primary goals. If attention is paid to these end results, the rewards will inevitably come.

Perhaps the most important criterion in making these decisions, then, is which outcome measurements are in the best long term interest of the client. In many cases, the client's long term interest is better served by programs with the higher short term costs. In such instances, the higher cost program can be justified if there are outcome studies documenting a superior long term result.

A practice devoted to the best possible result for its patients should compile outcome information on programs vulnerable to cost scrutiny. A practice lacking sufficient documentation to support a recommended program or treatment, should endeavor to access the necessary information from the sources mentioned earlier, or network through industry contacts to obtain supporting outcome data.

Under the principle of client-orientation, the most important outcomes to measure would be:

1. Injury rates of employees
2. Length of time between injury and therapist intervention
3. Length of time between therapist intervention and return to work
4. The specific intervention performed
5. Return to work status:
   Same employer/same job
   Same employer/modified job
   Same employer/different job
   Different employer/same job
   Different employer/modified job
   Different employer/different
   Not reemployed
6. Reinjury rates of assessed or rehabilitated employees

General Approach to Analysis

Gathered and compiled on an ongoing basis, the data from these six measurements could then be correlated with Industrial Therapy programs and services that have been provided. For example, if the practice begins administering JPAs, comparisons could be made with injury rates before and after the assessments begin. If a companywide employee fitness program is implemented, a prepost analysis could be made with regard to employee injury rates, absenteeism, turnover, and productivity. In a similar fashion, monitoring data as a matter of course enables therapists to develop convincing support for specific programs, procedures, reimbursements, and marketing efforts.

Ongoing measurement and tracking can also be used as a means of accounting for variables. Was litigation involved? Did the client skip sessions? Did the client have a history of injuries? Did the client attempt to function above recommended levels upon returning to work? Isolating employees displaying these circumstances and comparing them to the rest of the data base can yield conclusions about the influence of variables.

Of course, employers will also be interested in such data as Workers' Compensation costs and ratings, costs of total injuries and injuries per worker, lost work days, litigation trends, and settlement costs. The Industrial Therapy practice may want to include these measures for purposes of marketing, but only in addition to, not in place of, the six employee-oriented outcomes that are the primary focus of the profession.

Procedural Standardization

To enable statistically reliable analyses and predictability, the set of variables to be monitored must be recorded using standardized measurement methodologies. Personnel should measure the same things at the same points in time using the same tools and procedures. Accurate documentation through consistent forms and recording procedures should be adhered to.

For example, Functional Capacity Assessments should be performed using standardized equipment and protocols. The people performing assessments should interject as little judgment and "tester error" as possible—a prerequisite to any sound statistical process. Finally, the information should be processed in a consistent, objective manner with a minimum of opinion or guesswork applied.

Industry Standardization

The formats in which data is collected and compiled should be merged with existing industry formats to facilitate comparisons to normative data. Where industry norms as to treatment and outcome are available, the clinic can predict outcomes with greater confidence. Formats should be consistent with:

> US Department of Labor categories
> Standard Census Demographic categories
> Standard PT and OT weight, distance, frequency, and time parameters

Data Collection System

Developing and implementing data collection procedures can be a complex process involving considerable trial and error before arriving at a system that meets the needs of the Industrial Therapy practice and its' referral sources. To assist in that undertaking, an example system is presented and discussed below.

There are four key phases in the return to work process where data collection is most important:
1. At program initiation
2. During the program—at least one interim assessment
3. Upon exit from the program
4. After return to work—at least one follow up audit

Boxes 3.1 through 3.4 on pages 40 and 41 list, for each of these collection points, the basic information that will most likely be required for future outcome studies or litigation purposes. Of course, the information listed pertains primarily to outcome study requirements. In some cases outcome information requirements overlap the medical, physical, and psychological information that might also be needed to manage the client's treatment.

As mentioned earlier, to ensure valid and reliable statistical analyses, information must be gathered using consistent methodology. To accomplish this, standardized forms and procedures should be used. In addition to formatting the information needs on forms, each staff person recording the information should receive training to properly ask the questions and record the responses.

The final issue is information storage; for easy and efficient access later and for statistical analyses. Of course, computer data base storage is the preferred method, so data runs and outcome studies can be implemented quickly and accurately.

Statistical Reliability

It goes without saying that statistical reliability increases with the number of cases in the data base. With a large enough data base, information from one company, department, job classification, or worker can be compared to industry averages. Such comparisons enable a better assessment of whether the entity or person is performing above or below norms, and to what degree further improvement might be expected.

For most Industrial Therapy practices, accumulating an adequate data base can take a great deal of time. Fortunately, data bases are emerging that can provide information useful for many of the purposes discussed above. Tying into these existing data bases, however,

B O X   3 . 1

Program Initiation Information

Personal Information
Name, address, phone numbers, Social Security number
date of birth, height, weight, left or right handed
Education level, marital status
Standard medical history profile and current status

Employment Information at Time of Injury
Job DOT code, Industry SIC code
Job type, years at job, salary or wage
Date last worked, length of time out of work
Employer, supervisor
Intention of returning to pre-injury job
Likelihood of returning to pre-injury job

Injury Information
Date of injury, whether job related
How it happened, diagnosis, affected body parts

Post Injury Medical Information
Physician(s) and other providers
Medical and other treatment previously received
Medical and other treatment receiving currently

Other Party Information
Source of referral
Insurance company, Vocational Counselor, Attorney
Litigation status

Assessment Information
FCA results
Job demands
FCA validity of participation

B O X   3 . 2

Interim Assessment Information

Heart Rate Information
Resting heart rate
Activity heart rate
Maximum heart rate (220—age)
Activity rate as % of maximum

Job Task Capabilities
% attainment of job demands and treatment goals

Behavioral Information
Pain or other reports, at what activities or weights
Tardiness and absenteeism record
Compliance and cooperation

Postural Information
Postures performing job demands or treatment
activities

B O X   3 . 3

Exit Information

Program Review
Start date
Goals at beginning
Medical and other treatment received
% attainment of job demands and treatment goals
Attendance record

Discharge Information
Date of discharge
Satisfactory completion, or reasons for noncompletion
Exit FCA results versus goals
Litigation status
Customer satisfaction review

Work Status
Employed, unemployed, referred for vocational training
If employed, job type
Full or part time
Same, modified, or different job
Same or different employer
Working below, at, or above exit recommendations
Employer and facility identification

BOX 3.4

Follow Up Information After RTW Six and Twelve Months Post Program Exit

Employee identification
Employer and facility identification
Program exit date, RTW date, elapsed days
Working or not
Job type
Full or part time
Same, modified, or different job
Same or different employer
Working below, at, or above exit recommendations
Litigation status
Injury incidence since RTW
Medical and other treatment receiving currently

---

necessitates using the same standardized equipment, protocols, and treatment procedures that were used in gathering the existing data. Otherwise comparisons would be unreliable and irresponsible.

SUMMARY

Pressure to increase productivity and counteract rising costs of healthcare, Workers' Compensation, lost work days, litigation, and regulatory oversight has focused a great deal of cost scrutiny on Industrial Therapy programs and procedures. This situation has brought about a growing demand for statistically reliable studies that enable quantified cost-payout analysis.

There are a number of published outcome studies that serve to substantiate the benefits of many aspects of Industrial Therapy. In addition to these available studies, however, Industrial Therapists should adopt their own outcome management program, both to further enhance their credibility, and to better tailor treatment to their specific client base.

It should become second nature to follow up with clients post assessment or treatment. By monitoring, measuring, compiling, and analyzing the follow-up information, Industrial Therapists can continue to serve the demand for cost-payout substantiation, while also supporting the programs and procedures that are in the best long term interest of the client.

REFERENCES

1. Anderle M: A Good Case for Early Intervention, *NRC News & Views,* National Rehabilitation Consultants, 1–2, 1990.
2. Bigos SJ, et al: A Prospective Study of Work Perceptions and Psychosocial Factors Affecting the Report of Back Injury, University of Washington, Seattle, Department of Orthopedic Rehabilitation Medicine, Dec 1989.
3. Cigna: Benefits of Employee Health Programs, 1991.
4. Survey: The Legal Profession: the rule of lawyers, *The Economist* 324(7768):54.
5. Hunt HA, Habeck RV.: The Michigan Disability Prevention Study, Kalamazoo, Mich., WE Upjohn Institute for Employment Research, 1993.
6. IRSA, The Economic Benefits of Regular Exercise, *The Assoc of Quality Clubs,* Boston Mass., 1992.
7. Key GL: The Potlach Study, KEY Method, Sept 1990.
8. Mahone DB: Job Redesign, Not Quick Fixes, Thwarts Many Back Injury Hazards, *Occup Health & Safety* 63:51, Jan 1994.
9. Mayer TG, et al: A Prospective Two-Year Study of Functional Restoration in Industrial Low Back Injury, *JAMA,* vol 258, October 1987.
10. Personnel Decisions, Inc., KEY Functional Assessment Preemployment Screening Battery as a Predictor of Job Related Injuries, Minneapolis, Minn., Jan 25, 1994.
11. Schwartz G, et al: An Employer's Guide to Obtaining Physical Therapy Services, American Physical Therapy Association, 1989.
12. Waite HD: Use of a New Physical Capacities Assessment Method to Assist in Vocational Rehabilitation of Injured Workers, 1987.

4

Data Collection and Use in Industrial Therapy

Ed Dobrzykowski

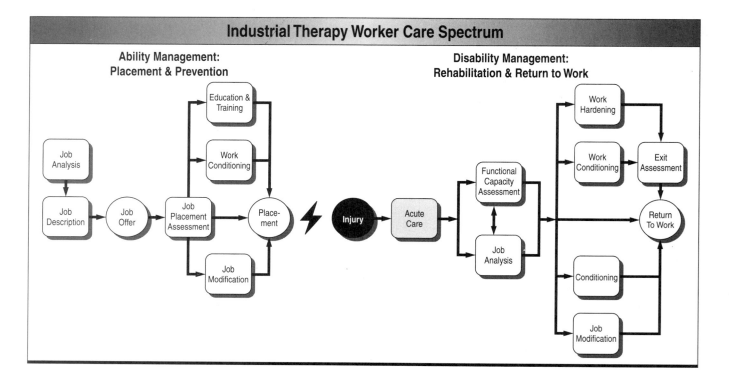

Industrial Therapy Worker Care Spectrum

Data collection involves capturing significant information before, during, and after injury and healing. The collection of data has proven to be an increasingly important component of Industrial Therapy.

This chapter will focus on the parameters for the collection and use of data in an industrial rehabilitation program, as well as the types of data that are most useful.

THE PURPOSE OF DATA COLLECTION

Data collection is undertaken to determine the relationships between treatment procedures and outcomes. This knowledge guides therapists who seek improved treatment procedures, and it documents for third parties that positive outcomes were not rendered by chance or random occurrence.

Clinical data measures in a rehabilitation program should be documented with the distinct purpose of absolute usage, after the program has ended. Unfortunately, much of the data traditionally gathered is of little relevance to our referral sources, employers, and payers (insurers); even measures demonstrating adequate *inter-* and *intra*-reliability are useless, if they are not understood.

Sometimes data is gathered because "that's the way we have always done it," or "we don't want to miss anything," or for "our protection" (defensive medicine position). New and more experienced therapists need to take a profound look at the types of measures available, and make sound judgments on data selection based upon customer requirements. Table 4.1 lists the major benefits of data collection.

Our thinking as therapists must undergo a paradigm shift, by asking ourselves first the question "which data measures provide the most useful information to our referral sources, insurance companies, clients, and to our own treatment planning and progression?" Then select measures with the ability to describe clearly the condition of interest and have predictive value.[1]

The growing collection and use of data in an Industrial Therapy program has become increasingly complex. A preponderance of data can be gathered during the process of evaluation and treatment of the injured client.

This information has two principal uses. First, much is learned about the client through the determination of their present physical capabilities and functional health status. Second, the data is then assimilated by the therapist to formulate a treatment plan, with the overall goal of maximizing a client's ability to return to safe gainful employment, as quickly as possible.

More accurate predictions of return to work can be made through combining information collected during the client's rehabilitation phase, by conducting a job placement assessment, with knowledge of an occupation's critical job demands, as determined by job analysis.

Legal Purposes

Data collection must also increasingly "stand alone" on its merits. Therapists should gather data, with the assumption that a high percentage of their clients' medical records have the potential to subsequently be deposed in a court of law. Indeed, in a recent outcome study of over 2,000 patients by Caremark Orthopedic Services Division in their Centers for Physical Therapy, 5% of patients at the time of their initial treatment date had already retained the services of an attorney.[3]

TABLE 4.1   Benefits of Data Collection

1. Evaluates relationship between treatment procedures and outcomes in order to determine the most efficient treatment.
2. Demonstrates to referral sources the effectiveness of therapy programs and treatments.
3. Identifies injury trends in the industry.
4. Supports depositions and court room appearances in the legal arena.

Depositions and actual court appearances by Industrial Therapists are becoming all too common. As the likelihood of future litigation increases with our clients, it is imperative that methods of measurement and data collection be chosen that meet all requirements ascribed to in this chapter.

In a court of law, medical records must be reliable, valid, and relevant to the worker's return to work. A patient's medical record is a legal document. When data is not recorded properly, it is inadmissible in legal proceedings. Data collection which is haphazard, inappropriate, or sketchy will ultimately be very embarrassing to the therapist presenting it to the courtroom.

Data will be admissible by the court if it has been objectively obtained and organized in a sequential manner, with measures substantiated by research and generally accepted standards of practice. The best advice is to be cognizant of the particular laws and regulations pertaining to medical and legal documentation in your own state of practice.

THE METHODOLOGY OF DATA COLLECTION

The initial assessment, treatment planning, and progression of care should involve clinical measures that can be obtained easily and rapidly.[2] Again, it makes sense to gather data with a defined purpose in mind.

Examples of Basic Measures

The Functional Capacity Assessment (FCA) is a key measure of the client's present physical capabilities, and allows comparison to the critical demands of the client's job. Although documentation of the assessment's comprehensiveness, and an organized and computer assisted method of FCA is lengthy, it will permit more streamlined collection of data and subsequent tabulation of results. The FCA is discussed in greater detail in Chapter 13.

Another example is the musculoskeletal evaluation performed by therapists at the initiation of industrial rehabilitation. The use of a standardized approach will allow more rapid data collection and ease in transcription.

General Guidelines

The types of data gathered will be a function of the therapist's academic and post-graduate training, and serve the needs of end-users. The data must meet the requirements for clinical assessment and treatment, while providing the customer with useful and meaningful information.

Data collection must also go beyond historical precedence or the perceived value to a customer. It must reflect the changing and evolving nature of health care and industry, such as the return to work status of clients seen in the program.

There are important factors to consider when determining the types of clinical measures to be utilized (Table 4.2): the type of event to be measured, the logical criteria of measurement (validity), the measurement's reliability, the event's stability, and the way in which measurements are to be used.[6] These factors warrant further discussion.

Reliability and Validity

The components of reliability and validity are essential to the accuracy of clinical measures. Reliability is the extent to which measurements consistently yield similar results. It is important to produce measures which exhibit intra-tester reliability (a positive statistical correlation of the same person measuring the same thing over time), and inter-tester reliability (a positive statistical correlation of different individuals measuring the same thing over time).[9]

The same person measuring the same event on different occasions should get the same result. Different people measuring the same event on different occasions should also get the same result.

Validity is the extent to which a method actually measures what the therapist purports that it measures. An FCA is valid only if its results accurately represent the person's true capabilities to perform job functions.

A further explanation of reliability and validity is beyond the scope of this chapter, and the reader is encouraged to review additional sources.[2,6,9]

DATA COLLECTION AND THE WORKER CARE SPECTRUM

The Worker Care Spectrum (see page 42) provides several opportunities for data collection, including job placement assessment, job analysis, rehabilitation, and whole body assessment. Keeping healthy workers injury-free and rehabilitating injured workers are the focal points of the Worker Care Spectrum. Data collection will be described during the phases of early (acute) intervention and Work Hardening.

Early Treatment Intervention

In the acute injury stage, it is important to begin rehabilitation as soon as possible. The remarkable success of many athletes returning to their sport activities quickly is often attributed to early, aggressive, and frequent treatment intervention.

The results in treatment of the "industrial athlete" should not be any different!

Accordingly, it is imperative that therapists record the time (days) from injury, to the initiation of rehabilitation. With this interval determined, a much better understanding can be made of the injured worker's profiles. For example, when this time period appears excessive (seeing the injured worker for the first time several months post-injury), reasons for delayed treatment intervention should be documented, and the delay should be related to the eventual outcome. This will permit more valid comparisons of outcomes among Industrial Therapy programs.

Other measures to consider in early intervention programs are the frequency and types of treatment provided. (Figure 4.1, A, B) Does providing daily treatment of the injured worker versus the traditional three times weekly approach, permit more rapid return to work? Which exercise regimens and specific modalities produce better outcomes?

Work Hardening and Work Conditioning

As the time accumulates from an injured worker's date of injury without return to work, physical deconditioning of the client and other psychosocial factors may hinder success and return to gainful employment. The measures ordinarily used in Work Hardening and Work Conditioning include:

1. Functional Capacity Assessment
2. Behavioral screen
3. Physiological assessment
4. Musculoskeletal evaluation
5. Job Analysis

The Functional Capacity Assessment is the cornerstone measure in the initiation of an Industrial Therapy program and a primary reference point for goal-setting and rehabilitation program design. A client's present safe physical capabilities are assessed in performing several different functions, including crawling, car-

TABLE 4.2 Considerations In Choosing A Clinical Measure

1. The type of event to be measured.
2. The measurement's validity.
3. The measurement's reliability.
4. The event's stability.
5. The way the measurements are to be used.

FIGURE 4.1 By testing the use of two different treatment procedures **A,** Ultrasound, **B,** Icing, and collecting outcome data, the therapist can document which procedure is more successful.

A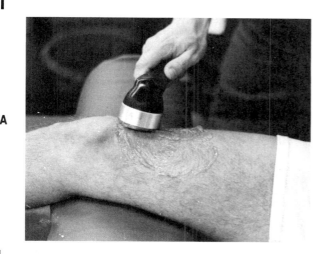

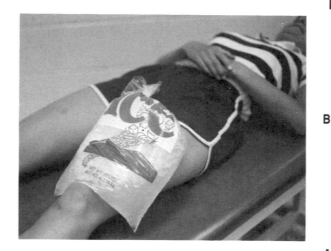 B

(From Prentice: *Rehabilitation Techniques in Sports Medicine,* ed 2, St Louis, 1994, Mosby.)

rying, walking, stair-climbing, and lifting at different heights (Figure 4.2).

Comparisons are made to the critical demands of the client's actual job. These work requirements can be ascertained through a Job Analysis. Alternatively, they may be referenced through listings provided for the United States Department of Labor by the National Institute for Occupational Safety and Health (NIOSH). This information is general and may not accurately reflect the intricacies of a client's occupational work demands. In this regard the usefulness of published job descriptions is limited.

The behavioral screen of the client is ascertained through one of several measurement instruments, such as the MMPI (Minnesota Multiphasic Personality Inventory) or Beck Depression Inventory. The successful treatment of many industrial clients may be prohibitive without appropriate behavioral intervention guided by these results.

For the assessment of behavioral status the skills of a clinical psychologist are strongly recommended, and they are required for accreditation in Work Hardening by the Commission on Accreditation of Rehabilitation Facilities (CARF). The psychologist's measures of a client's behavioral status enable the rehabilitation team to better plan and implement a successful program.

Moreover, by taking measurements in a consistent way each time, therapists may begin to compile norms for different job classifications. For example, construction workers may consistently exhibit a fear of returning to work and a high propensity for bore-

FIGURE 4.2 The Functional Capacity Assessment is used as a reference point for goal setting and program design.

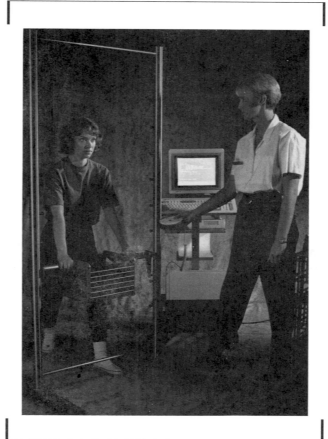

dom. Knowing tendencies such as these in advance, can help abbreviate the assessment process and improve the mix of program components for this job category.

The physiological assessment measures include heart rate, blood pressure, and cardiovascular risk factor screen. The heart rate is assessed at rest, during exercise, and particularly during job simulation tasks. Changes in heart rate should reflect the client's exertional levels. Blood pressure is assessed at rest. If baseline abnormalities are detected, or present in the client's history, blood pressure is also monitored during exercise and job simulation tasks. The cardiovascular risk factors (Box 4.1) indicate the client's personal devotion to health and wellness behaviors.

As the data base of physiological information grows, therapists can develop norms that enable them to sharpen their program's safe activity levels.

The musculoskeletal evaluation is performed by a Physical or Occupational Therapist. This evaluation begins with a review of case history information and the client's past medical history (Figure 4.3).

It also includes ratings of pain and functional abilities from the client's perspective (discussed in more detail later), joint range of motion and muscular strength measures, special muscle and joint tests unique to the evaluation of individual conditions, a palpitory exam, and a neuromuscular assessment. By measuring these factors before, during, and after rehabilitation, the therapist is able to accurately document progress and therapeutic outcomes. (Figures 4.4, *A, B, C*, page 49)

A Job Analysis is necessary for ensuring that all aspects pertinent to a client's occupation are known and considered in the planning and progression of the Work Retraining program. Job Analysis measures can be grouped into two main categories—1) the sequenc-

es of tasks, such as weights lifted, work height levels, and cycles of time, and 2) an ergonomic review.

The Job Analysis is performed by an experienced Industrial Therapist, Vocational Rehabilitation Consultant, or Ergonomist. The customers of the information gained in a Job Analysis include everyone who has a stake in the worker's successful rehabilitation, including members of the rehabilitation team, the claims payor, Workers' Compensation personnel, the line supervisors and human resource personnel. A further description of Job Analysis is provided in Chapter 7.

The Job Analysis, in combination with the Functional Capacity Assessment, behavioral screen, physiological assessment, and musculoskeletal evaluation is assimilated into a detailed Work Retraining plan for the client. The data collected must be useful in planning and managing treatment progression and in returning the client to safe gainful employment, as quickly as possible.

Collecting data is not remedial. It cannot transform a sedentary, smoking, overweight bricklayer with a low back impairment into a model of physical conditioning. However, it can be used to educate this client on the benefits of exercise, the perils of smoking, correct lifting and postural techniques, and injury avoidance and prevention.

The therapist must feel confident in answering the question: can the client safely perform the critical demands of their occupation? If not, the therapist must document the present capabilities and send the client back to the referral source with appropriate recommendations.

Computerized Measurement

There are numerous computerized measurement devices available which have been designed to aid the therapist in the rapid assimilation and compilation of client data for Work Retraining purposes. In addition to enhanced productivity, the computer's value lies in its potential for accuracy, its data storage capabilities, and its quick turn-around on comparisons with baseline measures for documenting progress. However, many computerized measurement devices are considered fairly expensive, and not all have had sufficient research completed to verify their reliability and validity.

Therapists are strongly encouraged to determine which measures are the most critical in their scheme of evaluation and most necessary for the provision of quality rehabilitative care. If desirable, a computerized device should provide these measures with sufficiently demonstrated reliability and validity.

BOX 4.1

Cardiovascular Risk Factors

- Smoker
- Family history of heart disease
- Male
- Non-exerciser
- Poor nutritional habits
- Hypertensive
- High stress level

Text continued on p 49.

FIGURE 4.3   This evaluation is one of the many joint specific evaluations termed "musculoskeletal evaluation." Each evaluation includes a review of case history information.

CAREMARK

Spinal Evaluation

Centers for Physical Therapy
and Affiliates

SPINAL EVALUATION:

Name: _____ Acct. #: _____ Age: _____

Diagnosis: _____ Date: _____ Dr.: _____

Date of Injury: _____ Occupation: _____ Working: Y   N

HISTORY:

_____

_____

_____

_____

_____

_____

_____

Medical History: _____

_____

Surgeries/Dates: _____

_____

Dental History: _____

_____

Test Results: _____

Condition: Improving: _____ Worsening: _____ Static: _____

Symptoms: Constant: _____ Intermittent: _____

Symptoms Aggravated By: _____

Symptoms Relieved By: _____

Functional Limits: Sit: _____ Stand: _____ Walk: _____

Previous Treatments: _____

_____

PAIN INTENSITY RATING:

1.

0 ½ 1 1½ 2 2½ 3 3½ 4 4½ 5 5½ 6 6½ 7 7½ 8 8½ 9 9½ 10

2.

0 ½ 1 1½ 2 2½ 3 3½ 4 4½ 5 5½ 6 6½ 7 7½ 8 8½ 9 9½ 10

3.

0 ½ 1 1½ 2 2½ 3 3½ 4 4½ 5 5½ 6 6½ 7 7½ 8 8½ 9 9½ 10

NO
PAIN

EXCRUCIATING
PAIN

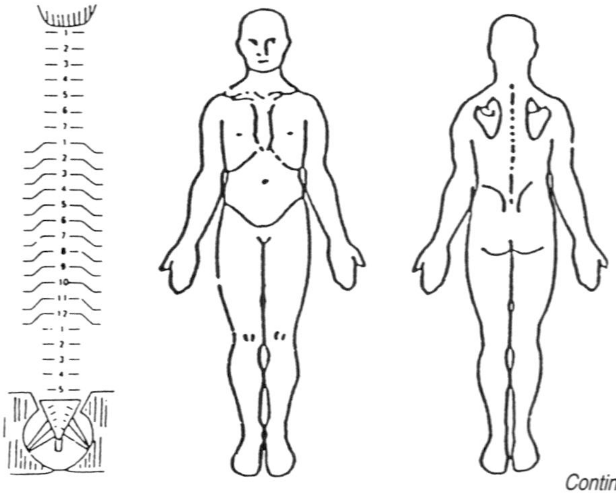

CM078-A (4-93)

Continued

(With permission from Caremark Orthopedic Services Division.)

FIGURE 4.3, *cont'd*

Name: _____   Acct. #: _____   Date: _____

Caffeine: _____ cups/day

Nicotine: _____ packs/day

ETOL: _____

Sleep: _____

Medications: _____

_____

_____

_____

_____

Preg/Comp.: _____

_____

_____

_____

SPECIAL TESTING:

Vertebral Artery (mod):   +   −

Alar Ligament: +   −

Sensory: _____

_____

_____

MMT: _____

_____

_____

Reflexes: _____

Max Mand Open: _____ mm.

SLR   R: _____ L: _____   Dural   R: _____ L: _____

Laseque R: _____ L: _____   Femoral R: _____ L: _____

Additional Findings: _____

_____

_____

_____

_____

_____

_____

_____

Contraindications: _____

_____

ASSESSMENT: _____

_____

_____

GOALS: _____

_____

_____

_____

_____

INITIAL TREATMENT: _____

_____

PLAN: _____

_____

_____

_____

_____

_____

P.T. Signature _____

FIGURE 4.4   Range of Motion (**A**), strength (**B**), and specific joint testing (**C**) should be measured before, during, and after rehabilitation in order to document progress and therapeutic outcomes.

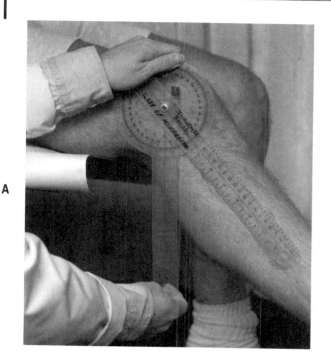

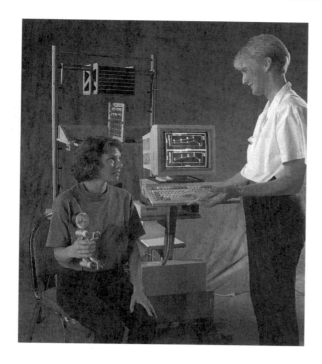

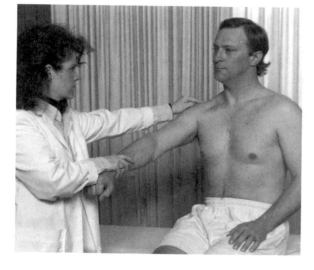

DATA COLLECTION AND CUSTOMER REQUIREMENTS

A variety of measurement instruments are presently available. In considering their use, it is important to keep in mind that the purpose of measurement is to produce truthful, valid data.[6] Astute therapists must reach a compromise between comprehensiveness and brevity, and attempt to gather data which is necessary not only for treatment planning, but more importantly, to meet referral source and other customer group requirements.

Traditional Measurements

Therapists are accustomed to the use of "traditional" measures such as joint range of motion, muscular strength, and disparate evaluative techniques. All of these measures comprise integral components of a client's Industrial Therapy program. However, the voluminous data which is compiled must relate to the critical job demands required by a client's occupation, and consider the specific requirements of each individual customer or end user.

The escalating costs to provide services in the Industrial Therapy setting must encourage each therapist to "rethink" techniques and measures traditionally performed, and concentrate on those measures which most aptly demonstrate the value of care, while providing the most useful information to the customer.

Customer Groups Served

The customers served typically include physicians, Vocational Rehabilitation Consultants, insurance companies, employers, and attorneys. Other customers interested in the measures include patients, families, psychologists, and counselors. These groups are expecting or demanding the documentable effects of treatment interventions. Although customer requirements within a group can overlap, it is imperative that an understanding is made of each individual customer's needs and their unique data requirements (Table 4.3).

The physician is a primary referral source to many Industrial Therapy centers. In a more acute injury situation, the physician desires information on measures of a client's muscular strength, joint range of motion, and performance in activities of daily living. Later, as the appropriate amount of healing time has elapsed and rehabilitation progress plateaus, the physician may request information on present funtional capacities for assistance in determining the client's impairment ratings and return to work decisions.

The Vocational Rehabilitation Consultant (VRC) is traditionally the case manager for the client. Frequent communication between the Industrial Therapist and the VRC regarding a client's progress is essential. Clinical information which is useful includes the client's present measures of physical capabilities and work levels, attendance record, and motivation level.

The VRC is interested in data that indicates accuracy and consistency of client results. Non-reproducibility can indicate lack of motivation or effort on the client's part to return to work in what Leonard Matheson has termed symptom magnification. Methods of determining the validity of a client's symptoms and behavior, such as the KEY Method Validity Index, are useful in planning and treatment modification. The VRC will also be very interested in the program's overall outcome and return to work statistics. For a more detailed description of the Vocational Rehabilitation Consultant's role, see Chapter 19.

The insurance companies and their adjusters are most interested in the documentation of continued client progress. In most cases, insurance companies are paying all of the bills associated with the injured worker, including medical expenses and the associated disability and compensation costs required by State law.

Typically, insurers will monitor the utilization rates (number of visits), charges per visit, and the total cost of services during the episode of care. Industrial Therapists should monitor these parameters as well.

Employers seek rehabilitation professionals who provide high quality care and value, and who diligently make attempts to understand and meet their unique requirements. The definition of quality care and perceived value will vary with each employer. They, too, will have interest in those service providers who are objectively progressing their employees and providing practical return-to-work information. This may include data such as the anticipated length of rehabilitation and projected cost.

It is also important to demonstrate and explain objective progress, in layman terms, so the employer clearly understands the benefits of procedures.

Additionally, data which is useful to employers include a client's physical capabilities, motivation levels, and attendance records.

Attorneys become involved for myriad reasons in an industrial injury case. They generally require information on their client's capabilities in meeting critical job demands, impairment ratings, and prognosis for assistance in case closure.

Forecasts of prognosis are generally made by the physician, although many Industrial Therapists assist the physician in this prediction. Attorneys may desire strength and functional comparisons to the uninjured side, if the patient has a unilateral extremity injury. Where available, they'll also want to make comparisons to preinjury measures from a job placement assessment.

Other customers, including the administrators of an Industrial Therapy center, will be seeking information on measures of utilization (number of visits), total treatment cost, client satisfaction ratings (described later), and return-to-work status.

These measures provide a mechanism for periodic program evaluation and trends in service delivery. In the future, these measures will likely be required, as an outcome data base becomes available. Reimbursement will become predicated upon a program's demonstration of acceptable outcome results.

THE MEASUREMENT OF PAIN AND FUNCTIONAL STATUS

In Industrial Therapy, there is an opportunity to measure a client's pain perception and functional abilities. Although an individual's pain perception is considered highly subjective, the measurement of pain can be performed in a reliable and valid manner.

There is general agreement that clients who have had variable levels of pain, lasting at least six months, are in a condition of chronic pain and may warrant pain management programs.

Although Industrial Therapy's main focus is restoring the worker's job function, pain perception can inhibit progress toward the goal. Accordingly, it is important to ascertain pain levels from the client's perspective. The measures of client pain can be supported or refuted by the therapist's observance of relational pain behaviors.

Pain Measurement Techniques

A measurement scale worth mentioning is the Pain and Impairment Relationship Scale (PAIRS).[8] The PAIRS consists of fifteen statements on pain and impairment, followed by a seven-point Likert scale rating the worker's degree of agreement, or disagreement with each statement (Box 4.2). Since a number of injured workers believe that they cannot return to work because of their pain, the PAIRS measures the extent to which they endorse this belief.[8]

Clients who demonstrate a PAIRS score reflecting abnormal and inappropriate attention to their pain and dysfunction may be more effectively treated in a pain management program than in Industrial Therapy.

Formulations of a visual analog scale are commonly used in pain measurement (Figure 4.5). The client is asked to rate their pain on a numerical scale of zero to ten, with zero representing the total absence of pain, and ten being unbearable, unrelenting, excruciating pain.

Pain can be assessed at rest, during activities of

FIGURE 4.5 Example of a visual analog scale.

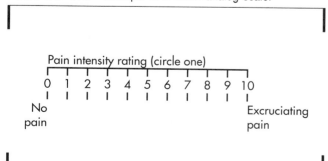

daily living, and during job simulation tasks. By monitoring this information over time, therapists are able to make daily program adjustments to accommodate the measured pain levels.

Another pain measurement instrument which has proven popular is the visual line scale (Figure 4.6). The client is asked to rate their pain in a similar descriptive

---

BOX 4.2

The 15 Statements on the Pain and Impairment Relationship Scale

1. I can still be expected to fulfill my work and family responsibilities despite my pain.
2. An increase in pain is an indication that I should stop what I am doing until the pain decreases.
3. I can't go about my normal life activities when I am in pain.
4. If my pain would go away, I could be every bit as active as I used to be.
5. I should have the same benefits as the handicapped because of my chronic pain problems.
6. I owe it to myself and those around me to perform my usual activities even when my pain is bad.
7. Most people expect too much of me, given my chronic pain.
8. I have to be careful not to do anything that might make my pain worse.
9. As long as I am in pain, I'll never be able to live as well as I did before.
10. When my pain gets worse, I find it very hard to concentrate on anything else.
11. I have come to accept that I am a disabled person, due to my chronic pain.
12. There is no way that I can return to doing the things that I used to do unless I first find a cure for my pain.
13. I find myself frequently thinking about my pain and what it has done to my life.
14. Even though my pain is always there, I often don't notice it at all when I'm keeping myself busy.
15. All of my problems would be solved if my pain would go away.

Patients check on a Likert scale beneath each statement whether they: Completely disagree; Disagree; Disagree somewhat; are Neutral; Agree somewhat; Agree; Completely agree.

TABLE 4.3 Data Customers and Their Requirements

Types of data	Industrial Therapists (clinical)	Industrial Therapists (management)	Office billing personnel	Employee	Employer	Physicians	Insurance company representatives	Vocational Rehabilitation Consultants	Family members	Attorneys	Accreditation agencies
Therapeutic evaluation results	X					X	X			X	
ROM Testing	X					X					
Muscle strength testing	X					X					
Treatment prognosis	X			X	X	X	X	X	X	X	
Anticipated length of treatment	X	X	X	X	X	X	X	X	X		X
Projected cost	X	X			X	X	X	X			
Functional capacities results	X			X	X	X	X	X	X	X	
Validity of participation	X				X	X	X	X		X	
Pre-injury capabilities	X			X	X	X	X	X	X	X	
Client progress documentation	X		X		X	X	X	X	X	X	X

Client motivation levels	X		X	X	X	X			
Performance in daily living	X	X		X		X	X		
Work capability levels at exit of program	X	X	X	X	X	X		X	
Number of visits		X	X		X	X			X
Attendance record	X	X	X	X	X	X			X
Client satisfaction survey results	X		X	X	X	X			
Impairment ratings			X	X	X	X		X	
Per visit charges	X	X	X	X	X	X			
Total case costs	X	X	X	X	X	X		X	X
Return to work success	X	X	X	X	X	X	X	X	X

FIGURE 4.6 Example of a visual line scale.

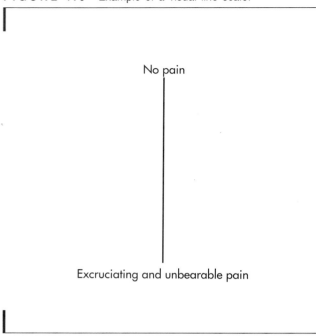

No pain

Excruciating and unbearable pain

manner to the pain numerical scale previously described through placement of a mark on a contiguous line.

Functional Status Measures

Several newer versions of assessment instruments have been gaining in popularity. Called functional status measures, they have been described by Deyo[5] to denote those questionnaires which assess a patient's limitations in performing usual human tasks of living.

The use of functional status measures allows a therapist to evaluate aspects of the client's basic functioning and health status, from the client's own perspective. The functional viewpoint unique to each client will become increasingly important in the future, as clients become more and more cognizant of the responsibility they have for their rehabilitation outcome.

One functional status instrument, the Short Form 36, or SF-36 (Copyright New England Medical Center Hospitals, Inc.) as it is commonly known, shows promise in assisting therapists with measures of client's perceived health functioning.[10] The SF-36 is completed by the client and includes one multi-item scale that assesses eight health concepts, including:
1. Limitations in physical activities because of health problems
2. Limitations in social activities because of physical or emotional problems

3. Limitations in usual role activities because of physical health problems
4. Bodily pain
5. General mental health (psychological distress and well-being)
6. Limitations in usual role activities because of emotional problems
7. Vitality (energy and fatigue)
8. General health perceptions.

The SF-36 is administered during the initial evaluation and at discharge, and results in a percentage score for each of the eight health concepts. Positive improvements in functional status can assist in the documentation of clinical results attributable to treatment intervention.

There are several other functional health status measures under development. In considering the use of a functional status instrument, five criteria are recommended for the evaluation of its utility, and hold true for all data collection measures:
1. Practicality—how much time is required both for the client to complete the questionnaire and for its administration and scoring
2. Comprehensiveness—what are the types of function or behavior considered
3. Reproducibility
4. Validity
5. Responsiveness—can an instrument detect changes over time, and will it detect subtle, but clinically important changes?[5]

DATA COLLECTION AND REASSESSMENT

After detailed baseline measures are compiled during the initial evaluation process, data must then be gathered at periodic intervals. The reassessment of the client must be methodical. The specific time interval for reassessment(s) will vary with the particular measurement instrument, client progress, and the nature of customer requirements.

With an acutely injured client, reassessment will be daily or weekly in the majority of cases. For instance, active range of motion measures of the affected joint(s) should be recorded daily. Strength should be recorded weekly.

Historically, manual muscle testing has been used by therapists, with measurements recorded as grades 1 through 5 or zero through normal. However, the reader is encouraged to investigate the use of hand-held myometers and isokinetic dynamometers, for assistance in recording measures of strength. Although all modes of strength measures have limitations relating to reliability and validity, the change in strength must be documented.

In a Work Hardening situation, clients are typically seen daily for rehabilitation on an outpatient basis. To adequately track progress and make indicated adjustments, it is important to daily record the client's hours of attendance, program completion, and consistency of pain reports and pain behaviors.

Physical performance (lifting abilities and cardiovascular endurance) should be measured weekly. At the time of discharge, therapists must complete a fairly comprehensive reassessment that can be relative to aspects of the initial evaluation. Particular attention must be paid to present lifting capacities and work level abilities.

DATA COLLECTION AND DISCHARGE

The length of time in a Work Hardening program, usually measured in days, is an important outcome measurement. A client usually completes a program in Work Hardening in about four weeks.[4] Additionally, an essential outcome measure is the return to work status of the client, which should be included in a summary of your program's results. Did the client return to their same job or a different job? On a full-time or part-time basis? These are measures of outcome, and are discussed further in Chapter 3.

Time in the Work Hardening program and return to work status should be kept at a minimum for industrial patients. Analysis of longer term follow-up information (post discharge measures of clients remaining at their jobs injury free) can document a program's overall effectiveness.

A successful case discharge in Work Hardening involves the client meeting their job's critical demands and returning to work, or maximizing their own physical capabilities with referral to a vocational specialist. Measures of the client's achieved work should be recorded at the initiation and completion of rehabilitation, and maintained as part of the program's evaluation.

The initial evaluation and assessment information should be compared with the reassessment and discharge data. The changes observed are not only important for recording an individual client's progress, but in a broader sense, to justify the existence and purpose of Industrial Therapy.

Key aspects of data collected (return to work status, length of time in the program, change in critical work levels) should be maintained in a log of all program evaluations. This information is not only useful for marketing efforts, it is demanded with increasing frequency by progressive payers.

DATA COLLECTION POST DISCHARGE

Client Satisfaction

Discharge planning increasingly involves measures of client satisfaction. An operational goal should be set to obtain information from each client following their discharge. The most accurate data is usually collected as close to the time of program completion as possible, although longer term follow-up (one year after discharge) has distinct marketing and accreditation implications. The results from the questionnaires should be summarized monthly, and action plans developed to make program adjustments addressing the lower scoring items.

Satisfaction questionnaires should be designed to measure the client's reactions specific to the rehabilitation program in which they participated. A sample patient satisfaction questionnaire designed for use with clients following early treatment intervention is shown in Figure 4.7, and one for Work Hardening is shown in Figure 4.8 on pages 57 and 58.

In each case, questionnaires should be carefully designed and tailored to help understand clients' perceptions of specific rehabilitation programs. For example, consistent ratings of home programs by clients as "below average" indicates a need to reexamine how the program is designed, communicated, or implemented.

A more comprehensive and elaborate mechanism for collecting client satisfaction data may be obtained with the assistance of an external consulting firm. Telephone interviews of randomly selected discharged clients can be conducted to evaluate several aspects of service provision, such as client and therapist interaction, quality of facility, individual involvement in goal setting, meeting customer requirements, and overall levels of client satisfaction. Although this method of measuring satisfaction measurement can be expensive, the distinct advantages are the elimination of internal bias, and the skill of the professional interviewer to effectively "probe" sensitive areas in more depth.

The collection of client satisfaction data is only valuable and useful when action plans are developed and implemented to improve lower scoring items. The use of bar graphs (Figure 4.9, page 59) to illustrate trends in satisfaction measures provides visual impact and demonstrates the importance to members of the rehabilitation team.

In the future, industry benchmarks of satisfaction ratings will be available and common, which will allow more accurate comparison of client satisfaction levels with different programs. It is probable that unsatisfactory ratings on a consistent basis will result in the

Text continues on p 59.

FIGURE 4.7 Sample of patient satisfaction questionnaire for use with clients following early treatment intervention.

CAREMARK

	Patient Questionnaire	Centers for Physical Therapy and Affiliates

Please take a few moments to complete this questionnaire. Your answers and comments are very valuable to us. Our goal is to provide you with the highest quality care at all times. Thank you for providing us with the opportunity to serve.

Location of Center _____   Today's Date _____

Please rate our service on the following (circle your response):

	Excellent	Good	Average	Below Average	Poor
Explanation of treatment program	1	2	3	4	5
Improvement in your condition	1	2	3	4	5
Confidence in your therapist	1	2	3	4	5
Consistency of your care	1	2	3	4	5
Written home exercise program	1	2	3	4	5
Overall professionalism of staff	1	2	3	4	5
Quality of equipment	1	2	3	4	5
Overall quality of care	1	2	3	4	5
Explanation of payment policy	1	2	3	4	5
Explanation of billing process	1	2	3	4	5
Understanding of monthly statements	1	2	3	4	5
Courtesy and helpfulness of staff	1	2	3	4	5
Convenience of scheduling appointments	1	2	3	4	5
Fairness of fee structure	1	2	3	4	5
Decor and cleanliness of Center	1	2	3	4	5
Adequacy and convenience of parking	1	2	3	4	5

How long did it take to schedule your first appointment?
    1 – 2 days   3 – 4 days   5 or more days   do not remember

On average, how long did you wait before each treatment visit?
    0 – 5 minutes   5 – 10 minutes   10 – 15 minutes   15 – 20 minutes   over 20 minutes

Would you recommend our service to a friend?   YES   NO

What did you like best about our service? _____

_____

_____

_____

What could we improve upon? _____

_____

_____

Your Name (optional) _____   Phone (   ) _____

Please deposit in the Patient Satisfaction box. If desired, see the Office Coordinator for mailing instructions.

Thank you for your time in completing this questionnaire.

JV-063-A

(With permission from Caremark Orthopedic Services Division.)

FIGURE 4.8 Sample patient satisfaction questionnaire for Work Hardening.

CAREMARK

Worker Satisfaction Questionnaire

Centers for Physical Therapy
and Affiliates

Name: _____ Date: _____

We would like to know how you feel about our program so that we can recognize areas that we need to improve. Please answer each question and provide additional comments as needed.

1. I was oriented to the program adequately and understood what was expected from me.

Strongly disagree	Disagree	Undecided	Agree	Strongly agree	Does not apply
1 __	2 __	3 __	4 __	5 __	N/A __

2. My assessment results and goals were reviewed with me.

Strongly disagree	Disagree	Undecided	Agree	Strongly agree	Does not apply
1 __	2 __	3 __	4 __	5 __	N/A __

3. I was shown ways to improve upon by body mechanics (sitting, standing, lifting, squatting, etc.).

Strongly disagree	Disagree	Undecided	Agree	Strongly agree	Does not apply
1 __	2 __	3 __	4 __	5 __	N/A __

4. I was shown how to properly care for my back or other injured body parts on the job and at home.

Strongly disagree	Disagree	Undecided	Agree	Strongly agree	Does not apply
1 __	2 __	3 __	4 __	5 __	N/A __

5. The program helped me to increase my strength, flexability, and endurance.

Strongly disagree	Disagree	Undecided	Agree	Strongly agree	Does not apply
1 __	2 __	3 __	4 __	5 __	N/A __

6. My program manager helped me to understand my program.

Strongly disagree	Disagree	Undecided	Agree	Strongly agree	Does not apply
1 __	2 __	3 __	4 __	5 __	N/A __

7. The work simulation activities were appropriate in relation to my job tasks.

Strongly disagree	Disagree	Undecided	Agree	Strongly agree	Does not apply
1 __	2 __	3 __	4 __	5 __	N/A __

8. The staff considered my suggestions regarding my program and was supportive.

Strongly disagree	Disagree	Undecided	Agree	Strongly agree	Does not apply
1 __	2 __	3 __	4 __	5 __	N/A __

9. The center was a pleasant environment and conducive to my rehabilitation.

Strongly disagree	Disagree	Undecided	Agree	Strongly agree	Does not apply
1 __	2 __	3 __	4 __	5 __	N/A __

Continued

FIGURE 4.8 *cont'd*

Worker Satisfaction Questionnaire (page 2)

Name: _____   Date: _____

10. My program at the center will help me return to work.

Strongly disagree	Disagree	Undecided	Agree	Strongly agree	Does not apply
1 __	2 __	3 __	4 __	5 __	N/A __

11. Group sessions were beneficial to me.

Strongly disagree	Disagree	Undecided	Agree	Strongly agree	Does not apply
1 __	2 __	3 __	4 __	5 __	N/A __

12. Vocational rehabilitation sessions were beneficial to me.

Strongly disagree	Disagree	Undecided	Agree	Strongly agree	Does not apply
1 __	2 __	3 __	4 __	5 __	N/A __

13. At the beginning of my program I felt:

No pain	Very little pain	Mild pain	Moderate pain	Severe pain
1 __	2 __	3 __	4 __	__ 5

14. Now that I am at the end of my program, I feel:

No pain	Very little pain	Mild pain	Moderate pain	Severe pain
1 __	2 __	3 __	4 __	__ 5

15. I was satisfied with the return to work program.

Strongly disagree	Disagree	Undecided	Agree	Strongly agree	Does not apply
1 __	2 __	3 __	4 __	5 __	N/A __

Do you have any other ideas or suggestions that might improve our present program?

_____
_____
_____
_____
_____
_____
_____
_____

Thank you for your participation in our program. Your comments and suggestions are greatly appreciated.

FIGURE 4.9 Sample client satisfaction ratings. The bar graphs represent the percentage who are satisfied with the program.

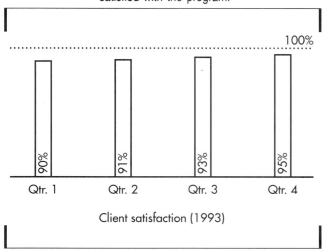

Client satisfaction (1993)

reduction or discontinuation of referrals from payers, as their influence grows in a managed competition environment.

Program Evaluation

It is valuable for data collection efforts to continue beyond the immediate time of discharge. An all-inclusive program evaluation scheme should involve longer term client follow-up, at time intervals approaching one year post-discharge. Many industrial programs make bona fide attempts to gather information at six and twelve months following client discharge, particularly in Work Hardening situations where clients are admitted to programs at varying time intervals following injury.

Measurements of the return-to-work results are of keen interest to administrators, payers, and accreditation services such as CARF. This information speaks loudly of a program's quality and success. As mentioned earlier in the chapter, it is important to include qualifying information such as the number of days from injury to program admittance, because this factor has significant impact on return to work success rates.

Client Motivation

The industrial therapy client will, in most instances, have a goal of return to gainful employment. However, the motivation to return to work and its timing will vary greatly from client to client. A prospective study by Bigos et al[1] showed that the most important factor in successful return to work was whether the client experienced positive work perceptions, mainly liking their job.

Therapists must understand the effects of client motivation in their measurements, and the overall "big picture" of a client's history and progress, for the production of useful, objective data and return to work recommendations.

THE FUTURE OF MEASUREMENT AND DATA COLLECTION

Baseline measures for employees in jobs with high risk of injury will become a normal facet of the pre-employment process. Industrial evaluation and rehabilitation will become more comprehensive and automated in nature. Predictive capabilities for return to work will improve through more reliable and valid measurement following an injury, and from relating this data to known baseline measures and features of many occupations.

There will be increasing specificity in clinical measures and work simulation tasks, through their applicability and comparability to actual job requirements and critical job demands. The science of ergonomics will continue to evolve and provide improved worker-job fit.

Data collection will become fully automated through use of computers, lessening the tedious burden and data-gathering redundancies of hand-written or transcribed records, while increasing the quality and reliability of the data. An additional benefit to the automation of clinical records will be the creation of large data bases of client information, for future study and analysis as we prospectively explore outcomes.

Continued cost containment pressures in healthcare will scrutinize resources available for rehabilitation of the industrial client. Ultimately, successful Industrial Therapy as measured by outcomes, will become the norm as acute injury cases are managed more aggressively and appropriately, returning workers to their jobs earlier with minimized risk of reinjury. There is the strong likelihood that Industrial Therapy cases will be reimbursed through capitation agreements and preferred arrangements with providers. This will require therapists to become more active as case managers, while completing only those activities critical to return-to-work success.

SUMMARY

Data collection before, during, and after rehabilitation is undertaken to relate treatment procedures to outcomes. Measurements should not be based on past practice, but on specific program needs. The major uses of this information are to improve program planning and success rates, and to document progress and outcomes for referral sources, insurers, employers, and in an increasing number of cases, attorneys and public sector agencies. In addition to enabling continuous improvement in the field of Industrial Therapy, the collection and analysis of data, documents for third parties that positive outcomes have not happened by chance or random occurrence.

REFERENCES

1. Bigos SJ, et al: A Prospective Study of Work Perceptions and Psychosocial Factors Affecting the Report of Back Injury, *Spine* 16:1, 1991.
2. Bohannon RW: Simple Clinical Measure, *Physical Therapy* 67(12):1845–1850, 1987.
3. Caremark Orthopedic Services Division, Caremark International: Outcomes Research, non-published data, 1992.
4. Caremark Orthopedic Services Division, Caremark International: Centers for Industrial Rehabilitation, personal correspondence.
5. Deyo RA: Measuring the Functional Status of Patients With Low Back Pain, *Arch Physical Medicine and Rehab* vol 69, Dec 1988.
6. Krebs D: Measurement Theory, *Physical Therapy* 67(12): 1834–1839, 1987.
7. Mayer TG: Functional Restoration of the Patient with Spinal Disorders. In Isernhagen S, editor: Work Injury.
8. Riley JF, Ahern D, Follick MJ: Chronic Pain and Functional Impairment: Assessing Beliefs About Their Relationships, *Arch of Physical Medicine and Rehab* 69: 579–582, 1988.
9. Rothstein JM, editor: Measurement In Physical Therapy, *Clinics in Physical Therapy*, vol 7, New York, 1985, Churchill Livingstone.
10. Ware JE, Sherbourne CD: The MOS 36-Item Short-Form Health Survey (SF-36), *Medical Care* 30:6, 1992.

5

A Day in the Life of an Industrial Therapy Practice Owner

Denise M. Miller
Linda M. Demers

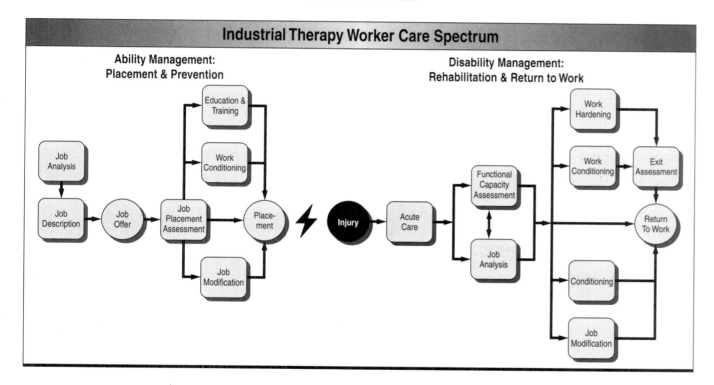

This chapter is a composite picture of an Industrial Therapy practice owner's typical day, based on numerous interviews.[3] The purpose is to give Physical and Occupational Therapists an idea of what life is really like when branching out into Industrial Therapy. It is written from the first person in certain portions to give the reader a better "feel" for the territory.

> *There goes that alarm clock again. 5:30 AM already? It seems like I just fell asleep a few hours ago. As a matter of fact, that's when I did go to sleep! I used to think owning my own practice would mean banker's hours and plenty of time on the golf course. Maybe someday, but right now I've got a challenging Industrial Therapy practice to run!*

An Industrial Therapy practice differs from a traditional Physical or Occupational Therapy practice in a number of ways. A key difference is that the Industrial Therapist has a greater degree of responsibility for their own referrals. Physicians still provide a percentage of the patients or clients, but many other players are becoming involved in referral decisions. Employers, Vocational Rehabilitation Consultants, Ergonomists, Occupational Health Nurses, Safety Experts, Case Managers, Insurers, and even Attorneys can be sources for referrals.

In order to ensure a viable share of the industrial referral market, the Industrial Therapist must do a great deal of networking among these rehabilitation team players. Developing strong relationships and a fertile referral network requires a great deal of time and effort over and above providing good therapy services.

> *Here's good news! After I left the office yesterday afternoon, we received six new referrals for acute care. The more involved we get in Industrial Therapy, the more acute care referrals we seem to receive. As our contact with employees broadens, referrals from their families, relatives, and friends are generated. We even get a greater share of physicians' referrals because they know their patients will be returned to work expeditiously and safely.*

The acute phase is where Industrial Therapy is most similar to traditional therapy. The Industrial Therapist typically has a one-on-one visit or evaluation with the injured worker lasting about 45 minutes to an hour. In this session traditional manipulations are administered such as manual traction, myofacial release, cranio/sacral positions, and other modalistic measures to decrease pain, increase movement and improve strength and flexibility.

While a number of traditional Therapist activities are now being performed by lower cost technicians, the acute care phase is where the Therapist's professional expertise remains essential, and reimbursements are sufficient to compensate the Therapist for priority attention (Figure 5.1).

The major differences in the provision of Industrial Therapy come after the acute phase of care. Then, the Industrial Therapist's focus on a safe return to work involves a number of activities unfamiliar to the traditional therapist. First, the Therapist typically administers a Functional Capacity Assessment (FCA) that measures the client's ability to perform a series of work-related tasks. These tasks are simulated to take into consideration the dynamic, real-world movements and resistances. Administering such evaluations usually requires additional training.

The Therapist may also perform a Job Analysis (JA) which catalogs all the functions of the job to which the client will return. This information can be used to develop written job descriptions. It can also be used in conjunction with the results of the Assessment either as a pre-hire or post offer tool.

Using the results of FCA and JA, the Therapist and client then set realistic goals for return to work. They also determine the components of care that will achieve these goals. Depending on the results of the FCA and JA, the therapist may also recommend that the employer modify the worker's job to bring demands within safe performance levels attainable through the Work Hardening, Work Conditioning, or Conditioning program.

Finally, Industrial Therapy is significantly more oriented than traditional therapy toward monitoring and measuring outcomes such as time out of work, total rehabilitation costs, percent of injured workers returned to work, and rates of reinjury. Outcome information is then related to assessment and treatment procedures to verify effectiveness, and to guide efforts toward future improvements.

Figure 5.2 indicates typical sources of revenue and their percentages to the whole.

FIGURE 5.2 Revenue sources.

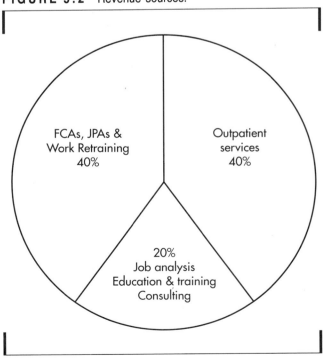

FIGURE 5.1 Workers in the acute phase of Industrial Therapy receive traditional physical and sports care such as modalities, range of motion, and strength training.

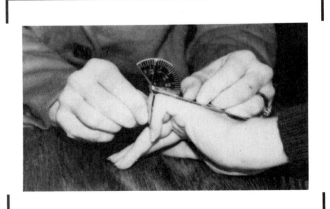

This morning we're going to use our new small parts assembly station for the first time. It is ideal simulation for a group of electronics manufacturing employees we've been treating. The employer wanted us to install real circuit board workstations in our facility. I had to convince them that as long as we simulate the postures and musculoskeletal functions involved, it isn't necessary to turn out real circuit boards. If we had to have actual equipment for each employer, we'd quickly run out of floor space and my therapists would have to become experts in each industrial process (Figure 5.3).

Work Conditioning and Work Hardening are good examples of the Industrial Therapist's involvement venturing into innovative areas, far afield of traditional medical care or traditional therapy. In these programs, the Therapist strengthens the clients' capabilities, using specialized equipment that simulates real world working conditions. Since job functions require dynamic body mechanics, job simulation has proven to be more effective than fixed position weight-training stations.[1]

The Industrial Therapist also strives to simulate the working environment and routine, requiring clients to punch in on a time clock, take standard breaks, and demonstrate proper work behavior, dress, and safe work habits.

Work Retraining centers typically include workstations that simulate small parts assembly, materials handling, construction sites, truck cabs, and heavy labor work stations. The nature of surrounding industries and injury rates typically dictates the type and quantity of workstations in the center. Some employers

prefer that Work Conditioning or Work Hardening be administered on-site using actual equipment, believing it to be the best context and the least cost option.

In some instances, the role of the Work Hardening center is to accommodate those cases in which on-site is not possible because of space, equipment or safety restrictions, or because of psychosocial issues related to the worksite (Figure 5.4).

The Industrial Therapist's role in the return to work process is as a member of a team. Team members are drawn from a number of professions and disciplines, brought together to address the diverse needs of injured workers. The emphasis for everyone involved, is on rehabilitating the whole person, not just the body part. Psychologists, social workers, Vocational Rehabilitation Consultants, and even family members can join the Industrial Therapist on the rehabilitation team.

All of these innovations in Industrial Therapy have not materialized simply because someone thought they would be a good idea. They evolved through experimentation, trial and error, and have been adopted because they increased the return to work rates, shortened the rehabilitation time frame, restored greater degrees of pre-injured function, reduced reinjury, or caused some other measurable benefit that justifies the invested costs. Industry executives face a growing number of challenges to maintain competitiveness, and keeping workers healthy and productive can play a major role.

As I look at my schedule for the day, it reads like the itinerary of an industrial engineer or consultant. I've got meetings with factory floor employees, plant managers, production engineers, and an attorney regarding a former client. In a way, although none of this is happening in a treatment room, I am nevertheless administering therapy services in every one of these instances.

The fastest growing and perhaps most important source of the Industrial Therapist's referrals is from the companies themselves, often at the Therapist's initiation. As employers attempt to take greater control over their health care expenditures, they become increasingly involved in deciding what services to buy and who will provide the services. Industrial Therapists must make sure this emerging referral influence is adequately covered in marketing efforts. The Therapist must make contact and nurture relationships with top management and middle managers. Both participate in deciding which Industrial Therapy programs and providers to use, so both must be given attention.

My first meeting today is to approve a new direct mail brochure designed to introduce our practice to 100 selected light manufacturers within a 30 mile radius of

FIGURE 5.3 A properly designed Small Assembly Station can simulate the postures and positions of a variety of jobs without the need for actual employer equipment.

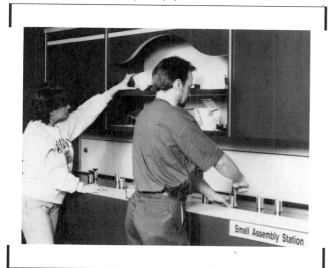

Small Assembly Station

FIGURE 5.4   Ideally, Industrial Therapists could offer employers the option of Work Hardening on-site (**A**) or in the Work Hardening center (**B**).

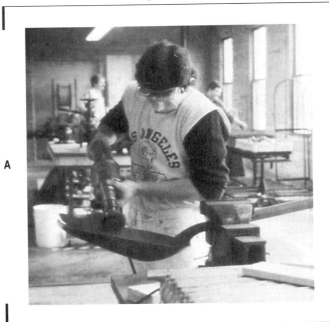

A

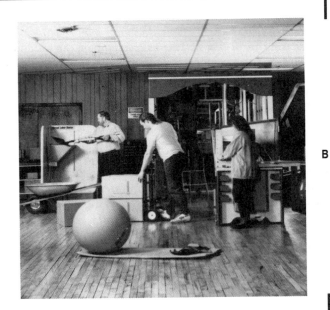

B

our Work Retraining facility. We went to the expense of color printing because, like it or not, cosmetics sells. Cosmetics sells? I never thought I'd be uttering words like that when I emerged from Therapy school propelled on an idealistic mission to heal the wounded and keep them well. It never occurred to me I'd be poring over and approving advertising materials (Figure 5.5).

The Industrial Therapist must become proficient at strategic marketing and one-on-one selling. With regard to strategy, the Therapist must carefully target prospects based on their potential demand for Industrial Therapy services, their fit with the practice's areas of specialization and strength, and the presence of competition.

The Therapist must then approach these prospects with a carefully orchestrated program of communications and personal selling, designed to move them from a position of knowing little or nothing about the practice, to signing the first contract for services. This process can involve many letters, special mailings, phone calls, and meetings over the course of six months to a year, and in some cases, several years to consummate.

In addition, once the contract is signed, the company may delay implementation up to six months, due to manpower or budgetary reasons. Because of these lead times, the Industrial Therapist must maintain a well-filled pipeline of prospects in various stages of the selling and implementation process in order to ensure a stable flow of revenue.

When I was going through college and then Therapy school, a driving fear was to avoid ever having to get a job as a salesperson. Now I realize that no matter what job you have, you're a salesperson. As a medical provider, you have to sell yourself to the patient to gain trust and a

FIGURE 5.5   The Industrial Therapist must become proficient at strategic marketing and personal salesmanship. Direct marketing is just one method of introducing a practice to employers.

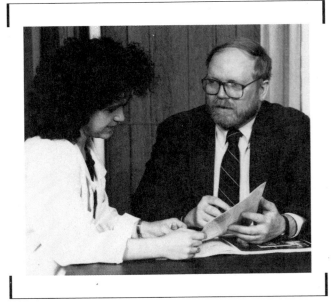

comfort level. That's patient relationships. As an Industrial Therapist, you have to sell the benefits of your services to companies who may not know they even need them. That's marketing.

Convincing prospects that the need exists and persuading them to purchase services makes personal selling one of the most critical factors in the success of an Industrial Therapy practice. The therapist must put forth factual, honest, straight forward communication in the process of carefully building trust.

Some therapists may initially view selling as outside their realm of capability. In actuality, however, this kind of face-to-face communication is not very different from the traditional bedside manner, except that it is administered across the desk of the corporate end-user. It is an indispensable part of helping the "patient" become comfortable with what is best.

Another challenge in communicating Industrial Therapy services is that the benefits are often intangible. Companies are used to spending money to acquire buildings or pieces of machinery. Many are uncomfortable with spending thousands of dollars on programs that they cannot see or touch. This underscores the need for the Industrial Therapist to package services and programs in ways that give them more tangibility.

Some measures that enhance tangibility are to give each program a descriptive name, use a visual schematic of each program's process that employers can see on paper, and ideally provide outcome studies that quantify the relationship between costs and bottom line impact.

I just found out that we lost a competitive bid for a Work Hardening contract to our arch rival in town. Sometimes it doesn't make any sense. I know their program is inferior. Our facility offers twice the resources of the competitor, including multiple upper extremity simulation stations to accommodate the company's higher incidence of cumulative trauma disorders. Furthermore, we presented definitive outcome studies, and they didn't. They do have a flair for selling!

In Industrial Therapy, injured workers come from commercial businesses. These businesses are used to being approached by vendors with a great deal of fanfare and flair. Accordingly, in marketing and selling activities the Therapist must give attention to two levels of consciousness—the rational and the emotional. The Therapist's equipment or program must not only be the best choice functionally and therapeutically, it must also *look like* the best choice, and the prospect must believe it is the best choice on both a rational and an emotional plane.

It is a common mistake in industrial marketing to think that approaching prospects with "iron clad" facts and arguments is all that is required to make the sale. Whether the purchase decision involves production line machinery or therapeutic services, it is a reality that a vendor or provider with inferior quality can still win a competitive selling situation. They can offset their deficits with emotional considerations.

Cosmetics, the right image, and personality can win the contract. Sometimes, Therapists have to sell themselves and be liked by the prospect before they will gain agreement as to the purchase of Industrial Therapy products or services. Other times, word-of-mouth, a credible reputation, and outcomes can help complete the selling process.

At 8:30 I've got to interview an applicant for the exercise physiologist position we've created. This person will join our Work Hardening team and also conduct Functional Capacity Assessments. In interviews, I've learned to look for enthusiasm and drive more than knowledge and experience. You can train an inexperienced employee. You can't teach enthusiasm and drive.

Industrial Therapists are beginning to hire a number of people who are not OTs or PTs to perform functions that, for a number of reasons, no longer require the expertise of a full-fledged therapist. This is especially true in specific methodologies where procedures such as Functional Capacity Assessment or Job Analysis have become increasingly standardized. As with any measurement or statistical discipline, refinements in methodology progress toward minimizing or eliminating "tester error" by standardizing the way tests are sequenced, instructed, observed, and recorded. As standardization improvements are implemented, the Therapist's presence at every step in the process is no longer warranted.

Standardized methodologies are making it possible for Exercise Physiologists, PT and OT Assistants, Athletic Trainers, and Kinesiologists to administer many or all of the components of certain Functional Capacity Assessments or Job Analyses. Therapists are able to attend to areas where their expertise is more critical, and perhaps more gainfully reimbursable. These personnel can also fulfill the roles of Work Trainer or Assistants to the Program Manager in Work Hardening and Work Conditioning.

Since Industrial Therapy involves a great deal of uncharted territory, Therapists must seek new employees who demonstrate the creativity and resourcefulness to solve problems in ways that may not be documented in any manual. New workers must be self starters with a natural inclination to forge ahead without being pushed or having all the steps specified for them. They must stretch and grow to fill the many needs that emerge as the practice evolves.

Figure 5.6 indicates the typical activities and time allocation of an Industrial Therapy private practice's owner, Program Director, and Exercise Physiologist.

> *The interview went well, so I've asked my administrative assistant to arrange follow up interviews with other employees. It is very important to build a harmonious atmosphere among the employees. My staff is often better than I am at telling whether or not someone fits in with the company culture.*

In Industrial Therapy, as in any enterprise, performance is a function of the people and the culture in which they operate. As to the people component, the secret to success is not for the Industrial Therapist to find perfect people, but to provide an atmosphere that brings out the best in those available.

Every person has strengths and weaknesses. To manage effectively, the Industrial Therapist must build a team in which people's strengths and weaknesses complement one another. Some employees have a grasp of the big picture. Others love delving into details. Some are creative. Others are numbers oriented. No one person has to be able to do it all, as long as the team as a whole, collectively possesses the knowledge and skills for success.

Regarding the cultural component, the goals have to be clearly articulated and the team has to enthusiastically embrace them. It is impossible for the Therapist to police everyone's commitment and productivity. It is

FIGURE 5.6   Industrial Therapy practice typical time allocation.

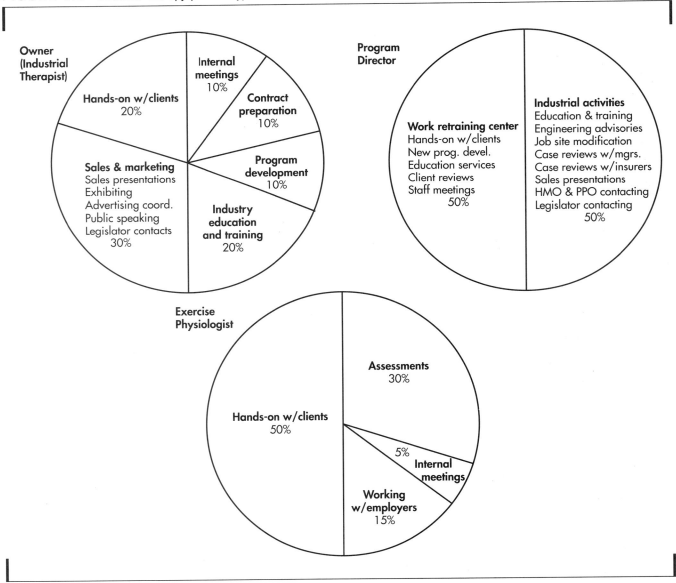

best to create an atmosphere that fosters self commitment and dedicated performance.

> *I'm due at the local bottling plant for a "tool box" talk with the line operators. This is an informal 15-minute meeting on the production floor, during a break, to discuss and review the back safety issues that I taught them in a recent six week series of on-site training sessions. I take off my coat and tie in the parking lot and slip on a sweater so that I don't come off as a surrogate of management.*

While providing services, the Therapist must wear many hats—to simultaneously be an advocate of cost control, quality standards, productivity, worker safety, and regulatory compliance. Where management and employees may see their interests in conflict, the Therapist must not take sides or pander to the prejudices of one or the other depending on which side is present. Instead, the Industrial Therapist must find common ground where both management and employees can achieve win-win outcomes, where safety and productivity are synonymous.

The Industrial Therapist must not be perceived as an advocate of employee interests, or of employer interests. Rather, the Therapist must be an advocate of the company's interests, designing programs to deliver results that benefit employees and employers mutually (Figure 5.7).

> *I used this particular "tool box" talk to discuss the idea of warm-up and stretching sessions before each shift. Many of the participants remembered being taught to perform such exercises prior to school athletics, and it made sense to them to do it before work activities. However, they were skeptical that management would ever allow it.*

Instituting an on-site, warm-up and stretching program is one illustration of this balancing act. The employees may feel it is simply another management idea that will go nowhere, or window dressing for regulatory compliance. Management may not like the fact that it takes away from production time. The Therapist must convince management, ideally through outcome studies, that the reduction in injuries more than offsets the production time lost. In fact, mini breaks tend to foster productivity by reducing fatigue and bolstering employees' energy and enthusiasm.

The Therapist must also convince employees that the sessions increase their job security, by both preventing injuries and helping to strengthen the company's financial position, necessary to maintain jobs.

> *I always try to touch base with the plant manager and staff whenever I'm in the building. This keeps their commitment to prevention on the front burner. It is also an opportunity to do a little pre-selling of other services I think they need. In fact, my first assignment here was a single Job Analysis that helped pinpoint the cause of high injury rates. On the basis of those findings, I've completed 33 Job Analyses covering every job in the plant.*
>
> *When injuries occur, I perform Functional Capacity Assessments and determine capability deficits by comparing the FCA results to those demands specified in the Job Analyses (Figure 5.8).*

FIGURE 5.8   Industrial Therapists should meet regularly with plant managers in order to monitor programs, trouble shoot problems, sell new services, and keep prevention a priority.

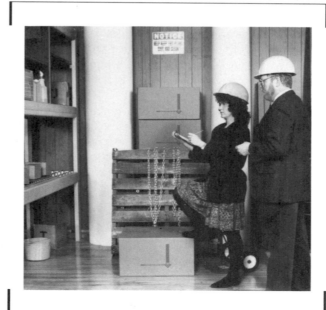

FIGURE 5.7   The Industrial Therapist must design programs that have mutual benefit to employers and employees.

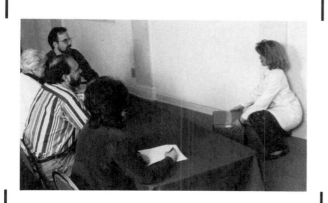

To gain company wide consensus and commitment to Industrial Therapy programs—whether oriented towards ergonomics, safety, fitness, or enhanced productivity—the Therapist must start with top management and work down. Presidents and Vice Presidents are always under a great deal of time pressure, and often want the Industrial Therapist to fix the problems without requiring their involvement. The Therapist must make these executives realize that without their active commitment, funding, and on-going support throughout the organization, the program will never become integrated with the culture, and it will gradually fade away.

The Therapist must impress upon management that once the program has been designed and launched, the company will run the program thereafter. The Therapist's role beyond that point is, on a regularly scheduled basis, to monitor progress, trouble-shoot problems, conduct follow-up sessions such as production floor "tool box" talks, and to periodically review cost and benefit outcome studies.

> *I take a few minutes to check out a small vacant office space just off the production floor. I've got my eye on it as a possible on-site clinic when it is justified by this company's use of our services. Satellite offices are proving to be an effective way to capture and maintain new contracts and diversify the industrial base. At this particular plant, we'll probably start with a half day staffing and develop it from there.*

Another key difference in Industrial Therapy is a growing trend toward Therapists providing services on-site. It minimizes the employer's production down time because employees do not have to travel to and from off-site locations. It also reduces or eliminates the Therapist's overhead costs associated with maintaining a facility. To facilitate this trend, equipment is being made portable, such as mobile Functional Capacity Assessment stations.[1]

There is also a growing belief that on-site settings are the best context for the Therapist to teach and instill safe workstyles. On-site is not always possible because of space, equipment, or safety restrictions, but Therapists who can offer on-site will gain a competitive edge over those who insist on remaining exclusively off-site.

In addition, there are advantages to the therapist appearing on-site regularly, under informal circumstances. It enables the therapist to develop a comfort level among the workers and union stewards that facilitates acceptance and cooperation regarding additional prevention and rehabilitation programs in the future.

> *While I'm at the bottling plant, engineering has asked me to advise with their installation of a new high-speed bottling line. When I first suggested they consider ergonomics in the design stage of tooling or installation, I could see the light bulbs go on. This significantly reduces the likelihood they'll have to retool or rip out an installation later on, to stem a rash of back or upper extremity injuries.*

To the uninitiated employer, "prevention" training may be nothing more than showing a video tape that fulfills the OSHA safety training requirement. Enlightened companies understand that safe behavior is an on-going process that must become integrated into the daily culture and routine of everyone in the company. In addition to implementing programs to achieve behavioral change, companies are also realizing the need to implement structural change.

The safest behavior may still result in injury if the tool, machine, or workstation forces the worker to use improper postures or body mechanics. The Industrial Therapist's involvement in the design of tools and workstations is an investment that can pay great dividends later on.

In most manufacturing operations, Therapists will find numerous opportunities to reduce the risk of injury by modifying existing tools and workstations and incorporating ergonomic principles into new tools and workstations. In addition, Job Analyses in combination with Functional Capacity Assessments or Job Placement Assessments (JPAs) can assist in preventing injuries by defining the worker's safe capabilities and modifying the job accordingly. For these reasons, companies represent a great deal of demand for Therapist services in ergonomics, JAs, FCAs, and JPAs.

> *My beeper indicates I've received the call I've been expecting from an attorney. Many of my colleagues dislike getting involved in legal matters, but I enjoy the challenge. They usually call in advance of the deposition to get a feeling for my responses to specific questions they have in mind. If they like the answers, they go ahead with the deposition.*

Some Industrial Therapists spend more time in legal proceedings than they may ever have imagined in traditional therapy. The reason for this is that there are still many variables and unknowns in Industrial Therapy, and the rule book is in the process of being written through regulations, legislation, and case law. Thus, there are numerous occasions to help one party sue or another party defend. Attorneys are taking advantage of these opportunities. Not unexpectedly, however, there is mounting evidence that when attorneys get involved, the return to work process lengthens, costs increase, and dissatisfaction on the part of one or more parties increases.[2]

Everyone involved in the rehabilitation process recognizes the advantages of win-win outcomes, and the hope is that they become the norm. In the meantime, Industrial Therapists will be called upon to give depositions or testimony on behalf of the plaintiff or defendant in legal disputes.

Sometimes Therapists are called as expert witnesses for cases in which they have no involvement. Other times, the case deals with patients they have evaluated or treated. In many instances, it is the attorney's objective to discredit the Therapist's professional judgment and expertise. In such situations, it is important for the Therapist not to take the interrogation personally, or get defensive. It is necessary only to concentrate on providing the most accurate and objective information possible. If that is accomplished, there is little else to worry about. Calm confidence shows in the delivery, often to the chagrin of the aggressive, cross-examining attorney.

Well, that Attorney liked my guidance on how to address the challenges to an assessment's findings. I'm sure he'll have additional questions as he puts his brief together. Beyond that, I doubt he'll need me, as the majority of cases I'm involved in are settled out of court.

That settled, I have a few minutes to practice my 11:00 presentation on the way back in the car. We're competing for a large employee fitness program contract with a local manufacturing subsidiary of a Fortune 100 company. Our equipment manufacturer has convinced this subsidiary's headquarters to mandate this particular brand of gear, but that doesn't mean we'll automatically get the contract.

It is becoming increasingly common for manufacturers of Industrial Therapy equipment to call on corporate headquarters in order to influence their subsidiaries' use of equipment or providers. For example, a manufacturer of fitness equipment may try to convince headquarters that fitness programs at every branch should be standardized. This uniformity would be accomplished by headquarters specifying this brand and mandate using only those providers who have the authorized brand of fitness equipment.

These providers are represented to corporate headquarters as a service "network" capable of delivering program uniformity at each local site. Theoretically, providers who buy the brand of fitness equipment should win the contract wherever there is a branch location. In this manner, the equipment manufacturer has served to "pull" demand for its products at the corporate headquarter level.

Although this marketing strategy provides an advantage, it does not guarantee the contract. The local management has often been contacted by other providers and may even have an existing provider relationship they do not want to sever. In addition, local managers are often reluctant to let headquarters call the shots for them, and headquarters may choose to fight more important battles than dictating the kind of therapy programs the plant should adopt.

As mentioned before, the Therapist must present the sale on both a rational and an emotional level to this prospect. The fact that the equipment is consistent with headquarters' desire to standardize, is only one part of the rational sell. Local management must be also convinced that the program is run by people every bit as proficient and *likable* as the incumbent provider.

In practicing my presentation to manufacturing and operations executives, I concentrate on eliminating medical jargon, being conversational, and talking about their needs rather than my practices capabilities. I try not to use slides or overheads exclusively, because they may distance me from the audience.

To appeal on an emotional level, it is helpful to make the presentation more intimate. The Therapist should try to create a feeling that everyone in the room is sitting on the same side of the table, discussing the company's problems and how they might be addressed. The Therapist must concentrate on listening rather than talking, and ask questions that help identify problems and solutions.

It is also important to clarify whether the solutions fit the company's mission, goals, capabilities, and culture. It is usually advantageous for the Industrial Therapist to invite prospects to visit their facility for final presentations, particularly if the facility and equipment are equal to or better than anything on the market. The visit also enables prospects to meet staff and reach a comfort level with the company's atmosphere and culture.

It's sometimes hard to tell how a final presentation went. Often, the prospects are committed to objectively reviewing the candidates and maintaining a poker face. Even when I'm "sure" we've won, we sometimes lose. Even the best among us are going to win only a certain percentage, so the best strategy is to make as many presentations as you can. It's a numbers game.

It is rare for Therapists to sign up a prospect in the final meeting of a competition for the contract. Companies are usually committed to an orderly, rational process. In some instances, they will take several months to make their final decision. This time period is viewed as a problem for some Therapists, and as an opportunity for others. It is possible for the leading contender to lose their position with the passage of time, and for the other contenders to capture the high ground through additional communication.

The specific approach the Therapist takes to this follow-up contact is critical. People do not generally appreciate being harassed over the phone. They also do not have time to read lengthy tomes in the form of a several page brochure or letter. Follow-up contact should be quick, easy to understand or read, and confined to as few critical points as possible. In addition, Therapists should always address what the prospect gets versus what the practice can do.

For instance, rather than saying something like "we have a broader range of equipment," the Therapist might say "each injured employee will achieve the highest possible productivity due to our broader range of equipment." It is not what you say, but how you say it.

> *One last thing to do today—a one-hour seminar with insurance adjusters on how they should read the results of our Functional Capacity Assessments. I used to think of them as an adversary, but we've mutually discovered common ground. If we do our job right and they do their job right, it's a win-win for everyone involved.*

With the growing pressure to control costs while avoiding litigation, insurance adjusters are looking for more objective, reliable ways of determining degrees of disability, the prospects for improvement through further treatment, and assurance that risks of reinjury have been minimized. Assessment tools are playing an increasingly important role in assisting these determinations.

It is important that providers and insurance adjusters are working from the same page, so Industrial Therapists are making efforts to educate adjusters on how to interpret and use assessment information.

> *One of the adjusters had an immediate problem that stimulated a spirited discussion. One of his clients, referred by a physician for Work Conditioning, was diagnosed as having "chronic recurring upper extremity pain" without significant objective clinical signs or findings. The person has been out of work and sedentary since the injury, and medical history indicates inconsistent pain reports.*
>
> *The discussion centered around how to determine if the client is misrepresenting the injury. The group consensus was that the first step should be an FCA that might indicate Invalid Participation (purposeful underperformance), and might also help set realistic goals that might include a Conditioning trial period prior to Work Conditioning or Work Hardening. Beyond that, a personality inventory such as an MMPI might also be worthwhile.*

In presenting to insurance adjusters, the Therapist must provide clear, straight forward communication, making sure to speak in the adjuster's language rather than medical jargon. A good technique in such sessions is for the Therapist to ask up front, what the adjusters hope to take away from the presentation, so that the content can be directed at specific areas of concern. The Therapist may find videos helpful, but they should be used sparingly and interspersed with verbal presentation and group discussions.

> *Four o'clock already! Time for our internal staff meeting. With so many new problems and challenges encountered daily, it's a good idea for everyone to share ideas and solutions weekly. We're going to talk about staffing the on-site office at the bottling plant, and set the focus for our upcoming presentation to the Chamber of Commerce. Sometimes we have outside speakers, or have staff members research a topic and give an inservice.*

Another weekly meeting involves the Industrial Therapy practice staff, sometimes termed "Staffings." These meetings deal with issues regarding client programs and progress. They are a good forum for discussing problems for which there may not be adequate answers in manuals, journals or magazines. For example, what should be done if alcohol is detected on a client's breath? How should the Therapist respond if a client asks whether they should get a lawyer? How should the Therapist counsel a client who is convinced the employer will terminate them upon return to work? How should frequent complainers or whiners be handled?

Problems such as these can spring up unexpectedly, and are better addressed in group discussions where everyone's knowledge and experience can be brought to bear on the situation (Figure 5.9, page 71).

In short, Industrial Therapy continues to be characterized by unpredictability and constant innovation. In many cases, the pressure to experiment and innovate is driven by the desire to save money through more cost effective treatment, or to increase productivity by reducing injury rates and expediting return to work. Therapists who find ways to fulfill these needs gain competitive advantages. Remaining sensitive to industry needs and staying abreast of new discoveries are important requirements for the success of the Industrial Therapy practice.

> *Tonight will feature another dinner eaten on the fly. I'm participating in a panel discussion at the Minnesota APTA. They're serving dinner beforehand, but I want to stop by our exhibit booth to see how things went today. The panel discussion will focus on a number of clinical issues and will involve the audience in brainstorming possible courses of action.*

FIGURE 5.9   Weekly staff meetings provide an opportunity to discuss problems, share ideas, plan for the future, and educate staff members.

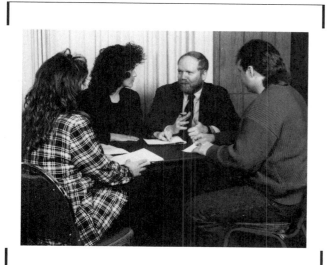

FIGURE 5.10   Trade shows are another avenue through which Industrial Therapists can gain awareness in the marketplace.

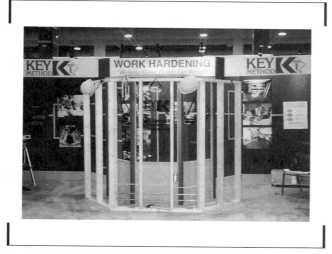

Ahhhh! Back home at last. What is it? 9:30? I feel like I accomplished a lot today, but also left a lot of loose ends. Better get some sleep. Tomorrow will be another exciting day.

Panel discussions at trade shows or conferences can be instrumental for Industrial Therapy practitioners to exchange ideas, and get feedback on their approaches to complex issues and challenges. For example, what is the best course of action when a Work Conditioning client begins to self modify their program without consulting the Therapist, or begins to "coach" other clients on their program? How should conflicts be resolved with unions when, for instance, recommended job modifications conflict with union rules? What should the Therapist do in the case of a Work Hardening client who is overperforming unsafely to meet job demands?

In most cases, solutions require both clinical and interpersonal skills. By bringing a variety of backgrounds and experiences to bear on issues, panel discussions tend to probe the complexities in greater depth and bring out broader creativity in exploring solutions (Figure 5.10).

Getting exposure through exhibiting at a trade show, making speeches, and writing articles are effective ways for Therapists to bolster their practice's exposure and credibility in the marketplace. In the process of seeking new referrals, it helps when the prospects have heard of the practice, and have a favorable impression. For this same reason, it is best for Therapists to precede the initial contact with a mailing of some sort—a brochure if it is affordable, or a letter at the very least. It is preferable to begin the conversation by referring to the letter or brochure that has been sent.

SUMMARY

The daily life of an Industrial Therapist differs from that of a clinical Physical or Occupational Therapist in many respects. Preventing injuries from happening is becoming as important as rehabilitating injured workers. In both instances, the amount of innovation brought to bear is venturing far afield of traditional therapy.

While referrals for traditional therapy still come mostly from physicians, Industrial Therapists can exercise more control over referrals by marketing directly to companies, and by building relationships with the many professions that participate on return to work treatment teams.

The Industrial Therapist works as much for the employer as for the employee, because prevention, wellness, productivity, and effective response to injuries are in the long term interest of both parties. The employer must maximize productivity per dollar of fixed and variable cost in order to remain competitive in the marketplace.

The employee must work safely and productively to ensure that the company, and the job, survive. Industrial Therapists' programs and processes impact each set of needs, whether administered in a clinic setting, Work Retraining Center, or at the employer's location.

In a number of ways, Industrial Therapists play an important facilitating role in helping management and employees seek their mutual interest and work cooperatively. First, Therapists must convince management that the programs and processes are good ideas—that the long term productivity and financial benefits will outweigh the costs. Then, they must convince employees to become committed to the programs' goals, and to follow through with appropriate behaviors.

Without top management's on-going encouragement and support, and without employees' whole-hearted commitment and participation, Industrial Therapy programs are destined to fail. Both parties must buy in, rationally and emotionally, and strive for win-win outcomes. The Industrial Therapist plays an important role in bringing this about, day after day.

REFERENCES

1. Reichley ML: Functional Capacity Assessment Unit Now Mobile, *Advance For Physical Therapists*, Oct 18, 1993.
2. Sachs BL, et al: Objective Assessment for Exercise Treatment on the B-200 Isostation as Part of Work Tolerance Rehabilitation, *Spine* 19:1, 1994.
3. Interviews with: Glenda L. Key, PT, Michael Melnik, OTR, Mary Beth Purdie, OTR, Keith Marmer, PT, Phil Moe, PT.

P A R T

II

Injury Prevention

CHAPTER

6

Ergonomics

Peter M. Budnick

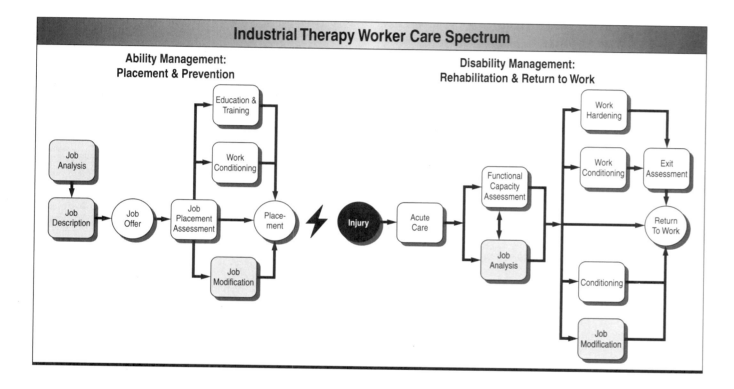

Industrial Therapy Worker Care Spectrum

Throughout the early industrial age, Western man was quite often forced to adapt himself, in some sense to subject himself, to the machine. To this day we have not yet completely reversed the relationship, for there is still much to be understood and much to be done in mastering our technological innovations.[2]

Humans design things for themselves to make life easier, more comfortable, and safer. Why, then, do we continue to adapt, or even subject ourselves, to technology created by us? Why do we not focus more closely on that most important parameter, the human being, when we design products, systems, and environments that interface with humans?

These are the perplexing philosophical questions that hit squarely on the topic of this chapter. You will not find the answers here, but with some luck you will achieve a greater understanding of complex issues that interplay in the design and analysis of living and working environments. You may also gain a new perspective on such issues, and pick up a few ideas applying to the problem.

First, some useful definitions are presented to clarify ergonomics and what is required of the qualified ergonomist. Next, the history of ergonomics is traced from its practical beginnings in the Industrial Age through today. This is followed by an overview of ergonomic principles and concepts, the building blocks of any successful intervention, analysis, or design effort.

The chapter closes with discussion of the essential elements of an ergonomics program that complements any organization committed to improving bottom-line concerns. This includes productivity, quality, and employee health and safety. It should be understood that this chapter is only a cursory review of some selected ergonomic topics. It should not be taken as a summary of the profession, which becomes immediately clearer as you read the definitions in the next section.

What is Ergonomics?

The word "ergonomics" originates from the Greek words *ergon*, meaning "work," and *nomos*, meaning "laws." Literally, ergonomics means the "laws of work." Depending on one's viewpoint, ergonomics can be either a science or an applied technology. For example, Wilson[10] views ergonomics as both a science and a technology, implying the need for data collection, analysis, application, and evaluation of application. He puts forth this broad definition (originally reported by Christensen et al, 1988):

> That branch of science and technology that includes what is known and theorized about human behavioral and biological characteristics that can be validly applied to the specification, design, evaluation, operation, and maintenance of products and systems to enhance safe, effective, and satisfying use by individuals, groups and organizations.

In contrast, Oborne[8] believes "ergonomics rests squarely in the applied domain . . . its sole purpose is to relate some kind of working system to the operator's abilities." Oborne does discuss the importance and role of scientific investigations, ". . . or at least the results and implications of those investigations . . . ," and makes a case for conducting those studies in a naturalistic environment, rather than a laboratory setting.

A qualified ergonomist must possess knowledge from a variety of traditionally separate disciplines. The origin in the study of work, an emphasis on productivity, more recently within the health and safety community, the use of engineering and psychological modeling concepts applying to the human, all constitutes the extensive training to an ergonomics expert. In the absence of learning by actual experience, such expertise is afforded by a combination of graduate training at an accredited institution and practice.

To stem the inevitable bandwagon of enthusiastic, if uninformed, self-proclaimed ergonomics experts, the Board of Certification for Professional Ergonomists (BCPE) has been established "to provide a formal organization certifying qualified practitioners of ergonomics" (BCPE, 1993).

From this point forward, assuming the success of the BCPE, professional ergonomists must achieve certification by passing a certification exam designed to test the breadth of one's knowledge of the various subject areas that constitute ergonomic expertise. The BCPE defines an ergonomist as follows:

> Ergonomics is a body of knowledge about human abilities, human limitations and human characteristics that are relevant to design. Ergonomic design is the application of this body of knowledge to the design of tools, machines, systems, tasks, jobs, and environments for safe, comfortable and effective human use.
>
> The board certifies practitioners of ergonomics, not ergonomics researchers or theoreticians. A practitioner of ergonomics is a person who has; (a) a mastery of a body of ergonomics knowledge, (b) a command of the methodologies used by ergonomists in applying that knowledge to the design of a product, system, job, or environment, and (c) has applied his or her knowledge in the analysis, design, testing and evaluation of products, systems, and environments.

The Glossary of OSHAs "Ergonomics Program Management Guidelines for Meatpacking Plants,"[9] discussed in the ergonomics program section later in this chapter, provides yet another definition of an *ergonomist*, or *professional ergonomist*:

> . . . a person who possesses a recognized degree or professional credentials in ergonomics or a closely related allied field (such as human factors engineering) and who has demonstrated, through knowledge and experience, the ability to identify and recommend effective means of correction for ergonomic hazards in the workplace.

Presumably, the OSHA ergonomics standard, reportedly to be completed by the end of 1994, will include a definition that may differ from these. BCPE notes that "ergonomics" is regarded as synonymous with "human factors" and "human factors engineering." This is a source of confusion among practitioners and lay people alike.

Ergonomics is often used to refer to the applied science focusing on the physical aspects of human work and capabilities, such as strength, size, and posture. More specifically, this might better be termed "industrial ergonomics." "Human factors," or "human factors engineering" is often taken to refer to the psychological aspects of humans, such as decision making processes, perception, mental loading, and behavior. However, the names are used synonymously, and ergonomics is generally more recognizable to the public.

Perhaps it was said best by Laughery[7] in his discussion regarding the name of the Human Factors Society: The Society represents a discipline that has two names, and the one we are not using—*ergonomics* —has become better known and more widely recognized than the one we are using—*human factors*. The

Society has since changed its name to Human Factors and Ergonomics Society.

To confuse the matter more, you may encounter terms like "human engineering," "human performance engineering," or "industrial psychology," which describe specialized approaches to topics that generally fall under the ergonomics umbrella. Reviewing the history of the field may shed some light on how and why such a variety of people and specialties have come to use the term "ergonomics" to describe themselves and their profession.

The debate over what ergonomics is, what knowledge constitutes ergonomic expertise, and who should rightfully practice ergonomics, will surely continue well into the future. While this author concedes a bias toward an engineering approach, materials covered in this chapter should indicate that a reasonable approach to ergonomics will often require a multidisciplinary perspective. Frequently, such perspective is not available through one individual expert, and is not feasible because of the financial burden a large team of experts presents.

History of Ergonomics

One way to understand the history of ergonomics is to view it in the context of technological development. Writing from the perspective of studying and improving human performance, Bailey[1] notes that early human concerns with gathering food, protection from the environment, animals, and other people probably provided the motivation for the first tool developments.

Improving performance meant improving the odds of survival for individuals and groups. With humble beginnings using sticks and stones to fashion tools, human technology has progressed to the complex systems and machines we depend on today. Fueling this progression, especially since the industrial revolution is a complex web of economics and human knowledge, each of which play a significant role in the development of ergonomics.

Kantowitz[5] classifies four levels of technology by focusing on the contributions made by humans and machines to the total system, in terms of power and control. At the lowest level, the human supplies both power and control. Pushing/pulling a cart, lifting and carrying, using a shovel, and using a manual hand tool (Figure 6.1) are examples of the first level of technology.

At the second level, the machine supplies the primary power, while the human retains control. Operating a punch press, a powered nut-runner, or welding (Figure 6.2, page 78) are examples of second level technologies.

As technological complexity increases, the third

FIGURE 6.1 Power Mechanic by Lewis Hines. This famous photograph illustrates the first level of technology where the human supplies power and control.

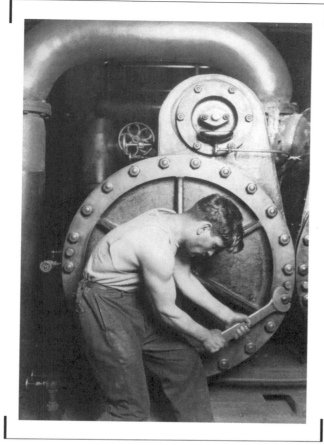

(From George Eastman House.)

level of technology exists when the machine supplies both power and information, but the human still controls the operation. The paper-making plant shown in Figure 6.3 on page 81, is an example of this level. At the highest level, the machine supplies power, control, and information, and the human role becomes one of monitoring the operation, intervening only when necessary.

The cockpit of a modern airplane while on autopilot (Figure 6.4, page 79) is one example of the fourth and highest level of technology. Conceivably, there is a fifth level of technology in which the machine provides power, control, and the ability to monitor itself and make intelligent decisions in the complete absence of human intervention. To date, there is no such machine.

Bernardino Ramazinni is often cited as an early recognition that exposure to "certain violent and irregular motions and unnatural postures . . . by which . . .

FIGURE 6.2 This welder illustrates the second level of technology. The tool supplies power while the human controls it.

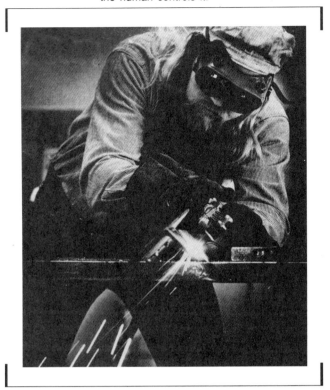

(Michael C. Hayman/Photo Researchers.)

FIGURE 6.3 A paper-making plant illustrates the third level of technology. The plant supplies power and information but the human is still in control.

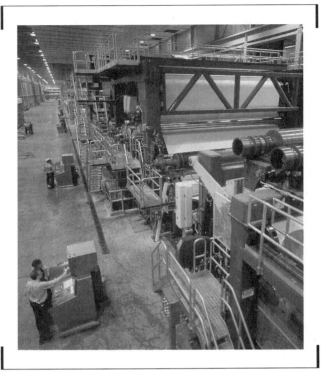

(Courtesy Westvaco Corporation.)

the natural structure of the living machine is so impaired that serious diseases gradually develop . . ."[3] He made this observation prior to the industrial revolution, while technology was primarily at level one.

Oddly, even as the industrial revolution expanded the levels and impacts of technology on individuals, little has been done, until recently, to address the problem of Cumulative Trauma Disorders (CTDs). Chaffin notes that economics and the lack of basic knowledge concerning the mechanics of the human body is in part responsible for the slow development of ergonomics.[3]

Manual labor was inexpensive and easily replaced. The biomechanical knowledge that did exist was generally restricted to intellectuals, and rarely reached the commercial enterprises that could have benefited from it.

Near the turn of this century, an important link between labor and economics was made by Frederick Taylor.[6] Combining the practical experience he gained as a laborer with the theoretical knowledge he gained in studies of mechanical engineering, he questioned: "What is the best way to do this job?" He applied a scientific approach to study work (until that time, scientific methods had primarily been the tool of

chemistry and physics). His most famous study focused on shoveling while employed by Bethlehem Steel. Prior to his study, 400 to 600 employees spent most of their time shoveling a variety of materials. Each employee brought his own shovel, none were trained, and pay was $1.15 per day.

By varying the scoop sizes of the shovels, and thus their carrying capacity, Taylor determined that the maximum amount of material shoveled per day occurred when the material load was 21.5 pounds (for distances up to four feet and heights less than five feet). To apply this new knowledge, he had special shovel sizes purchased, each to be used for different materials being shoveled. From then on, employees were issued shovels each day; large scoops for ashes, medium for coal, and small for ore.

By studying the work, Taylor was also able to establish a standard amount to be shoveled per day for each type of material. After receiving training in proper shoveling methods, and being issued the proper tool for the particular material type, each worker that exceeded the day's standard received a 60% bonus above the day wage. Workers who were unable to achieve standards were put on a different job. Quite common today, these concepts of studying work, in-

FIGURE 6.4 The cockpit of a Boeing 757 jet illustrates the highest level of technology. When the autopilot is engaged the airplane supplies power, control, and information while the human monitors the operation.

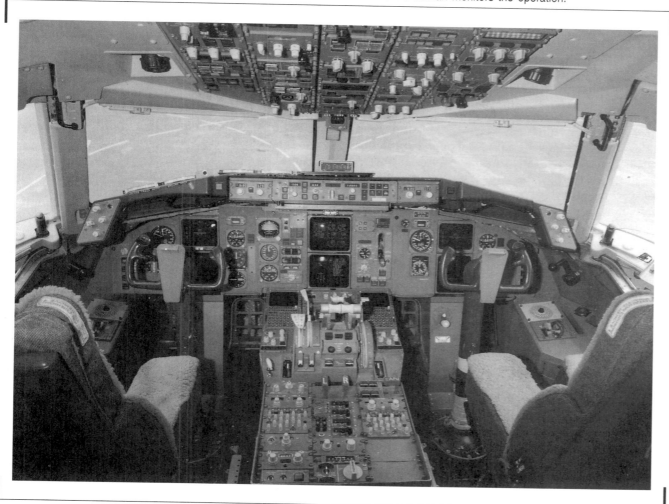

(Courtesy of Boeing.)

centive pay, and personnel selection were innovative in Taylor's era.

When Taylor's methods were applied at Bethlehem, the same amount of material was moved by only 140 employees (each making 60% higher wages). The material handling costs, including the cost of the studies, new tools, and the wage bonuses, was cut by half. "Taylorism," the idea that jobs should be designed by experts, and workers should just follow instructions, resulted in dramatic productivity improvements that contributed to equally dramatic increases in standard of living for many cultures. However, knowledge levels of individuals throughout society, not just the "experts," have increased since Taylor's time, and now employee involvement in the design of work, is an important part of successful ergonomics and successful organization.

Henry Ford, incorrectly credited for the automobile assembly line, made another important contribution to the economic worth of humans engaged in organized work.[6] (Random Olds had applied the assembly line concept in 1899, ten years before Ford. However, Ford dominated the auto building industry and held the public's eye.)[6]

By studying and controlling job and work design Ford made significant productivity increases. Through the use of assembly lines, Ford was supplying one half of the world's automobiles by 1924. An important factor in this success was his move to increase employee pay from $2.50 per nine hour day to $5.00 per eight hour day. He also established a $30,000,000 profit-sharing fund. Certainly, Ford made a significant amount of money himself, but his methods resulted in employees being more and more an economic factor in business and production decisions. On the other hand, this type of assembly method also exposed employees to highly repetitive activities, one factor associated with ergonomic hazards.

Frank and Lillian Gilbreth are credited with another important tool in the study of work: micromotion study.[1,6] The contributions they made in the study of micromotions laid the foundation for methods that are used to this day.

A key job in Mr. Gilbreth's construction business (he was an engineer) was bricklaying. He had learned bricklaying as a teenager, and later applied his analytical skills to study the trade in detail. Using micromotion studies, he broke the entire job into small subtasks, each requiring small motions or actions. With this detailed understanding of the job, he was able to optimize the motions required by humans to satisfy the job requirements.

Gilbreth also redesigned work methods, scaffolding, and standardized mortar consistency to reduce the number and extent of the motions required by the worker. When he was finished, he had reduced the number of motions per brick from 18 to 4.5. Using his new methods, bricklayers were able to lay 350 bricks/hour, compared to the previous record for similar work of 120 bricks/hour. What made this work so important was the job he studied; bricklaying had been performed for 3,000 years. Applying systematic study to the work, one man was able to generate a 300% improvement over the methods developed through experience for over 3,000 years.

After Frank Gilbreth died, Lillian continued his work on micromotion study, and the many small elements they recorded are called "therbligs," Gilbreth spelled backwards—almost. Therbligs form the basis for motion-time studies used to establish the time it takes to perform specific tasks. Many ergonomists use variations on the therblig theme to break a job down into its essential elements, for detailed hazard analysis and abatement. Lillian is also credited as the first person to develop process charts and symbols. Her charts were the forerunners of system developers' flow charts, and her symbols are some of the first icons to be used in business.[1]

After World War I, the Industrial Fatigue Board was set up in England. The board reportedly relied on objective measures to indicate evidence of fatigue in the workplace. Up until 1929, the board produced 61 reports.[1]

A series of productivity studies at the Western Electric Hawthorne plant were implemented in 1927.[1] After twelve years and five studies focusing on the relationship between workplace illumination intensity and productivity, many questions were left unanswered. These studies are remembered as the "Hawthorne effect." It may well be that change in

itself is responsible for some productivity increases, rather than the varied, specific parameters. The Hawthorne studies still debated today, are nevertheless important contributions to the study of workplace productivity.

So far in this discussion, the economic and scientific advancements detailed have been restricted primarily to the first and second levels of technology described at the beginning of this section. These developments fall primarily in the realm of industrial ergonomics, which you'll recall is only one aspect of the overall field of ergonomics, or human factors engineering.

After the depression in the 1930s, World War II spurred rapid scientific and technological advancements. During that period higher levels of technology became more common, and a shift in focus occurred in which psychological aspects of the human-machine interface became increasingly important.

The emphasis shifts, in part, to the study of the mind in the higher levels of technology, where humans exercise control over information and decision-making in complex machines and systems, rather than mostly physical control and power at lower levels.

No matter how much training, motivation, and personnel selection the militaries applied to their troops, accidents and catastrophes continued to occur. Human performance, or so it seemed, couldn't keep up with the technology. As Taylor reflected in 1957, "bombs and bullets often missed their targets, planes crashed, friendly ships were fired upon and sunk, and whales were depth charged." As reported by Bailey (1989—courtesy of the *American Psychologist*), Taylor further observed that:

> *Regardless of how much he could be stretched by training or pared down through selection, there were still many military equipments which the man just could not be molded to fit. They required of him too many hands, too many feet, or in the case of some of the more complex devices, too many heads.*
>
> *Sometimes they called for the operator to see targets which were close to invisible, or to understand speech in the presence of deafening noise, to track simultaneously in three coordinates with two hands, to solve analog, form complex differential equations, or to consider large amounts of information and to reach life-and-death decisions in split seconds with no hope of another try.*

For this author, two points stand out in this passage. The idea that the human be "molded" to fit the technology, and the idea that the technology required "too many heads." Using 20/20 hindsight, this author emphasizes a *match* between human and machine, rather than molding the human to the machine. If molding is to occur, it should emphasize the design of the system, not the human.

In practice, it is often a molding of the technology to fit human characteristics combined with a molding of human operators through training, selection, and motivation that constitutes an ergonomic approach.

The concept of "too many heads," as Taylor puts it, emphasizes an important divergence in the field of ergonomics. As technology entered the third and fourth levels described above, there became a pronounced need to focus on the mental, or psychological aspects of the human-machine interface. To this day, as discussed in the definitions section above, there has been confusion over terminology and "membership" in the field of ergonomics, with the psychological viewpoint generally using the name "human factors engineering," and the physical or biomechanically oriented viewpoint using the term "ergonomics." Today, the terms are, for the most part, interchangeable.

Since World War II, there has been a flurry of activity in studying human capabilities and limitations, and applying that knowledge to the design and evaluation of work and living environments. A variety of texts, journals, and organizations have risen to meet the challenge—too many to summarize here. Assuming that therapists most often interface with ergonomics in the industrial setting, this historical focus will conclude with developments that fall in that arena.

In particular, biomechanical modeling and the wider recognition of cumulative trauma disorders as a significant workplace concern, both industrial ergonomics topics, will conclude this discussion.

Chaffin provides a summary of epidemiological support for occupational biomechanics, which can be viewed as a supporting sub-specialty of ergonomics.[3] He notes that in the 1970s, for a variety of socioeconomic reasons, there was a realization that health and quality of life are greatly reduced for a large population due to acute and chronic musculoskeletal disorders. Since then, many industries have acknowledged this significant cost burden, in terms of degradations in bottom-line cost, and competitiveness factors, such as quality and productivity. Chaffin[3] summarizes a report published in 1978 by J.K. Kelsey:

About 20 million people in the United States had musculoskeletal impairments.

Musculoskeletal conditions ranked second to circulatory system diseases in total economic cost, and ranked first among all disease groups in cost attributed to lost earnings and non-fatal illnesses (about $20 million in 1972).

In the United States, at least 85,000 workers receive permanent disability allowances for musculoskeletal conditions each year.

Back injuries accounted for about one-sixth of all occupational injuries.

Since that time, these numbers have continued to rise, and awareness of musculoskeletal disorders has increased. OSHAs "Ergonomics Program Management Guidelines for Meatpacking Plants" begins with the following:

> In recent years, there has been a significant increase in reporting of Cumulative Trauma Disorders (CTDs) and other work-related disorders due to ergonomic hazards. CTDs account for an increasingly large percentage of Workers' Compensation costs each year, and they represent nearly half of the occupational illnesses reported in the annual Bureau of Labor Statistics (BLS) survey.
>
> Much of the increase in CTDs expose employees to increased repetitive motion and other ergonomic risk factors; some may be attributed to increased awareness— by industry, labor, and government—and reporting of these disorders.[9]

This passage covers the three main topics that have repeatedly surfaced in this historical perspective on ergonomics; economics, type of work, and human knowledge. Recall that early in the industrial revolution, workers, for all intents and purposes, were inexpensive and replaceable, and knowledge was often reserved by specialists outside of the commercial sectors that could benefit from it.

Consequently, little effort was directed toward the human machine interface early on. As technology developed and required new and different work roles from humans beyond simple physical power input and manual control, a more educated and conditioned work force was required.

Additionally, the costs required for selecting, training, keeping, and motivating a work force in higher level technologies increased the economic worth of employees in industry. Thus, as knowledge is disseminated to a wider population and the economic value of individual employees increases, so has the need for and knowledge about ergonomics increased.

ERGONOMICS PROGRAMMING

For better or for worse, the Occupational Safety and Health Administration (OSHA) has identified cumulative trauma disorders and the ergonomic risk factors that contribute to them, as primary enforcement targets. The meat-packing industries in particular have been singled out due to high incidence and severity of CTDs, culminating in OSHAs first step in producing ergonomic guidelines for industry.

The Ergonomics Program Management Guidelines for Meatpacking Plants (U.S. Department of Labor, Occupational Safety and Health Administration, OSHA 3123, 1991) sets outlines that summarize corporate commitments, program elements, detailed guidance and examples, some simple assessment tool exhibits, a bibliography, glossary, and a questions-and-answers section, thus providing a basis for those attempting to set up an ergonomics program.[9]

As this is written, OSHA is writing a standard which may appear within the year. The meatpacker guidelines are expected to serve as the basis for that standard. This section describes the basic elements of a successful ergonomics program, and remains consistent, yet not all inclusive, with the meatpackers guidelines.

Management Commitment

It cannot be stressed enough that the most important factor to initiate and sustain a successful ergonomics program takes clear and true commitment from management. That commitment should be evident at all management levels. When the corporate culture is such that all members are committed and dedicated to success, then that organization will benefit from an ergonomics program. In fact, an ergonomics program compliments and integrates well with other management initiated programs designed to enhance competitiveness, such as Total Quality Management (TQM).

In the absence of management commitment, an organization will remain in a reactive ergonomics mode, which will likely produce unforeseen, avoidable long term losses, degradations in quality, reliability, productivity, and efficiency, in addition to the commonly understood health and safety losses.

Employee Involvement

A successful organizational commitment will include employee involvement. Observations show that no matter how many experts and supposed experts parade through a workstation, the actual problems, and often the solutions, are left in the head of the person most knowledgeable with the area; the employee performing the task.

Employee involvement, in understanding and correcting ergonomic hazards, is a crucial part of the overall process, especially after employees have received training to recognize and correct such hazards. This fits well with the trend in American industry to "empower" the employees, and has been notably effective when employee team approaches have been implemented.

Ergonomic Program Elements

Once organizational commitments are made, the ergonomics program should be developed with at least these three elements; worksite analysis, hazard prevention and control, and training and education. These elements work in concert with existing organizational health and safety programs and a comprehensive medical management program.

Ergonomic improvements will often affect the workplace and design methods. Engineers and other product and process experts will also benefit the program.

The *worksite analysis* is used to identify existing hazards and conditions which may contribute to ergonomic risks. This includes confidential analysis of medical, insurance, and other injury-reporting records. This serves to identify tasks or work areas which require further hazard analysis and controls. This process is also used to identify low risk and light duty jobs, which should be shared with, and applied by, healthcare officials when injured employees are being reassigned to work.

Under no circumstances should a recovering employee be returned to a job that stresses the same body tissues and regions of the original CTD. The ergonomic hazard evaluation of specific workstations and tasks should identify the muscle and tendon groups and tissues that are stressed, and this information transferred to those in charge of work reassignments.

Following the worksite hazard evaluations are *hazard prevention and controls* consisting of one or more of the following; engineering controls, workpractice controls, and administrative controls. Personal protective equipment are not necessarily ergonomic controls in themselves, but should be selected and fitted so as not to contribute to ergonomic stressors. For example, improperly selected or fitted gloves can significantly increase grip forces. Braces, splints, back belts, and other similar devices are *not* personal protective equipment, and should never be used as such.

Engineering controls, where feasible, are the preferred means of controlling hazards in the workplace. Rather than seek minimum exposures to a hazard, engineering controls are used to minimize or eliminate the hazard all together by physically altering the work area. Administrative controls focus on reducing employee exposure to known hazards. For example, using job rotation, increasing the number of employees, providing rest pauses, and reducing production rates can reduce duration, frequency, and severity of exposure to ergonomic stressors.

Work practice controls are safe practices that are understood and followed by managers, supervisors and employees alike. Important elements in work practice controls include using proper work techniques, employee training and conditioning, regular monitoring, feedback, maintenance, adjustments and modifications, and enforcement.

It should be emphasized that each of these general elements should exist in an effective ergonomics program, but it is this author's opinion that only engineering controls actually minimize or eliminate ergonomic hazards.

Work practices, especially if they conflict with the most natural and efficient means of completing a task, may not be effective and may negatively affect production requirements. Administrative controls also come with expense, and may not always be adhered to under production demands. Engineering controls may be more expensive up-front, but they do reduce or eliminate hazards, and they do minimize additional costs in the long run, when injuries have occurred because of their absence.

The fourth major element of an ergonomics program, *training and education* throughout all levels of the organization, is crucial to success. Giving each individual the knowledge to recognize, understand the effects of, and ultimately the power to initiate control of ergonomic hazards will have long lasting positive effects.

A training program should include and be specifically tailored for the following generic organizational groups; all effected employees, engineers and maintenance personnel, supervisors, managers, and health care providers. Each plays an important role in the overall program, and each requires specific knowledge. Coordination among individuals in each of the groups is also required for success. The training should be conducted by qualified personnel with a broad understanding and expertise in the field of ergonomics, which includes extensive background knowledge in technical, health, and safety, as discussed in the introduction.

Both general and job specific training should be provided for effected employees. The general training should familiarize the employee with the nature of CTDs, the risk factors that may contribute to them, how to recognize and report such factors, any symptoms they may experience, and the steps each can take to prevent disorders.

Job specific training, at a minimum, should be provided for all new or reassigned employees. This type of initial orientation training is useful in teaching employees other job specific methods and concepts, which often compliments ergonomic training. As mentioned previously, sound ergonomics often improves other bottom-line organizational motives including quality, efficiency, and productivity.

The content of job specific training depends on the tasks required by the job. However, in general it should include instruction regarding the proper use, maintenance, and application of tools, jigs, and other process implements, the purpose of any safety equipment, and proper task methods to be used in the completion of the job requirements.

Important in this process, and ultimately the motivation empowering employees with such knowledge, is to instruct, allow, and encourage individuals to develop and implement safe and efficient methods, tools, and implements to meet the job requirements.

SUMMARY

The specialty known as ergonomics evolved through a complex mix of economics and human knowledge. As the marketplace increases the real value of individual employees and as accurate knowledge and information are widely disseminated throughout the population, more resources are made available to optimize the performance of employees.

Optimizing employee performance includes motivation, training, and compatibility with work station design. An ergonomics program which ensures input and communication between all involved parties and individuals is crucial when optimizing the human-machine interface. This type of organizational commitment and vision works well with similar competitive strategies, such as quality improvement programs. The benefits of such optimization efforts are reflected in increased productivity and quality. Employee safety, health, and comfort are also increased.

Ideally, ergonomics is applied proactively, beginning with the earliest design phases for product and process designs and carried on throughout the life of those products and processes. This is the most effective and efficient opportunity in terms of both cost and long term success.

In the absence of proactive ergonomics, a reactive approach may be required to control existing or unforeseen hazards. This is generally less effective and more expensive than proactive approaches, but still cost effective when potential losses related to employee injuries and reduced productivity and quality are considered.

The wide variety of knowledge required for an effective ergonomics approach requires either a qualified ergonomist with extensive training, or a team approach involving members with differing special skills. Knowledge of human physical and psychological capabilities and limitations, human anatomy, physiology, medicine, and engineering should be applied when devising an ergonomics intervention or program.

The abilities to apply scientific methodology and understand technologies used in industries are also required for successful ergonomics.

There are three general methods to reduce ergonomic hazards in the workplace.

- Engineering controls are used to reduce or eliminate a hazard through machine and system design or modification.
- Administrative controls, such as worker rotation, are applied to reduce individual employee exposure to hazards.
- Work method controls are applied to change employee behavior through training and rule-making intended to improve the interface between human and machine.

Engineering controls seek to eliminate the source of ergonomic and safety hazards through machine design (molding the technology to the human). *Administrative controls* seek to reduce employee exposure to hazards without affecting the hazard source. *Work practice controls* seek to reduce employee exposure by modifying employee behavior (molding the human to fit the technology).

Depending on the extent of the hazard and its associated costs, some combination of these controls might be applied. It must be emphasized that work practice controls will not be effective in reducing employee hazard exposures when the enforced work methods conflict with the normal and natural, most expedient methods to complete a task, especially when incentive compensation is in effect.

Economic and technical feasibility certainly play a large role in ergonomic hazard reduction. This author advocates the elimination of hazard through design, or a molding of technology to fit the human, as preferable to molding of human to fit technology. Realistically, a combination of the two extremes is required, however, adapting technology to the human seems much wiser in the long term.

REFERENCES

1. Bailey RW: *Human Performance Engineering: using human factors/ergonomics to achieve computer system usability,* Englewood Cliffs, NJ, 1989, Prentice Hall.
2. Cartier-Bresson H: Man and Machine, photographs by Henri Cartier-Bresson, IBM World Trade Corporation, 1969, Davis-Delaney-Arrow.
3. Chaffin DB: *Occupational Biomechanics,* ed 2, 1991, John Wiley & Sons.
4. Board of Certification in Professional Ergonomics: Certification for Ergonomists and Human Factors Professionals, an introductory pamphlet, Bellingham, Wash, 1993.
5. Kantowitz BH: *Human Factors,* 1983, John Wiley & Sons.
6. Konz SA: *Work Design: industrial ergonomics,* ed 3, Worthington, Ohio, 1990, Publishing Horizons.
7. Laughery KR: Should HFS Change Its Name?, *Human Factors Society Bulletin* 35(1) Jan, 1992.
8. Oborne DJ: Tipping the Balance Towards Ergonomics. In Lovesey EJ, editor: *Contemporary Ergonomics 1991,* Proceedings of the Ergonomics Society's 1991 Annual Conference, London, 1991, Taylor & Francis.
9. US Department of Labor Occupational Safety and Health Administration, *Ergonomics Program Management Guidelines for Meatpacking Plants,* OSHA 3123, 1991.
10. Wilson JR: Framework for ergonomics methodology, In Wilson JR, Corlett EN, editors *Evaluation of Human Work: practical ergonomics methodology,* London, 1990, Taylor & Francis.

CHAPTER

7

Job Analysis

Jane O'Callaghan
Sharon Switzer–McIntyre

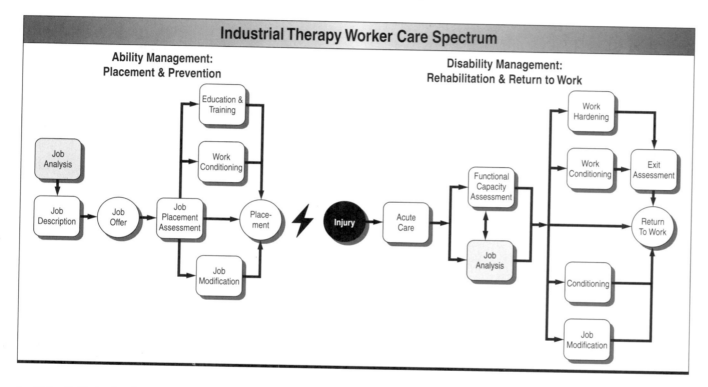

"*Manifold is the harvest of diseases reaped by certain workers from the crafts and trades that they pursue. All the profit that they get is injury to their health, that stems mostly, I think from two causes. The first and most potent is the harmful character of the materials that they handle, noxious vapors and very fine particles, inimical to human beings, inducing specific diseases. As a second cause I assign certain violent and irregular motions and unnatural postures of the body, by reason of which the natural structure of the living machine is so impaired that serious diseases gradually develop . . .*"

Bernardino Ramazinni,
De Morbis Artificum
About Diseases of Workers, 1700[15]

The need to analyze job demands was first recognized in the early eighteenth century in Europe. The first

cause of injury identified by Ramazinni (noxious vapors and very fine particles) has fallen into the realm of the contemporary industrial hygienist.

The second cause (violent and irregular motions and unnatural postures) constitutes an area in which Industrial Therapists often function. Carpal tunnel syndrome (Figure 7.1, page 86), repetitive motion problems, cervical strains, low back pain, and degenerative disc disease are all examples of problems referred to by Ramazinni and treated by Industrial Therapists, today, in clinical practice.[15] It is not enough to treat these problems in the clinic. They must also be treated on the job site as there may be a mismatch between the worker's capabilities and the workplace demands.

During the 1990s, the United States and Canada passed legislation that increased the rights of workers to demand safe working conditions, established the rights of injured workers to return to work and ensured

85

FIGURE 7.1   Carpal tunnel syndrome, the epidemic of the high-tech '90s.

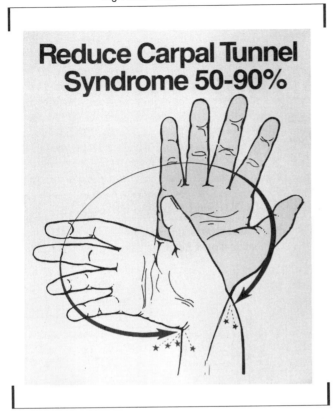

FIGURE 7.2   Teaching workers safer work styles is one of the most valuable Industrial Therapy measures.

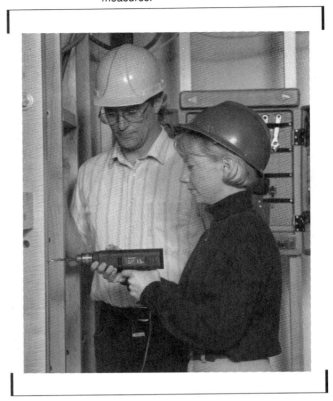

equitable employment for the disabled. These laws have made job analyses a legal requirement for employers as part of their efforts to provide safe working conditions, to return injured workers to the job and to accommodate people with disabilities (Figure 7.2).[1,4,8]

Industrial Therapists, using their acquired skills and expertise in the understanding of disabilities, injuries, and physical demands analysis are in an ideal position to assist organizations in conducting Job Analyses. The results of a Job Analysis are useful in many aspects of the Worker Care Spectrum—for matching workers' functional capacities with the job; for making hiring and job placement decisions; for identifying and correcting risk exposure; for determining Work Conditioning or Work Hardening goals; and for designing a modified job to ensure a safer return to work. It is therefore suggested that the Therapist develop an approach for concise analysis of job demands.

Since the 1700s, systems have been developed to meet a variety of objectives with respect to re-organizing a workplace to improve safety and for predicting the physical requirements of any job. Job analysis in the past has been subjective, estimation oriented and not always performance related. Recently this has changed due to the recognition of value in Functional Assess-

ments, and in response to changing legislation in the United States (Americans with Disabilities Act, 1992) and Canada.

Numerous lists, tables, charts, and scales which differentiate the various demands to be considered have been developed. This chapter describes one comprehensive approach to understanding and analyzing the demands of a job.

THE ANALYSIS CONTINUUM

Job Analysis (JA) is often the first step or the foundation for most aspects of Industrial Therapy, whether it is for a new hire or rehabilitation purposes. The term Job Analysis refers to the total analysis continuum of which Job Demands Analysis (JDA), Task Analysis (TA) and Ergonomic Evaluation (EE) are subsets.

Depending on the complexity of the job to be analyzed and the purpose for the assessment, there may be one or several types of analyses completed (Figure 7.3). In all cases it is beneficial to review the job description, whether written or verbal, to gain an understanding of the purpose of the job and how it fits into the organization. The goal of the analysis must be

FIGURE 7.3 The Analysis Continuum.

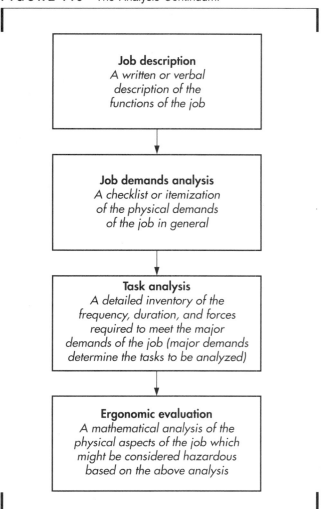

Job description
A written or verbal description of the functions of the job

↓

Job demands analysis
A checklist or itemization of the physical demands of the job in general

↓

Task analysis
A detailed inventory of the frequency, duration, and forces required to meet the major demands of the job (major demands determine the tasks to be analyzed)

↓

Ergonomic evaluation
A mathematical analysis of the physical aspects of the job which might be considered hazardous based on the above analysis

(Reprinted with permission from TOC Inc., 1993.)

FIGURE 7.4 The scope and budget of a Job Analysis is determined through discussion with the employer.

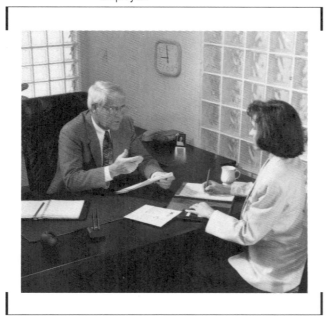

to have an inventory of the global demands of a job for Job Demands Analysis to be adequate. If there is concern regarding specific tasks within a job, then a Task Analysis will also be required. When there are identifiable risks that need to be investigated and can be measured mathematically then an Ergonomic Evaluation is conducted.

Appendix I, at the end of the chapter, outlines a comprehensive Job Analysis process. It includes an example form to fill out, a step-by-step methodology to follow, and a brief description of what is covered in each step. Not all situations will call for or cost-justify the fully-comprehensive process. Job analysis can be as comprehensive or as abbreviated as the company's needs and budget require. The Therapist must tailor the analysis to meet the needs of the situation. The scope and budget for the Job Analysis should first be discussed with the employer, payer, or both (Figure 7.4).

DEFINITIONS

Job Demands Analysis

A Job Demands Analysis (JDA) is an objective and systematic procedure to identify the demands of a particular job.[2,15] The demands of a job can include; basic physical demands (lifting, carrying, pushing, and pulling), mobility requirements (walking and climbing), sensory and perceptual demands (hearing and vision), vocational requirements and environmental conditions (exposure to heat, cold, and vibrations). Each demand is considered separately and in combination with other job components.

The word *objective* is key to this definition. A Job Demands Analysis is incomplete if it is based solely on subjective input. Although one cannot discount the importance of the subjective information, a comprehensive JDA should validate the subjective findings with objective data that is reliable and reproducible. Thus, it is imperative to collect data for a JDA from several sources.

Task Analysis

During the JDA, individual tasks that are essential, frequent, or potentially high risk are identified. Subsequently, a Task Analysis (TA) is conducted. The TA measures in more detail the frequency, duration, and forces generated.

When a JDA identifies that lifting of "X" pounds "X" number of times is potentially a high risk, a TA would be performed. In a TA you would measure the height lifted, the distance carried, the weight and frequency (Figures 7.5 and 7.6).

Thus, a TA provides a detailed picture of the demands placed on the worker by a particular task.

Ergonomic Evaluation

Tool and job redesign issues may be identified while performing the Job Demands Analysis and Task Analysis. These components may require Ergonomic Evaluation.

Ergonomic Evaluation is a mathematical analysis of any aspect of a job that is identified during the JDA, as "hazardous" or of "risk" to the worker.

Job Demands Analysis, Task Analysis and Ergonomic Evaluation are all areas of the study of work activities and do not include workers. The evaluation of worker capability is defined as a Functional Capacity Assessment. This measures an individual's capacity to sustain performance in conformance with the defined job demands analysis (see Chapter 13).

FIGURE 7.5 A hand held data recording device facilitates accurate record keeping during the Job Analysis.

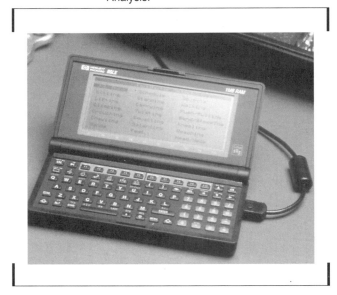

FIGURE 7.6 **A,** Reach; **B,** Lift; **C,** Turn; **D,** Carry. Job analysis involves breaking job tasks into components.

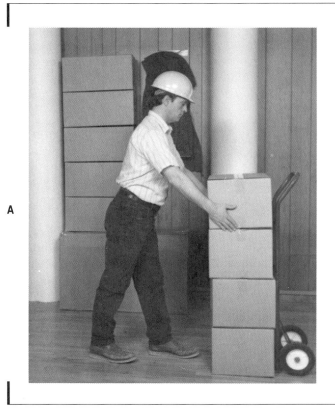

A

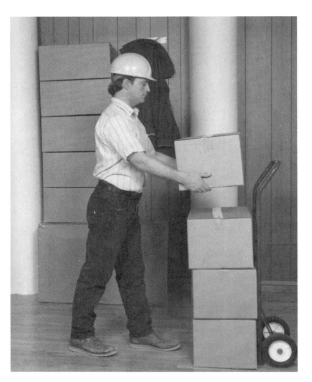

B

FIGURE 7.6, *cont'd*

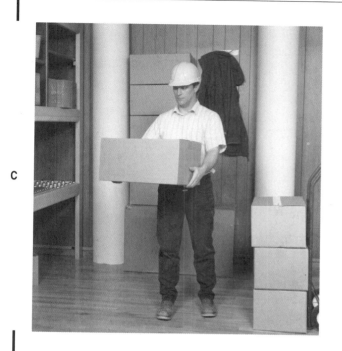

C

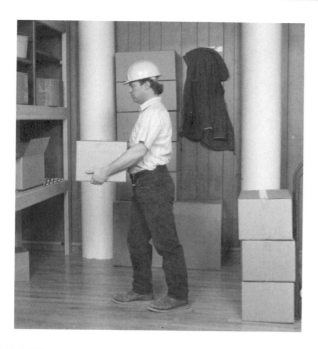

D

PURPOSES AND APPLICATIONS

Job Analyses are valuable to the worker, management, and the Therapist in many ways. The following section describes some of the ways a Job Analysis can be beneficial in Industrial Therapy.

Worker and Job Match

A Job Analysis can be useful during the hiring process, providing detailed information regarding the job to a prospective employee. In order to ensure nondiscrimination when conducting pre-placement medicals, the specific demands of a job can be compared objectively and systematically to a diagnosed medical condition ensuring appropriate placement. Furthermore, the job demands can be used to quantify strength, endurance, range-of-motion, and other physical factors required by a job. These measures can aid in the development of tests that are appropriate for evaluating applicants (Figure 7.7, page 90).

Assume that a visually impaired, diabetic person applies for a receptionist position. Organization ABC has done a job analysis and the applicant has the education, work experience, and expertise to do the job but is unsure whether the applicant can meet its physical demands. A Functional Capacity Assessment is implemented. Recommendations suggest that accommodations including a braille computer, high lighting, and a work station redesigned to facilitate a specific weakness on the right side, the applicant could do the job; that is, the applicant would "match the job."

There are other applications of the Job Analysis that ensure the worker and the job are appropriately matched. (Figure 7.8, page 90) These are:

- Rehabilitation requirements
- Job modification
- Reasonable accommodation
- Training and injury prevention programs
- Job and tool design and redesign

Rehabilitation Requirements

A basic understanding of the job and its demands assist the treatment team in setting specific and realistic rehabilitation goals with the worker. A JDA provides the baseline for comparison of the worker's current level to the demands of the job. This subsequently facilitates objective decision-making as to whether or not the worker is rehabilitatable to that particular job. Additionally, the Job Analysis can be used to set the attainable performance level prior to a worker returning to their job.

FIGURE 7.7 Worker/job match.

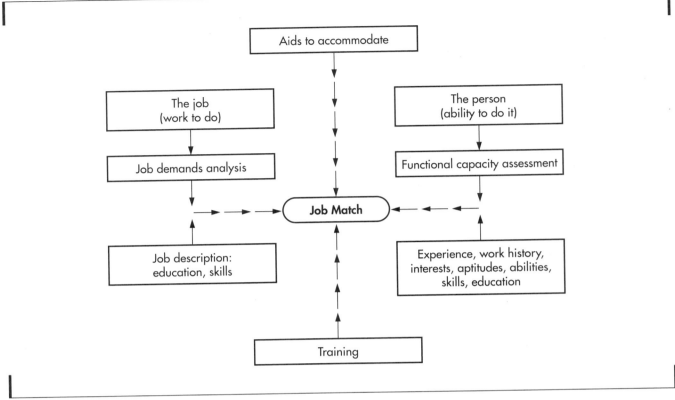

FIGURE 7.8 The job is matched to the worker through Job Analysis and Job Placement Assessment. **A,** Job Analysis; **B,** Job Placement Assessment; **C,** Job is modified to match the worker.

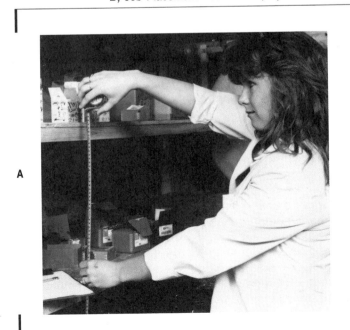

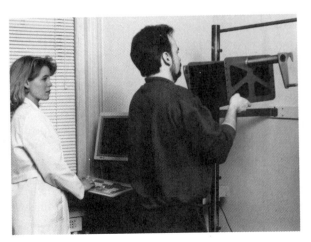

FIGURE 7.8, *cont'd*

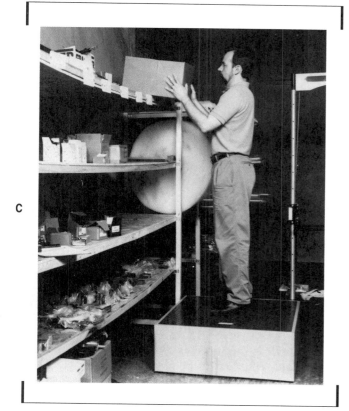

C

Job Modification

Through the job analysis process, specific aspects of a job that exceed the individual's work capacity, or present potential hazards can be identified. This baseline of information permits the Industrial Therapist and other members of the team to reduce risks by modifying the hazardous aspects of the critical tasks. Through job modification the worker can gradually, yet progressively, return to work in their fullest capacity. Clear guidelines should be developed to ensure that the worker returns to full capacity in a reasonable amount of time.

Reasonable Accommodation

In order to accommodate an individual, the specific mismatches between the job demands and the abilities of the individual need to be identified. According to the Americans with Disabilities Act (ADA) in the United States, the Workers' Compensation Board (WCB), and Human Rights Legislation in Canada, employers must provide reasonable accommodation for disabled employees unless such accommodation causes the employer "undue hardship" (ADA, 1992; WCB Act, 1990).[1,19]

Reasonable accommodation entails making facilities and jobs accessible to, and performable by disabled employees. Job restructuring, scheduling, workplace modifications, and other adjustments are required to accommodate the disabled individual. Employers and employees are advised to familiarize themselves with the appropriate legislation.

Training and Injury Prevention Programs

In order to ensure that workers receive adequate training for a job, it is essential to know the demands of the various tasks involved. Once the requirements of a job are quantified, training programs can be designed and implemented to inculcate the required abilities.

Injury prevention programs that do not consider the specific demands of a given job may not assist in reducing the injury rate. Back schools that do not focus on the specific lifting parameters of the target audience may not show statistically significant results, in reducing the incidence of back injuries.

It is apparent that in order to develop effective injury prevention programs within a given setting, one must have a clear understanding of the demands of the jobs on the workforce. This applies for all injury prevention and wellness programs ranging from back education programs and cumulative trauma workshops to nutrition and smoking cessation programs.

Job and Tool Design and Redesign

To effectively redesign jobs and tools a JA may be performed on the new job and equipment. New production lines without thorough analysis may lead to costly worker problems and additional equipment changes.

As an example, one client of the authors' practice had two employees on the production line who complained of upper extremity pain and fatigue. New chairs and air guns were supplied for these employees. Two months later the same employees had complaints of wrist and back pain. When the situation was reanalyzed, it was determined that the entire production line required redesign, and the initial fix represented unnecessary expense.

BENEFITS OF A COMPREHENSIVE JOB DEMANDS ANALYSIS

Once the Job Analysis has been performed the reports are available to match the worker to the workplace. With a better match, the potential benefits can include

FIGURE 7.9 The transition from a range-of-motion goal to a job performance capability goal. **A,** Teaching lifting out of job context; **B,** Teaching lifting in job context.

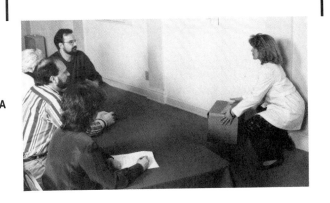

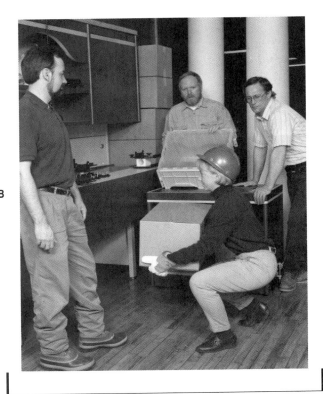

ing the work environment, and improved cooperation between management, the union, and labor.[17]

Job Analysis can improve communication with outside medical practitioners. Rehabilitation goals can be targeted through recognizing the demands of the job (Figure 7.9). This will ensure that the worker's return to work is safe and timely, eliminating the consequences of prolonged periods of absence.

THE PROCESS

The Job Analysis process involves a review of the job description, collection of all necessary equipment and documents, observation of the job, completion of the Job Demands Analysis form, discussion with the major stakeholders, specific tasks analysis, and written reports (Figure 7.10). Stakeholders include all the people who have a vested interest in making the process successful.

Following is a step by step guide of how to perform a Job Demands Analysis and a Task Analysis.

Step 1: Review the Job Description.   Review the job description, whether it be written or verbal. This provides an overall view of the job and how it fits into the organization.

Written documents such as job descriptions, Workers' Compensation Board claims, health benefit utilization records, and injury prevention procedures provide an insight into injury types and rates within an organization.

Step 2: Collect The Necessary Equipment.   Collect all the necessary equipment and forms (Figure 7.11). Box 7.1 lists the tools and equipment that you may find useful.

Step 3: The Job Demands Analysis—Observe, Measure, and Document the Job.   On-site observation is imperative when conducting a JA. The observer must witness the performance of all tasks associated with a given job, any variances that may occur from one work station to another, and any changes that may be due to environmental conditions. Cycle periods of the task will be determined by the time required to observe a particular job. Often between one and eight hours is sufficient.

Some jobs will however have components that are performed infrequently, obliging the observer to return to the job site a number of times. Observation includes the objective measurement of forces generated, distances traveled or reached, frequencies of occurrence, postures assumed and durations of various activities. These measurements are clearly outlined in Appendix I.

an improvement in productivity and morale. Equally important is the potential for a general improvement in the well-being of the workers, through a reduction of work related physical and psychosocial discomfort, overall improvement in the workers' health and thus a reduction in the incidence of occupational related disabilities.[6,8,14,17]

Hallmarks of a satisfied and motivated workforce may include a reduction in absenteeism rates and labor turnover, a reduction of personnel complaints regard-

BOX 7.1

Tools and Equipment

Special clothing:	To comply with organizational requirements for clothing and footwear.
Paperwork:	To record all the data. Clip board, pen/pencil, and appropriate documents (Job Demands Analysis form, graph paper, and writing paper)
Tape measure:	To determine reach distances, heights, and widths.
Force gauge:	To measure weights as well as push/pull forces.
Torque wrench:	To determine pull or turning forces on rotating parts such as steering wheels, bolts, and screws.
Pedometer:	To measure longer distances which are normally associated with pushing, walking, and carrying tasks.
Level:	To measure slopes particularly of walking and working surfaces.
Goniometer:	To measure joint angles of workers and working angles of equipment.
Stopwatch:	To measure precise intervals of time for calculation of task duration and of cycle frequency.
Grip dynamometer:	To measure the force required to close a hand around an object and squeeze firmly—gripping tools, squeezing wire cutters, etc.
Event counter:	To accurately count the number of repetitions of a specific event or cycle within a specified time period.
Camera or video camera:	To visually record and document critical information that can be reviewed again at a later date. Check the organization's confidentiality agreements and camera restrictions.

FIGURE 7.10   The process model.

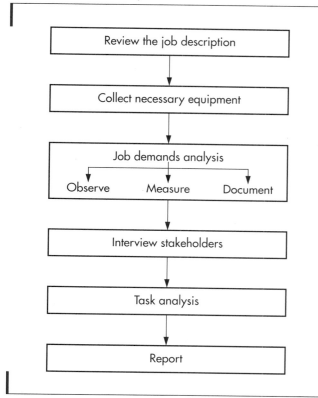

Review the job description

↓

Collect necessary equipment

↓

Job demands analysis

Observe   Measure   Document

↓

Interview stakeholders

↓

Task analysis

↓

Report

(Reprinted with permission from TOC Inc., 1993)

FIGURE 7.11   Equipment for a Job Analysis.

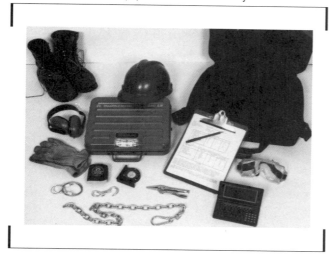

The Job Demands Analysis Form includes a brief written job description and comments related to all aspects of the job. The essential tasks of the job should be highlighted to indicate where specific task analyses might be required. An essential task is a fundamental physical demand that the worker must be able to perform unassisted. Questions which can assist the Therapist to identify essential tasks may include the following:

- Does the position exist in order to perform the task?
- Does performing the task make use of more than 50% of the worker's total daily work hours?
- Does the task require the worker to have specific expertise?[10]

While assessing the job, keep in mind that the picture being drawn is a very general one, yet it is the precursor to focusing on specific tasks and potential hazards of the job.

Step 4: Interview Stakeholders.   Subjective information regarding the job to be analyzed can be obtained by conducting interviews with the major stakeholders (those who see that their self-interest is involved in the situation). These stakeholders are individuals who may have valuable contributions to make and could be representatives from; upper management, middle management, line management, the work force, occupational health and safety, and the union.

Interviews are conducted only on completion of the Job Demands Analysis in order to maintain objectivity and to reduce the chances of being biased by the general attitude of the organization. The observer must bear in mind that each location will have its own managerial and political hierarchy that must be considered.

The Job Demands Analysis Form should be reviewed with the major stakeholders to ensure that they are in agreement with the findings, and that all components of the job have been observed in the correct context (Figure 7.12).

FIGURE 7.12   Subjective information from stakeholders complements the objective Job Analysis data.

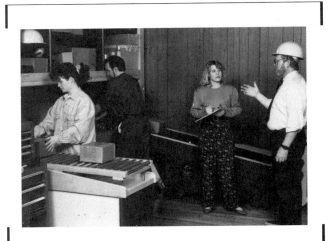

Step 5: Perform Task Analysis. If it is deemed appropriate to proceed beyond the global picture provided, perform a task analysis. Independently assess the tasks, using the guidelines provided in Appendix I for each task. If there are areas that require assessment beyond the expertise of an Industrial Therapist, recommend the appropriate consultant. If a job contains ergonomic hazards which may require equipment redesign, recommend an ergonomist.

Step 6: Report and Recommendations.   Once the job has been observed, measured, analyzed, and documented, the information is gathered into a report. The format of the report should be negotiated with your client prior to beginning the JA process. It is important that the client's receive information in a clear format. Reporting formats may differ depending on the reason for the JA. Recommendations for ergonomic evaluation, work station redesign, training, accommodation, and job modifications may also be included in this report.

A three-tiered approach to the report is recommended. First include your actual Job Analysis forms. The completed Task Analysis forms, along with the Job Demands Analysis form, should be filed together, making all the information regarding a given job accessible to all stakeholders. Second, if required write a narrative description of the findings with a summary statement. Third, if you have been invited to make recommendations as a result of your JA, the following section is offered as a guideline.

Review the report and recommendations with the major stakeholders to ensure all team members understand the findings. This review could take the form of a meeting where the Therapist presents the findings and recommendations. As a result of this meeting, a set of actions may be developed if follow-up is required.

Signatures of the major stakeholders also ensures that the report has been reviewed and accepted (Figure 7.13).

MAKING THE RECOMMENDATIONS

The Job Analysis process may result in a recommendation to modify the job to match the worker's capabilities, or to provide a transitional job that the worker can perform safely while completing rehabilitation to the original job. The following explains the kinds of recommendations that might be made in these two major categories.

Job Modifications

Recommendations for accommodations or job modifications can be classified into five general types:

FIGURE 7.13 Signatures of major stakeholders ensures that the report has been read and accepted.

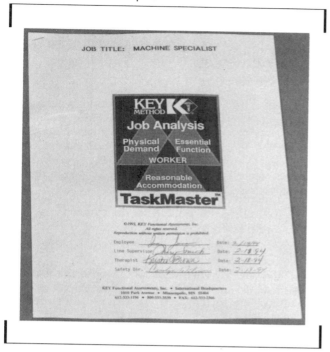

FIGURE 7.14 Modifications in the workplace can fit the job to the person.

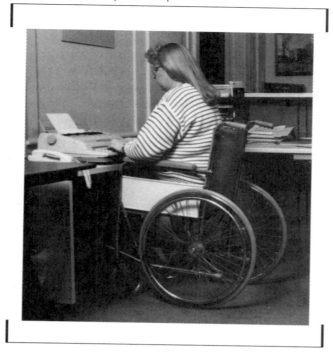

1. Physical Accommodations. This list is endless and would be different for each particular work setting. It encompasses not only the actual work station, but may also include products that are unique to the individual (Figure 7.14).

- Height of a desk to accommodate a wheelchair
- Adjustable desk height to accommodate a sit/stand requirement
- Ergonomically designed chairs allowing for adjustable back support
- Changing the distance workers must reach to access equipment or tools
- Providing a motorized scooter for those employees who cannot walk long distances
- Arm or wrist support for repetitive tasks
- Rearranging office furniture
- Materials handled can be bundled in smaller weights or more manageable box sizes

2. Environmental Adaptations. Attention to the impact the work environment may have on an employee:

- Temperatures that are either too warm or too cold can be adjusted mechanically or with the use of room dividers
- Loud noises can be diminished with head sets or acoustical room area enclosures

3. Work Site Modifications. Site accommodations will not only accommodate the worker's need, but can be beneficial to the entire business:

- Ramps and easily opened doors are necessary for wheelchairs but also benefit older workers, delivery, and sales people
- Elevators labeled for people with and without vision
- Restrooms with grab bars, large enough for wheelchairs
- Flooring—highly polished floors are hazardous to people on crutches, and too rich a carpet pile is difficult for wheelchairs

4. Job Restructuring. Job restructuring may lead to a redesign of a production line or the entire operation of a unit.

- Unnecessary task procedures can be identified
- Reassigning tasks to make the greatest use of individual's skills results in accommodation as well as increased efficiency

5. Work Activities Modification. Work activity modifications are changes to the general work requirements.

- Altering arrival and departure times to assist with transportation needs

• Dividing rest and lunch breaks into more frequent, shorter rest periods

RETURN-TO-WORK TRANSITION

In some cases, a worker can be returned to the job assignment at the end of rehabilitation without the need for any interim lower demand work. In others, there is need to provide meaningful productive activity while the worker is acquiring the strength and capability to assume the ultimate job assignment. This ultimate job may be the exact job they had prior to injury, or a modified version of it.

Transitional Modified Job

In building up to this job, the worker may be given a *transitional modified job*, defined as any job, task, or function that a worker who temporarily suffers from a diminished capacity may perform safely without risk of reinjury, exacerbation of disability, or risk to others. The work must be productive and have value to the worker and the organization.

The goal of transitional modified work is to maximize the work contribution and rehabilitative progression of the employee. A transitional modified job is determined in the same way a long term modified job is designed. The first steps are typically a Job Demands Analysis and a Functional Capacity Assessment of the worker.

The Transition Process

Transition to the job assignment is the same whether the worker is going to a permanent or temporary transitional job.

In rehabilitation, a Job Analysis system that can compare the physical demands of the job with the physical capacities of the worker is preferred over one that does not lend itself to both tasks.[6,7,13] Therefore, in communications with the physician, occupational health nurse, or benefits representative the same form can be used to report the Functional Capacity and the Job Demands Analysis. The form may require slight modifications.

The return-to-work transition process includes:

1. Prepare the job and task demands analysis.
2. Determine the worker's functional capacity.
3. Determine the tasks which may be within the worker's capabilities. Compare the job demands analysis with the worker's functional capabilities to determine if their major limitations are related to strength, mobility, work environment, or work conditions. Then identify a task that does not require demands in areas of limitations. For example, if strength is

the injured worker's major functional limitation, then modify the job by altering or eliminating strength demands.
4. If the worker is being assigned a transitional job, the Therapist typically offers modified work in the form of a progression by hours and by tasks. For example:

Week # 1   2–4 hours   most appropriate tasks

Week # 2   4–6 hours
Week # 3   6–8 hours
          Tuesday, Thursday
Week # 4   6–8 hours   progress tasks

5. Identify how the tasks of the job which the employee is unable to do currently, will be addressed (provide an assistant).
6. Prepare a new Job Demands Analysis to describe the work assignment.
7. If it is a transitional job, discuss the modified work and the progressed or stepped hours with the worker.
8. Advise the worker that a copy of the Task Analysis will be sent to their physician and, if on Workers' Compensation or Long Term Disability (LTD), a copy to the benefit carrier.
9. Prepare a cover letter to the physician explaining the organization's work program and the commitment to rehabilitation. If the program involves transitional work, clearly outline the progressed/stepped approach and the demands of the transitional "modified" work that has been offered.
10. Copy the demands analysis and cover letter and send to the insurance carrier involved.
11. Keep all pertinent information in a disability management file for each person.

SUMMARY

The Job Analysis approach eliminates much of the guesswork involved in dealing with an injured or ill employee. Guesswork is costly; it costs the employees days or weeks of idle time when they could be back at work, it creates pain and delay of recovery if they are sent back to certain tasks too soon, and it results in lost time to the employer, decreased efficiency, and increased disability insurance costs.[15]

By using the information provided in the Job Analysis any employee, physician, Industrial Therapist, counselor, placement officer, or employer who is called upon to make a decision regarding "fitness for work" will know specifically what that work involves. A decision based on concrete facts will be a much better decision than one based on guesswork.

REFERENCES

1. Barlow WE, Hane EZ: A Practical Guide to the Americans with Disabilities Act, *Personnel Journal,* June 1992.
2. Eastman Kodak Company: *Ergonomic Design for People at Work,* vol 1, New York, 1983, VanNorstrand Reinhold.
3. Eastman Kodak Company: *Ergonomic Design for People at Work,* vol 2, New York, 1986, VanNorstrand Reinhold.
4. Ilmarinen J, Suurnakki T, Nygard C, Landau K: Classification of municipal occupations, *Scand J Work Environ Health* 17(suppl):12, 1991.
5. Isernhagen SJ: *Work Injury: management and prevention,* Rockville, Md, 1988, Aspen Publishers.
6. Isernhagen SJ: Functional Job Descriptions, *Semin Occupat Med* 2(1): 51,1987.
7. Jacobs K, editor: Industrial Rehabilitation, *WORK* 1(1),1990.
8. Judy B: Job Accommodations and JAN, *Employment Relations Today,* 121–125, Summer, 1988.
9. KEY Functional Assessments Inc., Job Analysis Training Program, vol 2, Minneapolis, 1992.
10. Kittusamy NK, Okogbaa OG, Babu AJ: A Preliminary Audit For Ergonomics Design In Manufacturing Environments, *Industrial Engineering* 47–53, July 1992.
11. Leamon TB: Ergonomics: a technical approach to human productivity, *National Productivity Review* 331–339, Autumn 1987.
12. Milas GH: IE'S Role In Implementing The Americans With Disabilities Act, *Industrial Engineering* 36–39, Jan 1984.
13. Pheasant S: *Ergonomics: work and health,* Gaithersburg, Md, 1991, Aspen Publishers.
14. Schulenberger, CC: Ergonomics In The Workplace: evaluating and modifying jobs, *Occup Medicine,* 7(1):105,1992.
15. TOC Consulting, O'Callaghan J, Switzer-McIntyre S, Toronto, Ontario, Canada.
16. Wilson JR, Corlett EN editors: *Evaluation of Human Work: A Practical Ergonomics Methodology,* London 1990, Taylor & Francis Ltd,.
17. Woolsey C: Job descriptions in Writing: Required? No. Useful? Yes, *Business Insurance,* 10, July 1992.
18. Workers' Compensation Board Act, Bill 162: Revised Status of Ontario, 1990, Printed by the Queen's Printer for Ontario, April 1990.

APPENDIX I

Job Analysis Process

This Appendix outlines a comprehensive Job Analysis process including an example form to fill out, a step-by-step methodology to follow, and a brief description of what is covered in each step.

The Job Demands Analysis Form (Figure 7.15) includes the complete breadth of factors that might be measured or assessed. In cases, such as lifting, carrying, and pushing, the measurement techniques are easy to understand and quantifiable. In others, such as dust, vapor fumes, or radiant energy, the measurement techniques are more difficult to perform and quantify. Often, the Therapist learns onthe-job, how to make the difficult measurements and assessments as a result of performing many Job Analyses.

As mentioned earlier in the chapter, not all situations will call for, or cost-justify, the fully-comprehensive process. Job Analysis can be as comprehensive or as abbreviated as the company's needs and budget require. The Therapist must tailor the analysis to meet the needs of the situation. The scope and budget for the Job Analysis should be discussed up front with the employer, payer, or both.

COMPLETING THE PHYSICAL DEMANDS ANALYSIS FORM

Instructions for each section of the Physical Demands Analysis form are clearly outlined in the following section.

Job Title

Indicate the actual title of the job to be assessed.

Job Description

Include a brief description of the job as outlined by the organization as well as the DOT (Dictionary of Occupational Titles) or the CCDO (Canadian Classification of Dictionary of Occupations).

Physical Demand Level

The United States Department of Labor's Handbook for Analyzing Jobs (1972) provides an excellent framework for identifying the global physical demand characteristics of a job.

The physical demand characteristic is an overall assessment of the major tasks of the job. These physical demand characteristics can be used in the job description to highlight the global physical demand profile of the job. The physical demand characteristics are divided into five degrees of strength. These five degrees of strength are defined as:

1. **Sedentary.** Lifting 10 lbs maximum and occasionally lifting and/or carrying such articles as books and small tools. Although a sedentary job is defined as one which involves sitting, a certain amount of walking and standing is often necessary in carrying out job duties. Jobs are sedentary if walking and standing are required only occasionally and all other sedentary criteria are met.
2. **Light.** Lifting 20 lbs maximum with frequent lifting and/or carrying objects weighing up to 10 lbs Even though the weight lifted may be only a negligible amount, a job will be in this category when it requires walking or standing to a significant degree, or when it requires sitting most of the time, but entails pushing and pulling of arm and/or leg controls.
3. **Medium.** Lifting 50 lbs maximum with frequent lifting and/or carrying of objects weighing up to 25 lbs.
4. **Heavy.** Lifting 100 lbs maximum with frequent lifting and/or carrying of objects weighing up to 50 lbs.
5. **Very Heavy.** Lifting objects in excess of 100 lbs with frequent lifting and/or carrying of objects weighing 50 lbs or more.

Specific Vocational Preparation (SVP)

The level of vocational preparation required for a job provides insight into the complexity and training needs of a given job (Box 7.2, page 102).

FIGURE 7.15 Job demands analysis form.

Job Demands Analysis Form

Job title					
Description					
Physical demand level:					
Vocational Preparation	Unskilled	Semi-skilled		Skilled	
Physical demand	Not at all	Occasionally (less than 1 hr)	Frequently (1 - 3 hrs)	Major demand (more than 3 hrs)	Comments
Strength Lifting					Max wt / Usual wt
Carrying					Max wt / Usual wt
Pushing					Max wt / Usual wt
Pulling					Max wt / Usual wt
Fine finger work					Max wt / Usual wt
Handling					Max wt / Usual wt
Gripping					Max wt / Usual wt
Reach above shldr below shldr					Max wt / Usual wt
Mobility Neck motion					

continued

FIGURE 7.15, *cont'd*

Throwing					
Sitting					
Standing					
Walking					
Running/jumping					
Climbing					
Bending/stoop					
Kneeling					
Crawling					
Twisting					
Balancing					
Sensory/perceptual Hearing					

Vision: far
     near
     color
     depth					

Perception					
Feeling					
Reading					
Writing					
Speech					
Work environment Inside work					
Outside work					
Hot/cold					

FIGURE 7.15, *cont'd*

Humid					
Dust					
Vapor fumes					
Noise					
Proximity to moving objects					
Hazardous machinery					
Sharp tools					
Radiant energy					
Thermal energy					
Slippery					
Congested worksite					
Chemicals					
Vibration					
Jarring					
Conditions of work Traveling					
Work alone					
Interact with people					
Operate machinery					
Irregular hours					

There are generic forms similar to the one presented here. Practitioners tend to adapt forms to their needs.

BOX 7.2

Level	Training time
1	Short demonstration only.
2	Anything beyond short demonstration up to and including 30 days.
3	Over 30 days up to and including 3 mo.
4	Over 3 mo. up to and including 6 mo.
5	Over 6 mo. up to and including 1 yr.
6	Over 1 yr. up to and including 2 yrs.
7	Over 2 yrs. up to and including 4 yrs.
8	Over 4 yrs. up to and including 10 yrs.
9	Over 10 yrs.

SVP skill level:

Unskilled	SVP = 1 & 2
Semi-skilled	SVP = 3 − 6
Skilled	SVP = 7 − 9

BOX 7.3

Frequency of Activity Scale:

1	Not at all:	Never
2	Occasionally:	Less than 1 hour
3	Frequently:	Frequent repetition— for 1 to 3 hours daily
4	Major demand:	Maximum ability required— frequent repetition for more than 3 hours daily
5	Comments:	May include examples of activities, unusual activity periods, outstanding demands, or other considerations.

Frequency Designations

Referring to the "Frequency of Activity Scale" provided in Box 7.3, an "X" is placed in the column indicating the frequency with which the factor is required. Frequency indicates the actual time spent incorporating that factor, and not the entire time span over which the factor may be periodically incorporated (In order for "lifting 50 lbs weights" to be considered "#3 − Frequently" there must be frequent, repetitive lifting of a 50 lb weight for 1 to 3 hours daily and NOT just 2 or 3 episodes of lifting over a 1 to 3 hour period).

On the other hand, a factor may be rated as "4 − Major demand", if it is required to fulfill a major function for which the job position was created to address (if delivering mail for one hour a day is one of the major functions for which the position of "Office Clerk" was created, then walking and climbing stairs may be rated as "4 − Major demand").

The "Major demands" will guide you towards identifying the essential tasks of the job. Once the major demands or essential tasks have been identified and formalized, then task analyses can be performed. The task analysis focuses on the specific demands of each task identified as a "major demand."

Strength

Strength measures provide objective data on the forces generated in a given job or task. When indicating the weight, both maximum weights required to be moved in the job and the usual weights are recorded (50 lbs may be the maximum weight ever required to be moved, but the usual weight to be moved is 30 lbs).

FIGURE 7.16   Measuring lifting.

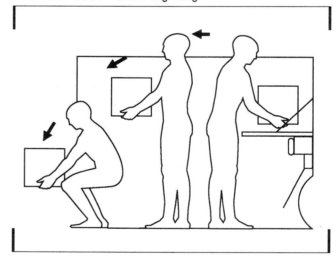

Lifting.   Raising objects from a lower to a higher position without the use of mechanical hoists. Also, lowering objects, as in lifting objects off a truck and lowering them to the ground in a controlled manner (Figure 7.16).

The following lifting rates are used to define frequencies for the United States Department of Labor as per the United States Department of Labor's Handbook for Analyzing Jobs (1972).

Seldom:	1 lift every hour
Occasionally:	1 lift every 30 minutes
Frequently:	1 lift every 2 minutes
Major demand:	1 lift every 15 seconds

For a JDA identify frequency and weight of lifts. For a TA add the height of the lift and distance moved.

FIGURE 7.17 Measuring carrying.

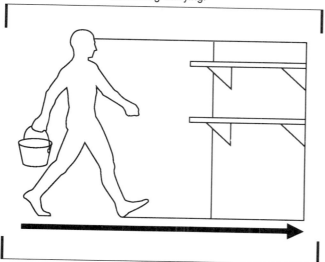

Carrying. Moving while supporting an object; transporting objects. Identify the frequency and weights for a JDA. If it is a TA, measure the distance the weights are carried (Figure 7.17).

FIGURE 7.19 Measuring pulling.

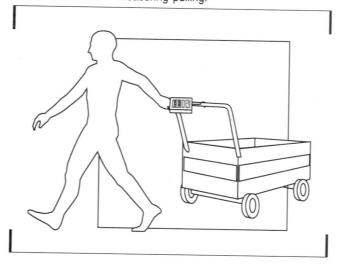

Pulling. Applying traction force, as with pulleys, heavy doors, dragging equipment, etc. For a JDA, measure frequency and weight pulled. For a TA, add distance traveled and forces generated (Figure 7.19).

FIGURE 7.18 Measuring pushing.

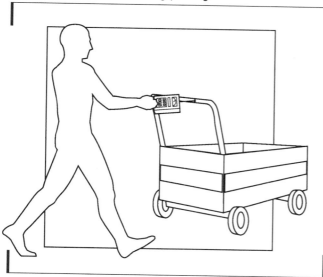

Pushing. Applying pressure force, as with carts, trolleys, shoveling, using a pneumatic drill, etc. For a JDA, measure the frequency and weights pushed. For a TA, add distance traveled and forces generated (Figure 7.18).

FIGURE 7.20 Measuring fine finger work.

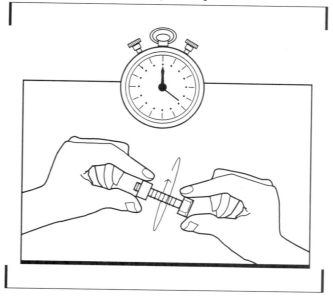

Fine Finger Work. Using speed and dexterity as in typing, dialing, manipulating fine nuts and bolts, planting seeds, etc. For a JDA, identify frequency and weights. For a TA, add actual repetitions and weight (Figure 7.20).

FIGURE 7.21 Measuring handling.

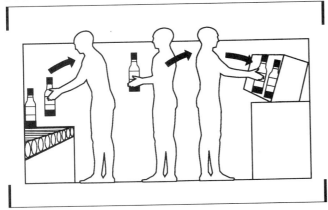

Handling. Using one or both hands to hold and pick up objects; to gather together (sorting papers, filing, managing tools). For a JDA, identify frequency and weight handled. For a TA, measure one versus a two hand activity, frequency of each and weights of objects (Figure 7.21).

FIGURE 7.22 Measuring gripping.

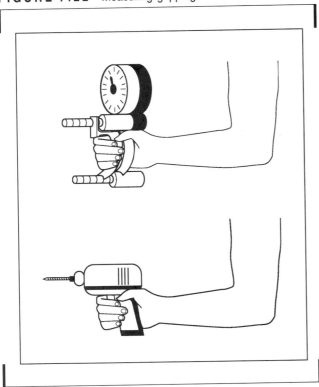

Gripping. Closing the hand around an object and squeezing firmly (gripping a hammer, squeezing a wire cutter or stapler, etc.). For a JDA, identify frequency. For the TA, measure frequency and forces generated (Figure 7.22).

FIGURE 7.23 Measuring reaching.

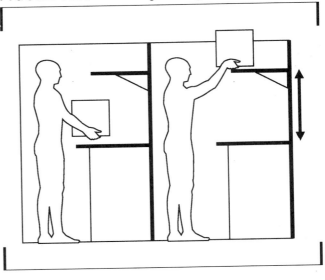

Reaching. Above shoulder level—stretching out the arm, either at or above the level of the shoulder joint.

Below shoulder level—stretching out the arm forward or laterally, below the level of the shoulder joint. For JDA, measure frequency and weight of the reach. For a TA, measure frequency, distance, and weight of the reach (Figure 7.23).

Mobility

Mobility measures provide information pertaining to the flexibility required to perform given jobs and tasks. For a JDA mobility is measured using the frequency scale. For a TA measure specific range of motion, duration, and distances for the appropriate components.

FIGURE 7.24 Measuring neck motion.

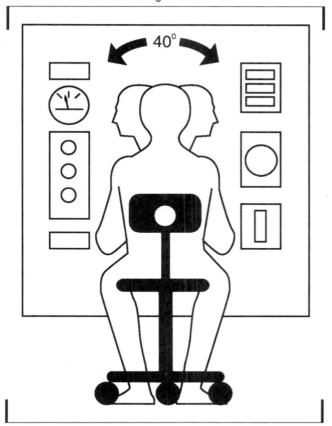

FIGURE 7.26 Measuring sitting.

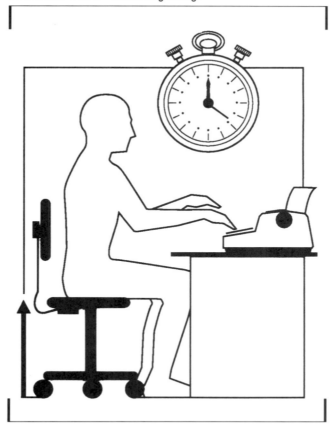

Neck Motion. Moving the neck through a significant range of motion, either in flexion and extension or rotation (Figure 7.24).

Sitting. Maintaining a seated posture on a chair, stool, vehicle seat, etc. (Figure 7.26).

FIGURE 7.25 Measuring throwing.

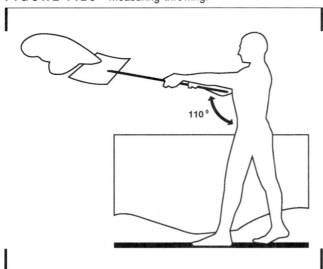

FIGURE 7.27 Measuring standing.

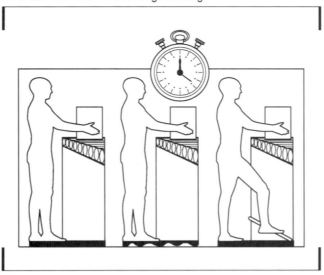

Throwing. Tossing snow with a shovel, pitching fertilizer bags into a truck, etc. (Figure 7.25).

Standing. Remaining in a stationary upright position (Figure 7.27).

FIGURE 7.28   Measuring walking.

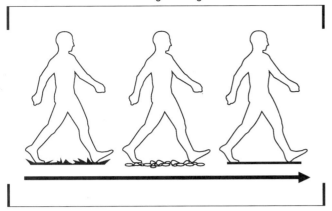

Walking.   Ambulating over a variety of flat surfaces, but does not include climbing (Figure 7.28).

FIGURE 7.30   Measuring running.

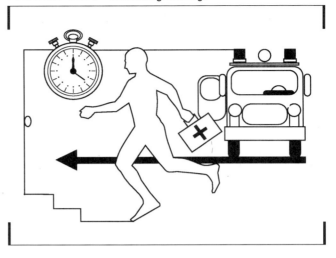

Running.   Ambulating rapidly; as when avoiding sudden danger (Figure 7.30).

FIGURE 7.31   Measuring climbing.

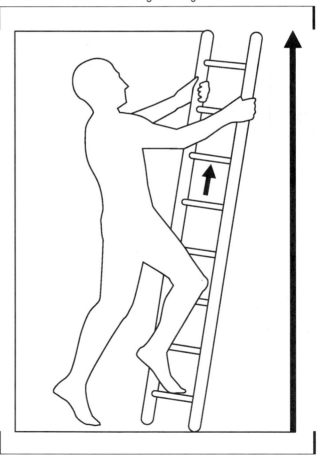

Climbing.   Ascending stairs, ladders, inclines, etc.; specify the type of climbing under "comments" (Figure 7.31).

FIGURE 7.29   Measuring jumping.

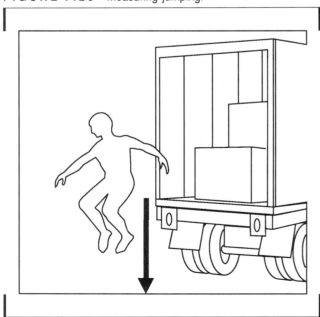

Jumping.   Jumping off truck beds, etc. (Figure 7.29).

FIGURE 7.32 Measuring bending.

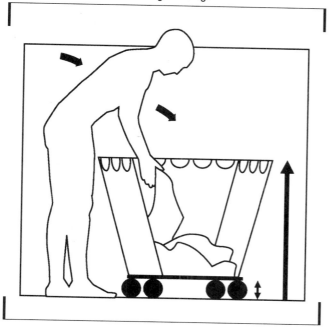

Bending/Stooping. Job requires flexion at the waist, it may be repetitive as in sweeping or continuous as when leaning over while standing and working at a low table; specify in comments section (Figure 7.32).

FIGURE 7.34 Measuring kneeling.

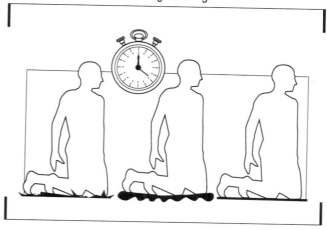

Kneeling. Touching one or both knees to the ground to support the body (Figure 7.34).

FIGURE 7.33 Measuring crawling.

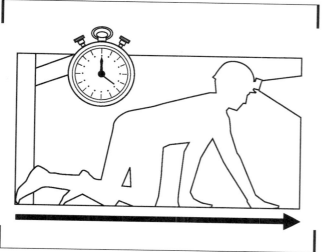

Crawling. Moving while on hands and knees (Figure 7.33).

FIGURE 7.35 Measuring twisting.

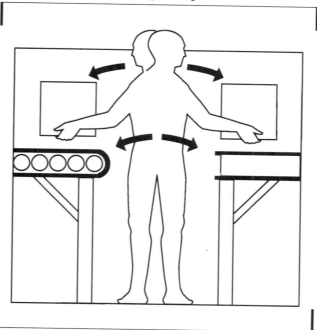

Twisting. Turning the upper body at the waist while lower body is stationary (Figure 7.35).

FIGURE 7.36 Measuring balancing.

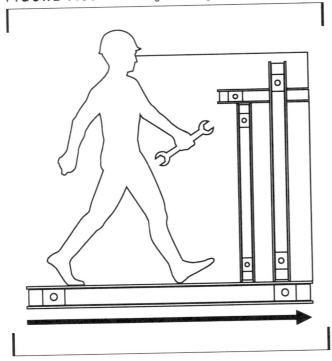

Balancing. Maintaining body balance while on a ladder, scaffold, etc. (Figure 7.36).

Sensory/Perceptual

The sensory/perceptual measures provide a picture of the sensory/perceptual demands of the job or task. These do not require specific measures at the JDA level, observation notes are sufficient. At the level of a TA, recommend the appropriate specialist.

Hearing. Conversation: face to face or on telephone. Other sounds—horns, buzzer, alarm bell, motor sounds, etc.

Vision. Far—Seeing objects in the distance (beyond arm's length).
Near—Seeing objects within arm's length.
Color—Noted only when objects cannot be differentiated by anything other than color (e.g. wires).
Depth—Seeing in three dimensions: necessary for judging distances, thicknesses, etc.

Perception. Ability to deal with spatial concepts such as "above, below, behind" and to accurately perceive the position of objects in relation to oneself and other objects. Necessary for performing directional tasks, using a pattern, lining up numbers, etc.

Form. Ability to discern subtle discrepancies or details in form and shape (e.g. shapes of drill bits, automotive parts, etc.).

Feeling. Only noted when touch is the primary means of differentiating between items or gaining information to dictate action (judging consistency of soil, and smoothness of surfaces).

Reading. Deciphering and comprehending written language.

Writing. Manual writing as opposed to typewriting.

Speaking. Speaking face-to-face or over a telephone or 2-way radio.

Work Environment

The work environment measures are solely to provide the Industrial Therapist with some insight into the environment. Subjective observation is adequate for this section. If observation indicates that the worker is subject to an unhealthy situation, recommend further analysis by the appropriate specialist.

Inside Work. Inside a building (shop, office, garage).

Outside Work. Includes outdoors but in a vehicle enclosure (i.e. truck cab).

Hot. Work in hot temperatures, either inside or outdoors.

Cold. Work in cold temperatures, either inside or outdoors.

Humid. Work in damp or excessively humid conditions (outdoors in rain, inside a tropical greenhouse, or in a wet underground excavation).

Dust. Exposure to significant airborne particles in the worker's environment.

Vapor Fumes. Irritating odors and chemicals, smoke, or exhaust fumes.

Noise. Exposure to noise above a normal office level.

Proximity to Moving Objects. Working in vicinity of moving objects, machinery, or vehicles (overhead cranes, forklifts).

Hazardous Machinery. Working with or near machinery with dangerous moving parts (chopper, snow blower, paper shredder, grinding wheels, saws).

Sharp Tools.   Exposure to sharp blades or cutting surfaces, other than scissors.

Radiant Energy.   Exposure to rays as from a photocopier, prolonged sun exposure, or X-ray equipment.

Thermal Energy.   Exposure to open flame or hot surfaces which could result in burns.

Slippery.   Refers to predictable work environment (icy, muddy, or oily surfaces) and not irregular occurrences such as water spills in an office environment.

Congested Worksite.   Allows little room for body movement because of limited area or cramped storage quarters.

Chemical Irritants.   Exposure to chemicals which could cause skin or eye irritation.

Vibration.   Continuous vibrating motion affecting the total body or specific limbs (riding in a vibrating truck cab, using a hand held grinder).

Jarring.   Sudden abrupt motion to the total body or specific limbs (abrupt motion experienced in a backhoe cab, sudden movement of a control lever).

Conditions of Work

The conditions of work identify some of the psychosocial demands involved in the job or task. These may be important when considering a rehabilitation or job re-integration process.

Traveling.   Working from home base in various locations.

Work Alone.   No one else in the immediate working area.

Interact with the Public.   General public or members of other departments, in person or by phone.

Operate Equipment.   This includes office equipment, vehicle, tools, and machines.

Irregular/Extended Work Hours.   Work which may be subject to changes in regular routine of work hours, or which may require extended work hours on certain occasions.

8

Job Placement Assessments and Preemployment Screening

Douglas H. Frey

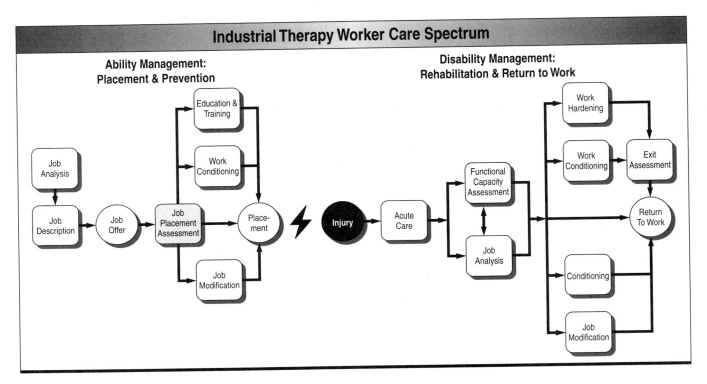

Industrial Therapy Worker Care Spectrum

Health care professionals who are regularly associated with industry are confronted daily by many issues and questions, including the following:

- The continuous significant rise in health care cost to individuals, families, employees, and employers
- Increased job related injuries, time off, and reduced work efficiency and productivity
- The increased work force volume necessary to meet job expectations and consumer demand
- Employers' increasing desire to provide a safe, efficient and regulatory-compliant work environment
- Employers' desire to promote employee satisfaction coupled with mutual goal development and fulfillment

- The need to hire the right employee for the right job, or make appropriate changes for rehiring or direction to other job positions
- Matching the right prospective employee to the appropriate positions within the company, by accommodating expected physical performance difficulties and proficiency demonstrations
- Reducing the cost of unanticipated and unknown preexisting injuries and difficulties following the hiring of a new employee
- Enhancing the parameters of the industrial screening process and the efficiency of evaluation during the interview and hiring process
- Compliance with the Americans with Disabilities Act (ADA) and Occupational Safety and

Health Administration (OSHA) regulatory guidelines and directives.

Evolution of Job Placement Assessments

Businesses and industries across the United States, and worldwide, have attempted to address these issues and concerns in many ways for years.[35,49] Many of the solutions they have developed fall under the general category of matching the capabilities of the worker to the demands of the job. A capable worker, functioning at safe levels, translates to reductions in injuries, disability pay, health care costs, lost productivity, and other ills.

To make better job-matching or placement decisions, industry and providers have sought ways to more accurately assess worker capabilities and job demands (Figure 8.1, page 114). Formerly an employment medical exam included chest x-rays and hernia tests to detect basic respiratory or physiological impairment. Then back x-rays were added, probably in response to the prevalence of industrial back injuries. Blood and urine tests were recently added to probe potential pathologies.

These traditional tests were valuable in identifying basic medical abnormalities, but often people who passed these general tests went on to become injured, or people who did not pass these tests went on to perform required job functions without injury.[8,17,18,21,31,34,38,39,40,44,48] In fact, studies have indicated that an x-ray has no predictive value with regard to job capabilities or injuries.[21,31,34,38,44]

As experience with industrial injuries accumulated, the value of performing functional tests gained acceptance. The earliest form were flexibility tests, such as the ability to bend down and touch the toes.[4–7,24,26]

Physicians and Therapists assessed back strength through force plate isometric tests. This measured the person's ability to pull upward from a standing position, bending forward at the waist, or squatting. With time, such isometric tests incorporated a variety of heights and positions to more completely encompass the back's multidimensional ranges. Such tests undoubtedly averted some problems, but their static circumstances were difficult to extrapolate to the dynamic job environment. Back problems and other industrial injuries continued.[3,10–15,22,28,29,30,46]

The next logical advance was to assess the person's capabilities using methods that replicate the dynamic nature of job functions. Physicians and Therapists began to test the person's ability to perform dynamic lifting, carrying, pushing, and pulling. These early forms of dynamic testing have evolved into what is today called Functional Capacity Assessment (FCA). A form of FCA used for the specialized purpose of job placement will be described in this chapter as Job Placement Assessment.[1,27,43,46]

CURRENT ISSUES

The compounding issues of cost, employee-employer dissatisfaction, and regulatory changes have recently pushed job placement considerations to the forefront (Figure 8.2, page 115):

Rising costs of insurance, health related benefits, long term disability and compensation payments call for new directions within the health care aspect of industrial management.[25]

Regulatory guidelines and changes have forced corporate management to reevaluate and revise their policies and procedures to satisfy these expectations. The Equal Employment Opportunity Commission (EEOC) and Affirmative Action guidelines have continually changed, and employer and employee must work together to effectively achieve satisfactory compliances.[2,19,23,32,33,41,47]

Litigation costs, court and trial delays, and their subsequent results have forced both management and workers to focus on improved understanding and attention to the often ignored parameters of the work environment.[25]

The ability to effectively analyze, criticize, and resolve these issues often means the difference between a company's success or failure. This in turn, can affect the direction of a nationwide economy and the financial stability necessary for continued prosperous growth.

Impact of the ADA

With the advent in 1992 of the Americans with Disabilities Act (ADA), the need for guidelines for appropriate interviewing and assessment of job candidates, prior to extending employment offers, has become critical. The ADA prohibits employers with 15 or more employees from discriminating against an individual with a disability, in hiring or promotion, if the applicant is otherwise qualified for the job.

The intent of the ADA is to ensure equal treatment for the disabled individual. Tests that focus on a disability or specific previous injury are barred, and decisions related to hiring must focus on self-limiting capabilities which affect actual job performance.

Accordingly, businesses must reevaluate their preemployment screening, hiring, recruitment, job assignments, and internal promotion practices to comply with the new standards. For a more extensive

FIGURE 8.1   The evolution of preemployment screening has included x-rays **(A)**, flexibility **(B)**, and strength testing **(C)**, with the most recent advance being dynamic testing **(D)**.

A

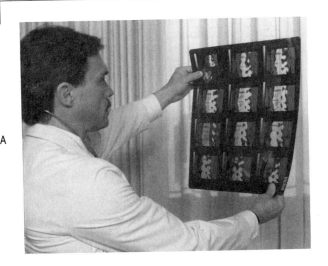

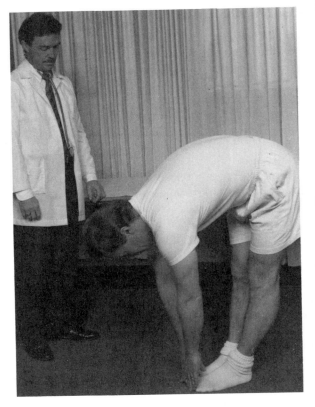

B

C

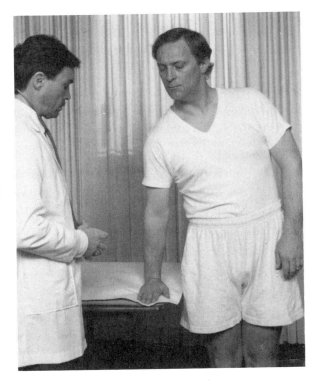

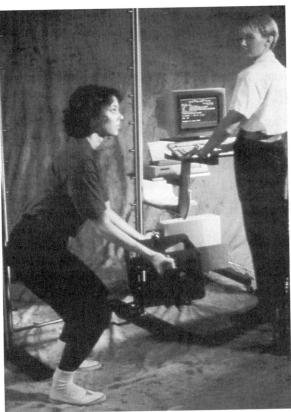

D

FIGURE 8.2 Factors, as reported by employers, which drive up workers' compensation costs.

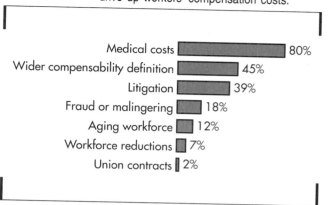

Medical costs	80%
Wider compensability definition	45%
Litigation	39%
Fraud or malingering	18%
Aging workforce	12%
Workforce reductions	7%
Union contracts	2%

(From Johnson and Higgins, subsidiary Foster Higgins: Survey on Workers Compensation, September, 1992.)

review of the ADA and its ramifications, see Chapter 22.[2,19,22,23,27,32,33,41,47]

The key to compliance with the ADA involves the concept of "essential functions"—those functions of a job that are necessary, not marginal or peripheral. Following enactment of the ADA, many companies have developed more detailed position or job descriptions, delineating essential and marginal functions of the job.

Under the "reasonable accommodation" section, ADA also requires that employers remove barriers which might inhibit a disabled person's performance of the essential functions of the job. An applicant for a job position must clearly possess the appropriate skills and experience to be considered for the job (Figure 8.3).

Under Title I regulations of the ADA, a preplacement screening is allowed once a conditional offer of employment has been made. However, the preplacement screening must be administered to all qualified individuals, be job-specific, and test the essential functions of the job.[2,19,22,23,27,32,33,41,47]

The right Job Placement Assessment process can provide companies with a standardized, valid, and defensible means to assess potential job candidates. Traditional employment exams that do not incorporate functional validity would not meet ADA requirements and regulations. Preplacement assessments based on an applicant's functional abilities and related to the essential functions of the job are the only kind of assessments allowed under ADA guidelines.

Conventional isometric, isokinetic, and static strength tests performed in a linear plane of motion are neither job-like nor functional, and do not accurately determine people's ability to perform essential job functions.

FIGURE 8.3 A job analysis provides essential function information that an employer can use to write a job description, establish reasonable accommodation, and perform preplacement assessments.

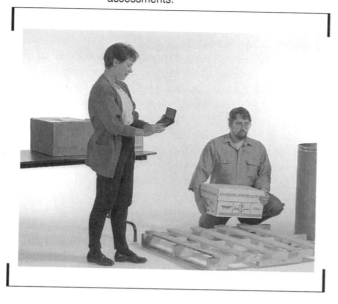

DESCRIPTION OF A JOB PLACEMENT ASSESSMENT

The foundation of many aspects of Industrial Therapy —accurate capability assessment, job placement, rehabilitation planning, progress monitoring, and risk-minimized return-to-work,—is the Functional Capacity Assessment (FCA). Preemployment job placement, however, requires only a portion of a full-blown FCA's information. Accordingly, preemployment job placement uses a scaled-back, specialized version of an FCA called a Job Placement Assessment (JPA) to objectively assess a potential employee's safe functional capabilities.[27]

The Job Placement Assessment, as identified within the Industrial Therapy Worker Care Spectrum (see page 112), fits very nicely into the area defined as evaluation and preemployment screening within the injury prevention phase. This area is extremely important in the future development and refinement of industrial standards to appropriately assess protocols for employee hiring, as well as continued proficiency within job responsibilities at given positions.

The Job Placement Assessment should fully comply with ADA, Equal Employment Opportunity Commission and Affirmative Action guidelines as a prescreening assessment. Since the JPA is a specialized version of an FCA, a close look at the words "functional capacity assessment" is helpful in understanding the advantages of a functionally-oriented assessment process:

Functional relates to a job applicant's ability to perform job-related functions, and since real work uses many body parts, the Job Placement Assessment encompasses the whole body's movement. It provides statistically based data on independent and interdependent work performance measurements.

Capacity refers to the candidate's capability to safely meet the physical requirements of the job for an eight-hour work day. This method of Job Placement Assessment relates specifically to the critical job functions of lifting, carrying, pushing, and pulling. In addition, weighted work load endurance and cardiovascular stress levels are measured by monitoring cardiac response for all analyzed activities.[27,36]

Assessment relates to the process of objective measurement and analysis of the applicant's capabilities. The Job Placement Assessment includes identification of body posture and mechanics throughout each activity, so safe lifting habits and potential injury risks can be evaluated.

Basic Features of a Job Placement Assessment

The Job Placement Assessment is typically a series of specific, objective, and standardized protocols followed in a consistent progression to allow for objective, accurate, and repeatable results. Standardization of variables like commands, verbal responses, weight loading protocols, notation of pain behaviors and reports, pulse rate variations and postural assessment protocol eliminate biased and subjective interpretations of the results. A JPA that incorporates standardized, reliable functional assessments assures compliance with existing regulations, while providing accommodations for further regulatory changes.

The Job Placement Assessment should allow for objective analysis and measurement of independent and interdependent tasks of job related activities. Most Job Placement Assessments generally measure three parameters of lifting—*above-shoulder* level, *desk to chair* height, and *chair to floor* height. In addition, most measure the ability to push and pull, carry, and perform endurance activities such as repeated stair climbing.

Some JPA's supplement these basic components with measures to include unique aspects of certain jobs. A JPA for fire fighters might include carrying weights up and down ladders. A JPA for ditch diggers might include digging below grade. The output

from a Job Analysis is typically used to determine such unique components.

While many unique job demands may warrant inclusion in the JPA, it is sometimes not necessary, other times not feasible to assess all the unique aspects of each job. The issue of necessity comes into focus when the risk of injury may be too small to warrant the assessment cost.

Feasibility may be an issue of prohibitive cost, physical impossibility, or lack of expertise on the part of the Therapist when faced with a particularly unusual assessment challenge. A job might require performing a number of tasks on the hearth of a blast furnace. Therefore, simulating the environmental heat becomes an important variable. In such cases, the options are to assess the functions on-site, find an alternative facility that can assess the function, simulate the function in a more feasible way, or reach an understanding with the employer that this particular function will not be assessed.

Coordination With Job Analysis

The findings of the JPA are most meaningful when they can be compared to a well analyzed inventory of an actual job's physical demands, as determined by a Job Analysis. In cases where a Job Analysis has already been performed, the Assessment Specialist should review the information either to ensure that all relevant capabilities are included in the JPA, or to determine what components should be added to cover unique job demands.

Where a Job Analysis has not been performed, the Therapist should recommend that it be incorporated as part of the total services required.

Benefits of Job Placement Assessment

When a worker's capability levels are safely matched to job demands, or the job is redesigned to enable safe performance, the results are less injuries, lower disability pay, lower health care costs, preserved productivity, and higher job satisfaction and morale. Case histories attesting to these benefits are accumulated, and some examples summarized below.

A Minnesota paper manufacturer instituted Job Placement Assessments (JPA) in September 1988 to help stem the costs of lost work days and Worker's Compensation claims. Two years later, experiences of the last 70 employees hired prior to the use of JPA's were compared to the first 70 hired after. The results indicated that JPA's reduced both lost work days and Workers' Compensation costs (Figure 8.4).

A state transportation authority has found that Job Placement Assessments pinpoint risk of injury to employees. Among 36 employees injured between 1985

FIGURE 8.4 Comparison of hirees of a Minnesota paper manufacturuer with JPA's versus those without JPA's.

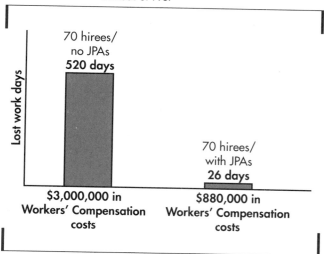

and 1992, 75% had already been categorized as "at risk" by JPA's performed when they were hired.

JPA Principles and Attributes

Therapists familiar with FCA's will recognize many aspects of JPA's. A number of therapy service organizations provide equipment and protocols for JPA's, and each has its unique features and benefits. However, there are some principles and attributes that are generally regarded as essential to a proper JPA, particularly with the advent of the ADA.

At a minimum, the JPA must:

Replicate job function with regard to postures, dynamic movements, and repetitions so that the observations, measurements, and assessments can be reliably translated to specific job performance capabilities.[19,23,27,36,41]

Require physical performance of job related functions (rather than self-reported or Therapist-judged capabilities and limitations.)[19,23,41]

Be objective, unbiased, and neutral so that tester differences or judgments do not color observation, measurement, or reporting of the results.[27,29,43]

Be standardized with regard to equipment, protocols, forms, and overall procedure so that the outcome is consistent, comparable, and projectable to real world job setting.[27,29,36,42]

Be multidimensioned in terms of variety of methods and components within each task to account for all relevant permutations of

posture, motion, resistance, and endurance that encompass safe capability parameters.[28,35]

Allow self limitation on the subjects of maximum resistance and fatigue points. This ensures greater safety and objectivity in opposition to the tester assigning those limits judgmentally or subjectively. (Subject overreporting can be ascertained afterwards by analyzing correlates of capability such as heart rate or blood pressure.)[9,20,28,29]

Allow comparability to normative data in the general population, and as a baseline for future FCA's in the event of injury.[29,50]

Be predictive of real-world safe, borderline, or at risk compatibility with job demands, which requires sufficient data base of validations for statistical projectability.[27,29,36,50]

Be legally defensible in any proceedings regarding liability for illegal discrimination or unsafe job placement, especially with regard to the ADA.[2,19,23,28,32,33,41,47]

Be ADA compliant in terms of relevance to "essential job functions", unbiased objectivity, and consistency from one subject to another.[2,19,23,27,32,33,41,47]

In addition to the above minimum principles, JPA's should adhere wherever possible and affordable to the following:[27,28]

Be adaptable to on-site testing at employer location if necessary, for convenience or unique simulation requirements.

Provide education or Work Conditioning qualifiers for determining measures to upgrade capabilities to job requirements.

Enable merging with Department of Labor categories of sedentary, light, medium, heavy, or very heavy.

Be Therapist friendly in terms of ease in administering the assessment and reporting of results.

Be cost and time efficient, prioritized toward the most valuable, relevant, and reimbursable information needs.

Allow for multiple candidate testing to economize on the Therapist's time.

JPA Guidelines

In addition to the above principles, a proper JPA should also incorporate the following procedural and reporting guidelines:

Allow recovery time between activities so that resistance or fatigue points are not influenced by previous exercise.[20,27]

Adhere to consistent instructions to minimize variability or statistical error incurred by differences in what is required by the subject.[27,42]

Adhere to consistent weight loading protocols to prevent influenced performance by differences in method, and when resistance is increased.[27,42]

Ensure accurate documentation through consistent forms and recording procedures.[27,36,42]

Provide user friendly reporting using terminology and visual aids that are easily interpreted and understood by management, supervisors, employees, insurers, attorneys, and other interested parties.

What Not To Measure

As measurement of functional and dynamic capabilities have replaced non-functional and static testing, it has become obvious that certain traditional or conventional measurements are no longer applicable. These obsolete measurements are:

- Standard goniometric ROM of joints
- Standard graded strength tests
- Traditional mobility and flexibility tests
- Static or isometric readings

In addition, it is not appropriate to attempt measuring factors outside the therapist's expertise, such as lighting or airborne toxins.

The above principles, attributes, and procedures have evolved considerably and will continue to do so in order to match with greater precision, worker capabilities and job requirements.

PERFORMING A JOB PLACEMENT ASSESSMENT

Scheduling and Preparation

The request to the medical facility for the Job Placement Assessment can originate from many potential referral sources: personnel and safety directors or managers, physicians, occupational health nurses, attorneys, claims adjusters, rehabilitation counselors, and other allied health professionals.

During the initial contact, facility personnel or the Assessment Specialist should secure all the information necessary to facilitate a comprehensive and concise Job Placement Assessment, without problems or inconvenience.

The information to secure from the referral source should include the client's name, address, and phone number, detailed job requirements, billing address, and reporting preference (mail or fax.) The informa-tion provided to the referral source should include the time, date, and location of the appointment, directions to the facility, expected duration of the assessment, report turn-around time, fees, and instructions for appropriate attire. All information should be appropriately verified between the requesting party and the Assessment Specialist.

The job candidate should also be fully informed about all aspects of the assessment, including time, date, location, and appropriate dress. The participant should understand how long the Job Placement Assessment will last. Dress should be casual and comfortable, including stable, well fitting shoes and loose nonrestrictive clothing to enable performance of the work related activities to be measured. The importance of the participant's attendance should be adequately stressed to both participant and referral source. The provider should also stress that group participants should control mixed-gender issues.

Overall, the facility personnel providing the Job Placement Assessments must furnish pertinent, necessary information to the referral source, with concern not to erode the nonbiased objective capabilities of the assessment process. Punctuality, preparation, and courtesy are critical elements the providing facility affords the clients, as well as the referral source. Efficiency and professionalism are critical to the acceptance of the service, and assure continued usage by current clients and future referrals.

Receiving the Participant

The arrival of the referred test subject signals fresh expansion of the Assessment Specialist's expertise and an ongoing opportunity for marketing of new and viable services available to industry within an area. Initial perceptions, understanding, and sincerity are critical elements for the development, refinement, and utilization of these services.

The initial contact between the referred participant and the Assessment Specialist is the most important factor dictating success of the venture. The specialist must greet the participant cordially and sincerely, realizing that this exchange sets the tone for the entire placement assessment.

Briefing the Participant

The participant should be given an overview of the Job Placement Assessment components and process. They should be shown all basic forms such as the data collection form, the report formats and documents, and the participant's authorization form to release the information to the employer and other designated parties.

The assessment location (clinic, office, hospital) may have integrated the protocols of the assessment process into computerized software, using standardized forms from the vendor of assessment equipment and protocols. These forms should be reviewed with the participant prior to the start of the evaluation process.

It is important to stress to the participant that the information derived from the assessment is strictly confidential. The summary, with appropriate recommendations, will be forwarded only to the requesting referral source, unless specified otherwise, or subject to authorization by the participant. The information noted and retrieved throughout the evaluation process will be discussed and reviewed with the participant thoroughly, following the completion of all parameters of the JPA.

The process should be reviewed with the participant. The participant needs to understand that the essential functions assessed must relate to activities in personal and working lifestyles. The overall purpose is to determine safe and productive parameters of these functions.

It should be stressed that the ability to participate safely at their highest level in these activities, is very important to successfully gain employment and to personal life. The client should also be informed that this will represent objective, nonbiased data relating to individual functional capabilities.

The Assessment Specialist should inform the participant that in order to effectively foster and maintain a nonbiased atmosphere conducive to the portrayal of objective results, the directions, and commands related to the evaluation process will be succinct, specific, and informative. Appropriate questions during the process should be answered very promptly, but without the specialist's personal suggestions or directions, to avoid interference.

Apprehension, fear, and insecurity are often felt by the participant. In most cases the prospective employee really wants the job and may try to overreach safe capability. These possibilities must be recognized and dealt with effectively by the Assessment Specialist to ensure proper analysis and participation during Job Placement Assessment. The introduction of the participant to the functional assessment process is very important to reduce apprehension, familiarize the participant with each of the anticipated testing protocols, and facilitates good cooperation, relaxation, and ultimate quality participation.

Performing the Assessment

As the participant enters the facility testing area, the therapist should observe and evaluate such factors as gait, body mechanics, postural control, and behavioral characteristics. Efficiency at handling the mechanics of postural control and behaviors should be noted while completing the employee information sheet and during preliminary discussions prior to commencing the evaluation process performance. The behaviors and characteristics noted will enhance the Assessment Specialist's ability to correlate other recorded observations and realize other possible limitations imposed upon the outcome.

When dealing with a group of job candidates, only one individual should be taken into the evaluation area at a time, avoiding any physical contact or visual observation of other candidates. This decreases individual competitiveness, allays an individual's apprehension, and markedly enhances the individual's comfort, reliability, and participation. This protocol is typically given high marks when referral sources review a clinic's Job Placement Assessment services.

The Assessment Specialist should carefully construct the sequencing of each of the evaluation functions, to appropriately interspace body areas used during each function and allow sufficient rest periods. Let the participants know that sufficient time will be allowed for rest between each performance of a functional activity.

Prior to the commencement of the evaluation procedure for each participant, the Assessment Specialist should record the resting heart rate. The assessor should secure subsequent heart rates from the same extremity used for the resting pulse, thereby ensuring conformity within the process. This procedure serves as a safety measure to avoid overexertion.

The assessor should use very precise, simple commands and responses at all times during the evaluation to maintain a nonbiased environment for the participant's performance. The Therapist should adhere to consistent guidelines regarding acceptable commands and directions to be used during performance of the JPA process. Commands should be concise and instructional, such as "lift the weight and walk from the yellow line to the blue line and back again."

The Therapist must consistently be aware of their vocal instructions' content and the mannerisms they choose to exhibit, so as not to influence the participant's responses, effort, or results. The judgment and ability to provide concrete and objective instructions greatly improves the authenticity of the Job Placement Assessment (Figure 8.5).

In performing the tasks—including lifting, carrying, and pushing/pulling—clients may or may not use good body mechanics. Accordingly, during the performance of each of the functional tasks comprising the Job Placement Assessment, the Assessment Specialist must employ excellent observation and visual skills, noting postural control, body mechanics, pain behaviors, and reports, as well as utilization of substitutional

FIGURE 8.5 The Assessment Specialist must employ excellent observation and visual skills in order to document postural control, body mechanics, and pain behaviors and reports during a Job Placement Assessment.

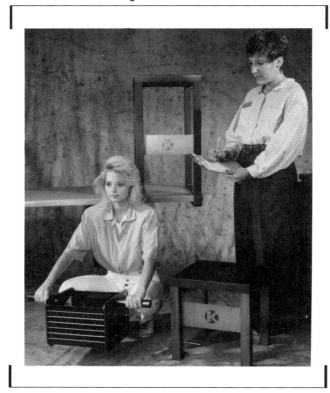

efforts during the completion of each of the requested tasks.

It is critical for the assessor to closely observe and note body mechanics such as stance pattern, flexion of hips and knees, gait, proximity to the unit being lifted, body part alignment performing the function (hand placement, functional, and body improvisations), shortness of breath, and endurance. Deficits, postural problems, poor body mechanics, and demonstrated deviations in performance must be noted for consideration at the completion of the Job Placement Assessment. Consistencies and inconsistencies noted throughout the process assist the Therapist in recommendations to both the participant and the referring source.

Weights achieved are recorded, noting difficulties or problems encountered, endurance problems, and excessive risks leading to decreased or reduced safety.

At the termination of the selected function, the assessor should record relevant information such as; the observed functional and behavioral mechanics, the elapsed time of the test, the starting and ending weights, repetitions, and any relevant verbal information from the participant. The participant should be

allowed sufficient rest time following the function's completion for recovery and pulse stabilization prior to advancing to the next desired functional task.[27]

The Therapist should review the results of the Job Placement Assessment with the participant prior to exit from the facility. This briefing would include a review of weights achieved, the performance observed, and the findings and recommendations to be forwarded to the referring source. The assessor may make general suggestions and comments regarding any workstyle modifications required in the future. Finally, as an overall guideline, it is important to conclude the assessment on a harmonious and professional note.

Reporting

When the participant has completed all functional tasks requested within the Job Placement Assessment, the Assessment Specialist should complete an overview report (Figure 8.6.) This report should include the employee's name, social security number, and position being applied for; as well as objectively detailing the participant's results of each assessed function.

Upon completion, the assessor should sign the report, and retain a photocopy as part of the permanent assessment record of the providing facility. The participant should also sign a statement on the report

FIGURE 8.6 The Job Placement Assessment Overview sheet details the participant's objective results and provides general recommendations.

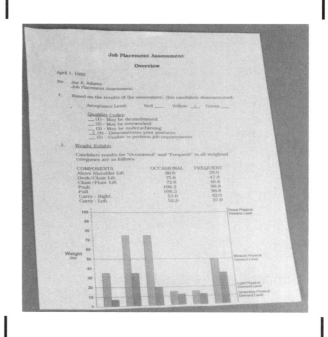

form or a separate document regarding whether they feel the resistances, repetitions, and other demands were at safe levels, unsafe, or "don't know."

All information forms associated with the employee's assessment should be retained as part of the permanent record, including the personal information form completed by the participant and the authorization for release of information prior to assessment. The compiled file represents the confidential and legal record of the Job Placement Assessment administered by the Assessment Specialist. This record should be checked closely by the Therapist and appropriately completed with all information prior to being permanently filed.

Once the client's overview report is completed, the company or referral source will be provided with the objective and concise Job Placement Assessment report. This report includes a narrative letter, graphics, and the Assessment Specialist's comments regarding the candidate's safe and productive work limits.

Examples of graphic formats are presented in Figures 8.7 through 8.9. Figure 8.7 compares the candidate's JPA results to the job demands, expressed in terms of the amount of weights involved in assessed activities. From Figure 8.7, it can be seen that the candidate performs above the job demands in every activity.

FIGURE 8.8   Comparison of the candidate's JPA results and job requirements with the physical demand levels (PDL) established by the U.S. Department of Labor.

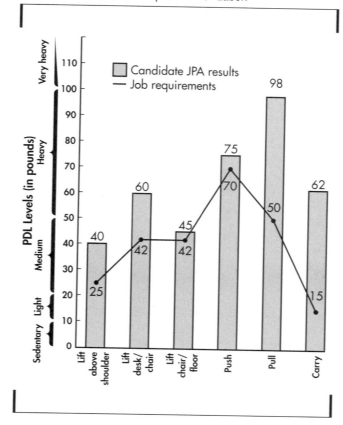

FIGURE 8.7   Comparison of the candidate's JPA results with job requirements. The candidate performs above the job demands in every activity.

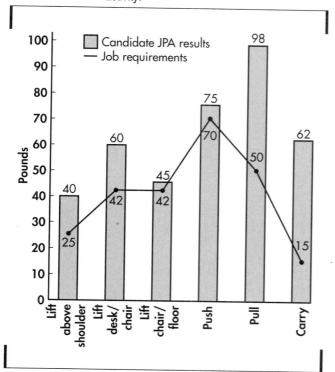

Figure 8.8 illustrates another way of expressing the candidate's capabilities—in terms of the physical demand levels (PDL) established by the U.S. Department of Labor. Figure 8.8 indicates that the candidate is able to perform in the "medium" range for the three lifting activities, able to do "heavy" pushing and pulling, but only "light" levels of carrying.

Figure 8.9, page 122 indicates that although a rehabilitated truck driver's FCA results are below the JPA norms for new hires, they are at or above the norms for injured truck drivers.[50] Without this information, therapists might have recommended additional, expensive Work Hardening even though the rehabilitation outcome was already above average. The more reasonable recommendation would be to return to work, while initiating a home conditioning program with the new hire levels as goals.

Reported recommendations and concerns may include the need for body mechanics education, general conditioning and strengthening programs, or suggestions relating to work environment modifications, which increase competency and efficiency in the employment field.

FIGURE 8.9 Comparison of a client's capabilities with other JPA and FCA results for truckdrivers.

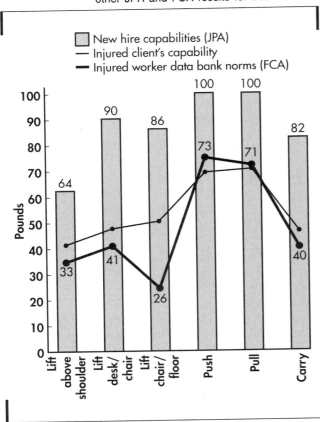

Some vendors of JPA equipment and protocols systematically collect and store all of the assessment findings in a computer data base, so that the results of each assessment can be comparable and predictive according to statistically valid norms.[51] With such data base supportive JPA's, the Assessment Specialist should take extra care in completing the assessment data sheet, thus maintaining the integrity of the data base resource for present and future analyses.

ADMINISTRATIVE ASPECTS OF JOB PLACEMENT ASSESSMENTS

Reimbursement and Billing Protocols

A designated representative of the providing facility should communicate the fee parameters to the referral source up front. Care should be exercised in establishing appropriate, competitive, and acceptable fee guidelines, taking into consideration comparable medical service fees, allotted third party payor allowances, and competitive fee scales within surrounding regional and state area.

Many providers of assessment equipment and protocols offer guidelines regarding fee ranges. Specific fee levels will vary widely based on regional economic conditions, but the order of magnitude is in the range of $50 to $100 per assessment, with a sliding scale downwards, if more than one person is assessed simultaneously. The facility's fee scale should be established and available upon request to all referral sources.

Fees should also be payable to the providing facility when clients fail to attend, or are inordinately late for the scheduled appointment. Cancellations may be made permissible if requested sufficiently in advance (24 hours). This understanding helps establish mutual respect and commitment on the part of the referral source, the referral client, and the providing facility. Contractual payment agreements are acceptable and are to be negotiated between the respective parties of the providing facility and the referral agency or source.

Marketing and Public Relations

Marketing Job Placement Assessments should be broadscale and continuous, and frequently reevaluated. The facility providing Job Placement Assessments must realize the large market that exists, and be careful not to exclude any particular potential referral group or source. Targeted groups may include industrial personnel and safety directors, human resource representatives, physicians, claims adjusters, lawyers, and Vocational Rehabilitation Consultants.

The marketing process must be carefully coordinated within the provisional facility, to make certain not to generate demand that exceeds the capacity of the facility and staffing. Strategic planning and coordination will help to establish the quality of services provided for referral sources.

Marketing may begin by positioning the JPA as a new, innovative, and beneficial service to the targeted group. There are a multitude of marketing techniques, including presentations, promotions, health fairs, brochures, career days, open houses, direct mailings, and media presentations. Avenues most appropriate to the selected groups should be used. The approach should be designed to achieve the highest level of acceptance and promote continued exploration and utilization. Marketing materials such as slide presentations, pamphlets, and marketing brochures are often provided by the manufacturer of equipment and protocols. Marketing events and programs are opportunities to provide additional information on the participating facility and to broaden the awareness and utilization of all the services rendered within it.

As an overall marketing strategy, it is important for the providing facility to establish and maintain an excellent level of service at all times. The facility must schedule requests for JPA's in a timely fashion, be punctual and effective in relaying information to designated recipients, communicate clearly and effectively, and continuously improve marketing efforts. Many facilities offer locker rooms where clients can change, toilet facilities, towels, refreshments, and continued education to the individuals. Such amenities upgrade the quality of the service provided and encourage continued use and growth.

SUMMARY

Because Job Placement Assessments are useful in addressing a number of issues faced by industry today —rising costs of injuries, increasing litigation, regulatory, and statutory compliance—the future applications are many, and its possibilities are only beginning to gain recognition and respect worldwide.

To effectively meet industry's evolving needs, JPA's must comply with OSHA, ADA, EEOC, and Affirmative Action guidelines. In doing so, they must be functional, objective, unbiased, standardized, projectable to the real world job environment, and statistically reliable. Over time, many of the traditional medical assessment approaches such as x-rays, isometric tests, and flexibility tests have proven to have little predictive relationship to job performance or injuries.

Job Placement Assessments afford industry the opportunity to significantly improve the quality of hiring practices and job placement. JPA's can give credible information and data for companies to reassess existing job descriptions. They can eliminate guess-work related to an individual's functional capabilities. In a growing number of cases they provide formula based predictive data on safe work capabilities. The accumulating track record, credibility, and useful applications of JPA's will significantly enhance growth and utilization in the future.

Job Placement Assessments can be a Therapist's introduction to providing other services like Work Hardening or Work Conditioning programs, back safety education, body mechanics education, job site analysis, and modification for the industrial setting. The success and growth of Job Placement Assessments is dependent primarily upon the Therapist's initiative, marketing skills, and excellence demonstrated in performance of the assessment process.

REFERENCES

1. Ayoub, MM, Mital, A, Bakken, GM, et. al: Development of Strength and Capacity Norms for Manual Materials Handling Activities: the state of the art, *Human Factors* 22:271–283, 1980.
2. Barlow, Wayne E, Hane, Edward Z: A Practical Guide to the Americans with Disabilities Act, *Personnel Journal* June 1992.
3. Battie MC, et al: Isometric Lifting Strength as a Predictor of Industrial Back Pain, *Spine* 14:141–147, 1989.
4. Battie MC, et al: The Role of Spinal Flexibility in Back Pain Complaints within Industry: a prospective study, Spine 15(8):768–773, 1990.
5. Bergquist-Ullman M Larson, U: Acute Low Back Pain in Industry *Acta Ortho Suppl* 170:1, 1977.
6. Biering-Sorensen F: A Prospective Study of Low Back Pain in a General Population, *Scan J Rehab Med* 15:71–96 (I–III), 1983.
7. Biering-Sorenson F: Physical Measurements as Risk Indicators for Low-Back Trouble Over a One Year Period, *Spine* 9(2):106–119, 1984.
8. Bohart WH: Anatomic Variations and Anomalies of the Spine: relation to prognosis and length of disability, *JAMA* 92:698–701, 1929.
9. Campion MA: Personnel Selection for Physically Demanding Jobs: review and recommendations, *Pers Psych* 36:527–548, 1983
10. Chaffin DB, Herrin GD, Keyserling WM: Preemployment Strength Testing: an updated position, *J Occup Med* 20:403–408, 1978.
11. Chaffin DB, Park KS: A Longitudinal Study of Low-Back Pain Associated with Occupational Weight Lifting Factors, *Amer Ind Hyg Assoc J* 34:513–525, 1973.
12. Chaffin DB, Andersson GBJ: *Occupational Biomechanics,* ed 2, New York, 1990, Wiley.
13. Chaffin DB: Functional Assessment for Heavy Physical Labor. In Alderman MH, Hanley MJ editors: *Clinical Medicine for the Occupational Physician,* New York, 1982, Marcie Dekker.
14. Chaffin DB, Herrin GD, Keyserling WM, et al: Pre-Employment Strength Testing in Selecting Workers for Material Handling CDC-99-74-62, NIOSH Physiology and Ergonomics Branch, Cincinnati, Ohio, 1977.
15. Chaffin DB: Ergonomics Guide for the Assessment of Human Static Strength *Am Indus Hyg Assoc J* 36:505–511, 1975.
16. Campion MA: Personnel Selection For Physically Demanding Jobs: review and recommendations, *Per Psych* 36:527–548, 1983.
17. Cushway BC, Mayer RJ: Routine Examination of the Spine for Industrial Employees, *JAMA* 93:701–704, 1929.
18. Diveley R, Oglevie RR: Preemployment Examination of the Low Back, *JAMA* 160:856–858, 1956.
19. EEOC: Technical Assistance Manual for the Americans With Disabilities Act, IV-5-IV12.
20. Ergonomics Guides: Ergonomics Guide to Assessment of Metabolic and Cardiac Costs of Physical Work, *Amer Ind Hyg Assoc J* 32(9):560–564, 1971.
21. Fullenlove TM, Williams, AJ: Comparative Roentgen Findings in Symptomatic and Asymptomatic Backs, *Radiology* 68:572–574, 1957.
22. Garg A, Mital A, Asfour SS: A Comparison of Isometric Strength and Dynamic Lifting Capability, *Ergonomics* 23:13–27, 1980.
23. Greenberg SN, Bello RP: The Americans with Disabilities Act: what you don't know can hurt you, *Occup Ther Forum,* June 1992.

24. Horal J: The Clinical Appearance of Low Back Disorders in the City of Gothenburg, Sweden, *Acta Orthop Scand* 118:9–109, 1969.

25. Johnson & Higgins, subsidiary Foster Higgins: *Survey on Workers' Compensation,* Sept 1992.

26. Karvonen MJ, Vitasalo JT, Komi PV, et al: Back and Leg Complaints in Relation to Muscle Strength in Young Men, *Scand J Rehab Med* 12:53–59, 1980.

27. Key GL: *Key Functional Assessment Policy and Procedure Manual,* 1984.

28. Keyserling WM, Herrin GD, Chaffin DB: Isometric Strength Testing as a Means of Controlling Medical Incidents on Strenuous Jobs, *J Occup Med* 22:(5)332–336, 1980.

29. Keyserling WM, Herrin DG, Chaffin et al: Establishing an Industrial Strength Testing Program, *Am Ind Hyg Assoc J* 41:730–736, 1980.

30. Kroemer KHE: Human Strength: terminology, measurement and interpretation of data, *Human Factors* 12:297–313, 1970.

31. LaRocca H, MacNab I: Value of Preemployment Radiographic Assessment of the Lumbar Spine, *Can Med Assoc J* 101:49–54, 1969.

32. Lorber LZ: Legal Report: the civil rights act of 1991, *Society for Human Resource Management* Spring 1992.

33. Lotito MJ, Allen JC: Legal Report: answers to commonly asked ADA questions, *Society for Human Resource Management* Summer 1992.

34. Magora A, Schwartz A: Relation Between Low Back Pain Syndrome and X-ray Findings, 2. transitional vertebrae (mainly sacralization), *Scand J Rehab Med* 10:135–145, 1978.

35. Park KS, Chaffin DB: Prediction of Load-Lifting Limits for Manual Materials Handling, *Prof Safety* 45–48, May 1975.

36. Personnel Decisions, Inc: *Key Functional Assessment Preemployment Screening Battery as a Predictor of Job Related Injuries,* Minneapolis, Minn, Jan 1994.

37. Randolf SA, Dalton PC, Limited Duty Work: an innovative approach to an early return to work, *AAOHN Jour,* 37:11, 1989.

38. Redfield JT: The Low Back X-ray as a Preemployment Screening Tool in the Forest Products Industry, *Occup Med* 13:219, 1971.

39. Rowe ML: Low Back Pain in Industry: a position paper, *J Occup Med* 11:161–169, 1969.

40. Runge CF: Preexisting Structural Defects and the Severity of Compensation Back Injuries, *Ind Med Surg* 27:249–252, 1958.

41. Silvestri SM, Zimic DL: An Employer's Compliance Checklist: a look at the practical aspects of compliance with the ADA, *Fed Bar News & Jour,* 39:1, 1992.

42. Snook SH, Irvine CH: Maximum Acceptable Weight of Lift, *Amer Ind Hyg Assoc J* 322–329 July-Aug 1967.

43. Snook SH: The Design of Manual Handling Tasks, *Ergonomics* 21:963–985, 1978.

44. Splioff CA: Lumbosacral Junction: roentgenographic comparison of patients with and without backaches, *JAMA* 152:1610–1653, 1953.

45. Stobbe T: Strength Testing, *Indus Erg,* An Arbor, University of Michigan, 1982.

46. Troup JDG, Foremen TK, Baxter CE, et al: The Perception of Back Pain and Role of Psychophysical Tests of Lifting Capacity, *Spine* 12:645–657, 1987.

47. U.S. Department of Justice, Civil Rights Division: The American with Disabilities Act: questions and answers.

48. Valkenburg HA, Haanen HCN: The Epidemiology of Back Pain. In White AA, Gordon SL, editors *Symposium on Idiopathic Low Back Pain,* St Louis, 1982, Mosby.

49. Wilson JR, Niegel: *Evaluation of Human Work,* 1991, Taylor and Francis.

50. Worker Data Bank, KEY Method, Minneapolis, Minn 1994.

9

Back Injury Prevention

H. Duane Saunders
Mark R. Stultz
Robin Saunders
Mark A. Anderson

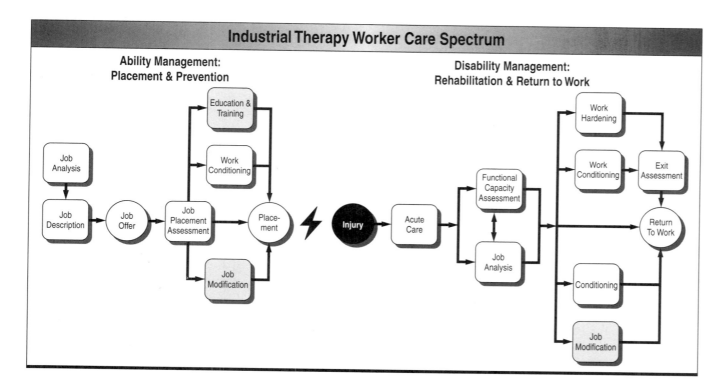

This chapter discusses how Industrial Therapy is working to ameliorate the impact of back injuries on industry, through innovative, enlightened prevention, and management strategies. The concepts presented in this chapter are for the practical and effective therapist, consultant, or future consultant who understands the problem of back pain and can implement positive solutions, or be a catalyst for change.

Economic Impact

Industrial back injuries and their associated costs have a dramatic and severe effect upon the financial viability of many companies and the costs of many products. In the U.S., the cost of low back injuries alone add an additional $1,800.00 to the sticker price of each automobile manufactured in Detroit.[27]

Consider the consumer preference for a car that costs almost $2,000.00 less than a competitive model with all of the same features! What an impact that would have on trade. The cost of these cars and injuries directly affect our personal, corporate, and national financial health.

The Back Injury Consultant

When Industrial Therapists become involved in back injury prevention and management, it is important for them to think of themselves as "consultants," not just therapists, because they must do much more than simply rehabilitate injured backs. They must also explore and address the company's attitudes and practices which can significantly affect the incidence and severity of these injuries.

Back injury consultants come from many different backgrounds, including health and fitness, medicine, ergonomics, safety, engineering, and business. There is a strong need for consultants who have the desire and ability to help companies succeed and compete, by reducing unnecessary and burdensome costs of low back pain.

The most qualified consultant, is the one who understands that the answer to the back injury problem does not lie in any one specialty area. Persons with a variety of backgrounds can become effective consultants when they take the responsibility to be competent in the areas that are traditionally outside of their discipline. The effective consultant is one who can draw from several other areas, to offer the variety of services necessary with a high level of comprehensiveness.

Traditional Solutions

After the costs associated with low back pain become apparent within an organization, consultants are frequently called upon to "do a back program" for them. This usually implies they are interested in a typical two to four hour group session where spinal anatomy, pathology, body mechanics, simple ergonomics, and exercise are presented, during obligatory, awareness raising sessions.

Although short term improvements are usually related to these back pain statistics after simple employee "training" sessions, programs of this type rarely foster healthy, long term organizational and behavioral change. When the costs of low back pain have fallen below the organizational attention threshold, awareness wanes and episodes of back pain are likely to approach pretraining levels.

When the associated costs again become apparent, there is a perceived need for another shot in the arm. Unfortunately, this safety program cycle repeats itself unnecessarily in many organizations, and clients may be sorely disappointed.

Enlightened Solutions

The consultant should respond to these clients by telling them that they can offer a much more effective intervention—one that helps them start a back injury prevention *process*. By using a process oriented approach, the goal of awareness is accomplished, while more importantly fostering the development of policies, practices, and procedures which facilitate the move from awareness to action.

Back injury consultants must become corporate

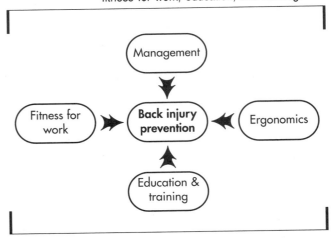

FIGURE 9.1 Back injury prevention is a process that incorporates management, ergonomics, fitness for work, education, and training.

catalysts to assure that a long term process orientation is in place prior to and after traditional training. Whenever they do not, the development of safe behaviors and practices is not fostered, and the programs offer only very short term effectiveness and awareness. A back injury prevention "program," ie training, is just one intervention of many within the back injury prevention process (Figure 9.1).

Intervention Strategies

It is important at the outset of a chapter like this to encourage readers, therapists, potential consultants, and experienced consultants, to take a comprehensive process-oriented approach to the prevention of back pain. Since the cause of back pain is multifaceted, the intervention approach must be multifaceted as well.

Back injury prevention is most effective when four primary and interrelated intervention strategies work in concert:

1. Management practices: Organizational management, Medical management, and Claims management
2. Ergonomics
3. Fitness for work
4. Education and training

If an intervention addresses only one of these areas without considering the others, the client has accomplished a short-term solution at best, and may have caused new problems.

If employees are given ergonomics awareness training but management's commitment to the process has not been obtained or verified, employees may become frustrated and antagonistic, and the ill-prepared consultant will have fostered an adversarial labor-management relationship.

Organizational management approaches place paramount importance on the actions and responses of the management team. If company management does not actively support the prevention process beyond mere lip service, attempts to take proactive steps will be futile. Strategies which help management develop a comprehensive, prevention-oriented philosophy and provide a way to handle injuries when they do occur are imperative. This role of organizational management in implementing effective policies and procedures will be discussed.

Medical management methods provide employees with knowledge about warning signs and symptoms, so that intervention can happen as soon as possible. Further, companies should secure the services of competent physicians and therapists, and encourage employees to see designated providers. Companies should be ready to implement modified duty, on-the-job Work Hardening, and ergonomic measures where warranted. These strategies will be discussed in more detail.

Claims management principles and practices should be understood and followed by company benefits personnel. There should be a formal written Claims Management Policy outlining the steps from point of injury, through acute care, then rehabilitation, and return-to-work. Regular communication with the injured employee and medical providers throughout this process is essential. A step by step approach to claims management will be described.

Ergonomics is also crucial, because it helps to provide a safer, more productive workplace as part of the overall prevention process. As this chapter will illustrate, ergonomics dovetails very well with the other injury prevention strategies. For example, ergonomic changes may help workers choose less risky behaviors. While the risk of injury has been reduced due to ergonomic modification supported by management, the remaining risk can be lessened through worker related interventions such as body mechanics training or instruction in the proper use of new ergonomic equipment. It will not be possible to implement changes successfully, unless management provides the support and means to do so.

Fitness for work is important to the overall preventive process. No matter how well a company performs in all other areas, injuries will still be a problem if members of the work force are not fit to perform the critical physical demands of jobs. Fitness is often a difficult area to address, because the ways in which individuals take care of themselves are usually outside company control. There are many things employers can do to facilitate on-the-job fitness to motivate and educate individuals to practice healthier lifestyles away from the job. This chapter will specifically evaluate the role of workplace exercise as a fatigue control measure.

Education and training is the vehicle used by consultants to provide the information necessary to implement an effective back injury prevention process. Everyone in the company—hourly employees, supervisors, and upper-level managers—must be part of the education and training process. Just as instruction in proper body mechanics is important for the hourly employee, information on the effects of management policies and practices is important to managers and supervisors. Educational programs should include these managerial issues.

Before embarking on the remainder of the chapter, it may be helpful to clarify the distinction between education and training. Simply put, education is the transfer of knowledge from one party to another. Training, on the other hand, involves the acquisition of new or refined skills. Education programs and training courses must be as action-oriented and skill-based as possible. If there is no difference after training, then the style or material was not effective or the approach to facilitating change was not comprehensive enough.

BACK INJURY PREVENTION STRATEGIES

Organizational Management

In this section, we will discuss the various actions that a company's upper management must take to create the environment in which active and effective injury prevention can thrive (Box 9-1). Not all the actions discussed are easy to implement. Many companies may initially resist the consultant's efforts to take a serious look at the effect management policies and attitudes

---

BOX 9.1

Management Strategies for Back Injury Prevention

1. Gain support from all levels of management
2. Establish manager accountability for the implementation and effectiveness of policies and procedures
3. Change manager attitudes by making them accountable for injuries
4. Establish and communicate work procedures and rules
5. Develop positive, open lines of communication between managers and employees to show that management cares about their employees' well being

have on their Workers' Compensation costs. Many companies want a "quick fix," such as a body mechanics training session or an ergonomic analysis.

It has been the authors' experience that successful injury prevention involves detailed consultation with management. A comprehensive plan to decrease the incidence and severity of injuries may require a willingness to change the corporate culture or the way the company operates.

Gaining Support

For a corporate back injury prevention process to be successful, management must support it. Although this fact seems simplistic, companies often need to be persuaded that they really can influence the rate and severity of work related injuries. It is frequently necessary to convince them that a proactive, organized effort on their part will pay dividends.

Top management is motivated by bottom line profit. If they can be convinced injury prevention will increase the profitability of the company, they will support it. There is good evidence that back injury prevention procedures, as described in this chapter, can reduce Workers' Compensation costs. It will be necessary to present this information to members of the management team to help them make the decision to implement effective interventions, policies, and procedures.

Getting department managers and supervisors to buy in to the program may be a different story. Often, managers and supervisors live within their own departments and have somewhat misguided ideas of their ultimate role with the company. A production manager or engineer, for example, may think their job is to produce quality products as quickly and efficiently as possible. If a new assembly line design or work procedure improves production by 5%, they will, of course, think it is a good idea and want to implement it as soon as possible.

What if the new design or procedure also increases the risk of back injuries? Department managers and supervisors need to recognize that they are not paid to simply produce, they are paid to help produce profits. Profit can be dramatically affected by changes in a company's or department's injury expenses.

The main question is "who pays for what?" The improved production may add to the apparent bottom line of the department, but who will pay for the associated increase in injuries? When production department managers are held accountable to a safety or Workers' Compensation budget, they will immediately see that increasing production at the expense of increased injuries is not necessarily a good idea. On the other hand, when the health and compensation department at corporate headquarters pays for the direct

cost of the injury, the production department manager may not consider the same factors in a decision to make a potentially negative change in the production process.

One of the goals of this process is to help department managers and supervisors to see the same bottom line as top management. One means of providing more information to department managers and supervisors is to charge Workers' Compensation costs back to budgets of the departments in which injury was caused. The injury thus becomes an expense item on their budgets, the same as raw materials. In this manner they will be factored into the efficiency formula, and department managers and supervisors will see that health and safety become production issues which affect bottom line profits.

Typically, top management support comes by way of funding work station modifications and other positive changes, and by the clear communication of policies and procedures, including written directives. All levels of the management team must be vocal and visible in their efforts to decrease and manage injuries. Management cannot simply give "lip service" to injury reduction, but must be seen as an active champion and facilitator of the entire prevention process.

Providing Authority

In addition to supporting the back injury prevention process, top management must provide authority for implementation, establish accountability for actions to be taken, and delegate responsibility to appropriate team members to put recommended policies and procedures into effect.

This may require a major shift in the current corporate culture. If management has done a good job of selling the program to department managers and supervisors, establishing accountability, and creating added responsibilities for certain team members the shift can be a smooth process.

Changing Attitudes Toward Work Injuries

Making department managers and supervisors accountable for the injuries occurring in their departments is an important step in helping the company to become more proactive and less reactive. The direct supervisor's attitude is particularly important because they are the most visible representative of management in the work environment. For this reason, training sessions relevant to the needs of the supervisor are important in helping them to understand the roles they play in preventing and managing back injuries. If the supervisor has misconceptions about the cause and effect of back injuries, an adversarial relationship can easily develop between the supervisor and the employees.

In an atmosphere of inadequate information and mistrust, these adversarial relationships can easily occur and undermine the effectiveness of the injury prevention process.

Supervisors should be aware that many back injuries occur gradually without any definite precipitating incident. In a work environment where the supervisor may be suspicious of episodes of back pain, the following thoughts may occur:

1. Why wasn't the injury reported when it happened?
2. How do I know this injury didn't occur at home?
3. How do I know the employee isn't trying to get out of work?
4. How do I know a back injury is real? I can't see the problem.
5. Doesn't everyone's back hurt at one time or another? Mine sure does, but I don't miss work because of it.

Without appropriate support and training, this supervisor can turn a minor problem into a major and expensive legal confrontation. In a study presented by Gunnar Andersson, at the International Society for the Study of the Lumbar Spine, the additional cost of involving an attorney in cases of low back pain was stated to be $26,000.[3]

When litigation can be avoided through the use of effective labor-management relationships, money can usually be saved. Injury reports, incorrectly handled, may lead injured workers down a long path that directs them toward disability. In the end, both the employee and the employer are losers.

Attitude change on the part of management and supervisors can dramatically affect injury severity. Three years after introducing a training program at American Biltrite, Fitzler, and Berger[12, 13] reported a 90% reduction in back injury claims, a 50% reduction in lost workdays and a ten-fold reduction in Workers' Compensation costs. The goal of their training program was to have managers and supervisors understand the causes and "commonness" of back pain and to simply accept back pain reports without exhibiting disgust or suspicion.

When reports of pain are addressed early and appropriately, the problems are much less severe, requiring fewer lost work days and are more amenable to simple changes in the job or work environment.

To avoid the problems described above, supervisors must be taught to do the following:

1. *Eliminate problem workers* before they have an injury. The Workers' Compensation system sometimes pays for the mistakes made because an ineffective employee evaluation system is in place. Workers who take advantage of their employers by demonstrating low productivity, poor quality work, and high absenteeism can be expected to take advantage of the Workers' Compensation system, too. Companies with an effective employee hiring and evaluation system eliminate many of these problems before they become major Workers' Compensation cases.
2. *Understand the nature of back injuries,* how they occur, and what causes them, in order to adopt a leadership role in preventing injury.
3. *Convey a positive attitude* when injury does occur. Supervisors should treat injured workers with the same respect they would expect if they were injured. Finding solutions is everyone's responsibility.
4. *Assume the claim is real.* Giving employees the verbal or nonverbal message of disbelief only makes the problem worse. Employees who feel they must prove disability, cost the company much more money in the long run.
5. *Solicit employee involvement.* Employees should be encouraged to provide input to the safety, ergonomics, injury prevention teams. Suggestions and ideas from workers need to be acted upon quickly, so they become part of the solution and to provide visible proof that good ideas from workers' are implemented. Good ideas stop coming in when they are not acted upon. An attitude of learned helplessness and lack of control may flourish, when employee attempts at involvement are ignored.

Establishing Work Procedures and Rules

Management must be aware of the messages their policies, procedures, and practices communicate to the workforce. Issues, as basic as poor housekeeping and lack of preventive maintenance, communicate a message to employees that safety is not really a corporate priority.

Similarly, unrealistic production standards or incentive pay systems do little to encourage safe work practices. Safety incentives that are tied to work days without injury tend to facilitate under-reporting of painful episodes. When an injury is finally reported, it is likely to be even more severe, requiring greater lost time and expense. Further, if these incentives typically apply to the work group as a whole, peer pressure not to report injuries can in many cases be tremendous.

When the risk inherent in jobs cannot be reduced or eliminated, job rotation can be a realistic, workable, and effective solution. Job rotation is best accepted when input regarding the development of the rotation schedule is solicited from affected employees. The consultant's role in this case is to guide the process and assure that employees are rotated among jobs that truly involve different physical stressors. While the physical benefits of a well-planned rotation scheme are obvious, reduced mental fatigue and improved quality may be an added result.

Work rules and procedures within a company need to be evaluated and communicated within the overall context of a safe work environment. Once communicated, it is the responsibility of the supervisor to ensure that these policies are enforced, and the rationale fully understood.

MEDICAL MANAGEMENT

Business and industry can rapidly improve work injury statistics through proper management of the injuries that do require medical attention (Box 9.2). Much of this change can be accomplished simply by teaching workers about back injuries and what comprises effective and noneffective treatment. This same information, of course, will help management and supervisors as they support and counsel injured workers ensuring they receive proper and timely care. Active involvement by management with the medical providers who actually treat injured employees is equally important. Management can be effective in the following ways:

1. Encourage early, aggressive treatment of reported injuries. When an individual reports an injury or the first symptoms of a cumulative trauma problem, management should encourage early, aggressive, conservative care. Acute injuries are easier to treat than chronic ones.

2. Find competent physicians and therapists. A company must find competent physicians and therapists with whom to work, if they are going to implement an effective medical management program. Company personnel must

actively seek physicians and therapists who emphasize reasonable ergonomic modification, exercise, education, and self-responsibility. Once secured, these providers must have a clear understanding of the company's expectations of them.

3. Encourage employees to see designated medical providers. Employers cannot afford to allow their employees to receive care from physicians and therapists who do not support their injury prevention and management philosophies. Workers' Compensation laws vary from state to state, and companies do not always have total control over employees' choice of health care provider. Experience has shown that companies with an organized, positive, and predetermined approach to injury management are able to direct most injured workers to the carefully selected provider.

4. Provide modified duty and on-the-job Work Hardening and make sure medical providers understand. It is essential that the company's medical providers understand the available return-to-work options and corporate philosophy, so that they will encourage the return of the injured worker to appropriate work as early as possible. Some experts believe return-to-work is the single most effective treatment that can be offered to the injured worker.[23] Management and all employees must understand that return-to-work is a treatment issue and not a production issue. There is considerable evidence that returning injured workers is cost-effective, even if little or no productive work is accomplished.[8,19,22,24,25] Coworkers provide one of the best sources of support, for individuals with work-related stress or strain.[16]

A common mistake made with modified duty return-to-work programs is that they have been used as the only method of treatment or rehabilitation. In such cases, the injured worker is likely to remain status quo for weeks or months at a time. The return-to-work process should always be associated with time limits and involve weekly or biweekly reassessments and updates by the physician and therapist. Because coworker relationships are so important to the return-to-work process, on-the-job Work Hardening programs are preferred to clinical Work Hardening programs when they can be appropriately structured.

5. Make sure medical providers consider ergonomic factors in the treatment plan. The medical provider must have basic knowledge of the interaction between the essential functions of the job and the employee's abilities.

BOX 9.2

Medical Management Strategies

1. Encourage early, aggressive treatment of reported injuries
2. Find competent physicians and therapists
3. Encourage employees to see designated medical providers
4. Provide modified duty and on-the-job Work Hardening, making sure medical providers understand it
5. Make sure medical providers consider ergonomic factors in the treatment plan

An ergonomic change may be the most important treatment. Even if the patient has symptom relief, return to the same job without ergonomic changes may cause the problem to recur.

CLAIMS MANAGEMENT

Worker injuries need to be managed as well as treated. The medical providers treat the individual, but the company manages the case. It is no longer appropriate to rely solely upon the doctor's opinion about the injured worker's care and medical management. Obviously, the Workers' Compensation insurance company will be involved in case management to some degree, but it is still necessary for company management to know medical management principles (if for no other reason than to make sure their insurance carrier is doing a good job) and to communicate concern to the employee while fostering a positive mental attitude (Box 9.3).

For this reason a corporate claims management philosophy should emphasize regular contact with an injured employee and effective communication with medical providers.

To accomplish these objectives, companies should have specific, written claims management policies. The policies should clearly outline a sequence to be followed every time there is an employee incident that may result in a lost time injury. The following list is an example of an appropriate claims management policy:

1. When an accident occurs, the supervisor determines the severity of the injury. If the injury cannot be treated by in-house first aid, the injured employee is provided transportation to the medical provider the company has selected. A standardized form is sent along with the employee. The form is to be used by the treating provider to clearly list the employee's restrictions and time frames.

2. Once the initial treatment is over, the company's standard form is completed by the treating provider and returned with the employee. Transportation is provided for the employee to return to the workplace.

3. The employee and supervisor meet to discuss the incident or injury and the restrictions if applicable. They determine how long the employee is going to be off work, if at all. If the case is complex or appears to involve extensive lost time, the supervisor and appropriate management personnel will be involved immediately, to plan the employee's return-to-work process.

4. If the employee must miss work, the supervisor or management representative will explain the employee benefits and rights under Workers' Compensation law. Complete details will be discussed about the weekly wage, when it will be received, who will be sending it, and how payment will be arranged.

5. The supervisor contacts the employee regularly during time away from work. These contacts are to make sure the employee is receiving benefits and adequate medical care, and to communicate that the employee is an important part of the organization. Whenever a contact is made, the discussion will always include mention of when the employee will return to work and what type of job will be available at that time.

6. A specific return-to-work plan will be developed for any employee who will be off work two weeks or more. It is the manager's and supervisor's responsibility to determine precisely what jobs are available for the employee within the restrictions that have been set forth by the treating physician. Part of this determination involves establishing a plan and submitting it to the treating physician for review.

7. Once the physician accepts the return-to-work plan, the supervisor meets with the employee to discuss the details and inform what work will be available and when.

8. When the employee, physician, and employer have agreed upon the return-to-work program, the plan is submitted to the insurance adjuster.

9. The facility's manager, the departmental supervisor, and appropriate management personnel will monitor the employee's work load while being on modified duty. They will be

---

BOX 9.3

Claims Management Strategies

1. Emphasize regular and effective communication with the injured employee and the medical providers
2. Establish specific written claims management policies, and adhere to them
3. Know and internalize medical management principles to make sure they are being followed correctly
4. Progress towards case closure when maximum benefit from medical treatment is achieved

certain the employee is performing tasks within restrictions. Progress toward release to full-time duty is discussed periodically with the employee.

10. Injured workers must not be allowed to continue ineffective treatment. If progress is not being made with a certain treatment approach, the Claims Manager must be proactive and ask the treating physician about other methods.

Case Closure Considerations

Eventually, the injured worker will achieve maximum benefit from medical treatment. Too often, cases go on and on, from one physician to another with very little progress, if any. The employee has probably achieved maximum benefit from available medical care if:

- There has been appropriate evaluation, treatment, and rehabilitation,
- The employee has received multiple medical opinions, and
- An unusual amount of time has lapsed since injury.

These employees may return to a permanent job within restrictions at the present company, or may have to be placed outside the company. Cases should be settled. Keeping the first one open that is progressing with no end in sight is damaging for both employee and employer.

Another case that must be settled is the uncooperative employee. When the employee refuses to cooperate with the treatment and rehabilitation plan, the case must be hastened to conclusion. Good communication between the company, the insurance adjuster, and the medical providers is critical to identify and manage these cases.

Positive Atmosphere

The key to long-term success in managing injured employees is developing a positive, open line of communication between the supervisor and injured worker. If an employee genuinely feels that management cares about his or her well-being, they will be more inclined to cooperate. A positive atmosphere is extremely important. The objective is to make the employee feel secure and welcome. Without this feeling, an employee is far more likely to seek legal counsel, which will only result in higher costs and increased frustration.

ERGONOMICS

Ergonomics is one of the essential components of an effective injury prevention process. Ergonomics, literally the study of work, has been classically defined as the science of designing workplaces, machines, and tasks with the capabilities and limitations of the human body in mind. By applying the basic principles of ergonomics, the company and its employees can make great strides toward a safer, more productive work environment.

The best ergonomist is the employee doing the job. A major aspect of an ergonomics program involves workers and front line supervisors in the process of performing a basic ergonomic analysis of their work areas. When management supports the ergonomic process and when the basic principles of ergonomics are understood, the employees can return to their workplace and implement appropriate changes or recommend possible solutions.

Worksite evaluation and redesign may also be performed by experts who are trained in industrial engineering and ergonomics. If specific problems are found that cannot be corrected by application of the basic principles of ergonomics, a company may hire an ergonomic consultant to redesign a particular job or machine. Even if major worksite redesign is impractical, simple and inexpensive modifications can often be made to greatly reduce the risk of back injury.

When conducting the ergonomic evaluation, it is important to note good examples as well as bad. Much of the information gathered during the ergonomic survey will later be incorporated into training sessions. As we will discuss, customization of training materials goes a long way toward encouraging attentiveness and interest.

Purpose of an Ergonomic Survey

It is important that a worksite evaluation or ergonomic survey of the work area is performed very early when undertaking back injury prevention. It is done for two purposes:

1. To familiarize the prevention team with the work process, tasks, and procedures so that any education or training courses can be customized to address specific problem areas.
2. To identify problem areas that should be redesigned or modified to prevent injuries.

The prevention team should be familiar with the company's injury records before worksite evaluation begins. This information can direct team members or outside consultants to specific areas requiring immediate attention.

Performing an Ergonomic Survey

Some basic design principles must be understood before performing a worksite evaluation. With these principles firmly in mind, worksite evaluation should begin by reviewing an activity or job which requires

FIGURE 9.2 Work surface heights that are too low **(A)** should be modified to ensure proper postures are encouraged **(B).**

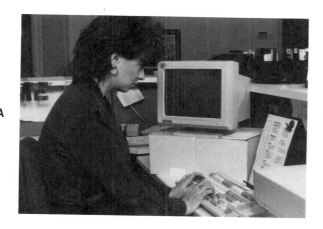 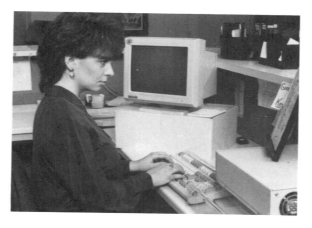

excessive physical demand, or one which has been responsible for one or more injuries or pain complaints in the past. All the jobs in the work area should then be carefully analyzed for potential risk factors.

Back pain can result from many different sources. It is important to consider more than just the heavy lifting jobs. Potential problem areas include:

1. *Work too low.* If the work is too low, an employee will be forced to stand or sit with the head forward, shoulders slightly rounded, and the low back in a forward bent position. Ways should be sought to reduce the need to bend forward. The work may be raised or tilted toward the worker. Ideally, the work station should be adjustable. The right work height also depends on the type of work:
   - Most work should be performed with the hands at elbow height, (Figures 9.2, *A, B*).
   - Light, precision work should be performed with the hands above elbow height,
   - Heavy work should be performed with the hands below elbow height.

   If the work surface height is not adjustable, fixed height work stations should be biased toward taller individuals. Shorter individuals may be accommodated by providing platforms to stand on (Figures 9.3, *A, B*).

2. *Work too high.* Continuously working at or above shoulder level can be very stressful. Tasks that cause the elbows to exceed a 45° angle away from the sides or front of the body should be modified. Attempts should be made to lower the work height or raise the worker. This can often be accomplished by using raised work platforms, rearranging storage areas, or by providing stair platform ladders that are safer than step ladders. A policy should be

in place, and enforced, such that ladders are returned to a fixed and predictable location to assure ready access to them (Figures 9.3, *A, B*).

3. *Work too far away.* Whether the worker is standing or sitting, repetitive or continued forward reaching at arm's length is very stressful. All work should be performed in a manner allowing efficient use of the arms, and shoulders, without creating a long lever arm that transfers excessive force to the neck, arms, and back. The least stressful work position involves working with the hands positioned between elbow and waist height, with the elbows held close to the sides and front of the body. In some cases, simply providing toe space under a work surface can bring the worker six to twelve inches closer to the work (Figures 9.4, *A, B*).

4. *Work activities in confined areas or that require twisting.* If there is limited space for employees to maneuver and move objects, they will often twist to accomplish the task. Repetitive twisting is one of the most damaging movements for the back. There should be enough floor space for the employee to pivot the feet when lifting or moving an item. In some cases, it helps to place items far enough apart so the employee must turn and step, rather than twist. Swivel chairs help workers who are sitting. Conveyors, chutes, slides, and turntables can be used to change the direction of material flow. When possible finished parts should be placed within 90° of the work area to limit excessive rotation. Allowance should be made for proper clearance through doorways and down aisles (Figures 9.5, *A, B*).

5. *Prolonged standing on hard, concrete surfaces.* The

FIGURE 9.3   Work surface heights that are too high **(A)** should either be lowered or the worker should be raised in order to prevent injury.

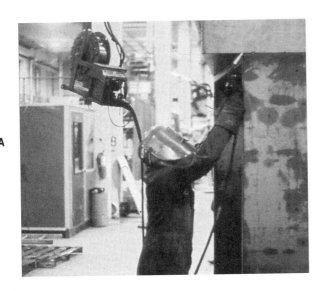

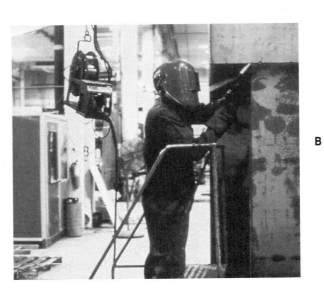

FIGURE 9.4   Excessive reaching should be eliminated **(A)** in order to avoid the excessive forces that are transferred to the neck, arms, and back **(B).**

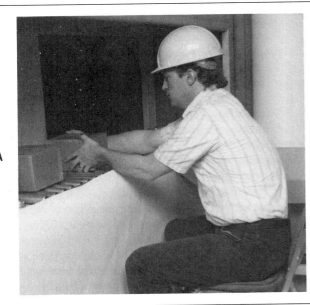

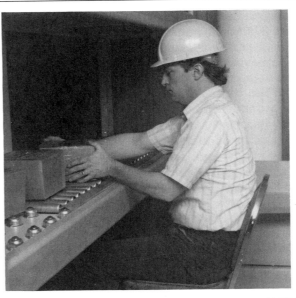

FIGURE 9.5 A, B, C   Work spaces should be modified to eliminate twisting movements.

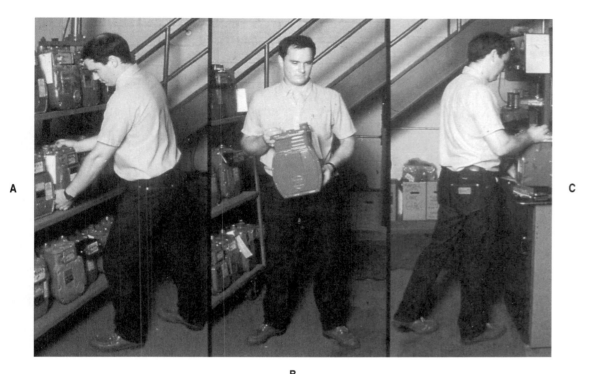

A

B

C

muscles of the low back work to maintain the standing position. Without occasional relief, these muscles become fatigued. A foot rail, box, or stool allows the worker to raise one foot and reduce stress. Rearranging the work so the employee alternates between standing and sitting tasks, or allowing a brief stretching break periodically throughout the day may also effectively reduce fatigue. Antifatigue mats, visco-elastic cushioned shoe inserts, shoes with leather uppers, cushioned soles and heels designed for work, also reduce strain on the legs and back (Figures 9.6, *A, B*).

6. *Sitting or standing in a static position for prolonged periods.* When work requires intense concentration or does not allow movement, the back can become fatigued or tense. It is important to provide some movement to relieve the stress that occurs. Work spaces might be rearranged to assure that people move periodically. Jobs that are designed to provide a variation between sitting and standing activities are less likely to be related to pain or injury because they facilitate normal joint and muscle movement.

7. *Sitting with the back unsupported* Sitting work increases pressure within the disc more than standing work. This effect becomes even more pronounced if the worker slouches forward to complete work. A high stool with no back or foot support is a common example of a work station that encourages the employee to assume a slouched position (Figure 9.7).

Chairs and stools should provide support for the lower back and pelvis and allow the feet to rest on the floor, or foot support, comfortably. The head, shoulders, and hips should all be aligned and supported in an erect, well-balanced position. Ideally, the chair adjustment controls should be easily accessed from the sitting position. The back support should be easily adjustable to enable control of its height, angle, and position relative to the seat pan. It should be curved to support the neutral, inward curve of the lower back. The height and seat pan angle should adjust easily to accommodate variations in the work tasks. The chair should roll and pivot easily and have arms and other special features if needed (Figure 9.8).

If the back support of the chair is flat, a rolled towel, small pillow, or cushion can be used to fit the inward curve of the low back. A variety of cushions and back supports are available for office chairs, automobile, and truck seats. Some truck and automobile manu-

FIGURE 9.6 A, B Back fatigue from prolonged sitting and standing can be decreased through work space modification and exercise.

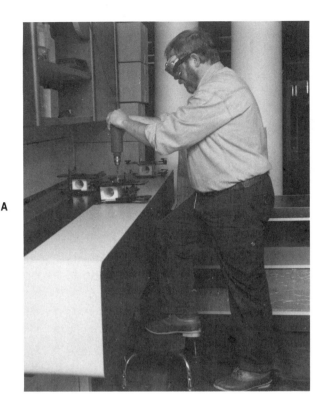

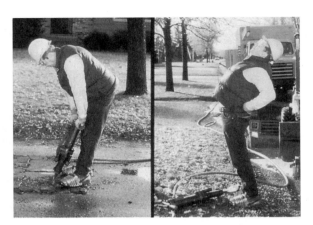

FIGURE 9.7 High stool with no back or foot support encourages the employee to assume a slouched position.

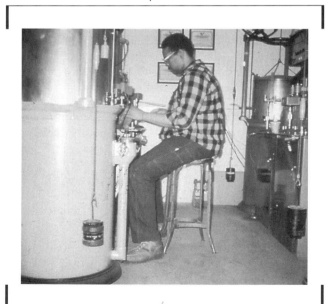

(From Saunders, HD: Self Help Manual For Your Neck, Minneapolis, 1986, The Saunders Group, Inc.)

facturers have made an effort to improve the seats in their cars and trucks. Advanced, air-ride truck seats are readily available, fully adjustable, and contoured to provide support to the lower and mid back.

8. *Frequent manual material handling.* Any time employees lift and carry objects, even when proper body mechanics are used, there is potential for a problem. Manual materials-handling tasks should be reduced or eliminated by usage of lift tables, lift trucks, hoists, work dispensers, conveyors, and similar mechanical aids when possible. To eliminate the lifting and reaching tasks completely, materials can be delivered to the worker by roller ball caster tables, automatic conveyor systems, or other means.

Four basic principles of task design for manual material handling should be followed:
- Minimize the weight or bulk
- Minimize the vertical and horizontal lifting distances
- Provide sufficient time for stressful tasks, and
- Work with, rather than against, gravity whenever possible

FIGURE 9.8 Chair which can provide proper support for the worker.

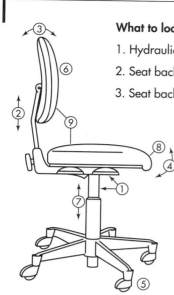

What to look for in a chair:

1. Hydraulic controls

2. Seat back adjusts up/down

3. Seat back pivots forward/backward

4. Seat pan tilts

5. Five caster-easy roll base

6. Seatback supports natural lumbar curve

7. Seat height adjusts

8. Waterfall seat front

9. Seat back and seat pan appropriate size for user

Additional features when needed:

- Arm rests
- Stool height with foot rests
- Self-locking casters
- Material/fabric appropriate for environment
- Casters for carpeted versus vinyl floors

(From Saunders, HD: Self Help Manual For Your Neck, Minneapolis, 1986, The Saunders Group, Inc.)

Many items used by companies today can be packaged in smaller boxes or containers. Some vendors may be able to ship products in bulk, so the only way they can be handled is by mechanical means. This type of shipment takes the entire process out of the workers' manual materials handling loop.

The factors below should be considered when ordering supplies. Boxes and bags of materials can be broken down and placed into tote containers with handles. This not only lightens the load, but also eliminates reaching all the way down to the floor to lift the container. Shelves should be arranged so that the heavier, more frequently used items are between shoulder and waist height, which is a more convenient height for lifting. The lighter, less frequently used items are placed higher. The rarely used items should be on the lowest shelves. Another idea uses baskets or storage pallets that can be tipped for easier access. Side opening baskets also help avoid excessive bending (Figure 9.9, *A*).

9. *Awkward or oversized loads.* Manual handling of an awkward or oversized load can be a dangerous task if not performed properly. Employees should be encouraged to ask for help or use an assistive device if they are unsure of their ability to handle a load safely. If a load is oversized and is being handled manually, repackaging the material, using mechanical assistance, or performing a team lift should be considered (Figures 9.9, *B*, *C*).

10. *Miscellaneous hazards.* Pieces of metal, paper, and liquid spills on the floor are all potential hazards for trips, slips, and falls. It is important, therefore, that the quality and regularity of housekeeping and maintenance is at acceptable levels. Absorbent material should be readily available to handle spills, and proper non-slip footwear should be worn.

Equipment which is improperly maintained may require more force or non-optimal postures to perform the job. Therapists and consultants should always note these conditions on an ergonomic survey.

FITNESS FOR WORK

Even when the worksite or work practices cannot be optimized, the condition of the worker can always be improved. The fitness of the worker can be approached from several perspectives. Exercises can be used to improve cardiovascular condition; increase flexibility and strength; promote relaxation; and control fatigue through position reversal and circulation stimulation (Box 9.4).

There is considerable evidence to indicate that people who are in poor physical condition and practice other unhealthy lifestyles are at greater risk of back injury.[2,6,7,10,18,21] Therefore, it seems logical that one important aspect of a back injury prevention program would be to help individuals identify deficiencies and attempt to help them improve their level of physical fitness. It is important to emphasize that many work situations are like athletic events. They require a

---

BOX 9.4

Benefits of Exercise

1. Improve cardiovascular condition
2. Improve flexibility and strength
3. Promote relaxation
4. Control fatigue through position reversal and circulation stimulation

FIGURE 9.9 A, B, C   Materials handling tasks should be reduced or eliminated by using mechanical aids, team efforts, or positioning modifications.

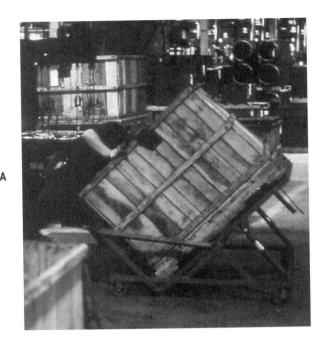

A

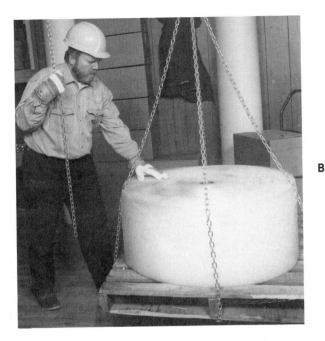

B

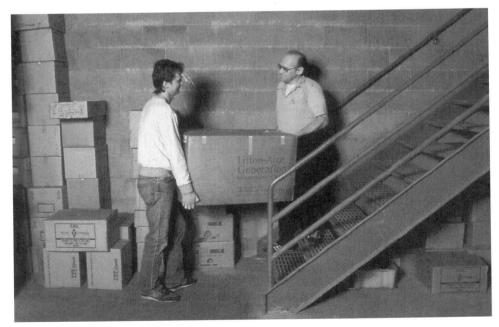

C

certain level of physical fitness, strength, and flexibility. Many people attempt to work at jobs that require considerable physical labor and involve stressful positions, but they make little or no effort to keep their bodies in the physical condition required to do these jobs.

It is true that most individuals work hard at their jobs, and it is difficult for many to concur on the need for exercise after already being tired from work. However, hard work rarely provides the intensity required to obtain an aerobic benefit necessary for cardiovascular conditioning. In addition, workers tend to use certain muscles and joints and not others. That is why many people can work hard all day, yet still have stiffness in some areas. An exercise program should emphasize the type of activity that is lacking at work.

Company Exercise Programs

A certain number of individuals will indeed be motivated to exercise on a regular basis through such an independent program. It is unrealistic to expect that every employee will be motivated enough to participate in a home exercise program. Some companies are taking the issue of fitness for work to a much higher level than simply teaching about it in an educational program. Many are actually encouraging exercise programs by subsidizing memberships to local health clubs or by setting up corporate fitness centers. Health center staff can help individuals to understand the exercise requirements for obtaining the aerobic, strength, and flexibility benefits they receive from exercise (Box 9.5).

On-the-job exercise is an important component of the total injury prevention process and has created a great deal of interest in industry. Many companies begin by offering voluntary exercise programs. In such cases, the company usually hires an instructor to provide exercise training. In companies where groups are formed, participants often volunteer to lead the sessions. On-the-job exercise programs are usually related to group flexibility and strengthening or to personal fatigue control exercises.

Mandatory exercise during work is currently attracting some interest and companies are experimenting with these types of exercise programs on a limited basis. If these programs prove to be effective, mandatory exercise during work hours may become a

popular way to reduce work-related back injuries. The obvious advantage to mandatory exercise is that those who are in poor physical condition and lack motivation to exercise on their own, can be required to participate.

Perhaps one of the most effective uses of mandatory exercise is to require participation by those who have had previous back problems, or have scored poorly on strength and flexibility tests or Job Placement Assessments. It is often easier to get these people to participate willingly after they have received training or have been evaluated objectively in company evaluation programs.

Importance of Employee Support

Even though mandatory, an exercise program can backfire if it does not have the grassroots support of employees. With this support, peer pressure can become an effective motivator to get all workers to participate. Companies should move with caution if they plan to implement a program of this sort without emphasis on employee participation in the decision-making process, regarding how and when these exercises should be performed and presented to the remainder of the work force.

The role of the supervisor is critical in fostering acceptance of the exercises. The effective supervisor can organize and participate in warm-up exercises before starting work, and lead or be an example in using fatigue control exercises throughout the work day, to reverse positions, stimulate blood flow, and reduce stress.

Exercise Frequency

While fatigue control exercise performed for short periods throughout the day appeal to our common sense, they are sometimes simply difficult to remember to do. When possible, consultants should consider connecting the performance of brief, twenty second exercise pauses every twenty minutes, (the "20/20 rule") to some of the following triggers:

1. When workers experience fatigue or work-related discomfort,
2. When properly-positioned posters or business-card size exercise reminders are seen,
3. When work tasks are completed on an interval based cycle such as filling a box, loading a pallet, or emptying a bin of supplies or raw material,
4. When a bell or buzzer sounds or music is played at a regular interval, and
5. When observing coworkers or supervisors performing the exercises.

In companies or departments of more than 200 employees, there should always be someone exercising to control fatigue at any one point in time.

BOX 9.5

Company Fitness Strategies

1. Provide exercise alternatives which may include:
   - Subsidized health club memberships
   - A corporate fitness center
   - On-the-job exercise
   - Mandatory exercise of previously injured workers.
2. Acquire and maintain employee support.
3. Emphasize exercise frequency.
4. Assess each employee and provide individualized exercise programs that are functional and biomechanically sound.

Individualized Strength and Flexibility Assessment

The strength and flexibility assessment results should give the employee an objective determination of their strengths and weaknesses, provide the necessary knowledge to correct any problem that may be found, and foster encouragement to take responsibility for their own wellness and safe work practices.

To achieve widespread acceptance of back strength and flexibility exercise programs, the assessment must be practical, easy to use, affordable, and comprehensive enough to include all appropriate exercises. It is common to find people who are strong or flexible in one part of their body, yet weak or stiff in another. These strengths and weaknesses are usually job related or may even be related to the type of exercise program in which an individual is participating (too many low back flexion activities and not enough emphasis on extension strength and flexibility). Assessments that test only one or two movements will usually miss these out-of-balance individuals.

Above all, a program of assessment and training in back strength and flexibility should be functional and biomechanically sound. Many back testing devices or machines are promoted as more objective or "scientifically based" than the simple assessment exam advocated by the authors. Moreover, therapists and consultants should be wary of devices that assess strength and range of motion in nonfunctional or inappropriate biomechanical positions. For example, measuring total range of motion from flexion to extension is of little value because a score of "normal" does not say anything about how well they can perform the job.

Lifting the trunk with the legs straight and the back in a flexed position is biomechanically unsound. Testing trunk flexion strength in the standing or sitting position requiring a concentric contraction of the abdominal muscles is also unsound. Industrial workers should not be tested in this manner for safety and practicality reasons. Only strength and flexibility assessment tests which are readily converted into corrective exercises that are easily performed at home or at work should be used.

Normal standards for range of motion and strength are lacking, and opinion varies about what constitutes normal range of motion and strength. Some opinions expressed in the literature are based on scientific studies, while others are based on experience and the particular bias of the author. For this reason, the authors recommend that the tester use well reasoned objectivity to determine acceptable levels of flexibility and strength, without becoming too technical.

The strength and flexibility assessment tests the authors recommend (Box 9.6) can be done at the work-

---

BOX 9.6

Strength & Flexibility Assessment Tests

TEST	SATISFACTORY RESPONSE
A. Lumbar Flexion (Figure 9.10, *A*)	Lumbar spine flattens to neutral during sitting toe touch
B. Lumbar Extension (Figure 9.10, *B*)	Ability to achieve test position with smooth lumbar curve
C. Lumbar Rotation (Figure 9.10, *C*)	Ability to achieve test position
D. Hamstring Flexibility (Figure 9.10, *D*)	Ability to achieve test position with 80–110° hip flexion
E. Hip Flexor Flexibility (Figure 9.10, *E*)	Ability to achieve test position with knee (on side of extended hip) flexed to 80°
F. Hip Joint Flexion Flexibility (Figure 9.10, *F*)	Ability to achieve test position with hip (on side of flexed hip) flexed to 125°
G. Squat to Stand Strength and Flexibility (Figure 9.10, *G*)	Ability to achieve test position and repeat correctly ten times
H. Shoulder Girdle Strength and Flexibility (Figure 9.10, *H*)	Ability to achieve and maintain test position (hands 9″ off floor) for 30 seconds
I. Back and Hip Extension Strength (Figure 9.10, *I*)	Ability to maintain test position for 60 seconds
J. Abdominal Strength (Figure 9.10, *J*)	Ability to maintain test position for 10 seconds (repeat with right and left twist)
K. Abdominal Strength (Figure 9.10, *K*)	Ability to maintain test position for 10 seconds
L. Quadriceps Strength (Figure 9.10, *L*)	Ability to maintain test position for 60 seconds

FIGURE 9.10(A-L)   Illustrations of strength and flexibility assessment tests.

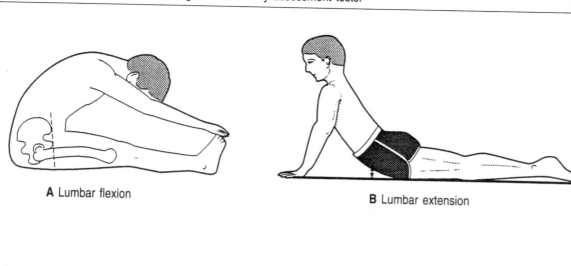

A Lumbar flexion

B Lumbar extension

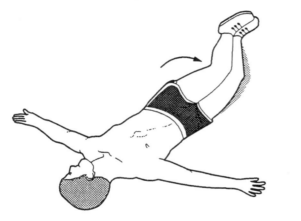

C Lumbar rotation

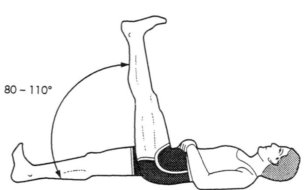

80 – 110°

D Hamstring flexibility

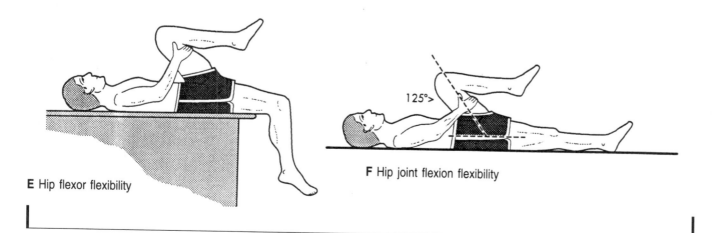

E Hip flexor flexibility

125°>

F Hip joint flexion flexibility

FIGURE 9.10(A-L)   *cont'd*

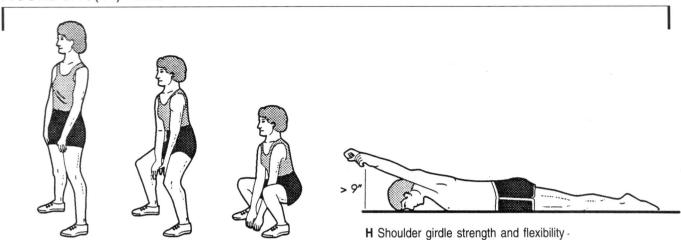

G Squat to stand strength and flexibility

H Shoulder girdle strength and flexibility

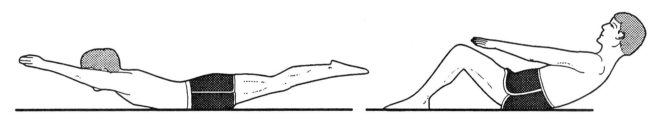

I Back and hip extension strength

J Abdominal strength

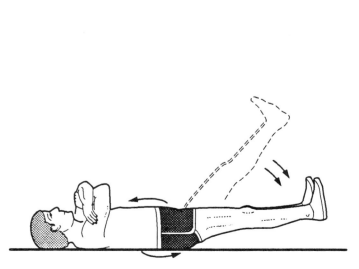

K Abdominal strength

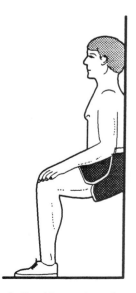

L Quadriceps strength

site, requiring less than one hour of each employee's time. One evaluator can assess and train a group of six to eight people per hour. No expensive equipment is involved. The test positions easily convert into exercises that can be done at home. The basic rule of thumb is that any exercise on which an employee's performance is less than satisfactory should be incorporated into that employee's overall fitness program. Some companies schedule regular follow-up evaluations to assess the employee's progress toward strength and flexibility goals. This method of follow-up helps to assure accountability on the part of the employee to begin and hopefully continue exercises and pursue a more healthy lifestyle.

EDUCATION AND TRAINING

There is much controversy about the effect injury prevention training programs can have on back injuries. Some studies show that back injury prevention training has no effect on injury statistics. These studies contain questionable standardization of methods, make faulty basic assumptions, and contain flaws in the experimental design.[9,17,26,28,31]

The effectiveness of back injury prevention training programs has been difficult to assess, partly because of the wide variety of topics the various training programs emphasize. Some programs emphasize training in exercise, rest postures, first aid, or body mechanics, while others concentrate on management training to effect attitudinal and administrative changes.

Case Histories

The earliest and most often cited study of back school effectiveness was that of Bergquist-Ullman and Larsson.[5] In this study, an educational program resulted in a 30% reduction in the time required to return to work after injury and a 50% decrease in the time required for recovery (14.8 days for the training group and 28.7 days for a placebo group). Johnson[30] reported that after injury prevention training, PPG Industries experienced a 70% to 90% reduction in injury rates and costs at two years.

Tomer, et al[32] reported a 67% reduction in back liability claims and 70% decrease in lost workdays after introducing back injury prevention training at Lockheed Missiles and Space Company. In a massive undertaking at Southern Pacific Transportation Company, 39,000 employees participated in training to reduce the incidence and severity of back pain episodes. The low back injury rate decreased 22%, and there was a concomitant 43% decrease in lost workdays two years after training was initiated.[28]

BOX 9.7

Results of Comprehensive Back Injury Prevention Process

Case	Results
Elk River Nursing Home	95% decrease in lost time back injuries over a two year period.
ADC Telecommunications	69% decrease in lost time back injuries.
Gross Given Manufacturing	22% decrease in lost time; 43% decrease in lost time injuries

---

In her study of eight different industries, Melton[20] reported a 40% decrease in lost work days with associated reductions in medical insurance premiums. Although an increase in the reports of lower back pain was noted, those reporting showed an 86% reduction in lost time days. Hultman, Nordin, and Ortengren[15] reported the effect of training upon postural changes observed at the worksite. Their results showed a 74% increase in the time spent in "safe" postures and a 54% reduction in time spent in "risky" postures, at three months post training. Examples of the authors' consulting experience as demonstrated in Box 9.7 indicates the positive results of implementing a comprehensive back injury prevention process for several clients of The Saunders Group in Minneapolis.[11]

Implementation

From this wealth of confirming data, it is clear that successful back injury prevention includes education and training. Effective dissemination of information is essential if the injury prevention process is going to succeed. While the content and style of presentation are critical, creating a relaxed and friendly environment can also help with acceptance and buy-in of the back injury prevention process. Simple things such as providing snacks and beverages during training are appreciated by most employees.

While many concepts regarding management's role in overall prevention training have already been discussed, a back injury prevention training program should never be offered to hourly employees without first obtaining management's commitment to the process. This commitment is gained through effective education of management personnel, making them aware of their important role in any companywide prevention process.

Selling the Process to Managers and Employees

Gaining total company support from all levels of management, typically involves a series of meetings in which the Industrial Therapist is selling their credibility and the program's benefits of initiating such a process.

The first such meeting often entails an informational "marketing" session with one or two upper middle managers, such as the human resources or safety manager. It is in this initial meeting that the foundation is laid for the principles on which all subsequent interventions and methods will be based.

This is the time to provide an overview of the recommended process based on an understanding of the corporate culture. When the initial contacts with the Therapist are satisfactory, the stage is set to request a buy-in meeting with upper level managers.

Before an upper level management meeting can take place, the initial contacts will have to "presell" the clinic or Therapist to convince these top managers to attend. These initial contacts must believe that the clinic or Therapist can help them achieve their goals before they will be willing to take highly paid personnel away from their jobs.

When possible, the upper level managers who attend this meeting should have decision-making authority, like the president or chief executive officers. This meeting should be relatively short and discussion oriented, lasting one hour or less. Frequently, the initial contact will introduce the clinic or Therapist and the basic concepts to be discussed. The Therapist's role as consultant is to provide a professional presence and fill in any perceived gaps in the managers' understanding of the overall picture. Ideally, the benefits of the process should be expressed in terms of productivity and quality, as these are concepts with which managers are comfortable. It is important, however, not to present too much detail, as this may tend to drag out the meeting and provide increased opportunity for dissension.

The managers should leave the meeting with an understanding of the current scope of back injury problems at their company and the resolution that the prevention program can bring. They should also have a good understanding of the critical role they play within the process, and a realistic expectation of outcomes based on the selected intervention methods and prevailing corporate culture.

After the management group becomes committed to the process, it is frequently helpful to make another presentation to the safety committee members and union leaders, when appropriate. It is during this stage that employees are encouraged to voice opinions on how the process should be laid out. The simple fact that they are allowed to be involved dramatically impacts the success of the process. People lend stronger support to things they help to create.

Some companies, because of their size or complexity, require selected individuals to become ergonomic advocates or group exercise leaders. When there is a need for this type of specified training, it should also occur prior to employee level training. When training is conducted in this sequence, the chosen advocates or leaders can be introduced during and incorporated into the employee sessions.

It is important that effective systems are in place, to respond to the increased employee interest and input that training is likely to foster. The best way to kill an otherwise effective process occurs when employee input is disregarded, or not responded to, in an effective or timely fashion.

Implementation of Training

After all of these important bases have been covered, employee training can begin. Upper and middle managers and supervisors should also attend training with hourly employees, even though some of the material will be redundant for them. Top management needs to be seen as active participants and facilitators of prevention, rather than passive observers.

A representative from the company's Workers' Compensation insurance carrier should participate in any educational programs presented to management and employees, so that the insurance adjusters handling the company's claims are well-informed about company philosophy and policies.

Although the amount and scope of information varies depending on the group focus, there is some information about back injuries with which everyone must be familiar so that everyone is working from a common base. This basic information is outlined in Box 9.8.

Although an educational program must be flexible to meet the individual needs of companies and institutions, a standard or model program should be developed. The basic program should consist of two to four hours of instruction by a qualified, experienced instructor. To achieve maximum effectiveness, no more than 30 participants should be included in each course.

Instruction should be carried out by means of an audio-visual program, instructor demonstration, and active class participation. Open discussion should be encouraged and time should be allotted to answer questions following the presentation. A ten-minute break for each hour of the presentation should be scheduled, with shorter stand-up breaks every fifteen to twenty minutes.

The session should start with a summary of the contents of the whole course. Two common miscon-

---

BOX 9.8

Back Injury Education and Training Program

Essential Elements

1. Establish an understanding of the scope of back injury problems
2. Instruct in anatomy and function of the spine
3. Discuss the common causes of back problems
4. Instruct and demonstrate what to do when an injury occurs
5. Emphasize the importance of a healthy lifestyle, good body mechanics, ergonomics, and fitness
6. Direct instruction toward attitudes, forcing the worker to recognize their obligation and self-responsibility to perform work tasks properly

---

ceptions about the way back injuries occur must be abolished at the outset. Participants need to understand that back injuries are **not** caused by a single event such as lifting a heavy weight (the back "going out"); and that even when there is no pain, a problem may still exist.

The participants should be instructed in the anatomy and function of the back, and the results of research and studies on the back should be presented where appropriate. The mechanical strain experienced in different positions and during different movements should be discussed. The relationship between the center of gravity and strain on the back should also be explained. The function of muscles and their influence on the back should be demonstrated. Unfavorable working postures, using real work place examples, should be analyzed in detail.

The pathology of back injury (muscle, ligament, disc, and joint) should also be discussed in relation to the above-mentioned stressful postures. Various methods of treatment should be analyzed and the body's natural capacity for healing should be emphasized.

The program should teach individuals what to do when a back injury occurs. Participants should be taught that self management of an injury is always more important than what the physician or therapist does. Likewise, participants also need to know that what they do for themselves before an injury occurs, such as exercising, using proper body mechanics, and making changes in the design of their workplace, is as important as what the employer does for them.

Even when a company makes every effort to

eliminate stressful tasks and heavy material handling, there will still be times when the employee will have to choose between safe and unsafe, which technique to use. The technique chosen has a great deal to do with potential for injury. Therefore, employees must be trained in the use of proper techniques and safe work practices. Opportunities to learn and practice these techniques with guidance need to be available. Optimally, this assistance is provided in the work environment to support what was presented in the classroom.

While many workers recognize how to lift and carry properly they do not take proper work procedures seriously. Instruction should be directed strongly toward attitudes, forcing the worker to recognize their obligation and self-responsibility to perform work tasks properly. Appropriate disciplinary procedures and accountability to use safe techniques should be secondary to the employee's internal motivation to change.

The participant should be encouraged to review their personal standards of fitness, nutrition, and stress control. The harmful effects of smoking and its relationship to back pain are also important to point out.[10,18] Participation in various types of physical activities and sports must be encouraged to improve psychological and physical tolerance to work demands and stresses. The participant will also benefit from information regarding proper nutrition as a foundation of good health.

Overweight people tend to be less active, and more readily prone to stiffness, which can foster an even less active lifestyle and even greater weight gain. It might also be pointed out that stress directly affects muscle tension, function, and potential for back pain. The participant could be trained to perform relaxation exercises that can be helpful in reducing stress.

At the conclusion of the program, the participants will benefit from a flexibility and strength evaluation and should follow an exercise program that will help them maintain a healthy back. This would include practicing proper body mechanics and posture techniques. Each participant should receive a booklet or pamphlet outlining the main points of the course. The booklet would also contain a section of general flexibility and strengthening exercises for the spine. Each of the exercises should be demonstrated and discussed in the class.

CASE STUDY

This case study illustrates the need to take a comprehensive look at the factors affecting a company's injury rate and the financial impact of those injuries. This case concerns an actual nursing home that retained the services of The Saunders Group, Inc. in Minneapolis.

The name of the nursing home has been changed to protect confidentiality.

Background

Sunnyvale Nursing Home is a typical 120 bed, long-term care facility in rural Minnesota. The workforce of 137 individuals is mostly young to middle-aged females. For many years, they had a back injury rate that was consistently above the Workers' Compensation average for their category. The high injury rate was causing a morale problem because the "healthy" nurses had to do most of the heavy work and at least two young nurse's aides had suffered considerable pain and disability from back injuries.

The Problem

The administration and board of directors of Sunnyvale expressed a genuine concern about the welfare of their employees. In addition, their Workers' Compensation insurance carrier had given them notice that their injury record had to improve or they would be transferred to the high risk insurance pool.

The high risk pool would double, or even triple their Workers' Compensation insurance rates, which would pose a real threat to the existence of the home as a viable business. The administration and board described it as a crisis. It was under these rather dire circumstances that they decided to undertake whatever measures were necessary to effectively reduce the number and severity of back injuries.

The Saunders Group, Inc. was selected as an injury prevention consulting firm to evaluate the situation, make recommendations and implement total injury prevention.

Toward A Solution

The nursing home had established a Risk Management Task Force consisting of a member of the board of directors, the nursing home administrator, the director of nurses, and the controller. The consultants met with members of the Task Force to be apprised of their perceptions of the problem. A written proposal was then presented to the Task Force outlining the process that came to be called the "Save Your Back Program." The proposal outlined the comprehensive nature of the program, the costs, the time commitment, and their individual responsibilities.

The first recommendation was to form a committee with which the consultants would work as the "Save Your Back Program" was implemented. This was done by expanding the Task Force to involve people significantly affected by the process, including front line supervisors, workers, and department representatives. In the case of Sunnyvale, it involved the physical therapist, the nurse responsible for employee training and education, and the Workers' Compensation claims manager from the human resources department. Several hourly employees were members of the committee. This was necessary to get first hand information from the people who were actually doing the work. It was also important for the hourly employees to feel involved with the program and know that they had input into the process as it developed.

A short presentation was given to the newly formed "Save Your Back Committee" incorporating in a general way, the four intervention strategies (management, ergonomics, education, and fitness) that would be involved as the process unfolded. During this meeting, the consultants tried to listen and learn from all the individuals involved to find out what they thought the problems were. This provided good understanding of the extent of Sunnyvale's problems. Many of the employees disliked the return-to-work program; there was considerable difference of opinion as to the quality of staff training and supervision; and most injured employees were receiving passive treatment, without any rehabilitation or education.

Following this preliminary orientation and gathering of information, a one day on-site evaluation was conducted with one of the nurses from the Task Force. The purpose was to find out about the ergonomic risk factors, work rules, education and training, staff responsibilities, and management of the injured and pre-injured workers. The on-site evaluation revealed major problems in all areas. Since it was uncertain whether Sunnyvale's supervisory staff could be educated and persuaded to support and carry out all the essential changes, these factors were included in the presentation to the Task Force. In addition to presenting the results of the on-site evaluation, policies and procedures were developed. Individual priorities, responsibilities, and authorities were established.

ON-SITE EVALUATION RESULTS

Management: Organizational Management

Early in the evaluation it became evident that Sunnyvale's supervisors were not aware that they had a responsibility for back injury prevention. This was evident throughout. It was difficult to get meetings with managers and supervisors, and few seemed to have any sense of urgency in making time available or keeping appointments.

To consultants, this indicated a lack of understanding in the very influential role that managers and supervisors play in the health and safety of their personnel. The supervisors apparently perceived their role to be primarily that of patient care, and did not realize the extent to which they could affect the problem at hand.

There was no formalization or continuity in specific patient handling and transfer rules. Supervisors could not provide any examples of written transfer instructions. Complete, organized information on specific, recommended patient transfer methods simply did not exist.

Management: Medical

Sunnyvale had a modified duty program that most of the employees disliked and felt was not working. The two common mistakes most often made with return-to-work programs were being made here. First, when an injured worker was returned to work with a lifting restriction, they were nevertheless assigned a full patient schedule. However, they were told to not do any heavy lifting, but to get help. This meant that the healthy nurses had double duty—their own heavy lifting and that of the modified duty nurse.

Understandably, this caused considerable resentment and confusion for the staff. The second mistake was that there was no time limit and no concurrent rehabilitation program to complement the return-to-work program. There was no process for the injured worker to get stronger and return to regular duty. The five primary care practitioners in the community were very busy and offered little time to communicate patient status with the claims manager at the nursing home. The three chiropractors appeared to be practicing traditional manipulative techniques with little or no evidence of patient education, functional training, or exercise. The two medical doctors were prescribing rest and medication followed by modified duty return to work without time limits. Physical therapy, or any form of rehabilitation (patient education and exercise), was not being initiated except in a couple of cases after employees had been off work for several months.

Several of the injured workers reported that they did not like to go to the "nursing home doctor" (an M.D.) because it usually meant waiting one or two hours. Often, without being examined, they were prescribed medication and rest or modified duty. These individuals reported that they preferred going to the chiropractor who could see them in less than ten minutes and who could actually do something.

Ergonomics

Problems were found with wheelchair locks, bed locks, and side rails that were difficult to manipulate. Beds were arranged in ways that made it difficult to transfer patients and adjust the beds. There was a need for more electric beds for the difficult care patients. Mechanical assist devices were available. However, there was no clear understanding of when and how to use them.

Education and Training

As is their usual and preferred approach, consultants gathered observations of both good and bad body mechanics. In this case, the day ended with many poor examples and few good examples. It was soon evident that there was little regard for proper body mechanics or proper patient transfer techniques. When a few basic ideas were demonstrated to the nurse's aides on the floor, it became evident that they had not had adequate training.

The apparent disregard for proper technique was present even though the nursing home had a physical therapist on staff. This therapist was ready and willing to be involved in employee training and injury rehabilitation. But with the few in-service classes on body mechanics and patient transfer she conducted attendance was voluntary, and only a few new employees attended. Few existing employees or supervisors participated.

Fitness

No one was performing exercises on the job to reverse the stressful positions that are inherent in the nurse's or nurse's aide's daily routine.

SOLUTIONS

To Management Problems

1. The nursing home administration and supervisors took more responsibility for improved communication with their employees. A critique system was initiated so that all employees had input into the injury prevention process. Policies were clearly communicated verbally and in writing.
2. Policies were established concerning who had responsibility to evaluate new patients and determine each patient's transfer and handling needs. Supervisors and employee representatives had input into the formation of the policy. Policies were then documented and were easily accessible.
3. Supervisors assumed more responsibility for observing the nurse's aides as they did their work. They became more proactive, helping

the aides with suggestions and individualized training. It became the supervisor's responsibility to make sure the aides in their department were trained and performed their jobs properly.

To Medical Management Problems

1. Written policies and procedures for dealing with injured employees (medical management) were established.
2. The consultants met with the medical providers, and received their cooperation in implementing an early return-to-work program that included a physical therapy evaluation and on-site rehabilitation. Sunnyvale claims managers and supervisors became more aggressive about asking for clarification and suggestions from the medical providers.
3. All employees involved in the early return-to-work program were carried as "extras" and were not assigned to patients who required care that was beyond their restriction.
4. Employees on early return to work were evaluated by the medical providers on a regular basis and their duties updated by the physician and Physical Therapist.

To Ergonomic Problems

1. A regularly scheduled maintenance program for all equipment was instituted.
2. A member of the board of directors who had attended the two sessions found 35 electric high-low beds in storage at a nearby hospital that had closed a wing. These were purchased at a reasonable price and used for some of the difficult patients.

To Education and Training Problems

1. Proper body mechanics and patient transfer techniques were taught to all employees, and the supervisors were made responsible to enforce that they were used.
2. Personnel were taught exactly how and when to use assistive devices.
3. Regular in-services and review sessions were scheduled for all nursing personnel regarding body mechanics, patient transfer techniques, and other back care principles.

To Fitness Problems

A class on exercise was conducted to show individuals how to evaluate their own need for exercise. Demonstration and practice time for exercises was allowed. Each employee was given an exercise manual and encouraged to do certain exercises on their own. Additionally, employees were taught fatigue control and relaxation exercises to reverse positions, stimulate blood flow, and reduce stress.

RESULTS

The Sunnyvale Nursing Home ended the previous year with 705 lost employee work days. The following year this figure dropped to only 39 lost work days. The comprehensive approach to analyzing the causes of the injuries and marshalling support from top management on down yielded the kind of progress that justifies the expense and effort.

SUMMARY

Back injuries are a costly expense that can heavily impact product pricing and affect U.S. companies' competitiveness in the global economy.

Preventing back injuries requires more than an event such as a body mechanics training session. It requires a process orientation that takes into consideration four basic intervention strategies—(1) management practices, (2) ergonomics, (3) fitness for work, and (4) education and training.

Management must participate in, support, and empower a companywide process to implement these strategies. *Ergonomics* must fit the job to the employee, enabling safe postures and motions. *Fitness* programs that render muscles and joints less vulnerable to injury should be encouraged by management and accepted by employees. *Education and training* help everyone acquire greater awareness and knowledge regarding proper prevention strategies, early warning signs of injury, and the mind set for early reporting and response when symptoms appear.

Because back injury prevention encompasses a broad range of disciplines, Industrial Therapists must think of themselves not simply as rehabilitating injured backs, but as consultants who facilitate cultural, attitudinal, and behavioral change throughout a company.

The consultant's tasks include the following:
1. Gain management support.
2. Perform worksite evaluation, recommend interventions, and use information gained to provide customized training.
3. Perform management training. Emphasize establishing authority, accountability, and responsibility to facilitate the prevention process.

4. Perform supervisor training. Emphasize openness to communication, facilitation, and enforcement of preventive principles.
5. Perform employee training. Emphasize communication, body mechanics, and exercise.
6. Help the company implement administrative policies that support the prevention process (realistic standards, appropriate reward structures, job rotation, and exercise breaks).
7. Help develop case management and medical management policies.
8. Help develop an employee feedback system, with an ongoing process of prevention awareness.

There remains much work to be done before process-orientated back injury prevention becomes widely accepted and accorded the recognition it deserves. As dramatic reductions in incidence and severity are achieved, employees, owners, and the public at large stand to reap abundant economic and societal rewards.

REFERENCES

Parts of this chapter have been taken from the book *Evaluation, Treatment, and Prevention of Musculoskeletal Disorders, volume 1*

1. American Back School, 5936 Swanson Dr, Ashland, Ky 41102.
2. Anderson C: Physical Ability Testing as a Means to Reduce Injuries in Grocery Warehouses, *Intl Retail Distrib Manag* 19(7):33–35, 1991.
3. Andersson Gunnar BJ International Society for the Study of the Lumbar Spine, 1992 Annual Meeting. Chicago, Il.
4. Back School of Atlanta, 1465 Northside Dr, NW–217, Atlanta, Ga 30318.
5. Bergquist-Ullman M, Larsson U: Acute Low Back Pain in Industry: a controlled prospective study with special reference to therapy and confounding factors *Acta Orthop Scand* 170: 1–117, 1977.
6. Biering-Sorenson F, "Physical Measurements as Risk Indicators for Low Back Trouble Over a One-Year Period", *Spine* 9:106–119, 1984.
7. Cady L et al: Strength and Fitness and Subsequent Back Injuries in Firefighters, *Jour Occup Med* 21:269–272, 1979.
8. Centineo J: Return-To-Work Programs: cut costs and employee turnover, *Risk Management* 44–48, Dec 1986.
9. Dehlin O, Hedenrud B, Horal J: Back Symptoms in Nursing Aides in a Geriatric Hospital, *Scand Rehab Med* 8:47–53, 1976.
10. Deyo R, Bass J: Lifestyle and Low Back Pain: the influence of smoking and obesity, *Spine* 14:501–506, 1989.
11. Educational Opportunities, A Saunders Group Company, 4250 Norex Dr, Chaska, Minn 55318.
12. Fitzler SL, Berger RA: Attitudinal Change: the chelsea back Program, *Occup Health and Safety* 35:24–26, 1982.
13. Fitzler S, Berger RA: Chelsea Back Program: one year later, *Occup Health and Safety* 52:52–54, 1983.
14. Gilliam T: A Two Year Prospectus: preemployment physical capability testing", Injury Reduction Technology, Inc, 110 Streetsboro St W, Suite 2A, Hudson Ohio 44236, Unpublished study.
15. Hultman G, Nordin M, Ortengren R: The Influence of a Preventive Educational Program on Trunk Flexion in Janitors, *Applied Ergonomics* 16(2):127–133, 1984.
16. LaRocco JM, Jones AP: Coworker and Leader Support as Moderators of Stress Strain Relationships in Work Situations, *Applied Psychology* 63, 629–634 1978.
17. Linton S J, Kamwendo K: Low Back Schools: a critical review, *Physical Therapy* 67(9):1375–1383, 1987.
18. McFadden J: Smoking May Be Significant Risk Factor in Failed Back Surgery, *Back Pain Monitor* 4:41–52, April 1986.
19. Mc Reynolds M: Early Return to Work, *Clinical Management* 10:10–11, Sept/Oct 1990.
20. Melton B: Back Injury Prevention Means Education, *Occup Health and Safety* 52:20–23, 1983.
21. Nachemson A: Newest Knowledge of Low Back Pain: a critical look, *Clin Orthop and Rel Res* 279:8–20, June 1992.
22. Nachemson A: Work for All: for those with low back pain as well", *Clin Orthop and Rel Res* 179:77–85, Oct 1983.
23. Quebec Task Force Study: Scientific Approach to the Assessment and Management of Activity Related Spinal Disorders, *Spine* 12:7S, 1987.
24. Ratzliff J, Grogrin T: Early Return to Work Profitability, *Professional Safety* 11–17, March 1989.
25. Ritzel D, Allen R: Value of Work, *Professional Safety* 23–25, Nov 1988.
26. Scholey M: Back Stress: the effects of training nurses to lift patients in a clinical situation", *Intl Nur Studies* 20(1):1–13, 1983.
27. Simmons EW: The American Back Society, San Francisco.
28. Snook SH, Campanelli R, Hart J: A Study of Three Preventive Approaches to Low Back Injury, *Occ Med* 20(7):478–481, 1978.
29. Snook SH, White AH: *Education and Training In Occupational Low Back Pain*, Pope MH, Frymoyer J, Andersson G, editors, Philadelphia 1984, Praeger Scientific.
30. Snook SH: *The Control of Low Back Disability: the role of management*, San Francisco, 1988, American Industrial Hygiene Association.
31. Stubbs DA, et al: Back Pain in the Nursing Profession: the effectiveness of training, *Ergonomics* 26(8):767–779, 1983.
32. Tomer G M, Olson C, Lepore B: Back Injury Prevention Training Makes Dollars and Sense, *National Safety News* (Jan)36–39, 1984.

10

Upper Extremity Injury Prevention

Michael S. Melnik

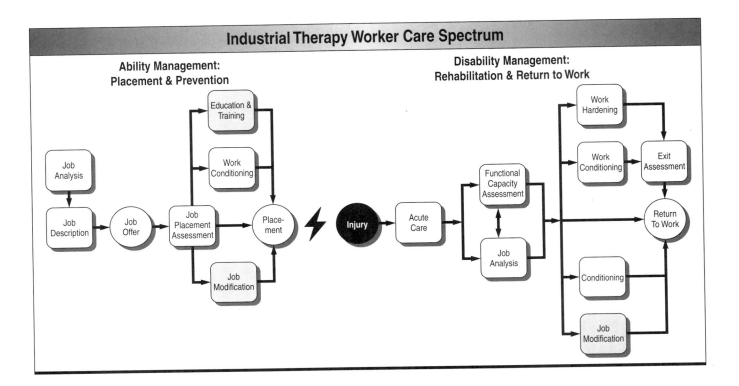

Industrial Therapy Worker Care Spectrum

Writing a chapter on the strategies for the prevention of cumulative trauma disorders is a challenging task. Articles that define and redefine risk factors, work practices that change with technology, a Worker's Compensation system that leaves industry and workers disgruntled and a medical management system that demonstrates inconsistency in methods collectively make cumulative trauma disorder prevention a highly necessary, but often complicated task.

This chapter will identify these disorders and discuss approaches used to address the problem. This will be followed by a description of the approach used by this author, which is, in essence, a compilation of techniques utilized by professionals across the country.

PROBLEM DESCRIPTION

Terminology

Cumulative Trauma Disorder is a term applied to a wide assortment of ailments that effect the upper body. More interestingly, these varied diagnoses, each with different pathologies, are grouped into a single category. This would be similar to grouping numerous types of back disorders into the category of "low back pain."

Understandingly, treatment for degenerative disc disease or a facet impingement should be treated differently than a muscle strain or disc herniation. In the same light, treatment (and prevention) of carpal tunnel syndrome would differ from the treatment of tendonitis or an ulnar nerve entrapment syndrome. In order for a diagnosis to be treated and prevented with specific methods it needs to be defined as a particular disorder.[38] For the purpose of this chapter, upper extremity disorders will be referred to as Cumulative Trauma Disorders (CTDs).

Types of CTDs

The CTDs most commonly observed in the industrial environment include, but are not limited to:

1. Carpal tunnel syndrome
2. Tendonitis
3. Bursitis
4. Raynauds syndrome
5. Cubital tunnel
6. Tenosynovitis
7. Trigger finger
8. de Quervains

These and other diagnoses are described in detail in a variety of publications.[11, 18, 21, 30, 47, 49, 56, 61]

Risk Factors

Each of these diagnoses have been associated with a variety of risk factors.

Posture/Position. Specific positions have been identified as contributors to a variety of CTDs. These include, but are not limited to ulnar and radial deviation, supination, wrist flexion and extension, external rotation of the shoulder, and awkward neck postures.[3, 4, 10, 21, 26, 33, 48, 61]

Force. Obviously, the greater the force, the greater the risk for a disorder. Whenever motor activity concentrates force on the muscles, problems can occur. The completion of tasks that require repetitive fine motor activity in the hands concentrates forces on the small muscles of the hand.[4, 6, 26, 54, 55] Force is also affected directly by position/posture. Many of the improper positions/postures mentioned above do not allow for efficient use of the body. This results in greater forces being applied to specific muscle groups while limiting the contribution of others.

Repetition. This is the multiplier of position and force. The greater the number of repetitions, the greater the risk of injury.[3, 4, 6, 54, 55, 61]

Vibration. Prolonged exposure to vibration has demonstrated a negative effect on both nerves and blood vessels, and is considered a contributor to "white finger," a disorder resulting in ineffective distribution of blood to the fingers due to vascular spasms (Figure 10.1).[3, 42, 54]

FIGURE 10.1 Tools that vibrate can affect nerves and blood vessels.

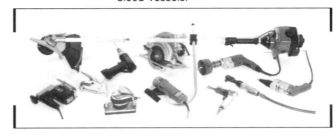

Temperature Extremes. A healthy upper body relies on adequate blood flow to and from the working muscles. Temperature extremes, such as the cold environment of meat and poultry processing facilities is thought to increase the risk of CTDs.[3]

Stress/Attitude. Stress can aggravate an already demanding work task, by increasing muscular tension and contributing to inefficient work practices.[5, 9, 12, 46, 71, 75]

Direct Pressure. This can be caused by a tight watch or wristband, or by resting a forearm on the edge of a work surface. This pressure can restrict the flow of nutrients to the working muscles and slow the flow of by-products away from this area.[61]

Gender. There is evidence that there are hormonal factors in females that can increase the likelihood of CTDs. Having a hysterectomy may also increase risk.[80, 81]

Previous Injuries. A fracture or dislocation can impinge on tissue and contribute to a CTD.[11, 47]

Disease. Certain diseases, such as diabetes, can effect circulation to extremities and thereby play a role in the development of CTDs.[11]

Physical Stature. The stature or size of an individual. Smaller dimensions of the carpal tunnel or other anatomical structures that encompass nerves and blood vessels, while still not fully understood, may be a contributing factor.

It is important to note that additional risk factors are not yet fully understood or defined. This is demonstrated by numerous individuals who develop symptoms in the absence of, or with minimal exposure to, the above mentioned risk factors. There are also those who respond well to new and innovative treatment approaches that focus on nontraditional causes of CTDs. Many writings focus on neck musculature as a major factor in the development of CTD symptoms in the arms and hands.[3, 48]

If it were as easy to eliminate the risk factors as it is to list them prevention would be simple. The prevention equation becomes more complicated when attempts are made to quantify common risk factors such as posture, repetition, force, and stress. There is no data that accurately predicts the length of time in specific postures, or minimum number of repetitions, or number of pounds of force that will cause symptoms in individuals. It is for this reason that the scope of prevention strategies has varied so greatly, and attempts to define specific ergonomic parameters has been such an involved and lengthy process.

Scope and Impact

The recognition of these disorders is certainly not new. Ramazzini first discussed them in 1717 by referring to cumulative trauma disorders as "the harvest of diseases reaped by certain workers from irregular motions in unnatural postures of the body." While the recognition of these disorders is nothing new, the concept of them as a "compensable" injury is.[64]

The Bureau of Labor Statistics reports an increase from 22,000 reported cases in 1979 to 45,500 in 1986. This number reached 147,000 in 1989.[16, 57] It is believed that these numbers may only be the tip of the iceberg due to lingering problems in the reporting system.[76] Regardless of the specific numbers, the business community is viewing this problem as an epidemic.[28]

There are several theories regarding the ongoing increase in CTDs evidenced over the last 20 years. A review of the literature indicates the following factors:

More Sophisticated Reporting and Recording of CTDs. This stems primarily from increased regulation of record keeping by the Occupational Safety and Health Administration (OSHA), the government agency responsible for establishing and enforcing workplace safety guidelines and regulations.[16]

Larger Fines for Companies Not Responding to CTDs. The fines levied by OSHA, have been in the millions of dollars. One ruling in 1988 charged a Philadelphia food company with more than 200 ergonomics violations and 170 record-keeping violations. In this instance OSHA proposed fines totaling $1.4 million.[34, 53, 68, 73]

Increased Public and Corporate Awareness. People have been exposed to these disorders to a great degree through the media[1, 64] and through employees' experiences. Employers have become more socially aware and responsible as a result.

Changing Physical Demands of the Job. Many work tasks in the past required using the large muscle groups through wide ranges of motions. With jobs becoming more automated, the motions required are increasingly confined to the smaller and weaker muscle groups of the hands and forearms (Figure 10.2).

Increased Job Specialization. The advent of the computer and other technical advances have increased the incidence of "one individual/one task" work environments. The "old days," when a worker would perform a variety of functions on the job, have given way to the modern workplace, where the more "specialized worker" performs a microcosm of the whole, often repeating the same movements in the same position all day.[16]

Increased Job Pressure. Stress claims are becoming more common, particularly in California where they have risen dramatically. According to a 1993 report by the International Labor Organization, job-related stress costs the U.S. $200 billion a year in diminished productivity, Workers' Compensation claims, absenteeism, health insurance, and direct medical costs.[25, 69, 71, 75]

Aging Workforce. In simplest terms, this means that people are literally "wearing out."[34, 64]

Individuals Exploiting the System. While specific numbers for this group are difficult, if not impossible, to determine it is assumed by many that there are a small number of individuals who attempt to take advantage of the system.

Poor Communication Between Industry and Medicine. Many medical practitioners still do not realize

FIGURE 10.2 The mix of workstyles has changed from heavy muscle groups to small muscle groups.

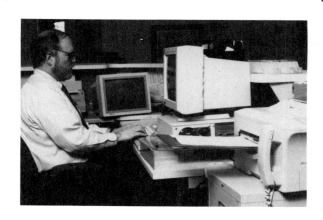

that the industrial environment is a magnificent laboratory for better understanding of the disorders they are treating. Too many individuals with CTDs are still being treated without considering the work or home activities that may have contributed to the disorder.

The Costs

It has been estimated that the costs of carpal tunnel syndrome range from $3,500 for non-surgical to over $30,000 for surgical cases, and over $100,000 if the employee is not successfully returned to work.[64]

These figures are the direct costs, and are considered to represent only a fraction of industry's overall costs. These direct costs include:

1. Workers' Compensation premiums
2. Medical costs
3. Lost time wages
4. Reserves—the money held by insurers to cover themselves against anticipated expenses.

Experts readily agree that there are numerous "indirect" costs associated with an injury that can make even a nominal Workers' Compensation case quite expensive. These indirect costs include:

1. Disruptions in production and quality
2. Administrative costs (processing the injury, hiring replacements, etc.)
3. Impact on morale
4. Training of replacements

Some industry experts calculate the indirect costs by multiplying the direct costs by four. In many industries it is as high as seven to ten times the direct costs depending on the work needed to compensate for the loss of an employee.

TOWARD PREVENTION

Background

In the past, industry was relatively immune to the financial impact of CTDs. An employee who suffered from CTD would either quit, continue to perform the job as best they could, or was fired. There were often people waiting in line for the position. Accurate reporting was not required by law, and training was a rarity.

This is no longer the case. OSHA has become a predominant force in industry, particularly in the meat and poultry sectors which now have specific regulations developed to reduce CTDs.[82] OSHA places special emphasis on accurate and timely reporting of injuries and training of employees. Unions have become significantly more sophisticated, not only in understanding and fighting for employees rights, but

in medical management and compensation issues as well.

The Americans with Disabilities Act (ADA)[35] puts additional pressure on industry to keep employees healthy and productive. Under ADA, being injured or disabled doesn't mean an employee can't work. Employers must now make adaptations or accommodations to fit the job to the employee's capabilities. Essentially, the days of the "disposable" employee are gone and industry must now focus attention and resources on aggressively addressing CTD problems.

The Role of Perceptions

It is well known that people approach problems based on how they perceive them. Perceptions impacting people's approach to CTDs include:

"It's not a real injury"

The way CTDs are verbalized by employees and observed by industry has lead many to the conclusion that such disorders are not real. CTDs are unique in being generally invisible, and are often reported by employees in vague terms. Moreover, CTDs have proliferated so rapidly, industry has not had sufficient time to understand what they are and how to deal with them.

Industry knows how to react to a typical slip, fall, cut, or back injury, where there is a recognizable incident and evidence of a damaged body part. Industry does not yet understand how to react to reports of "aching" or "tingling." An employee might tell a supervisor that after two hours on a specific job his or her hand "falls asleep," yet this same employee might be able to play softball all weekend with no problems. It's not surprising that many industries have reacted to reported CTDs with uncertainty or skepticism.

There are states that disallow CTDs as a work compensable injury and industries that deny that their work activities in any way could contribute to these problems.

In this author's experience nearly 100% of the employee population is familiar with the term carpal tunnel syndrome, while practically no employees are able to accurately define what it means. Lack of knowledge contributes to fear by all involved whereas knowledge leads to understanding and solutions.

"It's a medical management problem"

CTDs have fallen under the same medical management mind set as back disorders. "It's a medical management problem" means that CTDs are perceived as the responsibility of health care providers and not industry or its employees. The long-standing practice of focusing on post-injury medical management rather than preinjury prevention, although slowly changing, has perpetuated this belief.

What physicians often perceive as the solutions— "surgery" or "no repetitive work"—can be completely unacceptable to the worker. While the medical community does not personally place an inappropriate tool in a worker's hand or determine that an employee should complete 5,000 parts in a day, their awareness of the risk factors and their position as a primary care giver suggests they should assume greater responsibility for prevention of these disorders.

"It's a work style problem"

It has been documented for years that there are certain work postures that contribute to a CTD.[50, 64, 66] Though industry and the medical community have started to focus on behavioral modification to eliminate bad work styles, they've tended to overlook structural modification to eliminate bad workstation design.

Industry's initial programs for safe work styles have been largely confined to employee classes to correct behavior. In other areas, safety has been approached both behaviorally and structurally. For instance, to protect head and eyes, employees are not simply given classes on how to avoid trauma to these areas, they're also required to wear hard hats and safety glasses. Similarly, employees should not simply be taught safe postures. Jobs should also be redesigned to make risky postures more difficult, or in the best case, impossible to assume (Figure 10.3, A, B).

"It's a Workstation/Workplace design problem"

Addressing the problem from an engineering perspective has several benefits. First, it is the most objective method. Ergonomics, with its strong tie to engineering speaks to industry in familiar terms. It is becoming clearer that industry must take this approach as legislation regarding ergonomic standards develops.[20]

The problem for industry is the impact of variables that effect the success of an ergonomic approach. Ergonomically correct equipment is ineffective if employees use it improperly.

It's a work "stress" problem

Industry is increasingly being confronted with the issue of work related stress and its contribution to injury. Unlike the engineering approach, the psychosocial approach to injury prevention addresses aspects of work that have been neglected. A study by Boeing[9] made it abundantly clear that negative attitudes have a significant impact on increased risk of injury.

FIGURE 10.3 A, B A safer wrist posture can be achieved simply by changing the position or location of raw materials.

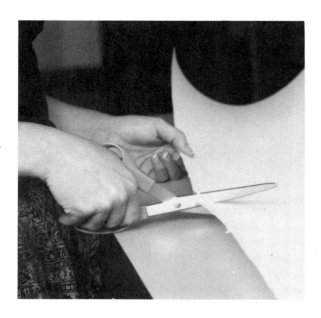

A

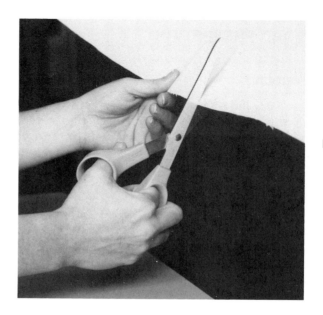

B

Changes such as extending more control to the workers[32, 53, 70] training supervisors in communication skills[25, 40, 44] and providing workers with incentives that encourage and reward safe work behaviors,[74] can positively effect an employee's sense of control and job satisfaction. Positive attitudes have demonstrated a positive effect on safety.

"It's a problem that is handled best my way."

Many involved with CTDs in any capacity tend to prefer dealing with the problem in their own way. A worker or patient who experiences a CTD will react based on "their" way of reacting to pain and disability, whether it's in their best interest or not. Similarly, management and supervisors will rely on their experiences to develop a means of effectively handling the case. Likewise, the medical community is accustomed to doing as they see fit.

Strong paradigms persist in the medical community. The approach, to date, has typically focused on treatment of the disorders rather than prevention. Treatment approaches vary greatly, ranging from splinting and stretching to surgery. Unfortunately, many in the medical community have subscribed to the belief that medical intervention alone is the answer to CTDs. There are individuals who have been told "if the problem gets bad enough, we'll operate."

Where prevention is addressed, the emphasis is primarily on the risk factors which directly impact the shoulders, arms, wrists, and hands. The process has been to eliminate the forces, minimize the repetitions, and alter the position of these segments. This approach has demonstrated an impact on reducing CTDs.

There is another body of evidence developing that suggests the medical community look at segments, such as the neck, that may also contribute to CTDs despite what appears to be limited involvement in a specific work task. Some of these later findings are the result of EMG studies that demonstrate a pattern of fatigue that begins in the neck and impacts upper body function.[27]

The history of CTDs and their rapid growth over the last decade should be viewed as an indication that effective communication between doctors, therapists, engineers, and employees is essential if the multitude of contributing factors is to be addressed.

A worker or patient may need to come out of their comfort zone and take on more self responsibility 24 hours a day to effectively identify risk factors and reduce symptoms. Managers and supervisors may need to recognize that this disorder is real and is attributable to many of the work tasks in the company.

The medical community has to evaluate methods and be willing to admit that they don't have all the answers, and consider job redesign, worker retraining, job rotation, stretching, warming up, and an ongoing dialogue with industry to effectively impact this process.

Issues To Resolve

The literature is replete with articles that outline methods that can alleviate the problem, and many of these approaches claim success.[8, 16, 37] If programs have demonstrated success and can save a company thousands or potentially millions of dollars, why aren't all industries implementing these programs?

The number of companies ready to become actively involved in aggressive injury prevention programs is minuscule, compared to those who do not yet fully understand the scope of the problem, have no idea that there is something they can do about it, or are unwilling to invest in change.

The issues that arise when a company begins to think about implementing a program include:

- How does a safety director justify program costs to the employer, particularly if the company is not profitable, the funds for the program are not available, or available funds are allocated to areas considered a higher priority?

- How can a supervisor with poor communication skills and lacks compassion for the employees be motivated to become actively involved in the company's program? What if the supervisor has no idea how to deal with this situation or how to justify spending money in this area?

- If the employee's attitude toward new work methods is, "I've done the job this way for 25 years. I'm not going to change now!" how do they learn to see that change is truly in their best interest?

The critical issue underlying all these questions is; How does a company implement change? Workers' Compensation costs, medical management costs, pressure from OSHA, and costs of lower productivity and poorer quality are being felt by industry and they are being forced to confront these issues.

Developing a Prevention Process. The first step in implementing an effective CTD program in industry is to recognize the paradigms that exist and build a program that addresses them on an ongoing basis.

Injury prevention consultants must be aware of the myriad factors within industry that minimize the chances of starting a program and reduce the program's chances for success.

Identifying Attitudes

One of the factors inhibiting change is attitude, often expressed through one or more of the following statements:

1. We're different; this program won't work for us.
2. We can't afford this program.
3. We'll only be telling people how to have (or fake) the problem.
4. We don't have the time for a program.
5. Our problem isn't really that bad.
6. We have union issues.
7. Not everyone is in favor of the program.
8. We don't want (or know how to) change.
9. We want a program on paper, but not in the plant.
10. We're profitable. Why change?
11. We don't want to turn this place into a clinic/gymnasium.
12. We're insured for these problems.
13. We already have a program.
14. If symptoms appear, we send them to the doctor.
15. Most of these people are fakers anyway.
16. These people have a bad attitude.
17. We have enough training already.
18. Hurry up, do your program and get out of here.
19. We've tried a program like this before. It didn't work.

Altering Paradigms

It is the exploration and response to these and other issues that will determine if the consultant is able to begin a program and whether or not the program will be given the opportunity to run its course, gain momentum, and become a permanent fixture in the company. It is not possible to alter paradigms overnight. A consultant must be aware that they exist in all businesses, and strategies must be developed during the preparation phase of any program to best deal with these issues as they occur.

The best way to alter a paradigm is to recognize where it originates and what purpose it serves. Many paradigms work against the success of a program, the company, and its employees. Innovative companies utilize a variety of techniques to alter these and many of the other paradigms that perpetuate negative attitudes. These include:

Work teams
Job rotation
Incentive programs (profit-sharing, recognition)
Cross-functional teams/task forces
Equitable medical management strategies
Human relations programs
Employee assistance programs
Formal training programs

A consultant who finds none of these in place may realize that initial efforts should be directed toward helping the industry to recognize the need for at least some of these strategies.

IMPLEMENTING PREVENTION

Table 10.1 outlines an Upper Extremity Injury Prevention Program in terms of the activities, the people involved, and the purpose of each component. With this table as a beginning reference, we will now examine each aspect of the program in detail.

Meeting with Management

Meeting with management is the first step in implementing an effective process. At this point the consultant is no longer selling a program. This meeting is an important time to identify roles and responsibilities related to the program. The "players" who will ideally be active in the injury prevention process include:

Management—the financial backing and overall leadership

Supervisors—the "in the trenches" support of the program and the primary reinforcement for the employee population

Employees—self responsibility is the key to a successful program

Unions—it is important to involve them at all stages of program development, implementation, and maintenance

Vendors—will they be willing to put the parts in 50 lb bags rather than 80 lb?

This meeting must address the purpose of the program and management's concerns. Management is often concerned about the program teaching employees how to fake CTDs, and will send droves of employees to the clinics. Since some employees may have already experienced symptoms, there might be an initial increase in genuine CTD reporting. The insurance company should be alerted to this possibility so that any increase in reported CTDs will be interpreted properly. Early reporting represents an increase in awareness and an opportunity to intervene before problems become more severe and costly.

As a consultant, it is important to provide clients with both guidance and autonomy. Consultants provide companies with tools to develop, implement, and maintain a program. Providing too much may make a company place the responsibility for the program's success solely on the shoulders of the consultant. If a

TABLE 10.1   CTD Prevention Program Components

ACTIVITY	WHO IS INVOLVED	PURPOSE
Meet with management	Management, union representative	Define needs/goals
Evaluate losses and review medical management strategies	Management, medical personnel, insurance representative	Establish baselines, target specific areas
Supervisor orientation	Supervisors	Enlist support, address questions and concerns
Worksite evaluation	Supervisors, employees	Familiarize consultant with work tasks, gather information for education/job modification
Management/supervisor education	Management, supervisors	Provide fundamentals of injury prevention to help delegate responsibilities
Employee education	Employees, management, supervisors	Increase awareness
Development of task force	Management, insurance, supervisors, employees, union, medical representative	To distribute responsibility throughout the company
Ongoing activities	Everyone	To maintain program effectiveness
1. Task force meetings	As appropriate	
2. Employee tool box talks	As appropriate	
3. Monitoring of medical management strategies	As appropriate	
4. Development of an ergonomic program	As appropriate	
5. Development of job rotation system (if applicable)	As appropriate	
6. Development of stretching/warm-up program	As appropriate	
7. Development of return-to-work program	As appropriate	
8. Development of program support materials	As appropriate	
9. Symptom control	As appropriate	
10. Program evaluation	As appropriate	

consultant provides too little, the program's success is jeopardized.

Accordingly, the consultant must emphasize the participation of management, supervisors, and employees in making the program successful. The more details and possible roadblocks that can be addressed in this initial meeting, the fewer surprises or concerns surface as the program proceeds. Let management know that a successful injury prevention program has a very recognizable beginning and no recognizable end. It is a process, not an event.

Evaluating Losses

This is an important meeting to properly focus the program and justify the need for it. It helps to ensure that the program is developed to address the real causes of the problem. Although some departments demonstrate significantly more claims than others, this does not necessarily indicate physical causes. It may mean that there are issues between the supervisors and employees; it may be due to a night shift of less experienced employees, or it could be the "light duty" department simply reaggravating old injuries. In any case, reviewing the medical data provides the groundwork for outlining the process.

The indicators that help justify expenses and target the efforts include, but are not limited to:

- Injury and illness incidence rates
- Workers' Compensation experience
- First-aid cases
- Medical insurance claims

- Absenteeism rates
- Worker complaints
- Turnover rates
- Amount of overtime worked[39]

Reviewing Medical Management

This meeting is also an appropriate time to address the company's current medical management issues. The key reason a consultant is invited in for prevention is that the company has a number of workers currently disabled with CTDs, and doesn't know how to get them back to work. It will become clear through the evaluation of records, if the company's injury management problems at that moment should take precedence over the need for prevention. The company may have had only two reported CTDs in the last year, but the lost time associated with each case was far above what would be expected for the diagnoses.

This initial focus on improved medical management can be expressed as a form of prevention—"preventing" an acute disorder from becoming chronic or disabling. One of the best questions to ask management in this initial meeting is "what brought you to the point of asking for outside assistance?"

Supervisor Orientation

This portion of the program is critical. Without participation and support from the supervisors the process will never fully reach its potential.[32, 44] Consultants must know how to operate effectively in a supervisor's territory. A supervisor who is not comfortable with the program can undermine the effort. This orien-

FIGURE 10.4 Owning the equipment required to visit a job site can provide evidence of experience.

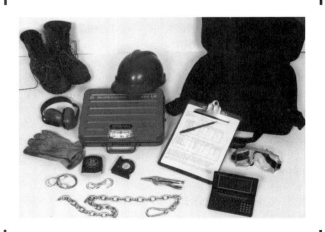

tation session is primarily focused on generating "buy-in." It is generally an hour in length, and provides an opportunity to outline the goals and components of the program. It allows the supervisors to have input, ask questions, raise concerns, and provide feedback.

Early supervisor orientation is much preferable to showing up in a supervisor's department for a worksite evaluation without having previously met or explained the program. This can create an awkward situation. Worksite evaluations are a designated time for evaluating the work. They are not the best time for personal introductions and program descriptions.

Worksite Evaluation

The details of Job Analysis at the worksite were covered in greater detail in Chapter 7, but some guidelines regarding the consultant's approach to injury prevention are important here.

In injury prevention, there are basically two formats for performing a worksite evaluation: an evaluation in preparation for an educational program; and an evaluation as part of an ergonomics program.

Worksite Evaluation for Educational Programs

In preparing for an educational program, the worksite evaluation serves two main purposes—1) it familiarizes the consultant with the job demands and work environment and 2) it familiarizes the consultant with the employee population.

It is important during this evaluation to find out as much as possible about the day-to-day operations of the facility. It is an opportunity to don a pair of gloves and do some of the jobs, if this is permitted; take slides or videos of individuals to use during the educational programs; and talk to the employees. It is also a perfect time to publicize the process.

In performing the worksite evaluation, the following principles should be adhered to:

1. All employees should be informed ahead of time of the visit and its purpose.
2. The consultant should have a hard hat, safety glasses, steel-toed shoes, and hearing protection available. It is best to own your own protective equipment (Figure 10.4). Walking into a facility prepared provides evidence of experience. Many companies provide a hard-hat with the company's name on it, which you may be able to keep if you are going to be making frequent visits. In addition, it is a great marketing tool when you go to other businesses wearing a hard hat that shows you have other clients. Just be sure it's not a company rival.
3. Talk with the employees. There is nothing

FIGURE 10.5 Some of the most valuable information comes from talking with the employees.

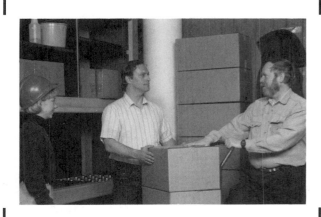

worse than watching an employee work, taking notes or pictures, and then walking away without talking with them. This is not only insensitive, but misses an opportunity for valuable information (Figure 10.5).

4. Review previous suggestions. It is important to find out from management and employees what previous injury prevention and job modification ideas had been suggested or attempted, how were they received, what worked, and what didn't. Often, helping a company is a process of building upon ideas and experiences from the past, or eliciting solutions from management and employees that are easy to unveil. Acceptance of ideas is generally stronger if they come from the company rather than the consultant.

  Sometimes a suggestion that has been rejected in the past is resurrected. When this happens, it's important to give credit to the employee who had made the suggestion originally. Otherwise the implementation of this change may not only be resented by the employee but even undermined. It is difficult enough to establish rapport with the employee population. Remember to review past suggestions, solicit their input, and give credit where credit is due.

5. Ask for permission prior to taking someone's picture. If a consultant sees an employee doing something they would like to get on video or film, they should explain to the employee why they would like to record it and request that they repeat the action.

6. Be observed by as many employees as possible. The consultant's presence in the facility adds valuable credibility to a program. It is important that the various shifts, particularly

evening and night, see that specific concerns are being addressed in this program.

7. Visit during more than one shift. Different shifts can be as different as snowflakes or fingerprints. Never assume that a visit during the daylight hours provides an adequate assessment of what happens at 3 o'clock in the morning.

8. Don't pretend to understand everything. Consultants are not experts in the day-to-day operations of a facility. The supervisors and employees are the experts at what they do, and you are in their environment. There are many variables and a significant history underlying what you may be witnessing for the first time. Do not be quick to judge or evaluate something just because it seems evident. The initial worksite visit is a time to keep the eyes open and ask many questions.

9. Take pictures or videos of the things that you plan to discuss in the educational program. Real examples from the employees' environment can assist them in assimilating the information while more effectively highlighting problems. These may include employees reaching and lifting, awkward wrist or shoulder postures, arms supported on sharp edges, or poor sitting postures. Videos are particularly valuable where jobs require rapid motions or subtle changes in posture. Overall, videos provide a "diary" of the visit for later evaluation away from what may be a loud and hectic environment. One caution: do not let the operation of the video camera take precedence over communicating with the employees.

10. Ask good questions. Asking employees and supervisors the following questions can increase insight and provide information that may not be observable (Figure 10.6, A, B):
    a. Is this a typical day?
    b. What is considered the most difficult job in the department?
    c. What is the job that most people like/dislike doing?
    d. Where do most of the injuries occur?
    e. How well do you feel safety is handled in your department?
    f. How is the maintenance in this department?
    g. What happens when something breaks down?
    h. Is this the pace people normally work (sometimes a consultant's presence can alter work behaviors).
    i. Are there ever any temperature extremes?
    j. What is the typical break pattern?
    k. Is there overtime? How much?
    l. How do you feel at the end of the day?

FIGURE 10.6 A, B   A Job Analysis involving loading the conveyor belt can vary depending on the time of day it is being conducted.

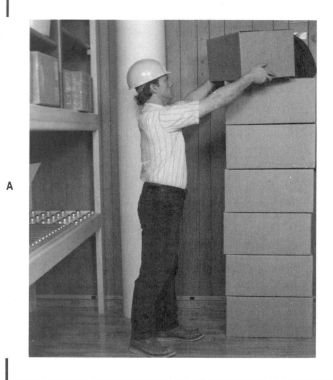
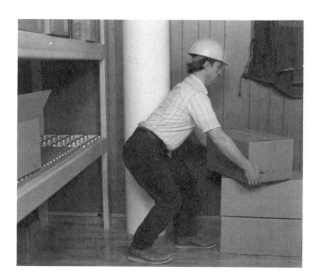

A

B

m. Where do you feel the most fatigue/discomfort?

11. Put relationships before details. Again, it is important to remember that in preparing an employee education program, becoming familiar with the employees and the overall operation overrides the need to amass details.

12. Focus on problems, not solutions. The consultant should not be over anxious to find solutions to the problems observed at this time, even if they seem obvious. He or she may not yet fully understand the operation or the modifications that are feasible.

   A punch press operator might be reaching above shoulder level to activate the machine. Although this motion might increase the risk of a CTD, the obvious solution of moving the controls to a more appropriate level may not be workable. The consultant may not be aware of the NIOSH standard which dictates that punch press controls must be located where an individual cannot press them accidentally or get their hands caught in the press. Having the controls overhead meets these guidelines. Having them at waist height does not.

   Possible engineering solutions include the use of light shields which cut the power to the machine if a body part breaks the plane of the shield, or activation switches that cut the power if they are not held for the duration of the cycle. There are numerous on-site and off-site experts who can work with the consultant to solve the problem once it has been identified. There are also several publications available to assist with this process.[13, 23, 33, 54, 74] The point is that the primary objective during a preliminary worksite evaluation is to fully evaluate the problems, not determine the solutions.

13. One of the simplest ways to perform a worksite evaluation is to divide it into two parts.
   a. Body position. First look at the person from head to toe, looking for postures or movements related to known risk factors. Begin with the neck and move downward through the shoulders, elbows, wrists, and hands. Do the same thing for the trunk and lower extremities.
   b. Physical environment. Look only at the physical layout of the job. This can include the heights, weights, and distances as well as pace. This method serves two purposes; first, it keeps the evaluator from missing something (a task appears to be very upper extremity intensive and as a result attention

is drawn away from potentially awkward or demanding lower body postures that are used to complete the task) and second, it helps the evaluator determine if the problem, as it appears, is a workstation design issue or an employee workstyle choice issue. Watching two different people work at the same station is also important in making this distinction.

Workstyle and Job Modification

When evaluating a job, it is important to differentiate workstyles from job design. This separation is most critical if the evaluator is a therapist with little or no engineering background, or an engineer with little or no therapeutic background. The expertise of most therapists is in the area of body mechanics and physiology. Engineers' expertise tends to be more in the area of machinery. Both are critical areas, and both need to be evaluated.

The focus here is "does the employee have an increased risk because of the way they choose to do the job, or because the job forces them to do the job a certain way, or both?"

Employee choice is often addressed behaviorally through training and development of alternative workstyles. (Figure 10.7, *A, B*) Job design is typically ad-dressed structurally through a process of ergonomic analysis and modification. These two methods are not mutually exclusive, and the evaluator needs to take both factors into consideration during an evaluation.

Further, ergonomic and workstyle approaches differ in broadness of scope. An ergonomics program, by definition, generally addresses the design of a job from the standpoints of work flow and physical demand on employees. Workstyle modification addresses a variety of factors beyond ergonomic issues, such as attitude/stress, preexisting disorders, body mechanics, and the medical management of employees.

As more health professionals become involved in the field of ergonomics, programs are becoming more comprehensive in nature. The assumption that any risk factor acts in isolation is incorrect, as has been confirmed by the documented interaction between job pacing and stress on CTDs.[5]

Industry needs to be educated as to the complex origins of injuries. Misconceptions persist, through the media and elsewhere, that injuries are the result of single incidents, and respond best to single-dimensional approaches such as ergonomics, bracing, surgery, training, or preplacement evaluations. The evaluator can begin to break down these beliefs during a worksite evaluation by documenting the contribution of several risk factors such as physical layout, employee work practices, housekeeping, and communication.

F I G U R E 1 0 . 7 A, B   There are a variety of ways workers might like to perform the job. The therapist is responsible for finding the best way.

A

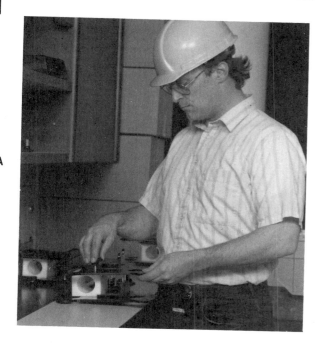

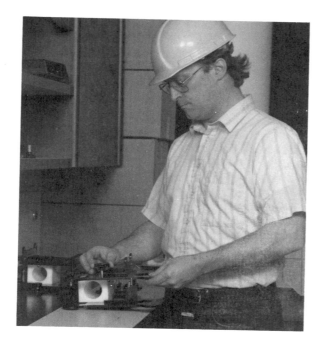

B

FIGURE 10.8 Ergonomic evaluation may include redesign of the workplace.

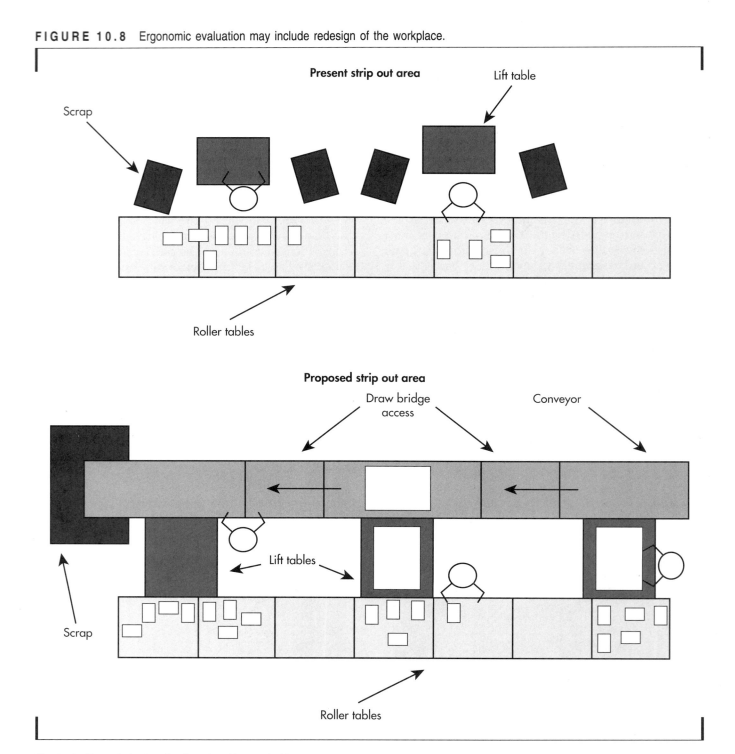

(Reprinted with permission from ErgoTech, Inc., Minneapolis, Minn.)

Worksite Evaluation Report

The report in preparation for an educational program should describe the purpose of the worksite visit, summarize the observations, and make general recommendations. A general recommendation may call for further in-depth evaluation of a process, or indicate that change is required. In contrast, a specific recommendation would describe in greater detail the particular changes that should be made.

The length of time to prepare the report for educational purposes varies greatly depending on the size of the facility, number of employees, locations, and number of different jobs. The primary goal is to get a baseline of information for the types of jobs and how they are performed, and to demonstrate to employees that you understand the type of work they do. This is essential in obtaining credibility as an instructor.

Worksite Evaluation for Ergonomics Programs

Worksite evaluation prior to an educational program may generate a report that includes general observations and recommendations, with a goal of job redesign it should involve a greater "engineering approach" and a much more detailed report, offering significantly more specific solutions.

A worksite evaluation for an ergonomics program is guided by the specific goals of the company and often focuses on one operation or department at a time. It goes into significantly more depth than the more "global" approach preceding an education program. The ergonomic-based evaluation also involves more active participation by a variety of in-house experts who are instrumental to the job evaluation and redesign process (Figure 10.8).

Ergonomics programs and parameters were described in more detail in Chapter 6 and in the literature.[17, 32, 50, 66, 78] Ergonomics has earned its place as a key component of an effective CTD prevention program. It has been reported with a great deal of frequency that position, force, repetition, and vibration, among other risk factors, contribute to increased risk of CTD.[3] Undeniably, these risk factors are often tied to the

worker's tools or the workstation design. A successful CTD prevention program would not be complete without addressing the risk factors associated with the physical environment.

There are numerous "holes" in the ergonomic solution when used in isolation. This means that ergonomics is not synonymous with the prevention of CTDs, it is a component of a comprehensive process. Some of the holes in this as a singular approach include;

- Was the change appropriate/physiologically sound?
- Does the employee take advantage of the change?
- Did the change move the problem to another body part?
- Is the change effective for all employees? (was a table raised and now is too high for an employee Figures 10.9, A, B).
- Does the change take into effect the 16 hours that the employee is away from work and quite possibly aggravating their condition?
- Does the change make it impossible to work in ways that can increase risk—or can an employees old habits circumvent these changes?

Part of the problem is in the terminology. As soon as this strategy is called an "ergonomics program" it is viewed as capable of standing on its own. The purpose of the ergonomics program needs to be established in order to put it into proper perspective. There are three basic reasons that ergonomics programs are implemented—1) to simplify a process; 2) to improve pro-

FIGURE 10.9 A, B It is important to analyze all job shifts to determine differences in people, job demands, and the environment.

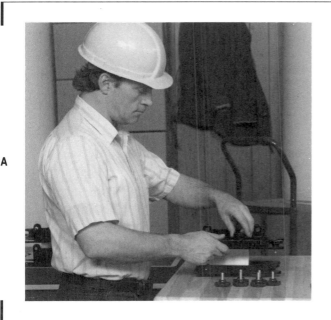
A

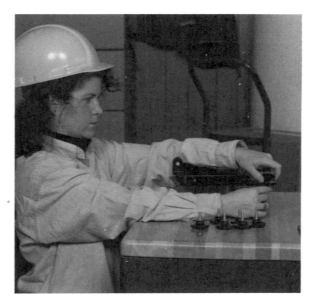
B

ductivity and quality; and 3) to reduce injuries; or perhaps all three.

Identifying these three categories improves the odds that critical components (such as education, stretching, and human relations programs) will be implemented. If a company says they want to simplify a process, ergonomics is certainly a part of this. So is additional training for employees. If they want to increase productivity and quality, ergonomics is also a part of this. So is an incentive program or an investigation of similar operations at other companies to learn their techniques.

Even satisfaction surveys sent out to customers can be a critical part of improving a manufacturing process. If a company wants a CTD prevention program, ergonomics is a part of the program, but so is training for managers, supervisors, and employees. So is the development of an Employee Assistance Program (EAP) and starting a stretching and warm-up program. Ergonomics is not a program, it is a piece of the process. Just as training and education are not programs, they are pieces of the process.

MANAGEMENT AND SUPERVISOR TRAINING

Background

In many instances education and training are only provided for the employee population. Management perceives that employees are the ones getting injured, so it is their behaviors which need to change. This attitude often contributes to a short-lived and ineffective prevention program. A successful program relies on contributions from every level in the company. The longevity of a program will depend a great deal upon management's commitment to ongoing support and supervisor's abilities to reinforce the program over time.

These kinds of sessions are enhanced if tools can be used and demonstrated to make certain points, or the classroom session can be combined with a visit to the facility.

Topics

The topics discussed in a management level meeting include some of the same information in an employee session, but additional topics address questions and concerns specific to management, including:

- Are these disorders real? How can we tell if our people are faking?
- What actions should we take when an employee says they hurt?
- What are our options for preventing CTDs?
- What changes are practical and cost effective?

While management may ask these questions in their own way, they form the basis for the management session which covers:

- History of CTDs/statistics
- Anatomy and biomechanics of the upper extremities
- Risk factors
- Medical management/return-to-work strategies
- Employee education and ergonomics programs
- Developing, implementing, and maintaining a CTD prevention program

Management and Supervisor Training

Both the management and supervisor training programs include methods for reinforcing new and improved workstyles by employees. The supervisor training program, in addition, includes specific methods for identifying and responding to risk factors in the work area.

The length of the management and supervisor programs will vary depending upon the scope of the process, management's willingness to be involved, and the instructor's judgment as to how much information is necessary and usable for each group. However, programs generally range from two to four hours.

Promoting Participation

Sufficient time needs to be spent addressing the critical importance of management and supervisors maintaining ongoing presence and support regarding the program. Providing an educational program for these individuals is relatively simple. Ensuring that they will use this information is the more difficult task.

It is important to inform these groups that the session is not the last time they will have access to this information or the consultant. Participants need to understand that the training program has not made them an expert, but rather, an active participant who now knows how to better take advantage of the consultant's skills, and how they can effectively and confidently participate.

Establishing a Task Force

Task forces can perform a variety of important functions.[56] This author develops them as an energy source for ongoing activities. Consultants generally do not have the time or energy to single-handedly manage a program, nor should they. Consultants generate the initial energy, enthusiasm, and ideas. Enthusiasm must be contagious and must be exuded by the company for the program to continue.

The consultant should also be aware that there may be preexisting committees, focus groups, or task forces within a company. It may be advantageous to tap into these groups rather than adding "another committee."

Ideally task force membership should represent a cross-section of company personnel, such as:

- Management representatives
- Supervisors
- Employees
- Union representatives
- Medical department representatives
- Outside consultant

In some companies individuals are elected to the task force or must qualify for this position by demonstrating a strong commitment to safety. The level of power this task force wields will be determined by management.

The function of the task force is best determined by the group, although the consultant can assist in this determination. It is important that the task force meet regularly and have goals. The frequency with which they meet and the goals they set need to be acceptable to all parties for it to survive.

Goals may include regularly scheduled educational programs, an active ergonomics program (which may require a different task force with a more specific focus), or simply responding to employee concerns by determining the most appropriate action to be taken (which could include bringing in an outside consultant).

It is generally advisable that a group remain stable in terms of its membership for at least six months. Otherwise there can be a loss of consistency. When membership changes are made, they should not be all at once, so that experienced members can set the pace for new participants.

PREVENTION EDUCATION

Background

Employee education in industry has not been well established. Despite the many potential benefits of training, a recent survey uncovered that 90% of the companies contacted do not formally train their employees.[40] In industry, education often consists of employees watching a 20 minute safety video and signing their name to a sign-up sheet. In such sessions, employees are exposed to information. How much they learn, internalize, or used is questionable.

The Nature of Change

It has been established that the reason people get hurt stems from either an unsafe environment or unsafe workstyles. Ergonomics addresses the environment, education addresses workstyles. A CTD prevention program attempts to elicit changes in behavior. It is

extremely important that consultants who teach in industry realize that education alone is not sufficient. Policies and procedures are also necessary to reinforce education. Workers are taught the dangers of trauma to their head or eyes, but many would not wear a hard hat and safety glasses if it were not mandatory.

Education is the instruction manual for an injury prevention process. It allows an employee to actively contribute, but it has no power except in presenting new choices and attempting to get employees to make them. Effectively getting an employee to choose new workstyles relies on two key factors; motivation to change and ability to change.

Motivation to Change

An important question when attempting to alter work behaviors is "what is in it for the participant?" A consultant or management may consider the important benefits to be improved health and well being, however employees may be motivated by material incentives or formal recognition for working safely.

In attempting to generate motivation, the consultant must assume the employee's point of view and imagine why they may be motivated to change the way they work. Few will be able to relate to the pain and suffering that is discussed. The consultant must be motivating.

The consultant might ask the participants what motivates them to stay healthy. In many cases they will respond openly. It is often family, recreation, or retirement aspirations. If this is the case, the speaker can focus some attention on these areas.

Gradually establishing rapport with employees, keeping expectations realistic, and progressing at a gradual and manageable pace, are successful strategies to generate motivation for a program. Enthusiasm, like boredom, is contagious. The consultant needs to generate as much motivation as possible, in a realistic sense.

Ability to Change

As a result of the educational program, employees may be motivated, but unable to change, due to deeply ingrained habits or physical constraints in the work environment. Sometimes, employees cannot change because the status quo returns after the program ends. This issue must be addressed early with management. If management does not commit to implementing change after the sessions, the effects of education will be short lived.

Despite this barrier, a program can still have impact if the consultant conveys that many of the changes after the class are the responsibility of the participants. One caution, however, is that false expectations created in a session can defeat the purpose of the program and potentially widen the gap between management and employees.

Program Principles

There are two issues that must be considered when putting together an educational program. One is "how you say it" and the second is "how they hear it." It is critical that both of these are taken into consideration as they will greatly impact the success of the program.

The most common method of educating employees is through lecture, discussion, participation, and demonstration. Consultants providing educational programs to adults will benefit from understanding how adults learn best.

Active Involvement. People learn best when they feel they are actively involved in the learning process. The more the learner can practice and project the information into real life situations, the more learning will take place.

A Climate of Respect. People learn best when there is a climate of respect and the teacher exhibits a sense of caring for each individual.

An Atmosphere of Trust. People learn best when there is an atmosphere of trust. This trust needs to be established early and is characterized by "unfreezing" a person's interactions through openness, honest negotiation, and problem solving.

A Climate of Self-Discovery. People learn best when they are helped to meet their own needs rather than having their needs dictated to them. Curiosity exists in every person. The skilled leader can bring out this natural curiosity in almost anyone.

A Non-Threatening Situation. People learn best when they have the opportunity to confront and challenge ideas without fear of consequences, and where error is accepted as a natural part of the learning process.

A Climate of Self Awareness. People learn best when they see themselves as they really are. Self-evaluation is of primary importance in the teaching-learning situation. Evaluation by others is secondary. Every opportunity for self-critique should be undertaken.[7]

Content Guidelines

An instructor should go through the program thoroughly before a presentation and critically evaluate all the information to be presented. If a message does not contain important and usable information, or it does not tap into an employee's idea of "what's in it for me?," it may be detracting from the program.

An effective way to determine whether the presentation is on track with the audience, is to break away from the subject matter for a few moments and ask the participants for feedback. If critical information is not discussed, the instructor may want to back up and reiterate the key points, or at least recognize the need to redesign the training to be more effective in future presentations.

Presenting effectively is no less a skill than manual therapy or designing a splint. The presentation itself is not the most important component related to the long term impact of the program, but it is important in establishing a relationship that will allow the consultant to develop rapport with the employees. It is for this reason that consultants who do public speaking learn to do so in a way that exemplifies as much skill as any other service they provide.

Program Content

There are different types of CTD prevention programs. There are those that are designed for high risk companies who may or may not already have symptomatic employees and excessive Worker's Compensation claims. There are also other programs for proactive companies with a lower risk, asymptomatic population to provide employees with general tips on topics such as posture and fitness. With the high visibility of CTDs today, it is wise to offer both types of presentations.

The low risk company's presentation generally carries a lighter tone, focusing less on risk factors and more on general "healthy upper body" concepts. The company with high risk or with existing CTDs present should have the following points included in its educational program, keeping in mind the "educate and motivate" concept.

Rationale for the Program. A brief discussion of the history of CTDs as they relate to the general population and the company specifically.

Anatomy and Biomechanics of the Upper Body. General descriptions of the basic structure of the upper body and the most commonly experienced disorders.

Instructors need to identify what is important and usable by participants. In this author's CTDs program the basic theme revolves around the "anatomical neutral" or "power position." The participants learn, through lecture and demonstration, that there are positions in which the body works most efficiently (Figure 10.10). As people work they are often either required, or choose, to move farther and farther out of

FIGURE 10.10 The body works most effeciently and handles force most safely from the anatomical neutral or power position.

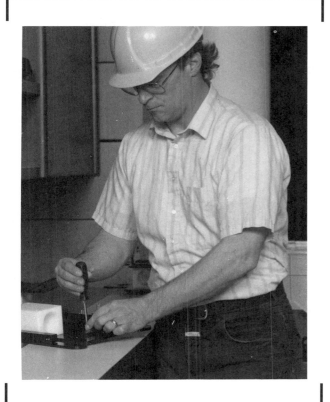

these neutral positions. These postures are then effected by the amount of force which must be generated in these postures, and the number of repetitions involved throughout the day. This theme of "anatomical neutral," position force and repetition is then perpetuated throughout the entire educational program.

Many companies are concerned about mentioning specific diagnosis, such as carpal tunnel syndrome or describing symptoms in detail. In most cases it is not necessary to discuss specific symptoms. The purpose of the program is to increase understanding of prevention techniques. It is not unusual, if symptoms are discussed, to find that questions begin centering on different symptoms the participants are experiencing as opposed to the goal of the program, prevention techniques.

It is advisable that the consultant generally discusses symptoms or carpal tunnel syndrome with management, before the program. This author has been specifically asked by employers to explain carpal tunnel syndrome to the employees. Everyone had their own definition and management wanted to eliminate mystery.

Other employers would like to focus strictly on the

"healthy upper body" and would prefer that any discussion of symptoms or diagnoses takes place outside the classroom. Whatever the consultant's philosophy is, the requests of the company must be respected. It is not unusual, if symptoms or diagnoses are not brought up by the presenter, for a participant to ask about carpal tunnel syndrome or a specific symptom. In this case it will have been beneficial to have discussed this with management before the program to ascertain how they would like you to respond.

Common Causes. In addition to the information that is widely understood about CTDs it is critical in this section that participants realize how much is not known and understood about these disorders.

Identifying a risk factor does not mean that doing one of these activities once in a while will cause a problem. It is also important to stress the "24 hour" factor that identifies home and recreational activities that contribute to the disorder (Figure 10.11, *A, B, C*).

One strategy is to address risk factors on a spectrum. For example take wrist flexion. On one end of the spectrum is full flexion or repetitive flexion. On the other is no flexion of the wrist. Too much flexion repetitively can increase the risk of a CTD. No flexion can cause loss of movement.

We also know that force is a risk factor on one end of the spectrum, but a lack of force can lead to atrophy on the other end. Somewhere in the middle is the maintenance of the muscle strength. It is important that employees do not think there are some things they can never do. This perpetuates the single incidence perception. Prevention is the result of balancing the risk factors and moderating the exposure.

Prevention Strategies. Instructors and employees can have fun with this section. This is a terrific opportunity for group participation and problem solving activities. If possible, you can have actual work tools available in the room. These allow for visual demonstration and concrete problem solving. If feasible, extend this approach to the work area to demonstrate how ideas can actually be implemented. It is important to stress the habitual nature of methods the employees currently use. This single session will do nothing to alter their behaviors until they put this information into practice.

Stretching/Warm-up. Many employees during the sessions ask questions regarding exercise programs. It is important to differentiate between exercise, warm-up, and stretching. An exercise program is designed to alter one or all the areas of strength, flexibility, and endurance. A warm-up program prepares the muscles and joints for work. A stretching program restores circulation and oxygen to muscles after sustained

FIGURE 10.11 A, B, C   The 24 Hour Factor. Wrist flexion or other stressful wrist positions can result from not only work activities, but round-the-clock activities.

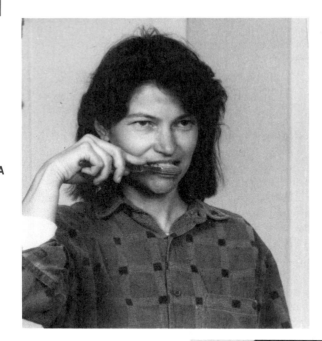

A

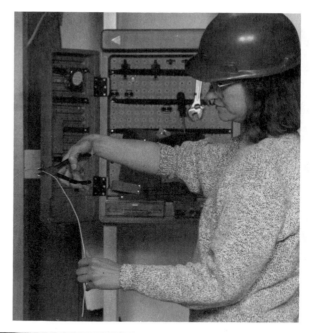

B

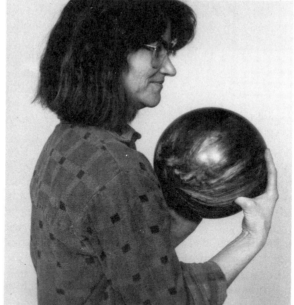

C

periods of work. Thus, muscles can be stretched to gain flexibility before work, or they can be stretched to "breathe" during the work day (Figure 10.12). A flexibility program requires an individual to take a muscle to a lengthened position, hold for 20 seconds and repeat three times. Stretching to let a muscle breathe can be done by taking a muscle to a lengthened

position for a few seconds. This type of stretch is called a "compensating stretch" instead of a flexibility stretch. In other words, the person is compensating for the work they have been doing in order to continue.

Studies have demonstrated the nature of muscle fatigue.[54] It has been shown that as muscle force increases, the ability to maintain a contraction over

FIGURE 10.12 On-the-job exercises that restore circulation and oxygen to muscles can help prevent CTDs.

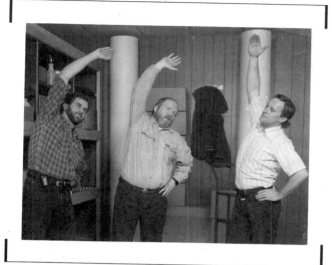

time decreases. In physiological terms this decrease in output is directly related to an increase of lactic acid build-up in the working muscle and an inability of oxygen to reach this same muscle. This is the process of fatigue. The work rest schedules developed by Rodgers[54] were designed to illustrate how often a person needs to let their muscles breathe in order to continue working. Some newer information shows that even at a 12% Muscular Voluntary Contraction (MVC) a muscle can fatigue in as little as 5 minutes of sustained effort.[79]

An additional concern to many is whether or not warm-up activities may contribute to the problem. Many programs promote flexion or extension of the wrist, both considered to be risk factors. There are a few things that need to be considered when addressing this concern.

First, generic warm-up or stretching programs for the general population in industry should not be viewed as "treatment." Those individuals who are symptomatic are instructed to abstain from program unless they have been evaluated by a medical provider, and the recommended stretches have either been approved, or replaced by ones that are more appropriate. There are numerous "healthy" and "normal" movements such as wrist flexion and extension that may be contraindicated for individuals with a preexisting condition.

Second, it may be appropriate to move the wrist into any position as a warm-up, if the person is going to be working in that position or moving in or out of that position during the day. What may be inappropriate is using a particular stretch as a compensating stretch if it moves the body part into the same position from which you are trying to compensate. Warm-up activities should be designed to make it easier for people to move into the positions they need to use. Compensating stretches should be designed to "open-up" and let muscles breathe that have been used in specific positions during the day.

It also needs to be recognized that the rate of muscle recovery for all individuals is not the same. This is particularly true for individuals in the moderate and advanced stages of cumulative trauma. EMG readings have demonstrated that some individuals' muscles have lost the ability to recover in a timely manner.[79] This may be the reason many employees will start work on Monday feeling all right, by Tuesday they are hurting, by Friday they can barely take it anymore and then they use the weekend to "rest up." The fatigue is accumulating over time.

Question and Answer. There should always be adequate time in an education session for questions and answers. It is also critical that the consultant anticipate potentially "difficult" questions and discuss the general nature of their answers with management, prior to the meeting. It is important that the presenter represents the philosophy of the management team and that statements regarding possible action on the part of management are in line with managements plans.

It is important for a presenter to steer clear of questions relating to an individual participant's symptoms or treatment. The participant may be testing to see if your response is similar to that of their medical provider or they may be genuinely curious. In either case it is best to respond by informing the individual that without an evaluation it would not be appropriate to respond, and it is important to keep questions focused on the material that is being covered. It is appropriate to inform the person that at the break or end of the class, you can discuss questions they may want to ask their medical provider.

Occasionally an employee will comment that management will not allow them time to stretch or learn a new technique because it takes too much production time. Therefore it is beneficial to discuss the most appropriate responses with management before the program. Inform the employees that management is aware of what is being presented to them, and management recognizes that while production is necessary, these other areas are important and they are willing to explore ways that stretching and new work methods can be incorporated into the job.

Ask management before a program, if they are willing to consider stretching, job rotation, and ergonomic changes. If the reply is negative, inform members that it will appear that all the responsibility of CTD prevention is placed on the employees. This may make employees question management's commitment.

In any event it is important to know management's position before facing the employee.

Regardless of the information presented, the presenter can expect that the information most likely to be remembered is that which affects an individual directly. It is not only important that there is time for questions, but also that questions are answered to a participant's satisfaction. This does not mean that significant time needs to be spent on a question. If a question is not appropriate for the class, a brief explanation of why it is not is given to the questioner. If handled appropriately, it will inform others with similar questions, in a fair way, that these questions are best asked at another time.

It is not uncommon to appear as if you are trying to be "politically correct" or an extension of management when answering sensitive questions. Inform the audience that you are there to give out information, not to set or change policy or enforce management or employee behavior. Questions should not be left unanswered. Unanswered questions demonstrate that management does not regard the information as important.[40]

Key Points

Having covered the general components of the session, there are key points that should be verbalized and reinforced repeatedly throughout every session. These include;

The Cumulative Nature of the Disorders. This will often be described relative to disorders people are familiar with, including heart disease and tooth decay. They happen gradually over time with little or no warning.

CTDs Are Not Contagious. This author presents a scenario where a person is sitting at their desk, while on their right is a person wearing a splint, and on their left is a person who is receiving cortisone shots. The person wonders how soon these disorders will invade his or her body.

Anatomical Neutral. The body's most efficient position.

Risk Factors. The risk factors for heart disease and tooth decay are discussed in order to get the audience to realize that any factor that is infrequent and isolated will probably not lead to a problem. Examine what happens if the risk factors are combined and the frequency increases. The same format is used to review the risk factors identified as contributors to CTDs and evaluated, relative to the activities performed by this audience both at work and at home.

Compensate. As expressed in the stretching program, one of the greatest contributors to CTDs is when people get in certain positions or apply forces without compensating for either of these. Compensating in

FIGURE 10.13 A, B   Changing work positions frequently ensures that forces are compensated during the day.

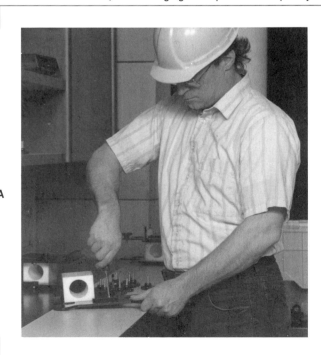
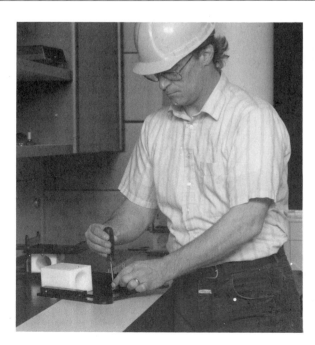

A   B

most cases means making frequent position changes during the day and stretching (Figure 10.13, *A, B*).

Twenty four hour risk factors.   The premise here is that the body does not care where a person is, it responds only to what they are doing. In this section daily activities such as brushing teeth and hair and recreational activities such as crocheting or card playing are evaluated in terms of how they may contribute to a CTD.

Personal Responsibility.   Self responsibility is emphasized throughout all phases of the program. In many cases it is appropriate to inform employees that regardless of the level of management activity relative to the program, there are things that an employee can choose to do that will minimize their risk at work and home. Everything in the presentation revolves around and supports these main points.

Testing

A company may want the instructor to provide a pre and post test. The instructor must be aware that this test may need to be adapted in companies where there are employees who are illiterate, have limited use of English, are visually impaired, or have another impairment that does not lend itself to this format. In addition, management needs to be aware that pre and post tests measure short term memory and that the test should be repeated in the future to determine the true retention of information. Industry also needs to be reminded that the results of a post test do not indicate the usability of the information presented.

The presenter may have employees fill out a brief questionnaire that provides feedback on their satisfaction with the educational program. This is valuable information in that it gives the presenter information that can be used to modify a presentation and, if the results are positive, can be used as a marketing tool with prospective clients.

Success Factors

Regardless of the talents of the presenter, their words and methods are only half of the equation of a successful session. Educating employees in a classroom setting relies on a variety of assumptions. These include:

1. The people you are teaching want to hear what you have to say.
2. The people you are teaching are capable of learning in this manner.
3. The instructor is capable of presenting the information in a way that makes sense to the participants.
4. The information presented is correct.
5. The participants will retain this information.
6. The participants can effectively utilize the information that is being presented.

Kilbom (1987) reported that when faced with a stressful situation, workers trained in alternative methods resorted to old work habits.[61] For example, an employee who has been instructed in a new method for holding a tool will return to the original method if they sense that attempting this new workstyle is slowing them down. This is particularly true if this is being called to their attention by supervisors or peers on a work line.

In many instances some or all of the above mentioned assumptions will not hold true and need to be dealt with accordingly. The best way to deal with them is to anticipate their existence. Experienced speakers learn to detect which ones are present and address them early in the program. It is important to develop "modes" of presentations that take into consideration various audiences. Teaching a class at the end of a shift often dictates a difference in energy level to accommodate for employee fatigue, or desire to go home now that the work is complete. The ability to make these changes is not book learned, or developed from patient contact, it requires practice.

Program Logistics

Ideally a program is no longer than 60 to 90 minutes. This is because of production issues as well as the ability to hold the employee's attention. Brief standing (and stretching) breaks should be given frequently and a five minute break should be given if the session approaches or goes beyond one hour.

These classes are generally held in any room the company deems fit for training. This is not always the most conducive to learning, but holding an audience in a distracting environment may win points for effort if the presenter can pull it off. Class size should be kept reasonable—groups of over 20 to 25 participants become more of a lecture and reduce the chances for active participation by the audience. All audiovisual equipment must be checked out prior to the program.

Attendance at these sessions, while focused primarily at employees, is complemented by the presence of supervisors and management. There are management sessions that preclude attendance of employees because of sensitive issues, but a mixed group for employee sessions is encouraged. This is particularly true for second and third shift meetings when management personnel are generally not seen.

This author asks to be introduced to the employees by the President of the company. If this individual is not available, then the next highest ranking official would be acceptable. Certainly the person in charge of safety should be present and speak on the session's importance, but someone from upper management can describe briefly management's commitment to the process. Bringing in management can break down the "us" and "them" mentality between employees and management.

MAINTAINING THE PROGRAM

Repetition

Repetition is one of the most effective learning tools. Consultants are often in awe how an employee can do their job "with eyes closed" and know where all controls are located, or know how much time has passed simply by the number of pieces being processed. This knowledge is based on repetition. Children learn to brush their teeth from hearing the message over and over each night before they go to bed. They do not attend a one hour seminar on the rewards of good oral hygiene and then choose to brush their teeth.

Repetition needs to be built into every phase of an effective CTD program.[63] Management needs to learn, and be reminded frequently to involve everyone in the process. Supervisors need to be reminded frequently to include safety in their evaluation of work practices and department meetings, and the employees need to be reminded constantly that they are a critical part of the process and are as responsible for their safety as is the company.

Supervisor Commitment

Management needs to realize that the reason supervisors are regularly informing employees to either work faster, or do better quality work, is because the supervisors are accountable to management for production and quality standards. If management believes that the prevention of CTDs is important, this needs to be conveyed to the supervisors in the same way.

Many companies are now developing specific protocols that dictate regularly scheduled departmental safety talks, standardize methods for dealing with ergonomic concerns raised by employees, and implement stretching/warm-up programs. These activities present the supervisors with a message on daily methods of operation; a message, if delivered regularly and enforced fairly passes from management to supervisors and from supervisors to employees.

Program Evaluation/Audit

The ability of a program to evolve is necessary for its survival. This ability can be built into the program design from the very beginning. Truly effective programs have a very recognizable beginning and no recognizable end. They are living, breathing entities that grow and change—or die.

This statement is not intended to give management the impression that they will never be rid of the consultant. On the contrary, reliance on the consultant should become less and less over time.

The question that best demonstrates this is "when will the prevention of CTDs no longer be of importance to this company?" If it will always be important, then it is necessary to build longevity into the process. This is the reason for a task force, and the ability to change needs to exist. Informing employees that each quarter the task force will gather feedback, make determinations on how the program is going, and take the necessary action to demonstrate that this process is alive.

Evaluating the program and finding out problems does not indicate that a program is not working and needs to be discontinued, it means that choices need to be made and action taken to improve the process. Employees should be informed that simply stating dissatisfaction with the program is not enough, they must provide some guidance for improvement. The most critical element is the ability to change. Rarely does a program have all the necessary pieces in perfect working order when it starts.

Policies and Procedures

Many employees cringe at the thought of more policies and procedures. That is because often the rationale for the policy has not been in sync with the reality on the floor, or the rationale has not been discussed beforehand with the employees. The policies surrounding a CTD program will be most effective if they are developed with employee input and participation.

The rationale for policies in this instance is to help the employees develop habits that will reduce the risk of injury. Exactly how the employees should be reminded of this policy (tool box talks, supervisor reminders, posters) is often best determined by the employees. Policies in many companies require participation in a stretching program, material handling methods, or the use of ergonomic equipment. The support and enforcement of these policies by supervisors and management is imperative. If there is one instance where a safety policy is circumvented or ignored for production reasons the policy will lose its power.

Moving Education Out of the Classroom. It is important to take the training out onto the floor where people are working. As was stated in an article by Rystrom and Eversmann, 1991,[56] "when education goes out into the workplace, it becomes training."

Tool box talks, also known as "Tail Gate Meetings" or "Shift Meetings" are brief sessions, generally five to fifteen minutes in length. They are provided by the

FIGURE 10.14   Popular "tool box" talks on production and quality issues can also include a review of CTD prevention measures.

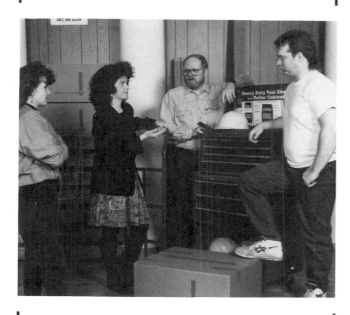

consultant, or more often a supervisor or employee. This format already exists in many industries for discussion of production and quality issues. These meetings provide an opportunity to review the key points of the CTD educational program and provide an opportunity for questions and discussion.

The critical factor is that meetings take place on a regularly scheduled and frequent basis. The consultant may conduct the first few meetings for a department and gradually involve supervisors and employees in handling sessions (Figure 10.14).

It is very expensive in many industries to take employees away from their jobs for extended periods of time. For this reason tool box talks are an excellent way to maintain interest and momentum in the process at minimal costs. The expensive part of a program is the down time associated with the classes. This issue is best addressed through frequent but brief meetings with employees.

STRETCHING AND WARM-UP PROGRAMS

Stretching and warm-up, discussed earlier in connection with education, are becoming the more widely recognized element of an injury prevention program. These factors vary greatly in scope but have demon-

strated success, particularly when incorporated in a comprehensive program.[14, 43, 52, 57, 60]

Attitude to Overcome

One of the biggest paradigms in industry that discourages them from becoming involved in this type of program is that stretching takes time, and time is money. This attitude persists despite the fact that the literature to date has not demonstrated that stretching programs slow down production. In actuality, companies have been able to maintain production standards, despite setting aside employee work time for participation in warm-up and stretching programs.[52]

Success Factors

The odds of a warm-up or stretching program being successful increase if the following are present:
1. Full management and supervisor support.
2. Easily implemented.
3. Does not interfere with production.
4. Employee participation in the development, implementation, and maintenance of the program.
5. The rationale for the program is easily understood.
6. Maintenance plan (program updates at tool box talks, consultant updating the stretches to keep people from becoming bored with the program, T-shirts, or other items that promote the program).
7. The program is fun (but not silly).

Getting management and employees to support the program comes through pointing out the benefits realized in other companies, explaining the concept and rationale clearly, then leaving it up to management and the employees to decide. These programs are generally much easier to implement and maintain if the desire and commitment are generated at employee level.

Once a decision has been made to implement a stretching or warm-up program there are a number of steps that, if taken, can increase the likelihood of a successful program. Following is an example of the stretching program format utilized by this author for a number of companies. The program is divided into three steps—1) program development, 2) program implementation, and 3) program maintenance.

Program Development

Prior to its beginning, a great deal of time and effort is put out to insure the program's success. A task force of motivated and interested employees from the department is organized. It is their responsibility to work

FIGURE 10.15   A company task force is charged with promoting and monitoring the program and eventually giving it a life of its own.

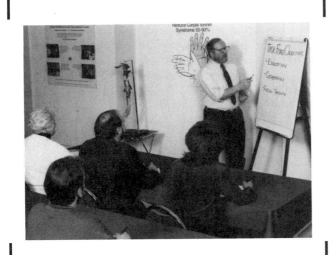

closely with the instructor, promote the program within the department, and monitor the feedback of their peers (Figure 10.15).

Program development begins with a task force orientation meeting. The orientation provides an introduction to the program, its rationale and proposed methods. The orientation offers the task force an opportunity to ask questions and discuss options that might improve the acceptance of the program.

During orientation, questions may be raised as to whether or not the program should be mandatory. A mandatory program may be faced with resistance. On the other hand, if the program is voluntary there could be limited participation. Many industries agree upon the program being presented to employees as a job function.

Evaluating the Worksite

The next step in development is worksite evaluation. The purpose for this is twofold; to introduce yourself to the employee population, and to gather information needed to customize the stretching program.

During the evaluation the type of work being performed is measured to determine movement and usage of muscle groups. Photographs (slides) are taken and customized for the employee orientation program. The consultant should talk with the employees about their jobs and solicit their input on the stretching program. Following worksite evaluation, a report is generated outlining the job demands and the most appropriate stretches. Documentation of the worksite evaluation is then formally presented to a stretching task force for their review.

Program Implementation

Program implementation begins with a one hour orientation for employees. This meeting is to introduce the program and provide them with the rationale and methodology for putting the program into place. A survey can be distributed to all employees during the program's developmental stage. A cover sheet provides them with some background information on the stretching program. The survey asks them questions regarding their interest in a program, discomfort experienced during the day, and other general information.

To address specific concerns during the class, this author recommends that the consultant has access to the results of the survey, prior to the initial employee session.

The orientation addresses basic anatomy, biomechanics, and how the body is effected by certain movements. The effects of work and the need for compensation for work demands throughout the day are also covered. The stretching program is introduced in a two part format—1) warming up first thing in the morning to prepare the body for work (Figure 10.16, *A, B*), and 2) stretching periodically throughout the day to allow the body to remain fresh.

The morning portion is formally organized and the periodic stretches are performed at the employees discretion. Each stretch is demonstrated with employees at the end of the session. Following the orientation, a date can be chosen for the official beginning of the program.

One of the companies this author has worked with determined early in the development of the program, that it should be fun and up-beat. To assist in this area, a cassette player was brought in and employees were encouraged to bring in music of choice while stretching.

Employees can choose to talk amongst themselves or listen to the music while stretching. A volunteer leader times the stretches. The leader is expected only to tell the employees when they should perform a different stretch. This is less threatening than having someone get in front of peers to demonstrate a stretch or answer questions about stretches.

The consultant should be present on two days during the first and second weeks, then one day per week for the following two weeks to insure that stretches are being performed properly and to answer any questions. Modifications or alternative stretches can be provided to those who experience undue discomfort or who had known disorders that precluded a specific stretch.

FIGURE 10.16 A, B   Stretching before work prepares the muscles and joints for the motion and stresses of job tasks.

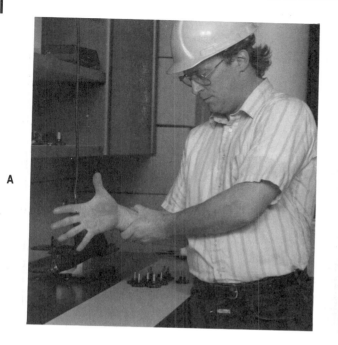
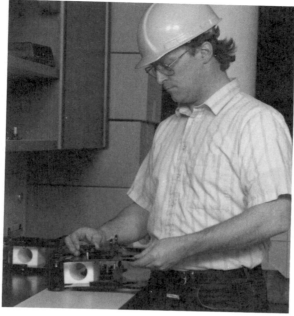

A

B

Warm-Up

You will note that the word "warm-up" is always placed next to the word stretching. Stretching is most effective when combined with a brief warm-up to prepare the muscles. For the first three minutes of a program the employees warm-up their bodies by marching in place, swinging their arms, and getting the blood circulating.

For most people in industry, the thought of seeing a group of workers marching in place and swinging their arms seems a little out of place. This may be the result, if the employees are not presented with the rationale for the warm-up. When presented properly the warm-up portion is readily accepted and has been described by many of the employees as a real "shot in the arm" to get the day started. In nearly all cases the acceptance of a new program is based largely on the method of presentation. Without an orientation to the employees and a forum to voice their concerns and ideas, the odds of program rejection are high.

All of the stretches in a program should be designed for either standing or sitting positions (Figure 10.17, *A, B, C*).

Program Support

To support a program, posters can be made and placed strategically throughout the facility. Some companies go as far as printing up sweatshirts to be distributed that display the stretching program title.

Individuals with preexisting conditions (shoulder problems, knee problems, etc.) should be identified, and precluded from the performance of certain stretches. A modification of a stretch or replacement stretch should be provided, and in extreme cases, have an employee consult the treating physician or therapist to provide them with alternative stretches.

Program Maintenance

The key ingredient to success is longevity. To insure longevity, meetings should be held with the task force on a monthly basis for the first few months to discuss follow up activities. This could then be extended to a quarterly meeting. Visits by the consultant to talk (and stretch) with the employees are scheduled for one or two mornings per month. This allows for observation of techniques and provides an opportunity to address questions that arise.

Ongoing Commitment

In one company several employees approached the manager requesting a stretching program for home use. A physical therapist was brought on-site to evaluate interested employees, ensuring that there were no conditions to preclude the performance of specific

FIGURE 10.17 A, B, C   Examples of stretches.

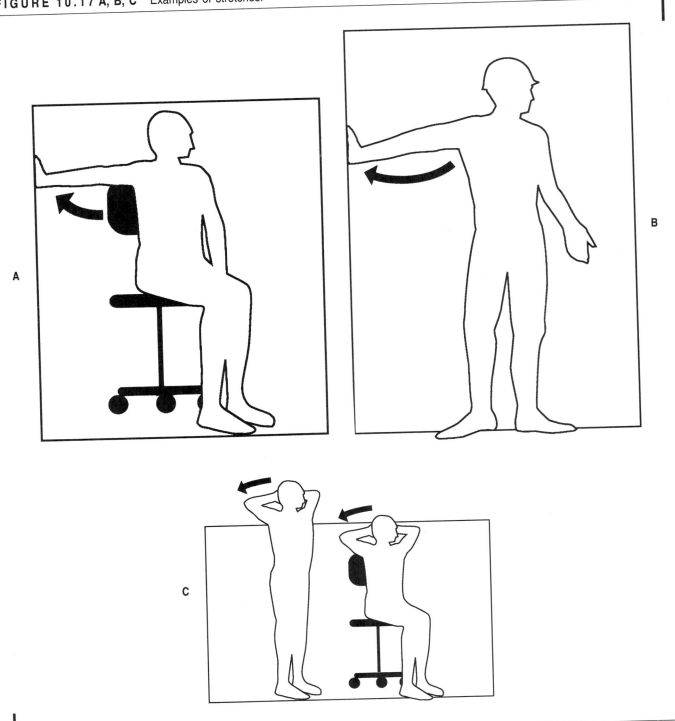

(From Innovative Systems for Rehabilitation, Minneapolis, Minn.)

stretches. Employees were told that information from their assessment would remain confidential and would not be shared with the employer.

Every employee in the department volunteered for assessment and to this date, (one year later) many still report participating in at least a portion of their home program. The assessments were made in the nurse's office at the plant, each one lasted approximately 30 minutes. As a result, a few employees were found to have conditions that warranted treatment. These individuals were encouraged by management to seek treatment, and were put on exercise programs that dealt specifically with their conditions. This preventive approach was foreseen by management as a cost effective way to curtail problems from becoming worse.

Program maintenance is supported by quarterly educational features which include one hour discussions on general health and safety concerns and focus on cumulative trauma prevention. A list of potential topics can be provided so that employees can choose the subjects of utmost interest.

Starting Time

An issue common to many companies is staggered starting times for employees. In this instance employees do not have the group leader to take them through stretches. At one company, the task force recommended that a tape be made that takes the participant through the routine. A tape of music is chosen by employees and the consultant can then ''dub-over'' instructions and timing of the stretches.

The program also encourages employees to perform stretches briefly throughout the day. Extra posters can be placed throughout the facility to remind employees and task force members to periodically stretch. The goal is for these activities to become habitual and eventually typical work behaviors.

ERGONOMICS PROGRAM

Ergonomics was discussed in great detail in Chapter 6, but some comments with regard to CTDs are important here.

Importance

It is difficult to implement an effective CTD program without incorporating ergonomics.[39] There are several ways to implement these programs and when ergonomic teams and longevity are developed into the program, greatest long term benefits are achieved.[22, 51, 58, 65, 77] The literature has reported minimal costs when ergonomic efforts have been implemented to substantially reduce incidence of injury.[24, 50, 56]

In instances where more expensive equipment must be bought, a thorough cost analysis can often justify the initial expense, through increased production and improved quality, as well as reduced risk of injury.[42]

Team Concept

Ergonomic programs work well when employee teams are established. Their role is to work with the consul-

tant to identify potential risks and develop strategies for eliminating or reducing these risks. There are systematic programs available on the market to assist industry with this process.[77] In many instances when this author is contacted, clients identify a risk factor and develop solutions. They call to verify whether the solution is in line with accepted ergonomic principles.

Important Considerations

Variables that can effect the success of an ergonomics program include:
- Perception (or reality) of the capital expenses necessary to make changes.
- How the changes are implemented. Were employees consulted on the changes, and if they were not, will they take advantage of them or ignore them because they were not consulted?
- Technical expertise of those working on the solutions.
- Does the solution truly impact the problem? It may simply move the problem to another part of the body (or to another person). It may not take into consideration the 16 hours of an employee's non-work day, that can significantly contribute to a CTD problem. It is those unknowns that need to be addressed in order to make the workstation design approach a complete solution.
- Incomplete understanding of ergonomic principles even by the experts. Ergonomics is still a relatively new science. Yet, industry and consultants grasp at bits and pieces and widely spread them, without fully questioning their impact.
- Is the maintenance/engineering staff available to make changes on a timely basis?

Role of Facilities Maintenance

It is very difficult to have a successful ergonomics program, or any type of effective injury prevention program without active involvement by the facility's maintenance department. Many changes relative to an ergonomics program entail either the repair of equipment, or slight modifications by facility maintenance people. It is also important that a format is developed to handle requests formally, so response time and prioritization of requests can be monitored. Many maintenance departments are already behind in their day-to-day tasks and can get bogged down easily when an ergonomic program begins. Companies need to be realistic in how much is possible and how fast it can be done. The maintenance department's involvement is essential in order to keep the ergonomic process from becoming bogged down with orders and lost requests for equipment repair.

MEDICAL MANAGEMENT PROGRAM

Regardless of the prevention efforts people will still get hurt. In addition, most companies already have employees off or on "modified duty" at the time they undertake a prevention program. It is important that the company has a systematic approach to dealing with these employees.

Detecting The Symptoms

Of particular importance is the need to understand how to react to an employee when they "ache" or are "sore." Most companies know what to do when the employee is bleeding. CTDs are now forcing them to recognize and react to "hidden" or "invisible" disorders. Many companies have aggressive but fair methods for dealing with these disorders. They include early detection, effective prevention, and management through screenings, splinting, and rotation programs.[8, 56, 62]

Controlling Symptoms At Work

Taking it another step is an innovative approach called Controlling Symptoms At Work (C-SAW).[27] This new process teaches either in-house medical staff or the employees themselves, methods of early symptom control that can be performed at the worksite. This program is based on evidence that links CTDs with fatigue and discomfort in the muscles of the neck, shoulders, and upper back.

Employees are instructed on methods to detect these conditions as early as possible, with the only symptom in most cases being fatigue, or mild discomfort. They are then instructed in specific stretching techniques and in the use of a thera-cane™, an instrument designed to allow the individual to apply pressure to knots, or trigger points that can develop in fatigued muscles.

The purpose of this program is to allow industry and employees to identify and eliminate symptoms as a part of the work day, avoiding increased lost time and medical intervention. This approach is based on surface EMG readings which demonstrate that progression towards cumulative trauma can be related to muscle dysfunction, beginning in the neck. This program was developed in response to a recognition that CTDs, carpal tunnel syndrome in particular, progresses in distinct recognizable stages. It was learned that while muscle fatigue is accelerated and recovery delayed in the earliest stages of carpal tunnel syndrome, impact in the later stages is significantly more pronounced and difficult to reverse.[26]

Return-to-Work Consultation

This is an extension of the medical management program. It involves a visit by the treating therapist when a previously injured employee returns to work. In this scenario the employee, the therapist, and the department supervisor all work together to insure a successful transition to the workplace. Recommendations are provided to the employee on methods to reduce aggravation of the injury.

The need and possibilities of ergonomic adaptation can be discussed and the supervisor can be informed on cues that should be given to the employee to help insure safe work practices. Other issues related to periodic icing, worksite stretches, or a splint schedule can also be addressed. This visit shifts the responsibility from the medical community to the employee and the industry.

Surveillance

Industry needs to regularly gather data regarding employees' experiences with symptoms or actual incidences of CTDs. This can be done through passive surveillance involving the review of medical data, or active surveillance which involves questionnaires or surveys. Samples of these can be found in the new ANSI Z365 proposed standards,[67] as well as in the professional literature.[21, 36] The standard is an attempt at establishing an objective method for dealing effectively with these disorders and is the combined effort of associations, employers, professional societies, researchers, insurers, academics, and individuals.[21]

Establishing the Team

The Industrial therapy team was discussed in greater detail in Chapter 2, but its role in preventing CTDs is important. It has become clear that the risk factors associated with CTDs and its costs are very diverse. It is therefore requisite that consultants understand that the ability to address these numerous factors is limited. Health professionals who consult with industry generally have expertise in the areas of musculoskeletal injury prevention and the medical management of these disorders. These individuals however, are generally less knowledgeable in dealing with some of the complex industrial psychology issues, Workers' Compensation laws and regulations, or the engineering aspects of job redesign. All these factors indicate the need to establish an effective team.

This team includes both on-site and off-site professionals who have talents necessary for the implementation of a truly comprehensive program. They can serve both as consultants, or as resources of information for situations that are beyond the expertise of the consultant. On-site experts include:

Managers
Supervisors
Employees
Engineers
Maintenance employees
Loss control director/safety director/risk
    manager
Union representative(s)
Medical personnel

The off-site team includes:

Risk management consultants
Ergonomists/engineers
Industrial psychologists
Workers' Compensation attorneys
Ergonomic equipment suppliers
Assorted clinicians
Insurance experts

REIMBURSEMENT

The fees commanded for injury prevention services vary greatly. They range, in fact, from no cost if provided as part of an insurance company's loss control program to hundreds of dollars per hour by consultants. Falling between these two groups are the services provided by hospital or clinic personnel who consult part time, primarily to maintain a relationship with business and industry in their community.

Due to the wide range of groups providing the service, it is difficult to outline a consistent fee structure. Insurance companies build the costs of a program into the premium they charge. Many hospitals and clinics will bill minimal amounts simply to maintain a foothold in companies that send them patients. It is primarily the independent consulting companies that command the highest fees.

The two main factors in determining a fee structure are—1) how much do you need? and 2) what will the market bear?

The first is often subjecture and the second can be learned from simple market research in your community. Keep in mind that it is best to have a set price for prevention services. Negotiation for long term, high volume activities is necessary, as it is difficult

to make a profit on those that are sporadic and short term.

When proposing services, it is appropriate to make statements regarding previous success. Predicting future success, and basing fees on a percentage of future savings can be a dangerous venture. Cumulative trauma, by its nature is the result of numerous risk factors, many of which may remain outside the realm of a consultant's control. While a consultant can potentially reap huge benefits by receiving a portion of savings, it is also possible that a consultant may end up with nothing to show for their efforts.

LONGEVITY EQUALS SUCCESS

The success of a program, measured in degree of participation, reductions in lost time injuries, incidence, and severity is determined to a large extent, by the length of a program. There is a phenomenon in industry this author identifies as the "Fatigue Factor." It is this phenomenon that determines whether or not a program will survive.

It is natural for people to resist change. Habits develop gradually so it only seems natural that changing habits would take time as well.

Management needs to recognize what has and has not worked for them in the past. Programs need to be designed with longevity in mind. Management needs to realize how employees react to programs that are started abruptly, and terminated nearly as fast. By going into this process with the idea that it will last for as long as the company is in business, companies will head into the process with a much more deliberate and thought-out approach of how to do this for the long haul.

Fatigue can destroy a well intentioned program. If a process is not thought out well, and there are no plans identified early for ways to react to problems or "glitches" in the program, then too much energy will be needed to keep it going. If the structure demonstrates the way business is conducted, there will be a greater likelihood of participation and success.

Employees are accustomed to seeing programs come and go. In some instances the consultant may be told by employees, "go ahead and start the program, but six months from now no one will be doing anything." This attitude should be addressed at both the management and employee level. Management needs to recognize the origin of this attitude and be willing to give some power and choices to employees to encourage willingness.

This author has told employees on several occasions that management is placing a lot of control for the program in their hands, they may then have to make some of the tough decisions. Employees are also informed that they are the ones who will determine its success or failure.

A company can make a person wear a hard hat or safety glasses, but the CTD problem has created a gray area. It is not easy to enforce a rule that tells employees "you will respect your body, you will minimize risk factors away from work, and you will stretch and change postures frequently throughout the day." These things have to happen at the employee level, and management needs to provide the financial support and professional guidance to help employees participate in this process.

Management needs to make the commitment to a CTD program by ensuring that the reduction of these disorders remains a priority. If a program's participation is limited, it does not mean the program should be ceased, only that it should be changed.

Once the decision is made to keep a program going, the only energy that needs to be expended by management is in methodology. Management in many industries start and stop programs so often that most of the energy goes into trying to convince employees that they are really serious about this program. Convincing an employee comes from maintaining a program over time, not from pouring more money into an elaborate kick-off.

SUMMARY

CTDs present a fast proliferating problem which causes, prevention, and treatment are only now beginning to be understood. Attitudes accumulated over many years do not change easily. Doctors, employers, and employees are in need of solid information and effective solutions. The consultant can be a catalyst, an educator, a motivator, and a facilitator to help industry gain control and start to manage this problem in ways that protect their financial well being, and serve the long term interests of the employee.

REFERENCES

1. Alters D: A Growing Pain in the Workplace, Star Tribune, Minneapolis, Minn, p 1D, March 8, 1992.
2. Americans With Disabilities Act: a technical assistance manual on the employment provisions. EEOC Office of Communications and Legislative Affairs, Washington, DC, January 1992.
3. Armstrong TJ, et al: Repetitive Trauma Disorders: job evaluation and design, *Human Factors* 325–336: 1986.
4. Armstrong TJ: Ergonomics and Cumulative Trauma Disorders *Hand Clinics*, 2(3): 553, 1986.
5. Arndt R: Work Pace, Stress, and Cumulative Trauma Disorders *J Hand Surgery* 12A(5): 866–869, 1987.
6. Astrand I: *Textbook of Work Physiology* ed 3, New York, McGraw-Hill, 1986.
7. Bates RE: Professional Selling Skills I, KEY method, (unpublished marketing course), 1988.
8. Berg DR, Ackerman E: Use of Vibrometry in Conjunction with Ergonomic Evaluation and Conservative Medical Management as an Ongoing Surveillance Program for Median Nerve Function, *Work Injury Manag* 1(5):7, Nov 1992.
9. Bigos SJ, Battie MC, Fisher LD: Methodology for Evaluating Predictive Factors for the Report of Back Injury, *Spine*, 16(6):669, 1991.
10. Board of Certification in Professional Ergonomics, P.O. Box 2811, Bellingham, Wash 98227–2811.
11. Bullock, MI: *Ergonomics: The Physiotherapist in the Workplace*, Churchill Livingstone, New York, 1990.
12. Cannon MPH, Lawrence J, et al: Personal and Occupational Factors Associated with Carpal Tunnel Syndrome, *J Occup Medicine* 23(4):255, April 1981.
13. Caplan SH, Champney PC et al: *Ergonomic Design For People At Work*, Eastman Kodak, vol 1 1983.
14. Clafin T: Woodmill Stretching Program Works For Fitness, Morale, Lower Costs, *Occup Health and Safety*, 60(11):34, Nov 1991.
15. Clarke J: Office Ergonomics: the wimp factor? *Occup Health*, p 234, Aug 1991.
16. Devlin P, editor: Cumulative Trauma Disorder: fact or fantasy, *Work Injury Manag*, 1(2):5, May 1992.
17. Devlin P, editor: Participatory Ergonomics, *Work Injury Manag*, 1(2):1, May 1992.
18. Dionne ED: Carpal Tunnel Syndrome Part I: the problem, *National Safety News*, March 1984.
19. Eversmann WW: Compression and Entrapment Neuropathies of the Upper Extremity, *J Hand Surgery*, 8(5B):759–766, Sept 1983.
20. Fernberg PM: Laying Down the Law on Ergonomics, *Modern Office Tech*, p 74, Oct 1992.
21. Fine LJ, Silverstein BA, et al: Detection of Cumulative Trauma Disorders of Upper Extremities in the Workplace, *J Occup Medicine* 28(8):674, Aug 1986.
22. Girling B, Birnbaum R: An Ergonomic Approach to Training for Prevention of Musculoskeletal Stress at Work, *Physiotherapy* 74:479–483, 1988.
23. Grandjean E: *Fitting The Task To The Man*, ed 4, 1988 Taylor and Francis.
24. Gross CM: Engineers, Safety Professionals Work On Total Ergonomic Quality, *Occup Health and Safety* 60(6):54, June 1991.
25. Hales T, Sauter S, Petersen M, et al: Health Hazard Evaluation Report, *NIOSH*, HETA 89–299–2230 p 25, July 1992.
26. Headley BJ: EMG Analysis: examining muscle activity in the workplace, *Occup Therapy Forum*, October 7, 1992.
27. Headley B: C-SAW, *Preventing Injury*, 2(1):2, Winter 1993.
28. Hembree D, Sandoval R: RSI has become the nation's leading work-related illness. How are reporters and editors coping with it?, *Columbia Journalism Review*, p 41, July 1991.

29. Hertz RP, Emmett EA: Risk Factors for Occupational Hand Injury, *J Occup Medicine* 28(1):36, Jan 1986.

30. Hozman R, Skosey JL: Differentiating Upper-Extremity Entrapment Syndromes, *Diagnosis* p 30, Sept 1987.

31. Johnson SL Ergonomic Design of Handheld Tools to Prevent Trauma to the Hand and Upper Extremity, *J Hand Therapy* 3(2):86, April 1990.

32. Joseph BS: Analysis of a Program for Control of Cumulative Trauma Disorders in the Auto Industry, *Ergonomic Interventions*, p. 133–149.

33. Joseph BS: Ergonomic Considerations and Job Design in Upper Extremity Disorders, *Occup Hand Injuries: Occup Medicine* 4(3):547, July 1989.

34. Joyce M: Ergonomics Will Take Center Stage During '90s and into New Century, *Occup Health and Safety* p 31, Jan 1991.

35. Kasdan ML editor: Occupational Hand Injuries, *State of the Art Reviews* 4(3), July 1989.

36. Katz JN, Larson MG, et al: Validation of a Surveillance Case Definition of Carpal Tunnel Syndrome, *Amer J Public Health*, 81(2):40, Feb 1991.

37. Key GL et al: *Reducing Symptoms of Carpal Tunnel Syndrome: a retrospective study of the key one-on-one intervention* KEY Method, Minneapolis, Minn.

38. Kilbom A: Intervention Programmes for Work-Related Neck and Upper Limb Disorders: strategies and evaluation, *Ergonomics* 31(5):735–747, 1988.

39. LaBar, G: Building ErgoLand, *Occup Hazards* p 29, Oct 1991.

40. LaBar G: Worker Training: an investment in safety, *Occup Hazards*, p 23, Aug 1991.

41. MacLeod D: *Strains and Sprains*, Minnesota Department of Labor and Industry, 1982.

42. MacLeod D: Competitive Edge: good ergonomics is good economics, *Preventing Injury* 2(3):14, Summer 1993.

43. Melnik MS: Implementing a Stretching/Warm-Up Program in Industry, *Preventing Injury* 2(1);8, Winter, 1993.

44. Minter SG: Creating The Safety Culture, *Occupational Hazards*, p 17, Aug 1991.

45. Morgan S: Most Factors Contributing to CTS Can be Minimized, if not Eliminated, *Occup Health and Safety* 60(10):47, Oct 1991.

46. Nathan PA: Hand and Arm Ills Linked to Life Style, *New York Times*, April 10, 1992.

47. NIOSH Criteria for a Recommended Standard: occupational exposure to hand-arm vibration, *NIOSH*, Cincinnati Ohio, Sept 1989.

48. Pronsati MP: Neck Muscles Play Part in Carpal Tunnel Syndrome, *Advance for Physical Therapists*, p 4, July 6, 1992.

49. Putz-Anderson V: *Cumulative Trauma Disorders: a manual for musculoskeletal diseases of the upper limbs*, New York, 1988, Taylor and Francis.

50. Rice VJ, Rice DM: Helping Hands, *Rehab Manag* 6(1):26, Dec 1993.

51. Rice VJ, Rice DM: Helping Hands: ergonomic Intervention offers employers a comprehensive approach to addressing upper extremity injuries, *Risk and Benefits Jour*, p 16, Summer 1993.

52. Rider BB: Cumulative Trauma Disorder Prevention: Is There a Lesson to Learn from Australia?: *WORK:* 2(4):67, Summer 1992.

53. Rigdon JE: The Wrist Watch: how a plant handles occupational hazard with common sense, *The Wall Street Journal*, September 28, 1992.

54. Rodgers SH, editor et al: *Ergonomic Design For People At Work*, vol 2, Eastman Kodak 1986.

55. Rodgers S: Recovery Time Needs for Repetitive Work, *Sem Occup Medicine* 2:19–24, 1987.

56. Rystrom CM, Eversmann WW: Cumulative Trauma Intervention in Industry: a model program for the upper extremity, *Occup Hand & Upper Extremity Injuries & Diseases*, p 489, 1991.

57. Sawyer K: An On-site Exercise Program to Prevent Carpal Tunnel Syndrome, *Professional Safety* p 17, 1987.

58. Sehnal JP, Christopher RC: Developing and Marketing an Ergonomics Program in a Corporate Office Environment, *WORK* 3(2):22, Spring 1993.

59. Smith RB: When Ergonomics Was Young, *Occup Health and Safety* 60(1):8, Jan 1991.

60. Sullivan JL: The American Society of Hand Therapists, *J Hand Therapy* 3(1):32, March 1990.

61. Tadano P: A Safety/Prevention Program for VDT Operators: one company's approach, *J Hand Therapy* 3(2):64, April 1990.

62. Thimm-Kelly SE: Control of Carpal Tunnel Syndrome, *Occup Therapy Forum* 6(9):1, March 1991.

63. Topf M, Preston R: Behavior Modification Can Heighten Safety Awareness, Curtail Accidents, *Occup Health and Safety* 60(2):43, Feb 1991.

64. Williams K: Doing Business with Carpal Tunnel Syndrome, *WORK* 2(4):2, Summer 1992.

65. Wilson PM: An Exercise and Job Modification Program in Industry, *WORK* 2(3):8, Spring 1992.

66. American National Standard for Human Factors engineering of Visual Display Terminal Workstations, ANSI/HFS 100 1988 Santa Monica, Human Factors Society.

67. ANSI Z–365: control of cumulative trauma disorders, National Safety Council, draft, June 1993.

68. CTD OSHA: OSHA briefs, *CTD News* 2(1):4, Dec 1992.

69. CTD LAW, *CTD News* 1(11):2, Nov 1992.

70. CTD LAW, *CTD News* 1(6):2, June 1992.

71. Does Stress Have a Price? *OSHA Up-To-Date* 22(6):3, June 1993.

72. Job Stress and CTDs, *CTD News* 1(6):1, June 1992.

73. Judge Limits OSHA Powers on Ergonomics, *OSHA Up-To-Date* 22(6):2, June 1993.

74. Member Profile: gross-given safety program attacks the root of high workers' compensation costs, *Perspectives*, Employers Association, Minneapolis, Minn, p 6, Summer 1991.

75. Rapid Rise in Stress Claims Strains System, *CTD News* 1(6):1, June 1992.

76. Repetitive-Motion Illness on Rise, Experts Say, *Los Angeles Times*, March 29, 1991.

77. Setting Up an Ergonomics Program, ErgoTech Inc., Minneapolis, Minn, 1991.

78. What Works for Companies Fighting CTDs?, *CTD News* 2(1):1, Dec 1992.

79. Hagberg, M: Electromyographic Signs of Shoulder Muscular Fatigue in Two Elevated Arm Positions, *American J Physical Medicine* 60(3):111.

80. Cannon L, Bernacki E, Walter S: Personal and Occupational Factors Associated with Carpal Tunnel Syndrome, *J Occup Medicine* 23:255, 1981.

81. Hirsh L, Thanki A: Carpal Tunnel Syndrome Avoiding Poor Treatment Results, *Post Grad Medicine* 77(1):185, 1985.

82. Ergonomics Program Management Guidelines for Meat packing Plants, U.S. Department of Labor, Washington, DC, OSHA.

CHAPTER

11
Employee Fitness Programs

Robert V. Volski

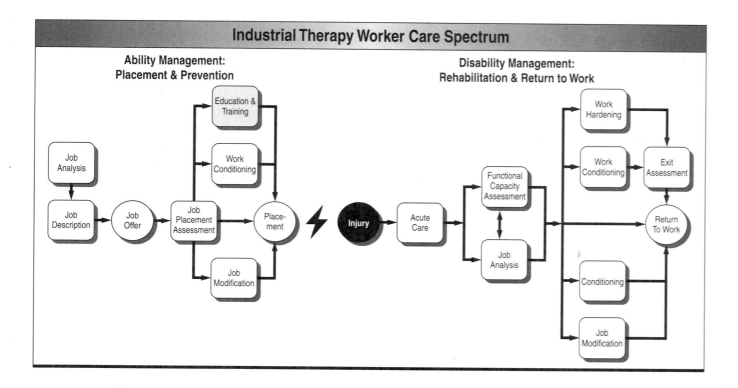

Industrial Therapy Worker Care Spectrum

The last 20 years have seen a tremendous change in the content of employee fitness programs. The growth in physical fitness concerns in the U.S. has been outstanding—a ten-fold increase in the last 20 years, according to the President's Council on Physical Fitness. In 1973, only 75 major corporations had physical fitness programs. Now the Fortune 500 Companies comprise a major share of thousands of companies that have physical fitness programs. Large corporations such as Xerox, Exxon, Mobil, Johnson & Johnson, IBM, Prudential Insurance, Control Data, Kimberly Clark, Sentry Insurance, Ryder System, and General Foods all offer some type of wellness program.[1]

This chapter is a working blue print of program design and content. What is the current "state of the art" in wellness programs? The answer is that there is such constant change and innovation, "state of the art" is a momentary point in time. Modern computer systems and software have streamlined overall program management while freeing staff for more specific "one-on-one" contact with the employee participant (Figure 11.1).

The evolving employee fitness center has been polished and expanded to include wellness and total health concepts. The benefits of an all-encompassing wellness program, as opposed to the traditional physical fitness program, are easily discerned. The latter exclusively addresses only the physiological components in the life of the participant, whereas the wellness approach addresses all areas of health and well-being in order to reduce risk.

Many companies have aggressively expanded their fitness programs to include other components such as family counseling, substance abuse counseling, and tests such as blood chemistries, cholesterol fractionation, and early cancer detection programs.

FIGURE 11.1   The employee fitness center has expanded from a traditional exercise approach to one that addresses all areas of health and well being.

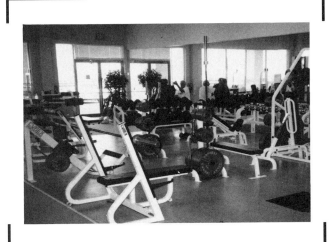

Another area that shows tremendous growth is fitness and physical testing in connection with employment and job placement assessment. Through this approach, a corporation can reduce risk in future health care expenditures for a specific job. This area is embryonic, but the real applications are significant.[14, 19]

PROGRAM DESCRIPTION

Fitness programs can run the gamut, from the small business with 20 employees that wants a home exercise program, to the larger company that can afford an in-house center with all the amenities. When expense must be minimized, fitness information and education materials can simply be distributed to all employees. This type of program does not require staffing and operational expenses are minimal. The outside provider of such a program may benefit afterwards from referrals for injury rehabilitation, as well as free publicity.

For the larger company that can afford a full in-house program, the provider must add staffing and programming responsibilities to equipment selection and program design. This type of undertaking is a much greater responsibility, but the rewards are greater on both financial and professional levels.

Program Types

Although there is a great variation in application and style of fitness programs, all programs can basically be classified into three categories:

1. *Company Reimbursed Programs*—reimbursed in full or in part, for use of outside programs and facilities (racquetball centers, YMCA, health spas).

FIGURE 11.2   A company must assess its fitness needs in order to determine which fitness program alternative is best for them; a company reimbursed program, a company sponsored program (**A**) or a company operated program (**B**).

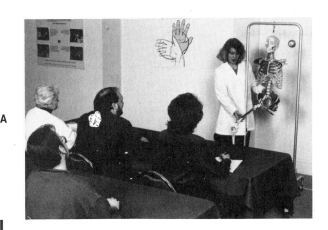

A

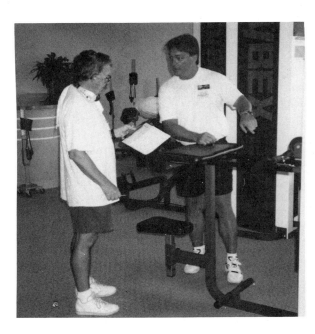

B

2. *Company Sponsored Programs*—sponsored and organized programs using an outside facility or vendor (softball programs at a county recreational facility or nutrition classes given by an outside vendor on company property Figure 11.2, *A*).

3. *Company Operated Programs*—with an in-house facility. These programs are more likely to be ''high tech—high touch'' versus recreationally oriented. Staff is either company employed or an outside firm is brought in to run the program (Figure 11.2, *B*).

Each of these program types has specific advantages, with the choice dependent upon company resources and commitment. Box 11.1 summarizes the advantages and disadvantages of each alternative.

Company Reimbursed Programs

This first category of programs has the advantage that the company, while not incurring any liability for possible injury that the employee may receive while exercising, still benefits from having physically fit employees. This type of program also enables the company to decrease its employees' health risks without the large capital expenditure that would be needed to have its own in-house program.

The use of outside facilities is advantageous when the company lacks sufficient financial resources to establish an in-house program, but wants employees to participate in some formal exercise program with structure and supervision.

In a recent survey of athletic and fitness clubs, 83% of those responding offered either special rates or services to corporations and businesses. The survey also indicated that one in five club members joined as a result of a company sponsored employee fitness program.[29]

The disadvantage of this type of program is that the company does not have direct control over the quality of service. The individuals who render the service are employees of the spa or health club and not responsible to the employer. Another disadvantage is that the employee may have to drive several miles to reach the facility. This can be a deterrent to long term use and hinder development of a fitness-oriented lifestyle.

Company Sponsored Programs

The second category of program gives the employer more control over the content and may allow better ''target population'' efforts such as hypertension management programs. For example, the American Cancer Society offers ''Stop Smoking'' classes that may be held on company property. Other vendors may be hired to

---

BOX 11.1

Comparisons of Alternative Company Fitness Programs

Company Reimbursed Programs
  A. Advantages
     1. Benefits from physically fit employees, without incurring any exercise injury liability.
     2. Smaller capital expenditure as compared to an in-house program.
  B. Disadvantages
     1. No direct control over the quality of service.
     2. Health club may not be conveniently located.

Company Sponsored Programs
  A. Advantages
     1. Employer has control over educational programs, therefore, programs can be company tailored.
     2. Vendor variety.
  B. Disadvantages
     1. Greater financial commitment than company reimbursed programs.

Company Operated Programs
  A. Advantages
     1. Increased employee participation due to location.
     2. Employer has control over program.
     3. Provides a site for research.
     4. Personnel recruitment drawing card.
  B. Disadvantages
     1. Financial commitment of start-up and operational expenses.

---

provide various types of programs, with the company picking up the expense. This type of program does require greater financial commitment from the company. The advantage here is focus and control. Specific areas of need within the company can be defined by a ''needs survey,'' and a program to address the problem can be designed.

Company Operated Programs

A company sponsored and operated in-house facility represents the greatest level of commitment. The company may choose to fund the program in full or in part.

Employee contributions can significantly defray the operational expenses of this program. In companies where the employee must pay to use the facility, their first impression is important. The preemployment tour becomes the functional point of sale.

The major advantage of an in-house program is increased employee participation. There is a much greater chance of continued use of a facility when an employee just walks downstairs. The habit of exercise as a normal part of the employee's day is an important part of compliance.

Pratt and Whitney Aircraft, in West Palm Beach, completed one study that indicated an 18 to 24 month payback of capital expense.[24] In this study, they looked at savings achieved by the company as a result of fitness and medical screenings done prior to program participation. Early screenings for detection of cancer and untreated cardiovascular disease saved the company real dollars. The savings due to the medical screening alone was enough after 18 to 24 months to offset the initial capital expenditure.

The in-house program, because it is easier to control and monitor, also offers a source for primary research in the area of physical fitness and related intangibles (effects on motivation and attitude). Variables are always the confounding factors in any research. The ability of in-house programs to control variables for the purpose of research is useful in evaluating improvements that enhance overall wellness.

Example Program Offering

Table 11.1 provides an example of a weekly schedule of programs that can be offered. Most of these classes can be taught by the program staff, while others such as smoking cessation or self defense might require an outside professional. All classes can be given in an aerobic room, if available, or in a company conference room.

The company fitness program can also be a good drawing card for personnel recruitment. Any preemployment tour through the corporation headquarters should include a visit to the fitness and wellness center. This will let the prospective new employee see that healthy living is a corporate commitment.

The disadvantages of in-house programs are the need for start-up capital and, to a lesser degree, the

TABLE 11.1 Health Promotion Classes

Employee Program Content	Monday	Tuesday	Wednesday	Thursday	Friday
Smoking cessation To assist the smoker to kick the habit		PM 60 min 8 Wks		PM 60 min 8 Wks	
Low impact Designed to spare the joints compression	AM PM 45 min		AM PM 45 min		AM PM 45 min
Stretching program Designed to improve flexibility		Noon 45 min		Noon 45 min	
Weight loss/control Designed to assist in proper eating and weight control		AM 45 min 6 to 8 Wks		AM 45 min 6 to 8 Wks	
Stress reduction and relaxation Coping skills will be taught	PM 45 min				PM 45 min

Self defense program
  For those interested in defending
    themselves; taught by a professional
					Noon
					60 min
					8 to 10 Wks

Healthy back
  For those in need of lifting for their
    job; proper biomechanics will be taught
			Noon
			60 min
			1 × mo for
			new employees		

CPR classes Will be taught by AHA certified instructor					

operational expenses, depending on how the program is funded. More and more companies are discovering that employee fitness programs are simply a part of good management policy, for in the end, what is good for the employee is good for the company.

Costs to the Therapist or Operator

Costs involved in the operation of a fitness center are usually broken down into capital expenses (for equipment initially purchased) and general operational expenses that pay the ongoing daily expenses.

With corporate contracts, most of the fitness space and equipment are always provided by the corporation. These are welcomed provisions because equipment is expensive and the square footage required for a fitness program typically far exceeds what is required for rehabilitation. The Therapist already has significant overhead without having to take on the additional cost associated with space and equipment.

Often, it is an effective customer retention strategy for the Therapist to provide the equipment used in the assessment of prospective participants. This costs the Therapist's clinic money, but acts as a barrier to competitive contractors because they would have to underwrite that expense.

The ideal arrangement is for the corporation to provide space and equipment and the Therapist to provide staffing and general operating expenses. The largest expense, for a Therapist operating a center or facility for a corporation, will be payroll.

Reimbursement as a Contractor

There are a number of approaches to billing and reimbursement. The most typical is to establish a monthly fee. This is derived by projecting payroll, operating expenses, and profit for the year and dividing by 12. If possible, a 10% contingency fee on top of the monthly fee protects against unexpected expenses and provides some extra flexibility to seize opportunities to upgrade or maintain a state of the art facility without having to obtain approval every time. Another common practice with many service contracts is to retain one or two months in advance in the form of a deposit that is refundable upon termination of the contract.

WHO NEEDS FITNESS PROGRAMS?

For many companies, the primary motivation for implementing a fitness program is financial. Many corporations faced with expensive operational costs, have already taken advantage of most external cost containment opportunities (cost of raw materials, manufac-

turing expense, and transportation). At some point, management turns to internal measures to enhance profits. Initially this may take the form of reducing the number of employees or decreasing payroll 10% across the board.[7,16,30] Recently, more and more companies are looking to fitness programs as a way to reduce health-related employee expenses.

In some corporations, the concern for wellness in the work place has expanded to include the reduction of risks in the total population.[1] Under the group insurance umbrella, dependents of the employee can also be health care risks. Those who do not live a safe and healthy lifestyle can increase health insurance payments made by the carrier.

Currently, many firms are self-insured, which means that disbursements come directly from the company's assets. In self-insured cases, corporations monitor health costs very closely. As a result, educational programs may be held not just for employees, but for their spouses and dependents as well.

BENEFITS OF FITNESS PROGRAMS

A well-planned and well-run employee fitness program goes beyond being a nice "fringe benefit" for employees. It becomes a bona fide financial benefit to the company as well. These benefits are summarized in Box 11.2.

The outcome studies that have been done to assess the benefits of physical fitness programs have indicated a number of benefits. Very little controlled research has been conducted to date, but this is expected to change in the near future as the benefits become more apparent.

BOX 11.2

Benefits of Employee Fitness Programs

1. Health care cost reduction
2. Decreased employee absenteeism, therefore, increased productivity
3. Stress reduction
4. Improved job satisfaction due to improved mood and self concept
5. Enhanced employer/employee relationship because the company has made a committment to the employee beyond the pay check

Absenteeism

Sick days cost employers money, and the higher the employee's level of management or position with the company, the greater the financial loss. Initial studies indicate that fitness programs do affect employee absenteeism.

Metropolitan Life found that 100 employees who participated in a fitness program averaged 4.8 sick days per year, compared to 6.2 days per year for the members in a control group who did not exercise.[31]

A study by Mesa Petroleum evaluated absenteeism of participants in their corporate fitness programs versus the national industry average. Fitness participants were absent an average of 1.6 days per year versus the national average of 3.4.[25] Although this was just short of two days difference, if multiplied by 1,000 employees, it can more than offset the cost of starting and operating a program.

The Association of Quality clubs compiled and reviewed the results of several studies comparing corporate fitness program participation to disability days. The results, summarized in Figure 11.3, indicate significant reductions in absenteeism among fitness participants. In the case of Du Pont the reduction was 14%, with total savings of 11,726 fewer disability days companywide.[27]

A geriatric hospital in Sweden monitored the absenteeism among participants who exercised during working hours and compared it to those who did not exercise during working hours. After 13 months, one member of the exercising group had been absent a total of 28 days, whereas 12 non-exercising members had been absent a total of 155 days due to low back pain.[13]

FIGURE 11.3 Reductions in disability days for employees who are in fitness programs.

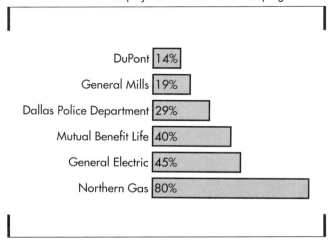

(From IRSA, The Association of Quality Clubs.)

FIGURE 11.4 British Columbia Hydroelectric employee turnover rate for those who participated in fitness programs and those who did not.

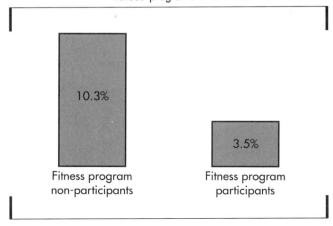

Tenneco, Inc., in Houston, showed a correlation between job performance and exercising. In the case of both males and females, absenteeism decreased with age among exercisers, and it increased in age among non-exercisers.[5] There seems little doubt that employee exercise is beneficial for the employer.

Employee Turnover

Studies now show that employee turnover and absenteeism can be reduced while improving employee morale and dedication. Tenneco found that fitness participants were 13% less likely to leave the firm than other employees. Tenneco also found that over a ten year period, it attracted a population of people more health conscious than average, and claimed that this provided an advantage over the competition.[5]

British Columbia Hydroelectric employees who participated in fitness programs revealed a turnover rate of 3.5% versus the company's average rate of 10.4% (Figure 11.4).[8]

Stress Reduction

Stress reduction has quickly risen to the top of the list of health-related employee programs. Individual employees have become increasingly concerned about on-the-job stress and are demanding corporate programs addressing this issue. Rigorous regular physical activity has been shown to reduce muscle tension, anxiety, blood pressure, heart rate, and the incidence of heart attacks.[25, 26] All are potentially stress-related symptoms.

It is clear that a program addressing the physical well-being of an employee could be expected to significantly reduce job stress and have an impact on the company's health care expenses.

Many companies now offer stress reduction classes comprising the mental component as well. Mental imagery and relaxation techniques dominate this approach. Mental imagery is the use of mental pictures to assist the body in relaxation. For example, during childbirth, the laboring mother is instructed to picture something pleasant at a time when the contractions get strong and painful. As part of a wellness program, the classes are usually taught by a professional or clinician with a behavioral modification background. Jacobsen's relaxation exercises have been well recognized for their ability to relax patients.[25,30] These techniques have been shown to reduce systolic blood pressure through a reduction in peripheral resistance. This approach has moved from the medical setting to the industrial wellness arena.

Health Care Cost Reduction

It is important to understand that you may not experience a bottom line impact on health care costs in the first year of a fitness program. Baun, et al, at Tenneco, estimate three to five years as the point at which the program's statistics begin to show cost savings. Yet other companies are making sharp turnarounds in health costs in the first year. The Scoular Grain Company reduced health care costs by over $1 million the first year of its fitness program, or $1,500 for each of its 600 employees.[29]

General Electric inaugurated a fitness program that reduced health care costs by 38% in 18 months. During this period, fitness participants' health care costs were $757, while non-participants' were $941.[27]

One strong area for potential savings is in group insurance policies. Information from the Health Insurance Association of America shows that firms with a fitness program cited no increase in insurance costs, while 15% noted a reduction in insurance costs.[33] The state of health in a corporate population can be an important consideration in the decision to implement a fitness program. Obviously, if the overall group is healthier, the insurance premiums, as well as lost work days, can be lowered.

The impact of unhealthy behaviors on health care costs was analyzed among 45,000 employees of Du Pont Company. The study compared health care costs of those exhibiting certain unhealthy behaviors with those who did not. The results, summarized in Box 11.3, indicate the extent to which unhealthy behaviors, including lack of exercise, increase health care costs.[6]

Focused screening programs are cost effective if they are targeted at the appropriate population. Many companies have done an effective job of targeting hypertensive employees by screening for hypertension then working to reduce it through exercise, weight control, medical follow-up, and if necessary, medications (Figure 11.5).

BOX 11.3

Analyzed Costs of Unhealthy Behaviors

Unhealthy behavior	Annual per person excess health care costs
Smoking	$960
Overweight	$401
Excess alcohol	$389
Elevated cholesterol	$370
High blood pressure	$343
Inadequate seat belt use	$272
Lack of exercise	$130

Improved Job Placement

There are additional benefits of having fit employees in occupations that make specific physical demands on workers. Physical fitness testing can be a component of

FIGURE 11.5 Focused screening programs such as hypertension screening are cost effective if they are targeted at the appropriate population.

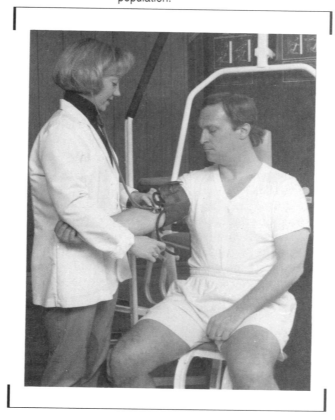

a physical agility test and can assist in matching the right person for the right job. Employees who are assigned tasks beyond their physical capabilities often experience difficulties in their jobs. Also, the lack of fitness in any given employee can result in substandard performance or even injury. The lower back is especially at risk in employees who have poor fitness and low aerobic capacity.

Employee Morale and Productivity

One argument for instituting a fitness program, which many employers may overlook, is that the presence of such a program shows the employee that the company has made a commitment beyond the paycheck. At Saatchi & Saatchi Advertising, morale was shown to improve in 75% of the fitness participants and productivity increased among 63%.[27]

NASA noted that participants in an exercise program demonstrated improved stamina and work performance, with enhanced concentration and decision-making powers. Exercise adherents were observed to work at full efficiency all day, whereas non-exercisers' efficiency decreased by 50% during the final two hours of the work day.[1]

Most fitness advocates will attest to programs being a very strong point in recruiting the best job candidates on the market. The President of Medical Affairs at Kimberly Clark Corporation, Robert Dedmon has stated, "It's been swell for us in recruiting. Other considerations equal, the program has helped sway the decisions of young people joining us."[18] *Time Magazine* has quoted a Xerox executive as saying, "Before I'd change jobs, I'd ask an employer if he had a gym."[11]

SETTING UP A FITNESS PROGRAM

Management Direction

Once management has determined to underwrite a company program, it is important that the direction and goals be clearly defined. Proper planning is the key to solid programs. Specifically, built-in monitoring of the program should be included in the original design. Cost/benefit analysis as well as program attendance rates should be considered. The program should have ongoing ways of using this data to modify and improve, thus maximizing employee satisfaction and adherence to the program.

The decision to begin a corporate fitness program or "Health Promotion Program," is often made by a financial executive. To these decision makers, the return on investment experienced by other companies can be a persuasive selling point. Box 11.4 summarizes the returns experienced by six major corporations.

BOX 11.4

Fitness Program Returns on Invested Dollars

Company	Dollars returned per dollar invested
Coors	$6.15
Kennecott	$5.78
Equitable Life	$5.52
General Mills	$3.90
Motorola	$3.15
Pepsi	$3.00

(With permission from IRSA, 1992).[27]

The offering of spin-off programs such as smoking cessation, nutrition, weight loss, stress reduction, self-defense, and the full range of related programs is also very conducive to program adherence.

Top management must support the program for it to have maximum impact and increase the chance of success. When the top personnel are exercising, this is the best testimonial possible.

Planning

Program design is like architecture—careful planning will improve utilization, scheduling, and logistics. Design is where the building blocks of the program's format are set. The fitness program design should be based on the facility's budget and on the population of the company, not just the numbers, but the type of workers. Are the workers in the company primarily white collar, or are they manual workers with heavy lifting responsibility in their job tasks?

If the company is manual labor intensive, the program should have a greater emphasis on cardiovascular stations—such as the treadmill, bike, rower, or stair climber. The needs of both administrative and manual laborers can be addressed at the same facility through the use of program modifications (Figure 11.6).

Space may be available in the company's main facility or at a separate location. Most companies start their program in the main facility and expand to a separate location. Many large companies hire outside contractors to run an in-house program. In competing for a contract to manage such a program, the Industrial Therapist may enjoy an advantage over other contractors, since the fitness program can be a second use of the space and equipment already in place for rehabilitative needs.

FIGURE 11.6 The fitness program design should be based on financial resources as well as on the company population and type of workers. Companies that have a large number of manual laborers should put a greater emphasis on cardiovascular stations.

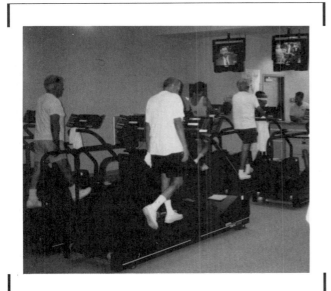

Some companies are ready to develop an in-house program and may be in the initial stages of goal setting and planning. Others have to be "sold" on the concept. Such companies may be aware of the benefits, but lack the requisite personnel to implement a structured program. In either case, the key is to try to assess management's motivation and commitment to the fitness concept. Do they really want an effective fitness program, or are they just going through the motions to satisfy the proponents of an in-house program?

The author once consulted on a job at a major employer's home office. Top management had invested thousands of dollars on equipment and capital for facilities, but neglected to staff the facility with fitness professionals. Instead, a current staff member who "used to play football" had been appointed to direct the program. Without professional planning and implementation, the considerable investment in space and equipment was not used to its optimal capacity.

Competitive bidding is often used to lower the company's operational costs. Some companies with multi-site operations will require on-site visits to all locations. This is costly and may not be practical unless there is a high probability of winning the contract.

With multiple-site relationships, doing a quality job on the first installation is critical. It is especially important to build a strong team to manage the facility

and develop the team concept. Any problems with the initial operation should be resolved before following through with another site or company.

Staffing

The next step is to evaluate existing staff to determine if it will be necessary to hire a fitness professional. This professional should demonstrate two essential capabilities. In the planning phase it is important to have a strong background in organization. For ongoing management, the program needs someone with the ability and personality to motivate employee participants. In addition, this person should be experienced in hiring, developing staff, with strong operational skills. Good design, effective motivation, and polished hiring and management skills will be strong allies in assuring high program retention rates.

The graduate degree candidate can be an asset, but it is important that they have practical experience. Well motivated undergraduate degree holders in adult fitness are well suited to working with the program participants, while the master's degree holder is better suited to program management functions.

Team building is important, and a multiplicity of talents is often necessary within the managerial setting of the fitness center. Staff members should be cross-trained for different responsibilities and duties, to keep things running smoothly when members are absent or other contingencies. Multiple responsibilities may include: booting up the computer system, scheduling new fitness assessments, closing the facility at the end of the day, substituting for an aerobics instructor, or taking a prospective new member on a tour of the facility. With some professional positions, cross-training is not possible, but within the fitness staff, it is good to promote and foster well-rounded capabilities.

Equipment

Equipment decisions are typically made in consultation with staff or a hired professional. The actual equipment purchases should be handled by a person with existing vendor relationships and the experience to develop new networks when price shopping. Often, the therapist can build profit into equipment procurement as compensation for providing this service.

The Starter Program

Companies with limited resources, or want to evaluate a "pilot" program can begin with a basic equipment package and space allocation. A "starter program" might use 1,080 square feet (30 feet by 36 feet) and the following equipment package:

Treadmill
Stationary bicycle
Rowing machine
Stair climber
Multi station strength training unit
Dumbbell rack with weights from 5 pounds to 25 pounds

The equipment would be placed along the walls to make room for an aerobic dance area. Such a facility would cover most of the scientific requirements for strengthening and aerobic conditioning for up to 200 employees, assuming efficient scheduling.

The Intermediate Facility

This scale of facility would be for corporations prepared to underwrite a more comprehensive program for a larger employee population.

An "intermediate program" for 1,000 to 5,000 employees might encompass the following equipment package:

4 treadmills
2 stationary bicycles
2 airdyne bicycles
4 rowing machines
4 stair climbers
1 versa climber
1 gravitron
Complete line of strength training stations (10 stations)
Dumbbell rack with weights from 5 pounds to 45 pounds
Stationary bench for weight lifting
Light weight set—mixed weights 300 pounds
2 abdominal boards

The square footage allocation for this program would be as follows:

Aerobic equipment	1,152 sq ft
Aerobic room	1,000 sq ft
Strength training equipment	360 sq ft
Rest rooms with showers (M & F)	960 sq ft
Storage	96 sq ft
Fitness assessment room	100 sq ft
Total space allocation	3,868 sq ft

OPERATING AND MAINTAINING FITNESS PROGRAMS

Assessment Process

It is important to assess each employee's abilities to participate in the fitness program, their safe level, and with their specific goals in mind. Each new participant should fill out a waiver of liability and a PAR-Q, or personal activities readiness questionnaire. Guidelines for testing and evaluation are available from the American College of Sports Medicine (ACSM).

If it is determined that the participant is on beta blockers or other medications that would alter cardiac output, a letter signed by a doctor should be required prior to testing. This letter should clearly state that the participant is able to take part in the corporate fitness program.

The staff member should proceed with physical assessment only when it is certain that the participant can be assessed safely. This includes body weight, height, resting blood pressure, resting pulse, body fat percent, submaximal bike or step test for cardiovascular assessment, flexibility assessment, and strength testing. If funding permits, pulmonary studies and blood work might also be included.

After the data is reviewed and participation is authorized, the employee is given a few minutes to discuss goals relative to the parameters indicated from the physical testing. If the goals are safe and realistic, a program is designed to achieve them.

After setting goals, the equipment is explained. Some people require more guidance than others, and they can be singled out for special instruction by the staff. If an unusual goal such as preparing for a 10K race is set, there may be a supplemental fee for the special staff attention required.

Management and Motivation

Practicing hands-on management is hard work in the beginning, but will be beneficial in the long run. It is also better to be proactive than reactive. The key measures of program success are employee attendance and adherence (Figure 11.7). The chances of achieving and maintaining good-to-excellent fitness are increased when these factors are maximized, which in turn yields targeted cost savings.

FIGURE 11.7 Fitness program success and cost savings are dependent upon employee attendance and adherance.

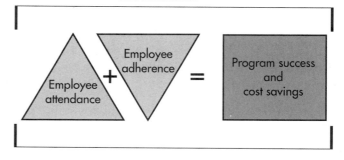

There are three types or levels of motivation that apply to preventative programs:

1. Purely voluntary
2. Monetary
3. Mandatory

Purely Voluntary

The purely voluntary is the least costly program, but requires an optimal level of self-motivation and self-discipline. Many programs give rewards for employee participation, such as mileage awards for bicycling, jogging, and walking programs (Figure 11.8). These rewards function as incentives, but the participation is still voluntary. One of the arguments against purely voluntary programs is that it attracts those who are already motivated towards fitness. These individuals are not the "at risk" groups that really need to get involved in a fitness program.

In one instance, a physical fitness program involving employees of Michigan State University used innovative motivation and reinforcement techniques to encourage participation. Participants were required to deposit $40 in an account that was progressively debited in the event of an absence. In this program, only 9% of the participants dropped out. Further, 98% of those who continued with the program exercised four or more times a week for 30 minutes or more.[6]

FIGURE 11.8 Award and incentives can be used to motivate employee participation in a fitness program.

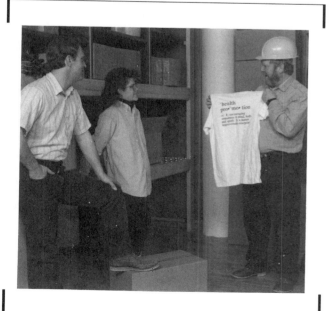

Monetary Incentives

Some programs use financial rewards to encourage and stimulate participation. Some companies give preestablished amounts for each mile run or pound lost. Others use prorated refunding of club memberships—perhaps up to 90% of annual membership dues, if the employee maintains a predesignated fitness level over a fixed period of time (one year).

Mandatory Participation

The mandatory requirement is more difficult to implement, because it is outside a company's traditional level of intervention in a person's life. Employers are often reluctant to cross this line. Additionally, if the program is on company time, employers may be concerned about the fitness sessions cutting into productivity. Notwithstanding that the program is mandatory, employees must be "sold" on its importance. If not, they will find ways to avoid compliance, and morale problems could surface.

Japanese programs of employee calisthenics have often been cited as an important reason why their productivity has so effectively penetrated world markets in the last 15 years.[9] Many American corporations are beginning to explore ways they might benefit from inaugurating similarly structured fitness programs. As more and more companies realize gains in employee dedication and productivity, the case for making fitness programs mandatory will be strengthened.

Legal Considerations

Many executives are wary of in-house fitness programs because of potential liability that could result from employee injuries. Exercise is like medicine. It must be used properly and in proper dosage to bring about a safe and effective change.

Generally, the outside contractor who operates the facility, manages the program, and motivates the employees should accept some liability for the project commensurate with their level of involvement and control. A $3,000,000 level of coverage would not be excessive. Coverage may be obtained through standard insurance channels, or through a professional association such as the ACSM.

One specific source for effective legal protocols to decrease the program's liability is *Legal Aspects of Preventative and Rehabilitative Exercise Programs* by David L. Herbert, Esquire and William G. Herbert, PhD, available through Professional and Executive Reports and Publications, Canton, Ohio.

Safety

Both employee participants and program staff should be made aware of potential risks and problems. Everyone should be sensitive to the need to comply with exercise prescriptions based on specific medical or physical problems or disabilities. Drills involving both employees and fitness center staff, in the event of medical emergencies or accidents, can be effective in quickening response, while contributing to a healthy level of awareness regarding possible problems.

Budget

The financial scope of the wellness or fitness center will limit the size of the facility. The overall quality of the program should not be severely restricted by budget. The components of a good wellness program are basic. As long as these are incorporated into the program, it will meet the needs of all members.

SUMMARY

The impact that a healthy work force can have on absenteeism, job satisfaction, stress, and health care costs is becoming increasingly recognized. Companies seeking to tap into these benefits must first acquire a strong commitment at the highest management levels. Initial involvement can start with little or no investment in space or equipment, simply by reimbursing employee participation in independent off-site health clubs or other facilities.

As management realizes that employee participation and continuity are the keys to success, companies are inclined to start moving these programs in-house and making them incentive-based or mandatory.

From the therapist's point of view, the "high tech" and "high touch" society that John Naisbitt spoke of in *Megatrends* is upon us, and nowhere is this more apparent than in the fitness and wellness area. New technologies are continually introduced to facilitate and monitor fitness progress. Operating the programs is becoming increasingly multidisciplinary and holistic in approach.

Considerable professional competition in this field stimulates the personal growth of many practitioners in a healthy way. Under the impetus of competition, practitioners often use technological and procedural innovation to differentiate their services and gain advantages. This in turn keeps the field ever changing and intellectually stimulating. The cutting edge of technologically-guided wellness is an exciting arena. Advancements are catalysts in bringing into the public spotlight, programs that heretofore have been viewed as ancillary to productivity.

REFERENCES

1. Association for Fitness in Business: Comparing Sponsored Employee Fitness Programs, 1991.
2. Pelletier KR; editor, *Ameri J Health Promotion*, March, 1991.
3. Bailey, NC: Reduction in Absenteeism, *Business and Health*, 1991.
4. Exercise Adherence in a Corporate Fitness Program. *Optional Health*, p 26, Jan 1985.
5. Bernacki, E, Interview, *Fortune Magazine*, Sept, 1989.
6. Bertera, RL: The Effects of Behavioral Risks on Absenteeism and Health Care Costs in the Workplace, *Jour of Occ Med*, 33(11):1119, Nov 1991.
7. Chaffin DB, Park KS: A Longitudinal Study of Low Back Pain as Associated with Occupational Weight Lifting Factors, *Amer Ind Hygiene Associate Jour*: 34, 513–525, 1973.
8. Cigna, Benefits of Employee Health Programs, 1991.
9. Cotter M: Corporate America Shapes Up, *Rehabilitation Management* 78:Aug, 1992.
10. Equal Employment Opportunity Commission, Civic Services Commission, Department of Labor, and Department of Justice. Adoption by four agencies of uniform guidelines on employee selection procedures. Federal Register, 43:38290–38315, 1978.
11. From Boardroom to Locker Room. *Time Magazine* January 22, 1979.
12. *Guidelines for Exercise Testing and Exercise Prescription*, ed 6, Philadelphia, 1989, Lea and Febiger.
13. Gundewall B, et al: Primary Prevention of Back Systems and Absence from Work: *Spine*, European Edition 18(5):587.
14. Hogan JC and Pederson K: *Validity of Physical Tests for Selecting Petrochemical Workers*. Unpublished Manuscript 1984.
15. Jacobsen E: *You Must Relax*, ed 4, New York 1957 McGraw-Hill.
16. Keyserlilng WM, Herrin GD, Chaffin, et al: Establishing an Industrial Strength Testing Program, *Amer Ind Hygiene Assoc Jour* pp. 41, 730–736, 1980.
17. Krusen F: *The Handbook of Physical Medicine and Rehabilitation*. ed 2, p. 426, Philadelphia, 1978, WB Saunders.
18. Lang JS: America's Fitness Binge, *U.S. News & World Report*, pp. 58–61, May 3, 1982.
19. Laughery RR, Jackson AS, Sanborn L, Davis G: Preemployment Physical Test Development for Offshore Drilling and Production Environments. (Technical Report). Houston, Texas 1981: Shell Oil Company.
20. Levy R: Fitness Fever: Everybody into the Company Gym, *Dun's Review* pp. 115–118, November 1980.
21. Newman JE, Beehr TA: Personal and Organizational Strategies for Handling Job Stress: a review of research and opinion, *Personal Psychology*, 32:1–44, 1979.
22. O'Donnell M: *Wellness in the Workplace*. New York 1984. Wiley & Sons.
23. Petren T, Sjostrand T, Sylven B: The Influence of Exercise on the Frequency of Capillaries in Cardiac and Skeletal Musculature, *Arbeitsphysiol.*, 9:376–386, 1936.
24. Pratt-Whitney Aircraft. Unpublished study. (1978)

25. Report on Mesa Corporate Health and Fitness Program, Mesa Inc, 1990.

26. Stoffelmayr BE, et al, A Program Model To Enhance Adherence in Work-Site-Based Fitness Programs, *Jour of Occ Med*, 34(2):156 February 1992.

27. The Economic Benefits of Regular Exercise, IRSA, *The Association of Quality Clubs*, p 6. Boston, 1992.

28. The Economic Benefits of Regular Exercise, IRSA, *The Association of Quality Clubs*, p 9. Boston, 1992.

29. This is Corporate Wellness, Wellness Councils of America, 1991.

30. Volski RV, Kadel KH: A Proposal for Physical Fitness Programs on Offshore Drilling Sites to Exxon Corporation, New Orleans, LA (1984) unpublished manuscript.

31. An Ounce of Prevention is Worth a Pound of Cure, or So Say the Proponents of the 'Wellness Movement', *The Wall Street Journal*, September 15, 1981.

32. White TH, The Danger From Japan. *The New York Times Magazine*, p 19 July 28, 1985.

33. Your Guide to Wellness at the Worksite. Health Insurance Association of America, p 6 1985.

PART

III

Returning The Worker To Productivity

12

Acute Care and Functional Treatment

Gary J. Smith

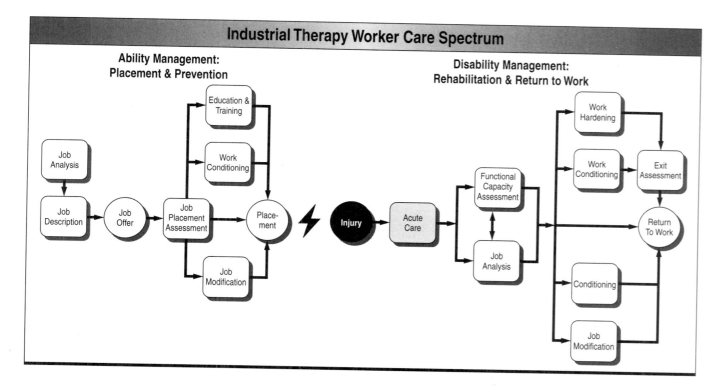

Industrial Therapy Worker Care Spectrum

Ability Management:
Placement & Prevention

Disability Management:
Rehabilitation & Return to Work

The acute care phase begins immediately upon injury and continues through the point at which pain and healing are stabilized. The worker is then able to begin the process of functional restoration. At this stage physicians still play a dominant role, but as time goes on, therapists become increasingly involved throughout the acute care process.

The purpose of this chapter is to explain this evolving role, and to provide practical information therapists can use to apply their expertise in this important phase of the rehabilitation process. The chapter will provide the reader with concepts of evaluation and intervention at the acute stage, that will assist the injured worker in a safe, functional, and rapid return to the workplace.

Importance of Early Intervention

One often hears of an injured athlete returning to competition in a very short period of time. Praise is lavished upon the athlete for the "mental toughness" and fortitude that allows for this quick return to function. How is this remarkable rehabilitation process achieved? The answer is suggested by observing the activities occurring at the time of injury. The injured individual is evaluated within seconds of the trauma, measures to decrease the amount of trauma are instituted immediately, and the individual begins functional activity as soon as possible. In reality, the athlete may not be superhuman, but only an injured individual who is receiving immediate and aggressive care, designed to allow for a rapid return to functional activity.

The injured worker will benefit from the same type of aggressive intervention and attention that is lavished on the valued athlete. In addition to being right for the worker, early intervention can also be seen to benefit productivity and global competitiveness over the long run.

When a worker is injured, the entire economic structure is affected. Decreased productivity, increased insurance cost, and increased medical expenses are only a few of the statistically documented costs of work-related trauma. A reevaluation of the medical model of intervention is crucial to reducing the $27 billion dollars spent annually on work-related musculoskeletal trauma.[21] A wealth of positive outcomes support the provision of early intervention to the injured worker.

PHASES OF WOUND REPAIR

Wound repair consists of three phases: the inflammatory phase, tissue formation, and remodeling. These phases are depicted in Figure 12.1 and discussed in more detail in text.

The Inflammatory Phase

In order for the Industrial Therapist to incorporate the concept of early intervention into the treatment regime, an understanding of the inflammatory response is necessary. The acute inflammatory response consists of vascular, cellular, and chemical reactions within the traumatized tissue which are required for wound healing.[28]

The signs of inflammation (redness, swelling, tenderness, heat, and pain) are caused by local vasodilation, fluid leakage into the extravascular space, blocking of the lymphatic drainage, distention of tissue from swelling and pressure, and by chemical irritation of nociceptors. The acute inflammatory response lasts from 24 hours to two weeks.[44] Therapist intervention, during the acute phase, requires the implementation of procedures and modalities that inhibit tissue reaction, diminish the leakage of fluid into the extravascular space, and enhance the lymph and venous return systems.

FIGURE 12.1 The three phases of wound repair: inflammatory phase, tissue formation, and remodeling.

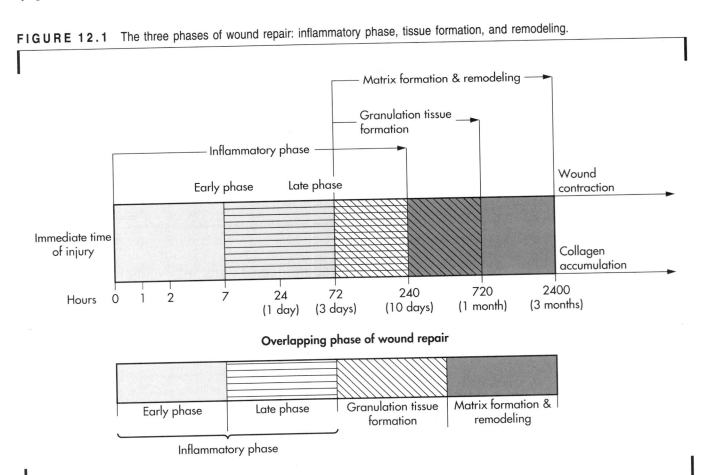

The Tissue Formation Phase

Between three to approximately twenty days following the injury, tissue repair becomes a predominant activity at the traumatized site.[44] During the repair phase, epithelial tissue and connective tissue undergo regeneration (termed reepithelialization and fibroplasia, respectively). These processes provide for wound closure and the reestablishment of the connective-tissue matrix, thus enhancing tensile strength to the wound site.[3,10]

During wound closure, a revascularization of the tissue occurs, allowing for the passage of nutrients necessary for healing. During the repair phase of wound healing, therapist intervention must be designed to accelerate the regeneration of injured tissue through movement and protection.

The Remodeling Phase

The final stage of wound repair is the remodeling phase. During remodeling, connective tissue becomes organized and provides tensile strength greater than that noted during the repair phase. The scar that is developed does not have the strength of normal tissue, and presents a diminished vascular system.[30] At this stage, functional activity must be designed to stress remodeling connective tissue, to provide for correct alignment of fibers to ensure the highest level of strength possible.[51]

As the above information reinforces again, it is of the utmost importance for acute care to be initiated immediately. If the tissue reaction to acute inflammation can be controlled and diminished within the first twenty-four hours, the entire process of healing can be enhanced. Without the limitations of swelling or pain, rehabilitation can begin much sooner, and the results of prolonged immobilization can be avoided. This shortened period of acute care allows the injured worker the opportunity to return to the work site in a shorter time frame.

THE TREATMENT PROCESS

Functional Orientation

When providing treatment, the Therapist must begin evaluation using the concept of function/dysfunction, rather than relying on the medical model of a diagnosis. The use of a Physical Therapy Diagnosis, a function-orientated diagnosis, is imperative in the treatment of work-related injuries. When dealing with the injured worker, a diagnosis of "low back pain" may not have practical meaning. The range of dysfunction of a client with low back pain can vary from the inability to get out of bed, to discomfort during rock climbing. Throughout the Therapist's evaluation, it is important to be aware of the medical diagnosis, and to develop a treatment rationale with the medical restrictions in mind.

The DEP Approach

A technique of documentation developed at the Department of Physical Therapy at Eastern Washington University[12] utilizes a functional method of note-taking and presents a hypothesis-based approach to Physical Therapy intervention. This technique is called the DEP Method (Data, Evaluation, and Plan).

After accumulating the information from the history and obtaining measurable data, the clinician hypothesizes a cause and effect regarding the dysfunction and suggests relevant treatment. Under the DEP approach, the Therapist states that "THE CLIENT IS UNABLE TO . . . (perform a function)" and proceeds to identify the cause of the dysfunction and indicate the therapeutic intervention appropriate to enhance the function. The therapy plan begins with the statement, "THE CLIENT WILL BE ABLE TO, . . ." and allows the clinician the opportunity to state how the treatment provided will cause an improvement in function. The use of a function-orientated diagnosis may be adapted into the standard S.O.A.P. (Subjective, Objective, Action, Plan) format with little difficulty.

Box 12.1 contains an example of the DEP format for documentation, using a Grade II ankle sprain for the trauma. A complete history and listing of measurable data is not included, and only an outline is provided. The use of such a tool enables the Industrial Therapist to document the "cause and effect" relationship of the care provided, and places the functional approach to a return to activity as the prime focus of care.

The central mission of the Therapist treating acute work-related trauma is to decrease the time of disability and expedite the return to function. In the author's opinion, based on twenty years of orthopedic experience, treatment for the acute aspect of the injury should be completed within six to eight treatments. Individuals differ, and the exact time-frame of care cannot be dictated without a complete evaluation of the client; however, it should be stressed that a controlled rehabilitation program must begin rapidly.

Extended use of modalities for control of acute inflammation and pain should be evaluated for effectiveness. The length of the rehabilitation process will differ from client to client, but a rapid and safe return to work is the primary objective.

The remainder of this chapter focuses on the approach used by the author in the treatment of acute injury. The care provided is aggressive, and initiated as

BOX 12.1

History:

First, basic background information is gathered, including:

- Pertinent information related to client (age, gender, etc.)
- Mechanism of injury
- Previous treatment and evaluation (x-ray, blood work-ups, MRI)
- Other information relating to the dysfunction

Measurable Data:

Then, the Therapist takes measurements that are important to the healing process:

- Pain levels as stated by client
- Client's statement of dysfunction
- Circumference measurements
- Water displacement measurements
- Range of motion
- Strength measurements
- Other pertinent measurable data

Evaluation:

The Therapist then identifies the cause of dysfunctions and indicates appropriate therapeutic interventions. For example, the Therapist begins with a particular dysfunction: The client is unable to walk five feet without pain.

Cause	Intervention
A. Pain	1. Ice
	2. High voltage pulsed current
B. Effusion	1. Elevation
	2. Pneumatic compression
	3. Compression stockings
C. Instability	Bracing
D. Weakness	Progressive strength and stabilization program

Plan: The client will be able to walk 30 minutes within six treatments as a result of Physical Therapy intervention to increase strength, to decrease pain, effusion, and instability.

rapidly as possible. Ideally, treatment should begin within one to two days of the injury. In the following treatment examples, attempts are made to document the interventions that have statistically demonstrated clinical efficacy. The amount of clinical research in physical therapy has recently increased, but there is still a great need for more. It is the responsibility of all practicing Physical Therapists to statistically substantiate the efficacy of treatment, to ensure that the intervention provided is the most effective.

TREATMENT PROGRAM IMPLEMENTATION

Prior to the implementation of a treatment program, the Therapist must address the most important aspect of care: the evaluation.

Without a comprehensive and consistent evaluation, the intervention most effective for the cause of dysfunction will not be implemented.

Outlined in Box 12.2, is an evaluation technique[31] that is adaptable for the assessment of any type of orthopedic dysfunction.

As may be derived from the partial list of special tests, determination of the site of injury is imperative. When dealing with the peripheral joints, such a deter-

mination is more easily achieved. Specific identification of traumatized tissue in the spine is much more difficult. Due to the depth and the close relationship of the spinal tissue, it is quite difficult to determine the exact site of trauma.

The initial scan of the lumbar and cervical regions will allow the clinician to determine the area of the body causing dysfunction. After the scan evaluation is complete, the Therapist is able to focus on the specific structure or structures involved and proceed with evaluation.

The tests listed in the preceding section are only a sample of those available for spinal evaluation. They are provided to assist the reader in determining the specific structures causing the dysfunction. References are provided to allow for more in-depth evaluation of techniques. *The Rehabilitation Specialist Handbook* by Rothstein, Roy, and Wolf and *Orthopedic Physical Assessment* by Magee provide an exemplary listing of testing procedures.[46, 31]

Use of passive movement, overstretching, and isometric contraction of the muscles are designed to determine whether the traumatized structures are contractile/non-contractile tissue, or are painful due to capsular involvement. Palpation and evaluation of joint play allow the clinician to determine the end feel of the joint under scrutiny.[28]

All peripheral joints should be evaluated in the same consistent manner. A sequence of procedures for evaluation of all peripheral joints is listed first. Special

BOX 12.2

Orthopedic Dysfunction Evaluation Technique Outline

History

1. Age
   Age related conditions need to be identified
2. Occupation
   A. May assist in the determination of mechanism of injury
   B. Posture related, repetitive trauma, over-stressed musculoskeletal system
3. Onset of dysfunction
   A. Immediate dysfunction
   B. Slow, progressive onset
   C. Locking, snapping sound
4. Previous occurrence of dysfunction
   A. Previous treatment (successful or unsuccessful)
   B. Site of initial pain
   C. Radiation of pain
5. Mechanism of injury
   A. Specific mechanism of trauma
   B. Cumulative trauma
6. Duration of dysfunction
   A. Determine pain level
      a. Acute pain
      b. Chronic pain
      c. Pain level (visual analog)
   B. Changes in pain
      a. Length of duration of pain
      b. Intensity
      c. Frequency
      d. Constant pain
      e. Pain related to function
      f. Pain associated with rest or posture
      g. Type of pain
         (1) Nerve–sharp, burning, nerve distribution
         (2) Bone–deep, "toothache," localized
         (3) Vascular–aching, difficult to isolate
         (4) Muscle–dull, aching, pain with function
   C. Joint dysfunction
      a. Instability
      b. Locking
   D. Circulatory deficiencies
      a. Triphasic colors of circulatory dysfunction
      b. Hair loss
      c. Changes in skin texture
   E. Additional medical information
      a. X-ray
      b. Medication (include any steroids)
   c. Previous surgery
   F. What dysfunctions are noted by the client?
      a. Unable to sit 30 minutes, sleep one hour, walk 20 feet, etc.
   G. What are the stated goals of the client?
      Goals of client may not relate to the goals of the clinician
   H. Be aware of litigation, Workers' Compensation, marital, or financial problems.

Observation

1. Note the client arriving into treatment area
   A. Gait
   B. Assistive devices
   C. Compare initial observations with information provided during the data collection period
2. Note posture of client
   A. Any deformities
   B. Postural symmetry
   C. Atrophy
   D. Note color and texture of skin
      a. Scars
      b. Signs of vascular dysfunction
      c. Areas of excessive stress (blisters, callous)
3. Crepitus/abnormal audible or palpable sounds in joints
4. Signs of inflammation (heat, effusion, redness)
5. Pain with palpation

Spinal Evaluation

1. Scanning examination of the cervical and lumbar region[7]
   A. Active movement of cervical or lumbar spine
   B. Passive movement
   C. Isometric manual resistance
   D. Active and passive movements of the peripheral joints
   E. Myotome evaluation
   F. Sensory test
   G. Reflex testing
2. Cervical evaluation
   A. Active movement (measure range of motion)
   B. Passive movement (measure range of motion)
   C. Resisted movement of cervical region (record strength of resistance)

Continued

BOX 12.2—cont'd

Spinal Evaluation cont'd

    D. Scan of the peripheral joints
      a. TMJ
      b. Peripheral joints of the upper extremities (record strength of resistance)
    E. Special tests
      a. Foraminal Compression Test (pain radiating into arm is positive for nerve root involvement)
      b. Distraction Test (decreased pain with distraction—positive nerve root involvement)
      c. Shoulder Abduction Test[8] (decrease in symptoms—cervical extradural compression)
      d. Maximal Cervical Compression Test[14] (positive with radiation to same side of rotation and extension)
      e. Tinel's Sign for Brachial Plexus Lesion[29]
      f. Vertebral Artery Test[32]
    F. Reflexes testing
    G. Cutaneous distribution
    H. Test for Thoracic Outlet Syndrome[31]
    I. Joint play movements[38]
    J. Palpation of cervical spine (note pain, abnormalities, asymmetries)
    K. Evaluation of the Temporomandibular joints
  3. Thoracic spine
    A. Active movement (measure range of motion)
    B. Passive movement (measure range of motion)
    C. Chest expansion (measure expansion)
    D. Resisted isometric movement (document resistance)
    E. Special test
      Slump Test[33]
    F. Reflex testing
    G. Cutaneous distribution
    H. Joint play movement[34]
    I. Palpation
  4. Lumbar spine
    A. Active movement (measure range of motion)
    B. Passive movement (measure range of motion)
    C. Resisted isometric movement (document resistance)
    D. Scan of peripheral joints
      a. Sacroiliac joint[27]
      b. Hip joints
      c. Knee joints
      d. Foot and ankle joints
      e. Leg length measurements recorded

    E. Myotomes to test strength of peripheral joints (record strength measurements)
    F. Special tests
      a. Straight Leg Raising Tests[47]
      b. Slump Tests[35]
      c. Prone Knee Bending Test[20]
      d. Femoral Nerve Traction Test[11]
      e. Quadrant Test[6]
    G. Reflexes
    H. Cutaneous distribution
    I. Joint play movements
    J. Palpation of the lumbar spine
  5. Sequence of evaluation for peripheral joints
    A. History
    B. Observation
    C. Evaluation
      a. Active movement (measurements recorded)
      b. Passive movement (measurements recorded)
      c. Resisted isometric movements (resistance measurements recorded)
        (1) Determine contractile or non-contractile
        (2) Evaluate myotome integrity
      d. Measurements to determine effusion or atrophy
        (1) Circumference measurements
        (2) Water displacement data, etc.
    D. Special tests
    E. Reflex testing
    F. Cutaneous distribution
    G. Joint play movements
    H. Palpation
  6. Special tests for the peripheral joints
    A. Shoulder special tests
      a. Anterior Drawer Test for the shoulder[15]
      b. Protzman Test for anterior instability[43]
      c. Apprehension test for anterior shoulder dislocation[18]
      d. Posterior Drawer Test for the shoulder[15]
      e. Norwood Stress Test for posterior instability[41]
      f. Posterior apprehension test[9]
      g. Test for inferior shoulder instability[15]
      h. Speed's Test (biceps test)[31]
      i. Supraspinatus test[31]
      j. Impingement test[40,19]
      k. Thoracic Outlet Syndrome Tests
        (1) Allen Test[2]

Continued

BOX 12.2—*cont'd*

(2) Adson Maneuver[1]
(3) Costoclavicular Syndrome Test[31]
(4) Roos Test[45]
B. Elbow special tests
  a. Ligamentous instability test[5]
  b. Test for epicondylitis[31]
C. Wrist and arm special tests
  a. Finkelstein Test[13]
  b. Brunnel-Littler Test[22]
  c. Ligamentous instability test[31]
D. Pelvic tests (sacroiliac joint involvement)
  a. Laguere's Sign[31]
  b. Supine-to-Sit test[42]
E. Hip special tests
  a. FABER or Figure-4 Test[31]
  b. Trendelenburg Sign
F. Knee special tests
  a. Abduction and adduction stress tests

(1) Full extension
(2) 20 to 30 degrees of flexion
b. Lachman Test[25]
c. Reverse Lachman Test[31]
d. Slocum Test[48]
e. Posterior (medial and lateral) Drawer Sign[23]
f. McMurray Test[37]
g. Apley's Test[4]
h. Tests for chondromalacia patella[31]
i. Patellofemoral Angle (Q-Angle)[31]
G. Foot and ankle special tests
  a. Anterior Drawer Sign[26]
  b. Talar Tilt[26]
  c. Thompson Test (sign for ruptured Achilles)[50]
  d. Homan's Sign (sign for thrombophlebitis)[31]

---

tests for the specific joint are listed under each joint section.

INTERVENTIONS PHILOSOPHY

The final section of this chapter describes some of the more common injuries related to musculoskeletal trauma and possible therapeutic intervention. The modalities suggested have demonstrated effectiveness in treatment and may be easily reviewed in the following texts: *Electrotherapy in Rehabilitation* by Gersh[16] and *Thermal Agents in Rehabilitation* by Michlovitz.[39]

The modalities and exercise programs presented are only suggested approaches to care. Other interventions may achieve success and should by utilized according to the skill level of the Therapist. Prior to the selection of modality, the clinician must examine the contra-indications and proper use of the modality. In the following review, the specific site of injury has been documented through a scan for potential pain referral.

Treatment Philosophy

Prior to the review of specific approaches to treatment of the acute injury, a brief discussion of treatment philosophy is needed. In the acute stage of treatment, the stated dysfunctions are provided by the client.

Objective documentation of the limits of walking, lifting, or any other dysfunction may not be readily accessible. High levels of pain, marked effusion, or limits of motion prohibit exact measurement of functional limits. Once the acute stage has passed, functional tests that mimic the specific job requirements must be incorporated into the rehabilitation process. Functional tests may include a Functional Capacity Assessment or specific activities that duplicate the job of the client.

The functional approach, as employed in Industrial Therapy, takes into account the requirements of a specific job. The common medical approach to an injury is to attempt to achieve complete rehabilitation prior to discharge. In a functional approach, it is vital to understand the needs of the client, and to match the rehabilitation process to those needs.

If an individual is employed as an assembly line worker, and the motion requirements of the shoulder joint range between 70 and 90 degrees of shoulder flexion, is it imperative to achieve 180 degrees of motion during rehabilitation? Ideally, all of our clients should obtain total recovery. Realistically, it is the responsibility of the Industrial Therapist to return the client to the work site in a safe and efficient manner. The functional goals assigned to the client must meet those of the job and the client to achieve an effective level of rehabilitation.

Finally, any increase or return of signs of inflammation is an indication that the therapeutic intervention is too aggressive. This is of prime importance in the rehabilitation process. If inflammation returns, the functional level of the client decreases. The Therapist must constantly monitor the client's response to care, whether at the acute stage or months into rehabilitation. Pain or an increase in symptomatology is an indication of trauma. The client can be protected during the rehabilitation process through an intelligent, progressive but well-monitored program. The

well-worn expression "no pain, no gain" should be replaced with the new phrase, "pain is your body's way of calling you a dummy."

INTERVENTION EXAMPLES

The following areas of treatment intervention are intended to provide Therapists with illustrations of how the foregoing principles and philosophies are

FIGURE 12.2 Exercise program for shoulder impingement.

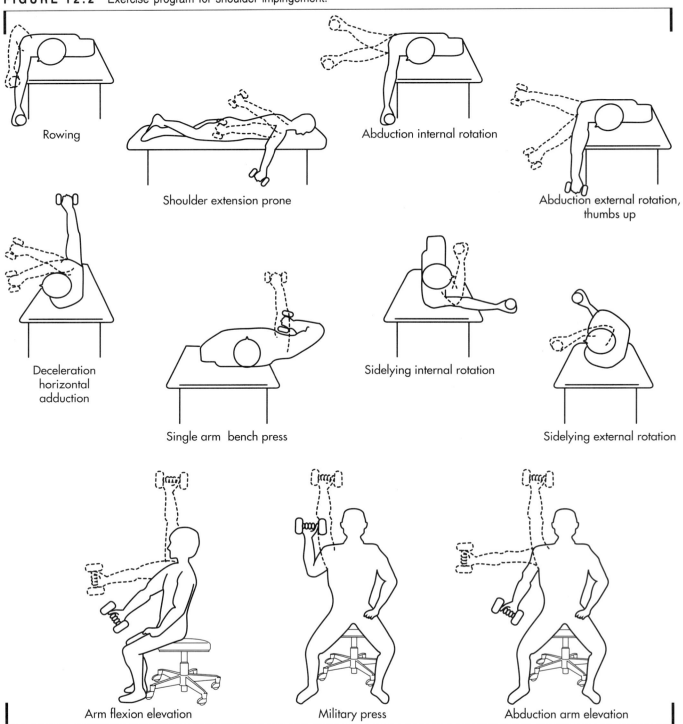

Rowing

Shoulder extension prone

Abduction internal rotation

Abduction external rotation, thumbs up

Deceleration horizontal adduction

Single arm bench press

Sidelying internal rotation

Sidelying external rotation

Arm flexion elevation

Military press

Abduction arm elevation

applied. The procedures and modalities outlined are in no way a complete listing of the tools available to the Therapist. The interventions listed do present procedures and modalities that have proven statistically effective in the treatment of acute musculoskeletal injuries.

Acute Shoulder Injury

Example A: Impingement Syndrome
Pain is noted with movement of the arm to shoulder height. Strength is diminished. Client works in a warehouse.

Dysfunction: The client is unable to lift boxes to shoulder height.

Cause	Intervention
A. Pain	1. Pulsed ultrasound
	2. Cryotherapy
B. Adaptive shortening of soft tissue	1. Capsule mobilization
	2. Stretching contractile soft tissue
	3. Postural instruction
C. Muscular weakness	1. Strengthening of postural muscles
	2. Strengthening of muscles of rotator cuff

Plan: The client will be able to lift 10 pounds to shoulder height within six treatments as a result of Physical Therapy Intervention.

A sample exercise program for shoulder impingement is illustrated in Figure 12.2.

Discussion. The prime objective in the care of acute Impingement Syndrome is initially to decrease the pain involved due to the mechanical dysfunction. It is imperative to address the cause of the impingement early in the care. It is important to insure that the capsule of the glenohumeral joint permits the correct arthrokinematics, and that the musculature of the entire shoulder complex is functioning correctly. Without the correct contraction sequence, the head of the humerus will not glide inferiorly and will subsequently impinge upon the acromium bridge.

Example B: Rotator Cuff Tear
Pain with resistance to muscle contraction of specific muscles of the rotator cuff. Diminished strength. Physical Therapy intervention is more appropriate after tissue repair is near completion. Level of activity depends upon the severity of tear. Client is a chef.

Dysfunction: Client is unable to lift pots and pans or mix food.

Cause	Intervention
A. Pain	1. Cryotherapy
	2. Interferential current
B. Mechanical dysfunction	1. Protection of injured structure
	2. Medical evaluation for surgical intervention
C. Muscle weakness	Tissue repair required prior to strength program

Plan: The client will be able to lift 5 pounds and mix food for 15 minutes within one month as a result of Physical Therapy Intervention.

Discussion. Correct evaluation is of prime importance when dealing with rotator cuff tear. No amount of exercise will heal a tear in this sheet of connective tissue; in fact, considering the physiology and the kinesiology involved in tissue healing, it is clear that active contraction will actually inhibit the healing process.

Strengthening activity to the torn rotator cuff must not be instituted until healing is complete. If surgical intervention is required, it is still necessary for healing to be complete prior to the implementation of physical stress.

Acute Elbow Injuries

Example A: Tennis Elbow (Lateral epicondylitis)
Client reports pain with any type of gripping activity. Pain is noted with resistance to active wrist extension or passive wrist flexion. Pain is noted with palpation of lateral epicondyle. Client is a carpenter.

Dysfunction: The client is unable to firmly grasp a hammer.

Cause	Intervention
A. Pain	1. Cryotherapy
	2. Pulsed ultrasound
B. Effusion	Iontophoresis
C. Mechanical dysfunction	Tennis arm band (epicondylar splint)
D. Soft tissue adaptive shortening	1. Soft tissue stretch
	2. Capsule mobilization
E. Muscle weakness	Progressive strength program

FIGURE 12.3   Strength program for lateral epicondylitis.

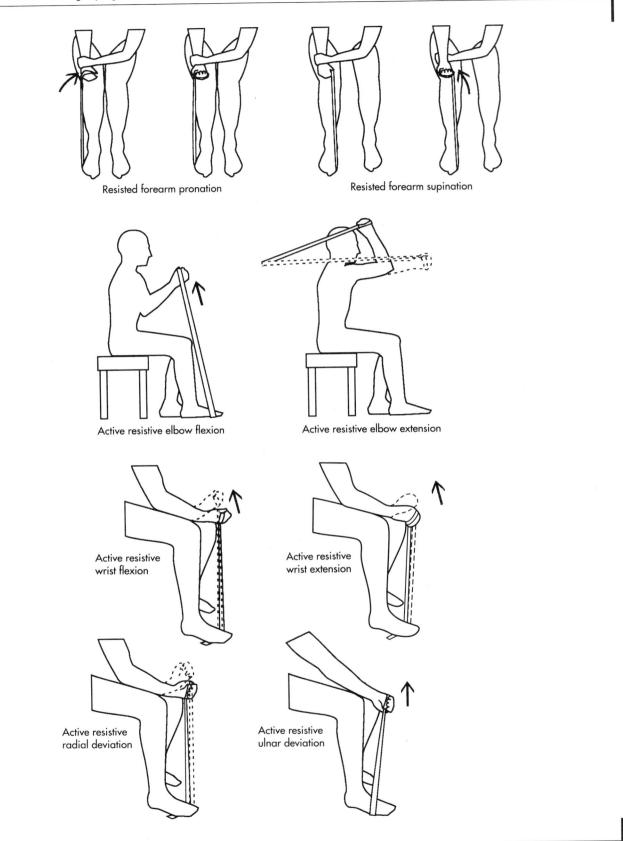

Resisted forearm pronation

Resisted forearm supination

Active resistive elbow flexion

Active resistive elbow extension

Active resistive wrist flexion

Active resistive wrist extension

Active resistive radial deviation

Active resistive ulnar deviation

Plan: The client will be able to hold and use a hammer for four hours within six to eight treatments as a result of Physical Therapy Intervention.

A sample strength program for lateral epicondylitis is illustrated in Figure 12.3.

Discussion. As with any peripheral dysfunction, it is necessary to rule out any spinal involvement. Lateral epicondylitis is difficult to deal with, and recovery may be prolonged. Rule out any nerve compression problems at the elbow if recovery is not progressing in the correct time frame.

Acute Wrist and Hand Injuries

Example A: de Quervain's Syndrome

Pain is noted with any attempt to use the thumb, as in attempting to use a pinch type grip. Pain also present with forceful supination and pronation. Client is a dentist.

Dysfunction: Client is unable to hold dental equipment for five minutes.

Cause	Intervention
A. Pain	1. Cryotherapy
	2. Pulsed ultrasound
B. Effusion	1. Iontophoresis
	2. Compression (sleeve or elastic tape)
	3. Splint
C. Adhesions	1. Transverse friction massage
	2. Gentle stretching
D. Muscle weakness	1. Gentle strength program
	2. Consider prolonged use of splint
	3. Evaluate job site

Plan: The client will be able to manipulate dental equipment for four hours within six to eight treatments as a result of Physical Therapy Intervention.

A sample strength and stretch program for de Quervain's syndrome is illustrated in Figure 12.4.

Discussion. The major difficulty when dealing with de Quervain's syndrome is that the individual plagued with this dysfunction normally requires repetitive use of the hand. Cumulative trauma is the cause of the pain and restriction. Treatment requires rest and protection. Functional splinting may enable some workers to return to the work site rapidly. If fine finger function and coordination are required, return to work may be delayed.

FIGURE 12.4 Strength and stretch program for de Quervain's Syndrome.

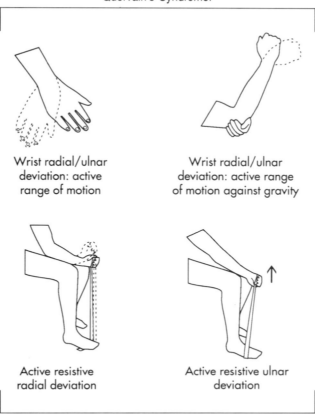

Wrist radial/ulnar deviation: active range of motion

Wrist radial/ulnar deviation: active range of motion against gravity

Active resistive radial deviation

Active resistive ulnar deviation

Acute Hip Injuries

Example A: Trochanteric Bursitis

Deep aching sensation. Pain with attempts to climb stairs. Pain noted with side-lying. Deep aching sensation into the L5 distribution (lateral thigh to the knee and to lower leg). Client is a house painter.

Dysfunction: The client is unable to stand on ladder for more than 10 minutes while painting.

Cause	Intervention
A. Pain	1. Cryotherapy
	2. Pulsed ultrasound
	3. Assistive devices for weight-bearing
B. Effusion	High voltage pulsed current
C. Soft tissue adaptive shortening	1. Capsular mobilization
	2. Stretching program
D. Muscle weakness	Gentle strength program when tolerated

Plan: The client will be able to stand on ladder for 45 to 60 minutes within six treatments as a result of Physical Therapy Intervention.

FIGURE 12.5   Gentle stretching and strengthening program for Trochanteric Bursitis.

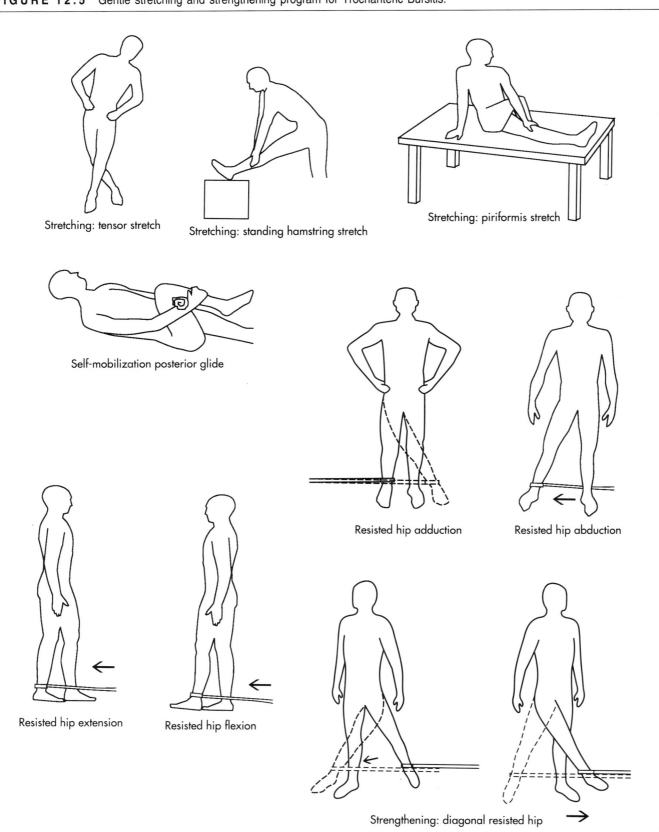

Stretching: tensor stretch

Stretching: standing hamstring stretch

Stretching: piriformis stretch

Self-mobilization posterior glide

Resisted hip adduction

Resisted hip abduction

Resisted hip extension

Resisted hip flexion

Strengthening: diagonal resisted hip

A gentle stretching and strengthening program for Trochanteric Bursitis is illustrated in Figure 12.5.

Discussion. The patient should be examined to rule out spinal problems or medical problems. As with any bursitis, some type of mechanical dysfunction is causing the inflammation. Unless this mechanical cause is discovered, success will be short-lived. Often, weakness in the muscles surrounding the joint, capsular tightness, or a structural problem (short leg, pronation) must be addressed prior to a return to work. The job site should be evaluated to determine if the dysfunction is due to a mechanical stress of the work involved.

Example B: Piriformis Syndrome

Pain radiating into low back and posterior thigh. Pain is noted with prolonged sitting. Client is a truck driver.

Dysfunction: The client is unable to drive truck for more than 15 minutes.

Cause	Intervention
A. Pain	1. Interferential current
	2. Pulsed ultrasound
B. Adaptive shortening of soft tissue	1. Soft tissue stretching
	2. Deep soft tissue mobilization
C. Muscle weakness	Strength program (stabilization)

Plan: *The client will be able to drive for two hours within four to six treatments as a result of Physical Therapy Intervention.*

A stabilization program for Piriformis syndrome is illustrated in Figure 12.6.

Discussion. The diagnosis of Piriformis syndrome is often missed in the medical evaluation. During the Physical Therapy evaluation, be sure to look past the medical diagnosis and relate the complaints to a musculoskeletal structure. If the Industrial Therapist is unable to duplicate the symptomatology by mechanically stressing the structures, the problem is not with the musculoskeletal structure. Further medical evaluation may be necessary. The Industrial Therapist's duty is to return the worker to the job site as safely and rapidly as possible. Improper diagnosis of medical or mechanical problems only delay correct intervention.

Acute Injuries to the Knee

Example A: Medial Collateral Ligament Strain (Grade II)

Client complains of pain with any rotational movement or walking on uneven terrain. Pain with stair climbing or valgus stress to the knee. The client is a farmer.

Dysfunction: The client is unable to walk in the fields of his farm.

Cause	Intervention
A. Pain	1. Cryotherapy
	2. Interferential current
B. Effusion	1. Pneumatic compression pump
	2. Compression sleeve
C. Joint instability	Knee brace for lateral/ medial stability
D. Muscle weakness	1. Closed kinetic chain stabilization activity
	2. Aerobic activity

Plan: *The client will be able to work in the fields of his farm for four hours within eight treatments as a result of Physical Therapy Intervention.*

A strength program for collateral ligament injury is illustrated in Figure 12.7.

Discussion. Many professions, farming in particular, do not allow the luxury of a long healing and rehabilitation program. It is very important for the farmer to be able to function as quickly as possible, with as few limitations as possible. Protective bracing and home strengthening programs will be more readily accepted than rehabilitation in the clinic. The financial stress of a family farm, or of any private enterprise, may require the owner to be present for much of the day. The Therapist should be aware of the requirements of the job and relate the rehabilitation process to those requirements. If it is necessary for the workers to be treated at the clinical setting, an adaptation of the clinic hours may be in order to provide the service. The Industrial Therapist should remain flexible in the provision of service to the injured worker.

Acute Ankle Injury

Example A: Acute Lateral Ankle Sprain (Grade II)

The client complains of pain with any type of weight bearing. Swelling prevents the use of shoes. Feelings of instability are expressed by the client. Client is using crutches. Client is a waitress.

Dysfunction: The client is unable to bear weight on ankle.

Cause	Intervention
A. Pain	Cryotherapy
B. Effusion	1. Elevation

FIGURE 12.6   Stabilization program for Piriformis syndrome.

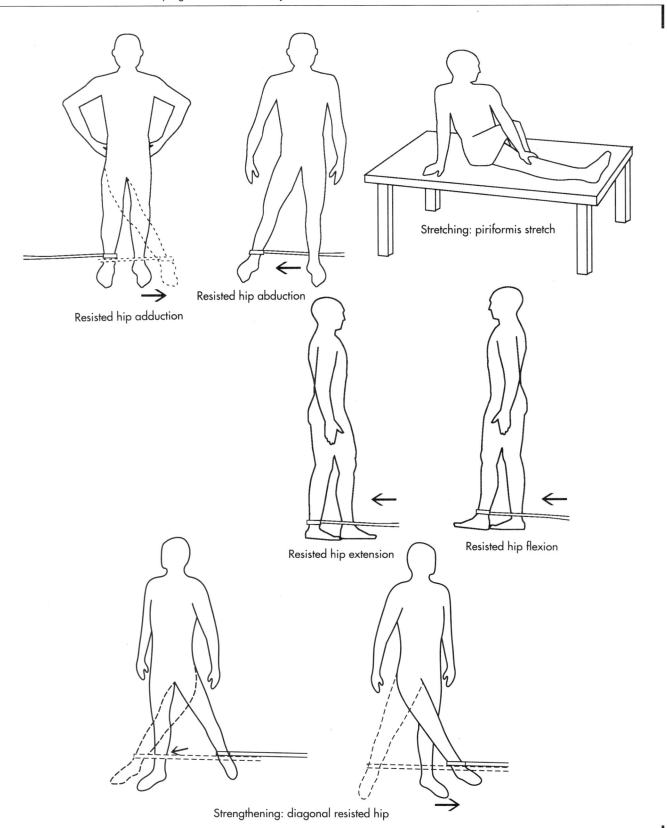

Resisted hip adduction

Resisted hip abduction

Stretching: piriformis stretch

Resisted hip extension

Resisted hip flexion

Strengthening: diagonal resisted hip

FIGURE 12.7   Strength program for collateral ligament injury.

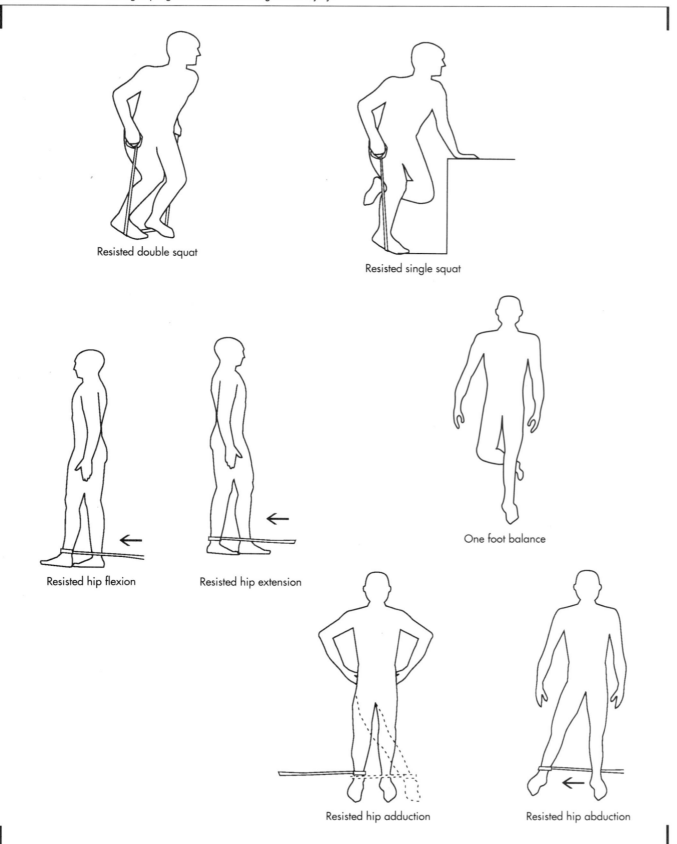

Resisted double squat

Resisted single squat

Resisted hip flexion

Resisted hip extension

One foot balance

Resisted hip adduction

Resisted hip abduction

2. Pneumatic compression pump
3. Compression stocking

C. Ankle instability — Ankle brace (non-elastic)

D. Muscle weakness
1. Stabilization exercise
2. Isotonic exercise program
3. Proprioceptive activity

Plan: The client will be able to work four hours within eight treatments as a result of Physical Therapy Intervention.

A sample rehabilitation program for acute ankle sprain is illustrated in Figure 12.8.

NOTE: Contrast baths or whirlpools, which require the leg to be dependent, are not utilized in extremities presenting marked effusion. Dependency of the limb would only further exacerbate the effusion,[36] and is not as effective as cold, elevation, and compression.[49]

Discussion. The most important aspects of care for the injured ankle are to decrease effusion and protect the ankle. Compression stockings, utilized any time dependency of the limb occurs, assist in preventing edema accumulating in the ankle complex. Active pumping and gentle strengthening activity assist in the muscle pump activity and decrease the edema. An ankle brace designed to provide stability prevents further trauma to the injured structures. The brace must be rigid enough to prevent inversion or eversion of the ankle but allow dorsiflexion and plantarflexion during gait. Elastic braces allow too much movement, and should not be utilized to provide ankle stability.

Acute Injuries to the Spine

Example A: Cervical Pain with Rotation
Auto accident during work. Pain is noted with rotation and extension to the side of injury (facet type pain). No radiation of pain into extremities. Client drives a taxi.

Dysfunction: The client is unable to rotate neck and head to back up while driving taxi

Cause	Intervention
A. Pain	1. Ice
	2. Interferential current
B. Mechanical dysfunction	1. Facet capsule mobilization
	2. Active range of motion exercise
C. Muscle weakness	Strength program (stabilization)

Plan: The client will be able to rotate cervical region to permit the client to back taxi up within four to six treatments as a result of Physical Therapy Intervention.

A sample rehabilitation program for the acute cervical injury is illustrated in Figure 12.9.

Discussion. With the acute trauma of an auto accident, radiographic evaluation must be provided by the attending Physician. An open-mouth view of the odontoid process insures stability of this vital structure. Evaluation of the Alar ligament and the vertebral artery is required of all cervical injuries.

Example B: Mid-Thoracic Pain
Client complains of mid-thoracic pain with prolonged sitting. No pain is noted initially, but with continued sitting, pain increases. The client is a secretary.

Dysfunction: The client is unable to sit for 45 minutes

Cause	Intervention
A. Mechanical dysfunction	1. Hot packs—tissue relaxation
	2. Capsule mobilization
	3. Self-mobilization
B. Muscle weakness	Progressive strength program
C. Decreased postural awareness	1. Educational program to improve posture
	2. Job site evaluation and modification

Plan: The client will be able to tolerate sitting for four to five hours within six treatments as a result of Physical Therapy Intervention.

A sample rehabilitation program for the mid-thoracic region is illustrated in Figure 12.10.

Discussion. Jobs requiring the maintenance of static positions for prolonged periods, such as a secretary, require the Industrial Therapist's intervention at the job site. An evaluation of the client's posture, the location of the computer, or how a telephone is held can lead to success in treatment. An adaptation as simple as using a telephone headset, as opposed to holding the telephone handpiece between the shoulder and ear, may allow the secretary to return to work.

Example C: Lumbo-sacral Strain (Grade I)
Client complains of pain with any type of bending activity. Pain is increased with sitting. Lifting from the floor increases pain dramatically. No radiation of pain into the legs. The client is a plumber.

FIGURE 12.8 Rehabilitation program for acute ankle sprain.

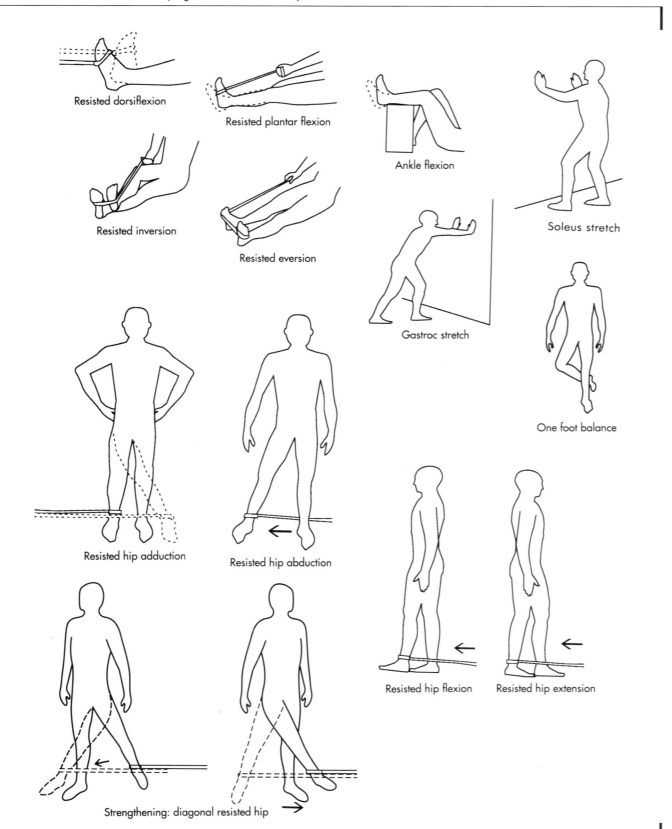

FIGURE 12.9   Rehabilitation program for acute cervical injury.

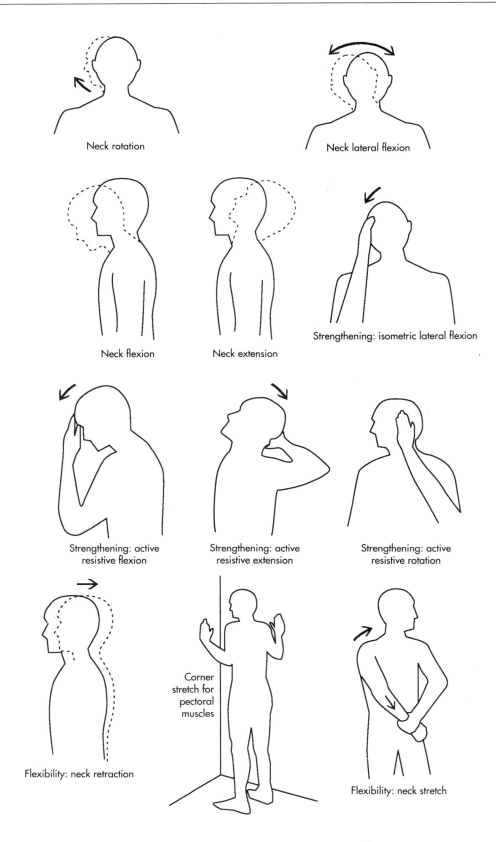

Neck rotation

Neck lateral flexion

Neck flexion

Neck extension

Strengthening: isometric lateral flexion

Strengthening: active resistive flexion

Strengthening: active resistive extension

Strengthening: active resistive rotation

Flexibility: neck retraction

Corner stretch for pectoral muscles

Flexibility: neck stretch

FIGURE 12.10   Rehabilitation program for the mid-thoracic region.

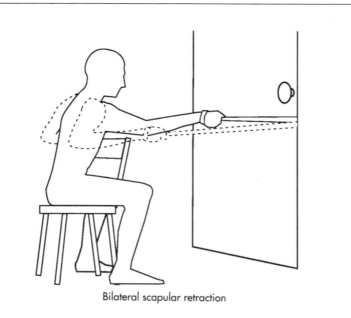

Bilateral scapular retraction

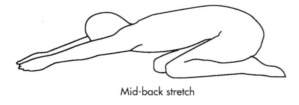

Mid-back stretch

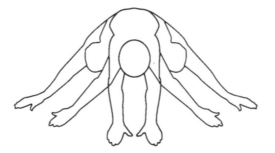

Mid-back rotation stretch

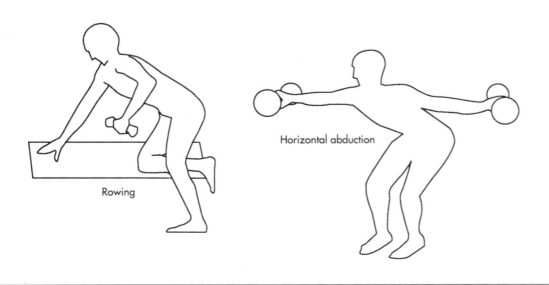

Rowing

Horizontal abduction

FIGURE 12.11   Rehabilitation program for the lumbo-sacral region.

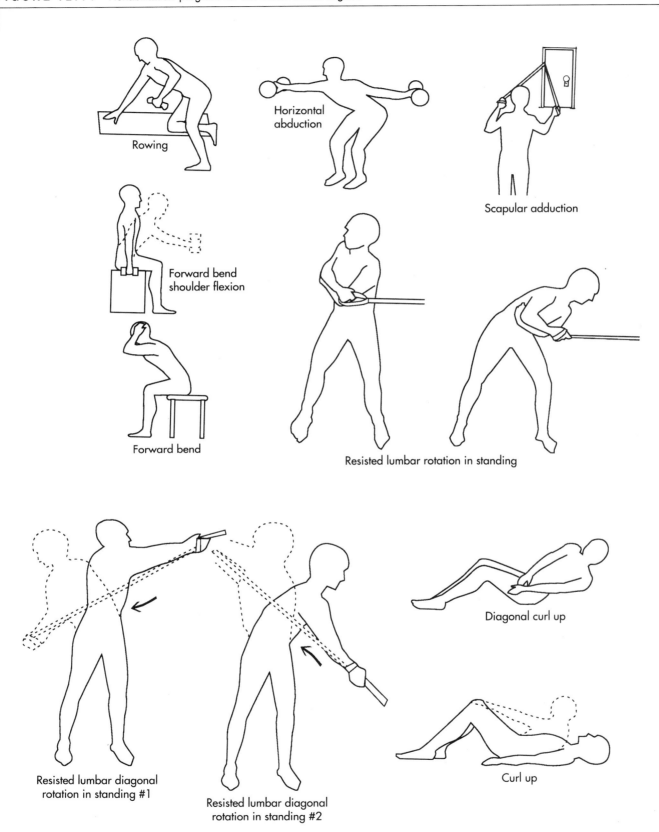

Rowing

Horizontal abduction

Scapular adduction

Forward bend shoulder flexion

Forward bend

Resisted lumbar rotation in standing

Resisted lumbar diagonal rotation in standing #1

Resisted lumbar diagonal rotation in standing #2

Diagonal curl up

Curl up

Dysfunction: The client is unable to lift 10 pounds from the floor.

Cause	Intervention
A. Pain	1. Interferential current
	2. Cryotherapy
B. Instability	Lumbar support
C. Muscle weakness	Stabilization program
D. Adaptive shortening of soft tissue	Stretching program
E. Lack of postural awareness	Back school

Plan: The client will be able to lift 50 pounds from the floor within six to eight treatments as a result of Physical Therapy Intervention.

A sample rehabilitation program for the lumbo-sacral region is illustrated in Figure 12.11.

Discussion. A client involved in a physically demanding job necessitates fitness levels to match those requirements. It has been the author's professional experience that the fit individual has fewer and less severe spinal injuries than the unfit worker. Levels of strength, aerobic capacity, flexibility, balance, and proper nutrition must be considered when treating any client with a work-related injury.

PRINCIPLES OF INTERVENTION

Monitoring

When dealing with the acute phase of the rehabilitation process, the Industrial Therapist utilizes input from the client and objective measurements to monitor changes from baseline information collected during initial evaluation. Once the acute phase subsides, a more in-depth evaluation of the functional levels of the client is necessary.

The acute phase of treatment passes so quickly that measurable data related to the goals of acute care can be monitored in an expeditious manner (the client is able to walk five feet without a crutch, or the client is able to lift three pounds to shoulder height). Range of motion measurements, strength measurements, or pain scales are all examples of measurable data that can be utilized in the development of information to monitor progress.

Stakeholders

One aspect unique to dealing with the injured worker is the number of individuals interested in the return to full function. Normally, the injured individual has family and friends to console and encourage a return to activity. When dealing with the injured worker, the Therapist must not only be aware of the client's family and friends, but the many other people involved at the work site with the worker.

The employer, personnel officers, insurance agents, vocational rehabilitation counselors, safety officers, union officials, and attorneys may all be involved in the care of the client. Open lines of communication, realistic functional goals, accumulation of measurable data, and documentation of changes in function are all crucial components of care provided to the various parties interested in the injured worker. Excellent rehabilitation is not always enough; documentation is mandatory.

SUMMARY

A therapist's role in the acute care phase post-injury is applying expertise to assist the injured worker in a safe, functional, and rapid return to the workplace.

If the client is not able to return in the time frame indicated by the initial evaluation, progression into Work Conditioning, Work Hardening, or retraining must be considered.

The most important concepts presented in this chapter are **early intervention, precise evaluation, and functionally-oriented treatment** of dysfunctions. From the phases of wound repair through the DEP approach to rehabilitation (Data, Evaluation, and Plan), it is imperative that the process focuses on an expeditious return to work.

Monitoring the process through accurate measurements of progress is a key element in any program. Measurements used in the normal medical model of care are only part of the information required for the comprehensive approach of Industrial Therapy.

The worker deserves the opportunity to receive intelligent, aggressive, and rapid care for any trauma received at the work site. Early intervention prevents the development of chronic dysfunctions and disabilities. The Industrial Therapist must work diligently to encourage early intervention through marketing programs targeting employers, Physicians, State Labor, and Industry Administrators.

The Industrial Therapist has the tools to decrease the excessive cost aspects of the industrial injury, and must utilize them to the maximum benefit.

REFERENCES

1. Adson AW, Coffey Jr: Cervical Rib: a method of anterior approach for relief of symptoms by division of the scalenus anticus, *Ann Surg* 85:839-857, 1927.

2. Allen EV: Thromboangitis Obliterans: Methods of Diagnosis of Chronic Occlusive Arterial Lesions Distal to The Wrist With Illustrative Cases, *Am J Med Sci*, 178:237-244, 1929.

3. Alvarez OM: Wound Healing. In Fitzpatrick editor: *Dermatology in General Med*, ed 3, New York, 1987, McGraw Hill.

4. Apley AG: The Diagnosis of Meniscus Injuries: Some new clinical methods, *J Bone Joint Surgery* 29B:78, 1947.

5. Carson WC: Congenital Elevation of the Scapula, *J Bone Joint Surg*, 63A:1199, 1981.

6. Corrigan B, Maitland G: *Practical Orthopedic Medicine* 1985, Butterworth.

7. Cryiax J: *Textbook of Orthopedic Medicine*, vol 1: Diagnosis of Soft Tissue Lesions, ed 8, Bailliere Tendall London, 1982.

8. Davidson RI: The Shoulder Abduction Test in Diagnosis of Radicular Pain in Cervical Extradural Compressive Monoradiculopathies, *Spine* 6:441, 1981.

9. Davies GJ, Gould JA, Larson RL: Functional Examination of the Shoulder Girdle *Phys Sports Med* 9:82-104, 1981.

10. Daly T: The Repair Phase of Wound Healing: Re-epithelialization and Contraction, In Kloth L editor: *Wound Healing Alternatives in Management*, Philadelphia, 1990, FA Davis.

11. Dyck P: The Femoral Nerve Traction Test with Lumbar Disc Protrusion, *Surg Neurol* 6:163, 1976.

12. El-Diny D, Smith G: A Functional Approach to Documentation, Eastern Washington University, Dept of Physical Therapy, Course on Documentation, Cheney, Wash, 1992.

13. Finkelstein H: Stenosing Tendovaginitis at the Radial Styloid Process, *J Bone Joint Surg* 12:509, 1930.

14. Foreman SM, Croft AC: Whiplash Injuries: *The Cervical Acceleration/Deceleration Syndrome*, Baltimore, 1988, Williams and Wilkins.

15. Gerber D, Ganz R: Clinical Assessment of Instability of the Shoulder, *J Bone Joint Surg*, 66B:551-556, 1984.

16. Gersh MR: *Electrotherapy in Rehabilitation*, Philadelphia, 1992, FA Davis.

17. Gungor T: A Test for Ankle Instability, *J Bone Joint Surgery*, 70B:487, 1988.

18. Hawkins RJ, Bokor DJ: Clinical Evaluation of Shoulder Problems. In Rockwood CA editor: *The Shoulder*, Philadelphia, 1990, WB Saunders.

19. Hawking RJ, Kennedy H: Impingement Syndromes in Athletes, *Am J Sports Med*, 8:151, 1980.

20. Herron L, Pheasant H: Prone Knee-Flexion Provocative Testing for Lumbar Disc Protrusion, *Spine* 5:65.

21. Holbrook T, Grazier K, Kelsey J, Stauffer R: The Frequency of Occurrence Impact and Cost of Selected Musculoskeletal Conditions in the United States, *Am Acad Orth Surg* 27B, 1984.

22. Hoppenfeld S: *Physical Examination of the Spine and Extremities*, New York, 1976, Appleton-Century Crofts.

23. Hughston J, Norwood L: The Posterior lateral drawer test and external rotational recurvatum test for posterior lateral rotary instability of the knee, *Clin Orthop Relat Res* 147:82, 1980.

24. Jahss MH: *Disorders of the Foot*, Philadelphia, 1982, WB Saunders.

25. Jonsson T, Althoff B: Clinical Diagnosis of Ruptures of the Anterior Cruciate Ligament: A Comparative Study of the Lachman Test and the Anterior Drawer Sign, *Am J Sports Med* 10:100, 1982.

26. Kelikian H, Kelikian A, *Disorders of the Ankle*, Philadelphia, 1985, WB Saunders.

27. Kirkaldy-Willis WH: *Managing Low Back Pain*, New York, 1983, Churchill Livingstone.

28. Kloth L, Miller K: Inflammatory Response to Wounding, In Kloth, McCulloch, J, Feeder J (eds) *Wound Healing: Alternatives in Management* Philadelphia, 1990, FA Davis.

29. Landi A, Copeland S: Value of Tinel Sign in Brachial Plexus Lesions, *Ann Roy Coll Surg* England 61: 470-471, 1979.

30. Levensen SM: The Healing of Rat Skin Wounds, *Ann Surg* 161:293, 1965.

31. MaGee D: *Orthopedic Physical Assessment*, ed 2, Philadelphia, 1992, WB Saunders.

32. Maitland GD: *Vertebral Manipulation* London, 1973, Butterworth.

33. Maitland G: The Slump Test: Examination and Treatment, *Aut J Physiother* 31:215, 1985.

34. Maitland GD: *Vertebral Manipulation* London, 1973, Butterworth.

35. Maitland GD: The Slump Test: Examination and Treatment *Aut J Physiother* 31:215, 1985.

36. McCulloch J, Hovde J: Treatment of Wounds Due to Vascular Problems. In Kloth L, McCulloch J, Feeder J editors: *Wound Healing: Alternatives in Management*, 191, Philadelphia, 1990, FA Davis.

37. McMurray TP: The Semilunar Cartilages, *Br J Surg* 29:407, 1942.

38. Mennell J: *Joint Pain*, Boston, 1964, Little, Brown.

39. Michlovitz SL: *Thermal Agents in Rehabilitation*, ed 2, Philadelphia, 1990, FA Davis.

40. Neer GS, Welsh RP: The Shoulder in Sports, *Orthop Clin North America* 8:583-591, 1977.

41. Norwood LA, Terry G: Shoulder Posterior and Anterior Subluxation, *Am J Sports Med* 12:25-30, 1984.

42. Porterfield JA, DeRosa C: *Mechanical Low Back Pain-Perspectives in Functional Anatomy*, Philadelphia, 1991, WB Saunders.

43. Protzman RR: Anterior Instability of the Shoulder, *J Bone Joint Surgery* 62A:909-918, 1980.

44. Reed B, Zarro V: Inflammation and Repair and the Use of Thermal Agents. In Michlovitz S editor: *Thermal Agents in Rehabilitation*, ed 2, Philadelphia, 1990, F.A. Davis.

45. Roos DB: Congenital Anomalies Associated with Thoracic Outlet Syndrome, *J Surg* 132:771-778, 1976.

46. Rothstein J, Roy S, Wolf S: *The Rehabilitation Specialist Handbook*, Philadelphia, 1990, FA Davis.

47. Scham SI, Taylor TK: Tension Signs in Lumbar Disc Prolapse *Clin Orthop Related Res* 75: 195, 1971.

48. Slocum DB, Larson R: Rotary Instability of the Knee, *J Bone Joint Surg* 50A:211, 1968.

49. Smith W: The Application of Cold and Heat in the

Treatment of Athletic Injuries. In Michlovits S editor: *Thermal Agents in Rehabilitation,* Philadelphia, 1990, FA Davis.

50. Thompson T, Doherty J: Spontaneous Rupture of the Tendon of the Achilles: a new clinical diagnostic test, *Anat Res* 158:126, 1967.

51. White A, Panjabi M: *Clinical Biomechanics of the Spine,* ed 2, Philadelphia, 1990, JB Lippincott.

CHAPTER

13

Functional Capacity Assessment

Glenda L. Key

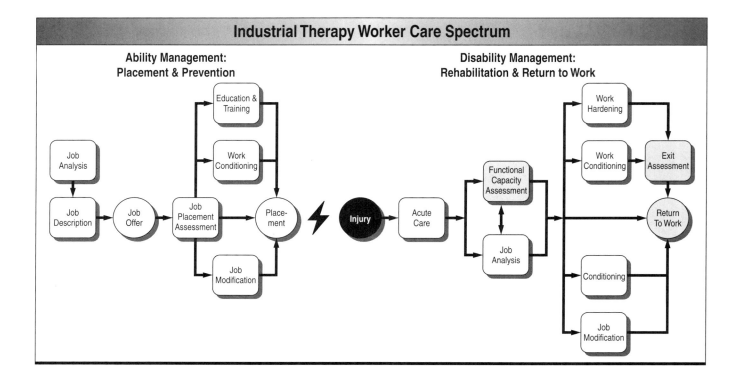

Industrial Therapy Worker Care Spectrum

Functional Capacity Assessment is a process of measuring, recording, and analyzing a person's ability to safely perform a number of job-related functions, such as lifting, lowering, pushing, pulling and carrying weights, climbing ladders and stairs, sitting, standing, bending, stooping, crouching, kneeling, crawling, and grasping. The assessment results are used at appropriate points in the Worker Care Spectrum to determine a worker's safe working levels for the purposes of job placement, injury prevention, and rehabilitation.

This measurement and analysis process involves physical capacity evaluation, work assessment, functional capacity evaluation, and functional capacity assessment. For the purposes of this book, the term Functional Capacity Assessment (FCA) is used.

FCA's role in Industrial Therapy has been steadily growing in importance in recent years. Increasingly, FCAs are used to assist in placement decisions, specify conditioning or job modification measures, and guide rehabilitation in the areas of goal setting, program design, progress monitoring, and return-to-work parameters.[69] While FCA's role is expanding, equipment design and assessment protocols have been evolving, guided by outcome studies and driven by the desire for greater accuracy and reliability.

If the recent past is any indication of the rate of change, this chapter represents only a snapshot of a point in time. For Therapists currently using FCAs or contemplating offering them in the future, it is helpful to know what the field of FCA looks like at present. It is also important to anticipate what it will be like in the future. One way to foresee future developments is to understand the underlying forces that have driven the evolution to this point, and those that will continue to shape FCA's.

This chapter will review those driving forces, discuss current issues regarding the design of equipment and protocols, describe the current role that FCAs play in the Worker Care Spectrum, and provide guidance for Therapists intending to utilize FCAs or to upgrade existing FCA services.

THE INFLUENCES SHAPING FCAs

There are a number of influences driving the growth and evolution of FCAs and the increasing demand for objective, reliable, valid data concerning a worker's safe capabilities.[10] Although there are a multitude of factors at work, the overall influences behind the evolution of FCAs are economic, environmental, and legal as indicated in Box 13.1. Within these overall influences, additional insight can be gained by examining the underlying needs of the key parties involved in injury prevention and rehabilitation: physicians, employers, vocational rehabilitation consultants, attorneys, insurance companies, therapists, and legislation.

Physicians

In the past, the objectives of medical intervention for injured workers were centered on medical outcomes. Anatomical and physiological findings were commonly used by physicians to categorize back injuries and make physical impairment determinations.[2,10] Treatment goals were expressed in terms of alleviated pain and swelling, restored range of motion and strength, and return to "normal" physiological functions such as heart rate, blood pressure, and blood count. The problems associated with using those measures were that they bore little relevance to functional capabilities. Two

workers with identical medical profiles may have considerably different safe capability levels.

As time went on, it became increasingly evident that meeting traditional medical criteria did not always correlate with meeting the job demands.[1] There remained a need to determine the safe level of the returning worker. Physicians relied on the worker's own assessment of capabilities. Often, the worker would overstate capabilities if they wanted to go back to work, and understate them if they did not. Physicians were bearing increasing responsibility for post treatment performance or reinjury, so it was only a matter of time before they would support more objective, valid and reliable methods of determining a worker's safe capabilities.

FCA's progressed into variables and contexts far afield from traditional medicine, and physicians became understandably willing to share return to work decision-making and responsibility, with people who were emerging as specialists in the functional assessment area. Orthopedic surgeons are trained in surgery, not in job demand fulfillment. It is easy to understand their willingness to sidestep an area of unfamiliarity, shift a portion of the liability, and avoid a great deal of the documentation involved in return to work assessment.

Presently, Physicians are realizing ever increasing benefits through FCAs. FCA methodologies are providing increasingly objective, accurate, and in some instances statistically reliable data for courtroom proceedings. In such settings, attorneys are more frequently requesting quantitative support for the Physician's treatment and recommendations. Some FCA's provide input into whether a patient is manipulating his or her injured status, or magnifying the severity of the impairment.[25,36,55] By gauging the patient's motivation or validity of participation, FCA's can help support the Physician's recommendations and allay suspicions of employers or payors as to the worker's honesty.

Employers

Quite regularly we learn that another large corporation is terminating hundreds of workers to cut costs and maintain a competitive position in the face of global competition. The layoffs make headlines, but employers are making every effort to save money and increase productivity. Skyrocketing costs of Workers' Compensation, health care, litigation, and lost productivity have brought the area of worker injury and rehabilitation under close scrutiny.

Each year, nearly 500,000 U.S. workers become injured and unable to resume their jobs for long periods of time. As few as half who enter the disability system eventually return to work. In 1985 the National

---

BOX 13.1

Overall Influences On The Evolution Of FCAs

Economic:	Environmental:	Legal:
Skyrocketing health care costs	OSHA & ADA regulations	Increasing litigation
Global competition	Tightening reimbursement restrictions	Increasing defensive medicine

Safety Council estimated the direct cost of work-related injuries totaled $16 billion.[23] Interestingly, it has been found that newer employees are more prone to back injuries than older employees (although older employees' back injuries are more costly).[9]

Employers have been implementing measures such as education and training programs, employee fitness, and ergonomic and job modification programs.[40,63] They have also been seeking ways to streamline return to work time frames and costs.[28,59] Accompanying the involvement of efficiency experts and financial people has been a growing demand for objectivity over opinion, validity over judgment, reliability over happenstance, accuracy over guess work, and science over art.

Regarding injured workers, employers are demanding quantitative support for the rehabilitation plan, reliable return to work dates, and precise assessments of the returning workers safe capabilities. To answer these needs, Functional Capacity Assessments have continuously progressed toward enhanced levels of objectivity, validity, reliability, accuracy, and science in use throughout the care continuum from injury to return to work.

Employers have also realized that in most cases, rehabilitating injured workers is preferable to hiring, training, and progressing replacement workers to comparable productivity levels.[5] Not only is the rehabilitation approach less costly, it sends a positive, morale-building signal to the workforce that the company stands behind its employees.[59]

FCAs enable employers, working with therapists, to more reliably determine the degree of functional restoration possible, and the rehabilitation plan's components and time frames. This facilitates a comparison of rehabilitation expense to the cost of replacing the injured worker.

The employer's legal and regulatory concerns are also driving the evolution of FCAs. With increasing encroachment of OSHA, employers need more reliable interpretations of safe work environments, work stations, and tools. Regarding the Americans with Disabilities Act, employers need more objective determinations of essential job functions and worker capabilities, so that hiring and placement decisions are defensibly nondiscriminatory and compliant with the legislation.[6,19,24,39,64,68]

Concerning litigation, statistically reliable supporting information has a distinct advantage over professional opinions, assumptions, or conjecture. For a more complete discussion of OSHA and ADA see Chapter 22.

Finally, in focusing on what the worker *should not* do, traditional medical assessments have often kept the injured worker on hold while costs accumulate. By focusing on what the worker *can* do, FCAs trigger a more proactive, goal oriented response to injury that is beneficial to the worker, employer, and the economy.

Vocational Rehabilitation Consultants

Vocational Rehabilitation Consultants (VRCs) play an important role in coordinating resources and people toward the goal of returning injured workers to gainful employment. The VRC facilitates communication and cooperation between the treating physician, therapist, employee, employer, insurer, attorney, and other members of the rehabilitation team.

Like a communication and information clearing house, VRCs must be in possession of accurate, reliable, timely information regarding the client's functional capabilities. They must know the realistic prospects for rehabilitation and reemployment, the presence of psychosocial factors, and the client's level of participation and commitment.

In addition to addressing psychosocial and motivational factors, some FCAs employ statistical means that determine whether the client is performing honestly. Formulas are used to detect malingering, exaggerating the injury, underperforming in the FCA out of fear of reinjury, or overperforming unsafely to disprove the injury.[36,55] This information can be invaluable to the VRC in avoiding misinterpretation of FCA results, allaying or confirming suspicion's, and developing proper rehabilitation goals.

Overall, with tighter controls over reimbursement to VRCs, there is an increasing need for ways to achieve case progression and closure more efficiently and effectively. FCAs are incorporating features and protocols to address this overall objective.

Attorneys

The attorney's job is to build as strong a case as possible against the opposing party, and to maximize the settlement amount. Statistically reliable supporting information wins over opinions, judgments, or guesswork in legal areas. When both parties have strong documentation, it becomes a question of whose information is more reliable. Where findings are in conflict, the FCA with the greater degree of statistical reliability and larger data base of validations will win. Analyzing improvements in capabilities, before and after rehabilitation, can also improve and refine treatment strategies.

Generally, a thousand validations *supporting* a finding will hold sway over 50 validations *disputing* that finding. A larger data base reduces doubt, strengthening the case for higher settlements.

Insurance Companies

In light of skyrocketing health care costs, increasing litigation,[32] tougher competition for policy holders, and the spectrum of more regulation, insurance companies are looking for ways to make premiums more competitive, while maintaining profitability. They are seeking measures that shorten the return to work cycle by streamlining or eliminating certain rehabilitation steps. They apply proven ways to restore a higher percentage of preinjury function, while lowering the rate of reinjury. They want to lower the incidence of fraudulent claims, reduce reserves, and keep the process out of litigation.

In response to these goals, FCAs are becoming better predictors of realistic treatment outcomes for the purpose of goal setting, program planning, and design.

Therapists

When the traditional medical model predominated, therapists played an important, yet subordinate role, to the physician's prescribed treatment program. As the need for more accurate determinations of returning workers' job capabilities increased, therapists were in an ideal position to assume this responsibility. Being experts in guiding rehabilitation after the acute care phase, it was a natural transition for therapists to pro-

vide more precise functional assessments. As functional considerations gained importance, therapists with functional assessment expertise were ideally situated to assume an expanding and influential role in what has become Industrial Therapy.

FCAs have been an important conduit to new areas of practice for therapists, they have also provided quantitative support for maintaining and expanding Therapists' involvement. By comparing FCAs to RTW outcomes, Industrial Therapists can provide quantitative support that Industrial Therapy components increase RTW percentages, reduce reinjury rates, and yield short and long term cost reductions.

Legislation

In the on-going effort to exercise increasing control over health care cost and potential waste or abuses, state and federal legislators are enacting a profusion of new laws. In effect these statutes require more objective determination of the patient's needs, and of the progress achieved by the health care services delivered. In many cases the legislation has established networks, coalitions, or alliances to oversee the practices of health care providers. Recent examples in Minnesota are Integrated Service Networks (ISNs) and Regulated All Payer Options (RAPOs).

Functional Capacity Assessment is well suited to providing the kind of objective defensible documenta-

FIGURE 13.1   The Functional Capacity Assessment has evolved out of the demand for objective, valid, and reliable data concerning an injured worker's safe capabilities. Physicians, employers, Vocational Rehabilitation Consultants, attorneys, insurance companies, Therapists, and legislatures are all influencing the evolution of FCAs.

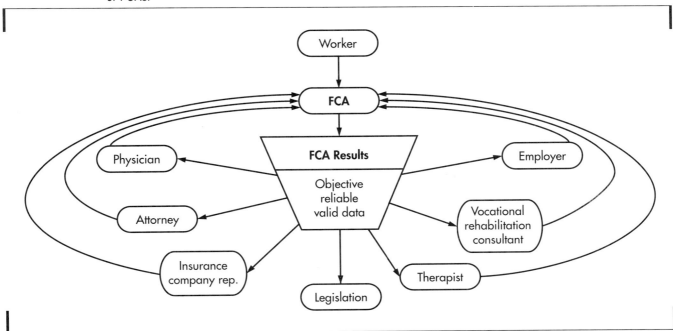

tion required to justify treatment procedures and substantiate reimbursement levels to these oversight organizations. FCAs are playing an expanding role in bringing non-discriminatory objectivity to job recruitment and placement decisions (Figure 13.1).[6,19,24,39,64,68]

The Needs Served By FCAs

The evolving influences of physicians, employers, rehabilitation counselors, insurers, attorneys, therapists, and lawmakers have collectively impacted FCAs to improve in the directions outlined in Box 13.2.

ASSESSMENT PRINCIPLES

As additional needs are recognized and the field of Industrial Therapy continues to evolve, there are a number of principles taking shape to which FCAs are adhering in order to fulfill the emerging requirements. To provide increasing levels of objectivity, validity, reliability, and predictability, the following principles governing FCA equipment and protocols are unfolding:

1. The assessment Therapist must be objective.
2. The equipment must be standardized.

BOX 13.2

Overall Needs
More objectivity and less judgment or prejudicial thinking
Greater validity in measuring what is desired to be measured
Greater reliability that the findings represent reality
Greater predictability that prognoses will hold true
Greater control over costs while maintaining quality

Placement Needs
More objective and accurate matching of workers' capabilities and essential job functions
More precise input into job modification requirements and options
Greater emphasis on what the healthy, disabled, or injured worker *can* do versus *should not* do

Prevention Needs
More accurate identification of each worker's safe capabilities, limits, and areas of risk
Better detection and input as to a worker's need for educational or conditioning programs
More reliable determination of safe work environments

Rehabilitation Needs
More reliable assessment of safe RTW time frames and capabilities

More timely information for planning and decision making
More reliable pre and post comparison for purposes of endorsing or modifying treatment components to streamline successful case progression and closure
More objective detection of manipulation, magnification, or malingering to confirm or allay suspicions
More dependable assessment of possible treatment outcomes

Treatment and Reimbursement Needs
Greater quantitative support for physicians' and therapists' treatment and recommendations
Greater quantitative support that treatment outcomes have not happened by chance or random occurrence

Legal and Regulatory Needs
More objective and accurate determination of essential job functions and workers' capabilities to perform them
More precise and defensible determination of reasonable accommodation options
More quantitatively supported legal positions versus opposing opinions
Deeper data base of outcome validations to win head-on-head data comparisons and ensure appropriate settlement amounts

3. The methodology must be consistent from test to test.
4. Information processing and reporting must be standardized.

Therapist Objectivity

For an FCA to meet the level of reliability, two different Therapists or Assessment Specialists testing the same patient, at the same point in time, should get the same results. Currently, FCA protocols differ in the degree to which the Therapist intervenes in the testing process and exercises judgment. Some approaches are based on the assumption that the Therapist's expertise and judgment are the only requirement in performing the assessment.

Other approaches seek to formalize and systemize the therapist's procedures as much as possible in order to reduce statistical variability caused by "tester error."

At whatever stage the Therapist is involved at present, market demand appears to be emphasizing increasing levels of statistical reliability.[37] Therapists interjecting opinions or subjective judgments in administering or recording tests create as much variability in the results as there is in the range of their subjectivity.

As a consequence, identical patients may test differently, or different patients may test identically. This not only weakens the reliability of normative data, it also risks inappropriate decisions when using the worker's test results for job placement, job modification, rehabilitation goals, plans, program design, and monitoring.

The therapist assumes greater liability when they interject opinions in obtaining or interpreting test results. In litigation proceedings, the Therapist who has used opinion in the FCA might have to defend professional credibility against a Physician's opinion or the client's word.

By incorporating more objectivity and statistical discipline into the assessment process, the Therapist's exposure is reduced, and his or her position is strengthened against other parties in any dispute that may arise.

Standardized Equipment

For the equipment to be considered reliable, a patient retested on the same equipment should generate same results. In addition, to be considered valid, the system should measure what it is purported to measure.

Equipment should be designed to accommodate a variety of hand position requirements. Different heights are required to accommodate standard lift activities, while other levels are required for special lifting, pushing and pulling, and other task activities.

Equipment must also be flexible to accommodate future test additions, modifications warranted by outcome studies, or changes in industrial requirements.

In the past, Therapists may have been comfortable making their own equipment or using slightly different equipment from one assessment to the other. Today, it is advisable to choose equipment that has already been proven reliable through a sizable database of outcome statistics, and to use this verified equipment in a consistent manner in all assessments thereafter. Otherwise, in a growing number of legal or reimbursement disputes, the FCA results and recommendations will lose out to more standardized and statistically supported protocols (Figure 13.2).

Consistent Methodology

Consistency in administering assessments is critical. Standardization is the basis for reliability, validity, and repeatability whether in equipment, instructions, analysis, or recommendations.[12,37] This is achieved more effectively if both the testing device and the protocol are safe, quick, and relatively easy to use.[45] Ideally, protocols should be written, verified wherever possible by outcome studies, and followed with acute consistency.

Instructions should be given in a clear, neutral, noninfluencing and nondemeaning manner. The completion point of each task should be determined objectively and in a consistent manner on each occasion. The information should be analyzed and reported objectively, using standardized methods and reporting

FIGURE 13.2 Standardized equipment, protocols, and training provide assessment consistency through repeatable, reliable, and valid data collection.

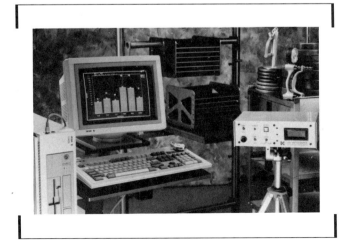

formats. All protocols must be in place and Assessment Specialists trained to assure accuracy and consistency of use.

Standardized Processing and Reporting

Assuming the issues of Therapist objectivity, equipment standardization, and methodology have been covered, the next important consideration is the method of processing the collected data. The Therapist may simply report the numbers at face value, temper them with experienced judgment, or process them through statistical functions. The trend clearly is to utilize various ways to apply science and statistics to the analysis of FCA information.[4]

By using final statistics to verify protocols and interrelate data, the relationships between FCA results and outcomes are becoming increasingly quantifiable and predictable. Reliance on judgment is being progressively reduced by the development of functions that yield statistically generated and supported conclusions.

Increasing quantification reduces the Therapist's exposure and provides stronger support for positions in legal or reimbursement disputes. Although there remains some resistance to the encroachment of science and technology, a growing number of Therapists are realizing the benefits of answering the demand for statistically supported assessment and treatment.

ASSESSMENT GUIDELINES

Keeping in mind the aforementioned general principles, it is possible to examine the application in those aspects of FCAs that are major determinants of whether results are objective, reliable, valid, and predictable. These critical aspects are:

- Instructing the client
- Determining the stopping point
- Demonstrating the tasks
- Translating the results to recommendations
- Determining validity of participation
- Verifying formulas
- Training assessment specialists

Instructions

The Therapist must give identical instructions on test components to all participants. Variations will render normative conclusions unreliable. If one individual is encouraged to terminate a task early and another encouraged to terminate it later, the basis for tying the data together is weakened. Without a consistent protocol for instruction, it is not clear what information is actually being gathered and normalized.

Each activity of the Assessment should have a specific instruction, dependent on how the data or information will be used. The Assessment Specialist should introduce all activities in a consistent manner. Different words can influence different results, so it is important to use the same instructions, word for word, with every assessment task.

The tone of voice and inflection must be neutral and nondemeaning, and body language should be controlled for consistency. The Assessment Specialist must be trained and given the responsibility to be consistent with each component across every evaluation.

It is also important to understand that consistency alone is only part of the equation. Otherwise, any instruction would suffice as long as it was used verbatim every time. Intuitively, there must be a particular set of words that surpasses all other options, in maximizing the validity and reliability of measurement. The superiority of one set of instructions over another can be established by relating assessment results to what the worker is actually able to do in the workplace.

Employing clearly defined, consistent instruction protocols, and diligent follow-up with clients in the work place, outcomes can be tracked to assess whether instructional protocols lead to accurate determinations.

Every vendor of FCA equipment and protocols has specific reasons why their particular instructions are most appropriate. The ideal way to evaluate instructions is through quantified outcome studies.[12] If one vendor uses judgment or logic to support their specific instructions, while another has statistically valid outcome studies, the outcome-verified instructions will be more useful in supporting recommendations.

A vendor without outcome verification will naturally argue that outcome verification is unnecessary, inappropriate, or unreliable. Where results are at issue, whether in court or in a reimbursement dispute, statistically reliable supporting information is more valid than opinions or judgments.

In the absence of follow-up verification through outcomes, the accuracy of the results involves subjective assumptions. This constitutes the same kind of return to work guesswork for which Therapists often criticize physicians.

In summary, regarding the manner of instructions, once drafted and verified through outcome studies, the Assessment Specialist must "do it the same way each time."

The Stopping Point

Since a Functional Capacity Assessment determines a person's limits, the protocol for determining the stopping point of each test is arguably the most important aspect of the assessment process. If the protocol artificially stops the client below the true capability that client may be wrongfully denied opportunities.

Similarly, the employer may unnecessarily incur expenses in work conditioning or job modification to correct a nonexistent deficit, if the protocol erroneously pushes the client beyond safe limits. That client may become injured in the assessment process, or be at risk in the workplace.

One can see lack of reliability in results, if one Assessment Specialist has the client stop when postured adaptations are first observed, while another stops the activity when the client suggests they discontinue. Clearly, no matter how the stopping point is determined, it should be consistent from one client to the other.

In determining when the client should stop, there are many instruction options:
- Stop when you can't do any more
- Stop when it starts to hurt
- Stop when you feel pain
- Stop when the pain gets so bad you cannot do any more
- Stop when you think you should stop
- Stop when you first start to feel anything
- Stop when I tell you to stop
- Stop after you have done as much as you possibly can

The importance of using a consistent method or instruction to standardize the stopping point is easy to realize. Choosing the best method, or instruction for reliability and validity is more difficult.

A precisely determined stopping point, in theory, would be the point at which the client is entering a level of risk. Currently, there is no infallible method for determining this exact point. There are two basic schools of thought on determining this pivotal judgment.

One supports the Therapist being in the best position to gather and process the information to determine the stopping point. The other (Park and Chaffin) supported by this author, holds that a system of sensors and central processor exists in the form of the client's central nervous system.[12,53] Receptors in the musculoskeletal system notify the central nervous system as to the degree of strain. This effectuates a safeguard against unsafe exertion or injury. All that is required is for the client to respond to and report the signals that the body is sending in order to determine the stopping point for themselves. Under this method, the Therapist must provide clear, consistent instructions to assist the client in reaching their own stopping point determination.

Whether the Therapist or the client determines the stopping point, each method affects reliability due to differences in how each Therapist or client receives and processes the information. The selection of one method over the other hinges on where the greater degree of variability exists.

Regarding variability in Therapists' judgment, studies have concluded that a significant amount of judgment involved in an FCA can lead to dramatically different findings.[67] As to the clients' ability to read their own body's signals, modern medicine has recently come around to the realization that the patient's input is among the most valuable information available in treatment or diagnosis.

Choosing the best method in selecting one vendor over another is something that each user of FCAs will ultimately have to decide for themselves. In reaching this decision, it is helpful to include the following considerations:

Outcome Statistics. These should be analyzed where available. They will help resolve which method or instruction yields the tightest relationship between assessment results and return to work outcomes.[12] When in doubt, go with the outcomes.

Therapist Exposure. When the Therapist decides the end point, they assume greater responsibility for the accuracy and the consequences. When the client makes the determination with the Therapist's instruction, the consequences are shared. In litigation, this reduces the extent to which the Therapist's position is pitted against client's word or a Physician's opinion.

The greatest exposure, is where the Therapist provides no direction regarding the end point of activity. The client may be an underachiever and choose to put forth very little effort, resulting in data that is far below their capability level. Or, the client may be an overworker and go so far as to reinjure themselves in the assessment, or on the job. The consequences are obvious.

In choosing a protocol, therefore, it is important to consider the implications in terms of Therapist exposure in legal or reimbursement disputes.

Therapist Expertise. Experienced Therapists conducting FCAs may be qualified to make accurate judgments as to the stopping point. The issue is the consistency from one assessment to another, and from one Therapist to the next. This very issue in many fields has given rise to more standardized methodologies to eliminate what is commonly referred to as "tester error." Standardizing a Functional Capacity Assessment system to avoid this, not only enhances validity, it also demands less expertise on the part of the administrator. When the FCA relies heavily on the Therapist's judgment calls, only the most experienced and highly paid Therapists are capable of conducting the FCAs. This may have implications for staff salaries, competitive billing rates, and reimbursability. In addition, when the most experienced Therapists must perform the FCAs, other practice needs get less of their attention.

Demonstration

Another important consideration is whether a demonstration of the activity should be provided before the client performs it. This decision needs to be made with each component of the assessment process. There are vendors of FCA equipment and protocols who argue for and against the Therapist demonstrating or intervening to modify the posture used by the client.

In any assessment, body mechanics are carefully monitored and documented. All assessment systems pay close attention to safety. For a growing number of assessment systems, however, "demonstration" does not equate with "safety," and is not always consistent with safety.

Those of us who advocate no demonstration[11,36,53] point out that the most accurate, reproducible findings are achieved by allowing the worker to use postures that are familiar and natural. Demonstrating or instructing the activity injects an artificial variable that overstates or understates the client's true capabilities. If the client uses the therapist-corrected body posture during a lift, the final level reached may be higher having used an "improved" posture.

It may also be lower if it is an unfamiliar posture, and the client's body has mechanically adjusted to a particular method. In either case, the Therapist's intervention creates greater variability in the determination of the client's true capabilities. Therapists often disagree on what the correct posture should be, which injects additional variability into the results[33,51,61] (Figures 13.3, *A, B, C*).

Although "safety" during the assessment is cited by some as the reason for postural demonstration, studies have shown that intervening to correct postures is not always safe.

The traditional concept for safe lifting (straight back/bent knees) is not the ideal posture for lifting some loads, and in some situations may be dangerous. Using the traditional lifting method for bulky loads can result in greater load moments on the lower back, place the quadriceps muscle at a severe mechanical disadvantage, and require greater expenditure of energy.[51]

Those who favor intervention believe that the client's capability should be assessed using only corrected postures. The inherent assumption is that since the correct posture has been demonstrated in the assessment, the client will use this posture upon return to work. Accordingly, the client's posture-directed assessment is assumed to be a more accurate expression of the client's true potential capabilities.

It is important to mention that even those of us who oppose demonstration for functional tasks, permit, and often require demonstration, if the activity is not a direct test of functional ability. One example would be in the use of dynamometers at various points throughout an assessment. To ensure consistency of performance, the Assessment Specialist may demonstrate the proper method of using the dynamometer so that variances in results are not a function of body or hand position[7,36,43,44,50,56,62] (Figures 13.4, *A, B, C*).

If demonstration or correction were to be provided for a functional task, another issue would arise as to when this intervention should take place. It is common that postures change as the load or the pain increases.[12,33,36,53]

Incorrect postures may be observed at the beginning of an assessment task, and may improve during the assessment without Therapist intervention. Alternatively, they may not appear until well into the task. Intervention comes at variable points during the assessment, bringing additional variability that could obscure the data.

Regarding the issue of the client's posture being corrected eventually, in some cases the musculoskeletal structure may be irreversibly adjusted toward the allegedly improper posture. In other cases, after postural instruction, the client may gradually revert to old habits. In either case, the recommendations based on Therapist-corrected postures may be inapplicable.

Safety should always be of primary concern, during the assessment and when the client returns to the work environment. During the assessment, postural concerns are mitigated by the fact that an incorrect posture of the client's choice does not necessarily make it an unsafe posture.[12,33,36,51,53,59]

In many cases, the client's musculoskeletal structure has adjusted to safely accommodate what may be judged as an "incorrect" posture. After the assessment, when the client resumes work, an overstatement of capability caused by postural adjustment during the FCA poses its own set of safety risks. As mentioned, even with in-depth education and training there is no guarantee the modified postures will be perpetuated.[15,46,53,57,58]

Liability issues must also be carefully weighed. Concerning injury during the assessment, while extreme postures may increase the risk of injury, modifying postures does not guarantee against it. And if an injury does occur during the assessment or upon return to work, the Therapist's exposure is greater, if the client was using the Therapist's choice of posture.

As to injury after the assessment, the increased variability caused by postural instruction increases the chance that recommended levels are overstated. This in turn increases the risk of injury upon return to work. Clients are more likely to allege inaccurate capabilities if the assessment posture used was not their own.

FIGURE 13.3 A,B,C   Postures that are corrected during an FCA may not transfer into the working environment, which affects assessment accuracy and Assessment Specialist liability.

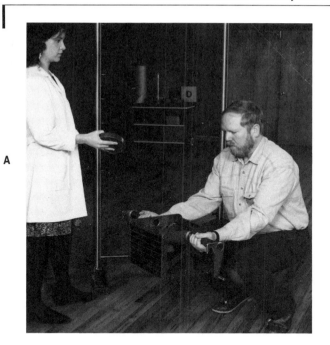
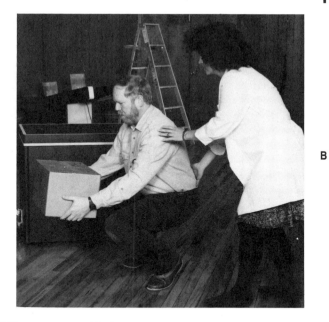
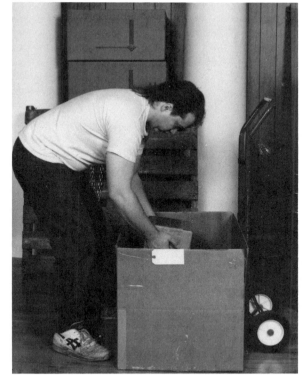

Allowing the client to use self selected postures during the assessment yields a more reliable translation to what will happen in the workplace. This approach also provides an opportunity for the Therapist to observe and note the postures that the client chooses to use. Observations may indicate the need for

FIGURE 13.4 **A,** Dynamometer reading 62 pounds; **B,** Dynamometer reading 73 pounds; **C,** Dynamometer reading 78 pounds. To ensure consistency of performance, the Assessment Specialist may demonstrate the proper method of using the dynamometer so that variances in results are not a function of body or hand position.

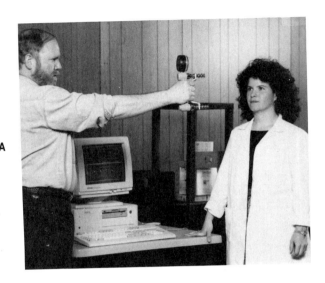
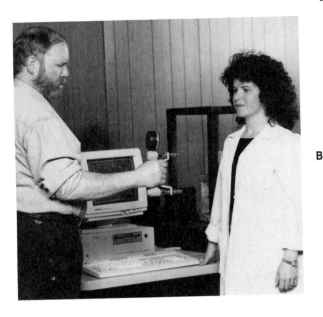
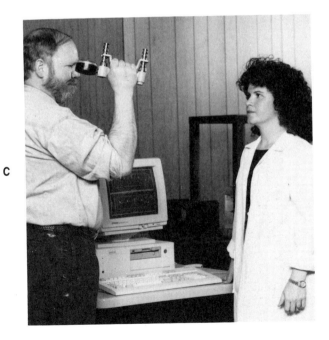

an education program or a strengthening exercise program. The duration of the Assessment allows for these postures of issue to be demonstrated frequently enough for the Therapist to determine the degree of this need.

In choosing the best method regarding instruction for posture, Therapists should carefully weigh the issues of objectivity, validity, reliability, predictability, safety, and liability. As time goes on, however, an increasing number of FCA protocols instruct against postural demonstration or intervention[11,36,41] in favor of standardization.

Translating the Results to Recommendations

The issues of processing all the information from an FCA, and deriving conclusions and recommendations that meet the need for objectivity, reliability, validity, and predictability are of growing importance.

FCA results can have substantial impact on the client's life. If the capabilities, as demonstrated in the FCA, do not meet the requirements of the job the client may be unable to work for a substantial period of time. If the FCA overstates capabilities, the worker may be at risk. It is important to make sure the recommendations are accurate and in the best long term interests of all parties involved.

The data collected from assessments consist of numbers that are the result of the clients actions during a given period of time, usually in a clinic. Lifting 60 pounds in a lab setting or clinic, however, may not translate directly to a 60 pound capability in the work force. There should be a process by which these numbers can be translated into return-to-work recommendations and the translation process itself must be accurate and reliable.[34,69]

The pressure to reduce time and expense has led this author and other therapists to seek ways to streamline assessment complexity and time frame. The basic goal of these efforts has been to identify the key measurements that predict return-to-work capabilities, and to develop algorithms that accurately translate this data into reliable recommendations. According to Webster's, an algorithm is a "predetermined set of instructions for solving a specific problem in a limited number of steps."[70]

Through much trial and error, validated by outcome statistics, therapists have been testing protocols and discovering algorithms that enable single-day four hour and even three hour assessments without sacrificing reliability. To accomplish this, the quantity and nature of musculoskeletal information formerly required has been streamlined, with some of it no longer applicable.

Musculoskeletal influences are now reflected in functional results and statistical correlations with outcomes. As the number of standardized case histories in data bases grows, and appropriate statistical analyses, FCAs are becoming increasingly efficient and reliable predictors of safe working levels and reduced risk of injury.[34,54]

Under some FCA systems, analysis requires the Therapist to apply judgment to the numbers. In this manner, when formulas are not available to translate raw data, the test activities have to be extended in frequency and duration in order to more closely replicate full work day demands. In most cases this requires extending the FCA beyond one day, and in some instances as many as six days.[61]

Without formulas, the analysis has to include more musculoskeletal testing in order to yield an accurate determination of the client's limits. In this manner, the assessment results can then be reported with more confidence.

Validity of Participation

Many employers, payors, providers, and people in general have been conditioned to be suspicious of injured workers. Although the percentages are lower than the perceptions, it is true that some injured workers exaggerate the symptoms to maximize settlement, or they attempt to artificially prolong the period of disability to avoid work. Understandably, the assessment results are more difficult to interpret if the client is misrepresenting, intentionally or unintentionally, true capabilities.

It is important, therefore, to make some determination of the client's forthrightness in performing assessment tasks.[25,52]

Statistical methods exist that enable quantitative, statistically reliable determinations. The results of all the client's individual FCA tests can be compared for internal consistency to detect whether the client is demonstrating true capabilities, underperforming, or overperforming.

This statistical validation is based upon the principle that a person's ability to perform one task is an indicator of the range of capability to perform another. For example, the amount that someone can lift correlates with how much they can push and pull. In addition, certain vital signs such as heart rate also respond normatively as a person approaches their exertion limits. By processing the results of thousands of FCAs, algorithms can be developed to establish the parameters within which measurements are internally consistent or inconsistent. These formulas can then be used to detect abnormalities in the results, and signal that a person is underperforming or overperforming in the assessment.[55]

Experienced therapists are able to detect some deception by observing kinesiological signals during the assessment process. FCA protocols predicated upon these judgment calls, stake their reliability on the assumption that all therapists will make these determinations with identical degrees of accuracy.

One vendor of FCA equipment and protocols has developed algorithms depicting the degree and nature of a client's consistency or inconsistency in performance levels. Those scale delineations are:[35,36,55]

1. *Valid participation,* which means the individual demonstrated full effort, and the results reflect safe capability levels.
2. *Invalid participation,* which means the individual consciously and intentionally demonstrated

less than full effort, and the results reflect less than full, safe capability levels.

3. *Conditionally valid participation,* which means the individual unintentionally demonstrated less than full effort, and the results reflect less than full, safe capability levels. However, the results do reflect the client's own perception of capability limits.[33]

4. *Conditionally invalid participation,* which means the individual demonstrated beyond what would be considered full, safe capability levels over long work periods. The results reflect more than recommended safe levels.

Such analyses can be instrumental in helping to resolve whether or not a particular injured worker is attempting to magnify or obscure the injury, or exploit the system. Figure 13.5 indicates the percentages in each category of participation found in a sample of 43,000 clients.

Whether validity of participation is determined by an algorithm or by the Therapist's judgment, it should never be taken lightly by the Therapist. Validity of participation can support or refute the assessment data presented by the client. While a great injustice is done when someone who is consciously manipulating for financial gain is not "caught," a greater injustice is done when someone who is giving full effort is not believed because of low capability levels. The importance of having an objective, reliable method of detection is paramount.

In selecting a vendor of equipment and protocols, it is helpful to weigh the following considerations:

Outcome Statistics.   Whether Therapist judgment or protocols are used, the methodology should be verified through outcome statistics in order to establish reliability. In the case of algorithms, if the determinations have not been validated, formulas may just standardize inaccurate information.

Therapist Exposure.   When making a judgment call regarding validity of participation, the Therapist assumes greater responsibility for accuracy and its consequences. In litigation, it may be the Therapist's judgment against the Physician's opinion or the client's word.

When the determination is based on a validated formula, the Therapist's position is considerably strengthened. The client's capabilities or honesty are not a function of the Therapist's judgments, but of statistically, reliable analyses of the data's internal consistency. If an individual is performing considerably below or above true capability, it will surface in the results of the algorithm process.

When algorithms are used, the Assessment Spe-

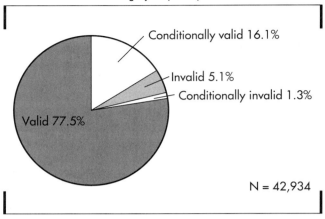

FIGURE 13.5   Percentages of FCA clients in each category of participation

Conditionally valid 16.1%

Invalid 5.1%

Conditionally invalid 1.3%

Valid 77.5%

N = 42,934

(From: Worker Data Bank, KEY Method, Minneapolis, 1994.)

cialist and the client share the responsibility. The Specialist has the responsibility to provide instructions while consistently and accurately documenting results. The client has the responsibility to be honest in their responses. The Therapist does not have to interject judgments that might inappropriately influence the client's results. In addition to limiting the Therapist's exposure in litigation, the client does not have to be "encouraged" to do more, so there is less chance of injury during the assessment.

Therapist Expertise.   It takes an experienced knowledgeable Therapist to make appropriate observations and judgments with consistent accuracy. A great deal of experience is not required to record key information and factor it into a validated formula. To determine the stopping point, relying on Therapist expertise only involves the more experienced and highly paid Therapists in the practice conducting the FCAs. The affect on salary structure, billing rates, reimbursability, and other priorities is obvious.

Verifying Formulas

Formulas can be established, based on protocols of the Assessment. It is imperative that the accuracy of these formulas be tested. If they are found to be inaccurate — if the client is not able to perform at the identified functional levels — the formulas must to be corrected and retested.

If subjects are initially able to perform at the originally tested level, they may also need to be tested at a higher level to ascertain whether the formula is too conservative. The formula would then result in sending clients out at levels considerably below full capability.

When establishing formulas to follow, it is important not to extrapolate from works of others, unless testing methods are identical. It is important to learn from others, but extrapolations can lead to inaccuracies and inappropriate use of published material. This underscores the need to carefully review the material from which formulas were derived.[17]

Training

To assure that all Assessment Specialists are performing the FCA in a consistent, standardized manner, policies and procedures must be written, a manual published, and a training process established. Assessment Specialists, whose role is to gather the most accurate data, should know and understand the purpose of the data and how it will be utilized. They must practice giving instructions in a consistent, non-influencing manner,[14] including tone of voice and body language. They must master the method of determining the stopping point of activities, whether on judgment or through instructing the client on making the determination.

Assessment Specialists must practice giving demonstration where appropriate and withholding it when necessary. They must learn to be observant, attentive, and accurately record critical observations and feedback from the client. To the extent these disciplines are thoroughly mastered, the results will be free of artificial variation caused by the Assessment Specialist.

ASSESSMENT PROCEDURES

Every commercially available FCA methodology is slightly different, and it is beyond the bounds of this chapter to describe each in detail. There are, however, procedures common to most, and a discussion of their nuances would be helpful.

Scheduling and Preparation

FCA referrals can originate from many sources, including the physicians and other therapists, companies, vocational rehabilitation consultants, attorneys, and insurance company representatives.[16]

To schedule the client, policies need to be established regarding who gets authorization for payment—the FCA center or the referring party. This may vary from one referral source to another.

Fees need to be communicated clearly including fees for a late show, no show, or late cancellation. It is fairly common that late cancellations and no shows generate 50% to 100% of the full fee.

Files must be prepared to collect scheduling information and medical history prior to the Assessment. It is helpful but not essential to review medical records prior to administering the FCA. In many cases, they are not provided in time.

The Assessment Specialist should remember that any notes left in the file can be subpoenaed and examined in legal proceedings. Any information that should not be disclosed to litigants or other parties should not be written down, even on stick-on notes.

Other information that will be helpful in preparation for the Assessment includes answers to questions referring to ability to read and write, primary language spoken, litigation status, date of injury, and primary diagnosis. This information enables clients to be assigned to Assessment Specialists based on areas of expertise. Clients with upper extremity diagnoses may be scheduled with the Occupational Therapist and back injured clients with the Physical Therapist.

Potential Problems To Anticipate

There are a number of problems that may arise during the course of the assessment. The list below provides a glimpse into some of the situations that should be anticipated, with strategies to resolve them being anticipated:

1. Clients showing up late.
2. Clients bringing family members with them—children that need caring for, or a spouse that takes a very active part in the influence over the client's participation.
3. Clients somewhat restricted by instructions from an attorney or family member.
4. Very emotional responses when results of Assessment are revealed if capabilities are much lower than expected.
5. Client's frustration or anger with the referral source or any of the members of the case.
6. Clients resisting participation through fear of reinjury.
7. Close to term pregnancies.
8. Referrals with diagnosis that are inappropriate for FCAs.
9. Physician's restrictions that are lower than client's full capability.
10. Referral sources pressing for their preconceived Validity Index.
11. Recommendations that will be withheld from the client by the referral source or case manager.
12. Clients making inappropriate advances to the Assessment Specialist.
13. Clients not finishing the Assessment.
14. Clients whose breath smells of alcohol.

Greeting the Client

When the client arrives for the FCA, they will have certain apprehensions and questions that must be addressed. Providing an orientation of the facility, the scheduled activities, and the purpose and use of the assessment is an important first step with each client. The Therapist should take care to:

1. Alleviate fears
2. Explain overall Assessment purpose and activities
3. Review expected duration
4. Introduce any overlying philosophies
5. Point out where refreshment sources are
6. Point out where bathrooms are

Components

Most FCA methodologies begin by gathering information on the client's medical history. Some also obtain psychosocial information through the MMPI (Minnesota Multiphasic Personality Inventory) or other psychological screens as an input into Validity determination and treatment recommendations.

This author incorporates musculoskeletal assessment into the functional components of the FCA. Formulas are then used to accurately correlate their results to outcomes. This is a departure from FCAs that still include a separate traditional musculoskeletal exam.

Most comprehensive FCAs include the physical activities specified by the U.S. Department of Labor. A list of 29 assessed activities is provided in Box 13.3. Descriptions of each are given in the text. The FCA may also include additional activities specified by job analyses.

Balancing

Definition: Maintaining functional balance in activities that might include toe walking, heel walking, braiding, and beam walking.
Assessment Decisions: Where to sequence within the assessment; which activities to assess; for what distance; whether to verbally instruct or physically demonstrate the activity, or both; to be compared with what other activities for consistency; to be the basis for what kinds of recommendations.

Bending and Stooping:

Definition: The ability to bend at the waist repetitively or in a static posture, in activities that might include the use of equipment.
Assessment Decisions: where to sequence within the assessment; whether to assess during another compo-

---

BOX 13.3

Physical Activities Typically Assessed in FCAs

Standard Assessed Functions

Balancing	Lifting above shoulder
Bending	Lifting desk to chair
Carrying	Lifting chair to floor
Cervical mobility	Pulling
Circuit board	Pushing
tolerance	Reaching
Climbing	Repetitive foot motion
Crawling	Simple grasping
Crouching	Sitting
Fastener board	Squatting
tolerance	Standing
Fine manipulation	Stooping
Firm grasping	Tool station work
Grip strength	tolerance
Keyboard tolerance	Walking
Kneeling	Work day tolerances

Other Functions*

Feeling	Seeing
Hearing	Talking

*If these are essential functions of the job, they can be assessed with specific supplemental tests of the traditional variety.

---

nent or assess separately, or both; whether to weight load activities, and with what progression; whether activity is static or repetitive, and with what duration or number of repetitions; whether to verbally instruct or physically demonstrate the activity, or both; to be compared with what other activities for postural consistency; to be the basis for what kinds of recommendations.

Carrying

Definition: Transporting an object while walking, with variations that might include unilateral carry on the right side, unilateral carry on the left side, bilateral carry, or a combination of the three.
Assessment Decisions: where to sequence within the assessment; which activities to assess; for what distance; heights of objects to be handled; where objects are to be picked up and set down; with what weight progressions and number of repetitions; whether to verbally instruct or physically demonstrate the activity,

or both; to be compared with what other postural changes, heart rates, and weight loads for consistency; to be the basis for what kinds of recommendations.

Cervical Mobility

Definition: Functional, real world movement mobility of head and neck, in activities that might include flexion, extension, and rotation, possibly including a variety of postures.

Assessment Decisions: Where to sequence within the assessment; which position activities to assess, whether to verbally instruct or physically demonstrate the activity, or both; to be compared with what other activities for consistency; to be the basis for what kinds of recommendations.

Circuit Board Tolerance

Definition: The length of time fine manipulation postures and forces using small tools can be tolerated continuously and throughout the overall work day, in activities that might include use of small screwdrivers, allen wrenches, tweezers, small files, needles, and other finger-held tools.

Assessment Decisions: Where to sequence within the assessment; which activities and tools to assess; performed with which hand or both hands; at what height of work activity; for what length of time; involving how many repetitions with each tool; within what range of acceptable postures; whether to verbally instruct or physically demonstrate the activity, or both; how to relate (through formulas or extrapolation) the test exercise to the real world job functions; to be compared with what other activities for consistency; to be the basis for what kinds of recommendations.

Climbing

Definition: Activities involving ladders or stairs, including ascending, descending, or both.

Assessment Decisions: Where to sequence within the assessment; which equipment to use; height and depth of steps; number of steps; whether to use railings or other assistive devices; whether to verbally instruct or physically demonstrate the activity, or both; to be compared with what other postural changes and heart rates for consistency; to be the basis for what kinds of recommendations.

Crawling

Definition: Moving on hands and knees, in activities that might include static posture, forward movement, backward movement, or all three.

Assessment Decisions: Where to sequence within the

assessment; which activities to assess; for what distances, or in the case of static, for what time period; how many repetitions; whether to verbally instruct or physically demonstrate the activity, or both; whether adaptations are acceptable or not; where and from what position the Assessment Specialist should observe; to be compared with what other activities for consistency; to be the basis for what kinds of recommendations.

Crouching

Definition: The ability to lower the body and lean over while maintaining a partial squat posture, in activities that might be static or repetitive while working on equipment as a distraction.

Assessment Decisions: Where to sequence within the assessment; which activities to assess; what posture to specify (feet flat, heels raised, feet parallel or staggered) or to accept if self selected; whether to assess during another component or assess separately, or both; whether activity is static or repetitive, and with what duration or number of repetitions; whether to verbally instruct or physically demonstrate the activity, or both; to be compared with what other activities for consistency; to be the basis for what kinds of recommendations.

Fastener Board Tolerance

Definition: The length of time fine manipulation, small assembly, finger and hand postures, and forces without tools can be tolerated continuously, throughout the overall work day, in activities that might include use of nuts and bolts, washers, twist caps and wires.

Assessment Decisions: Where to sequence within the assessment; which activities to assess; performed with which hand or both hands; at what height of work activity; for what length of time; involving how many repetitions of each activity; within what range of acceptable postures; whether to verbally instruct or physically demonstrate the activity, or both; how to relate (through formulas or extrapolation) the test exercise to the real world job functions; to be compared with what other activities for consistency; to be the basis for what kinds of recommendations.

Fine Manipulation and Simple Grasping

Definition: Using fingers with speed and dexterity, or squeezing lightly, with the right hand, left hand, or both, in activities that might include the use of nuts and bolts, small tools, wiring, or stringing.

Assessment Decisions: Where to sequence within the assessment; which activities to assess; performed with which hand or both hands; performed at what distance from the body; to be completed within what time frame, if fixed; involving how many repetitions; whether to accept assistive devices; whether posture is relevant or not; whether to include rest periods, and of what duration; whether to verbally instruct or physically demonstrate the activity, or both; how to relate (through formulas or extrapolation) the test exercise to the real world job functions; to be compared with what other activities for consistency; to be the basis for what kinds of recommendations.

Firm Grasping and Grip Strength

Definition: The ability and tolerance for squeezing firmly during a functional activity, or total grip strength, using the right hand, left hand, or both, in activities that might include multiple or single settings of a grip dynamometer or the use of tools.

Assessment Decisions: Where to sequence within the assessment; which activities to assess; performed with which hand or both hands; at what dynamometer settings; using which tools and whether they should be standardized; progressing torque, weights, and distances in what manner; how to observe performance changes that evidence cumulative trauma; whether to compute averages or analyze patterns; determination of normal performance; whether posture is relevant or not; whether to include rest periods, and of what duration; whether to verbally instruct or physically demonstrate the activity, or both; to be compared with what other activities involving what weights for consistency; how to relate (through formulas or extrapolation) the test exercise to the real world job functions; to be the basis for what kinds of recommendations.

Keyboard Tolerances

Definition: The length of time data entry postures can be tolerated continuously throughout the overall work day.

Assessment Decisions: Where to sequence within the assessment; whether to assign a fixed time frame or allow variable time frames based on completing activities; whether or not to measure keystroke pressure, speed, or accuracy; whether to test and retest for consistency; how to calculate consistency or inconsistency; whether certain postures should be corrected or not; to be compared with what other activities for consistency; to be the basis for what kinds of recommendations.

Kneeling

Definition: The ability to move while on knees or to perform work activities while on one or both knees, in activities that might include static posture, forward movement, backward movement, or all three.

Assessment Decisions: Where to sequence within the assessment; which activities to assess; for what distance, or in the case of static, what time period; how many repetitions getting in and out of the posture; whether to verbally instruct or physically demonstrate the activity, or both; whether adaptations are acceptable or not; to be compared with what other activities for consistency; to be the basis for what kinds of recommendations.

Lifting

Definition: The ability to raise and lower objects without assistive devices, in activities that might include lifting from desk height to above shoulder height, or lowering from desk to chair or chair to floor, with the right upper extremity only, left only, or bilateral.

Assessment Decisions: where to sequence within the assessment; which activities to assess; at what heights of origination and placement; of what size objects; with what weight progression and number of repetitions; whether to verbally instruct or physically demonstrate the activity, or both; whether adaptations or variations of posture are acceptable or not; to be compared with what other postural changes, heart rates, and weight loads for consistency; to be the basis for what kinds of recommendations.

Pushing and Pulling

Definition: Applying pressure or traction force to move objects, in activities that might involve pushing and pulling against static objects, or movable objects while standing in place or walking, using the right upper extremity only, left only, or bilateral.

Assessment Decisions: where to sequence within the assessment; which activities to assess; on what type of equipment; with hand placement at what heights; with what weight progression and number of repetitions; whether to verbally instruct or physically demonstrate the activity, or both; whether adaptations or variations of posture are acceptable or not; to be compared with what other postural changes, heart rates, and weight loads for consistency; to be the basis for what kinds of recommendations.

Reaching

Definition: Ability to extend arms up and out from the body with and without weight load, in activities that might include maintaining arms in an extended position, reaching to place objects at varying heights, or reaching to perform small tool activities such as wiring or nut and bolt assembly.

Assessment Decisions: Where to sequence within the assessment; which activities and tools to assess; whether to assign a fixed time frame or allow variable time frames based on completing activities; performed with which upper extremity or bilateral; at what height of work activity; for what length of time with each tool, and if dynamic, involving how many repetitions; whether to be weight loaded or not; to be compared with what other activities for consistency; to be the basis for what kinds of recommendations.

Repetitive Foot Motion

Definition: Ability and tolerance to use feet with speed and accuracy, in activities that might involve the use of pressure plates, foot pedals, bars, and resistance gauges, using the right, left, or both feet.

Assessment Decisions: Where to sequence within the assessment; which activities to assess; on what type of equipment; with foot placement at what heights; whether sequenced or performed in tandem; with what progression of resistance and number of repetitions; whether hip and knee motion are involved or feet isolated; whether to verbally instruct or physically demonstrate the activity, or both; to be compared with what other aspects within the same component and other components for consistency; to be the basis for what kinds of recommendations.

Sitting

Definition: The length of time continuous sitting, and overall work day sitting, can be tolerated.

Assessment Decisions: Where to sequence within the assessment; whether to assign a fixed time frame or allow variable time frames based on completing activities; choice of chair and other furniture; whether to verbally instruct or physically demonstrate the activity, or both; whether to include distractions and what kind; whether to include certain activities and exclude others; how to relate (through formulas or extrapolation) the test exercise to the real world job functions and work day tolerances; whether to test and retest for consistency; to be compared with what other activities for consistency; to be the basis for what kinds of recommendations.

Squatting

Definition: The ability to lower the body by flexing at the ankle, knee, and hip joints, in activities that might include the use of equipment to weight load the activity, or to facilitate it through distraction.

Assessment Decisions: Where to sequence within the assessment; which activities to assess; what posture to specify (feet flat, heels raised, feet parallel or staggered)

or to accept if self selected; whether or not to load with weights, and with what progression; whether to assess during another component or assess separately, or both; whether activity is static or repetitive, and with what duration or number of repetitions; whether to verbally instruct or physically demonstrate the activity, or both; to be compared with what other activities for consistency; to be the basis for what kinds of recommendations.

Standing

Definition: The length of time continuous standing and overall work day standing can be tolerated.

Assessment Decisions: Where to sequence within the assessment; whether to assign a fixed time frame or allow variable time frames based on completing activities; whether to verbally instruct or physically demonstrate the activity, or both; whether to include distractions and what kind; whether to include certain activities and exclude others; how to relate (through formulas or extrapolation) the test exercise to the real world job functions and work day tolerances; whether to test and retest for consistency; to be compared with what other activities for consistency; to be the basis for what kinds of recommendations.

Tool Station Work Tolerance

Definition: The length of time manipulation of tools with finger, hand, and arm postures and forces can be tolerated continuously, throughout the overall work day, in activities that might include use of wrenches, pliers, wire cutters, screwdrivers, sanding blocks, and clamps.

Assessment Decisions: Where to sequence within the assessment; which activities and tools to assess; performed with which hand or both hands; at what height of work activity; for what length of time; involving how many repetitions with each tool; within what range of acceptable postures; whether to verbally instruct or physically demonstrate the activity, or both; how to relate (through formulas or extrapolation) the test exercise to the real world job functions; to be compared with what other activities for consistency; to be the basis for what kinds of recommendations.

Walking

Definition: The length of time spent continuously ambulating over standard flat surfaces and during an overall work day, in activities that might include a walking circuit, treadmill, running track, or a combination.

Assessment Decisions: Where to sequence within the assessment; whether to assign a fixed time frame or allow variable time frames based on completing activities; whether to assign a speed or let the client self select; to be compared with what other activities for consistency; to be the basis for what kinds of recommendations.

Work Day Tolerance

Definition: The ability to tolerate a given number of hours of work in a day, based on a standard of eight hours per day.

Assessment Decisions: Where to sequence within the assessment; the test duration; which assessment components to include or exclude as part of the calculation; whether to weight components differently in the calculation, and what weights to assign to each; how to relate (through formulas or extrapolation) the test exercise to the real world recommended limit; how to verify accuracy through follow-up post-return to work.

Categories of Work

Relevant data is typically collected on three primary categories of work (Figures 13.6, *A, B, C*):

- Weighted activities
- Posture and tolerance
- Upper extremity activities

Weighted activities, generally considered materials handling, include three levels of lifting (above shoulder, desk to chair, and chair to floor), carrying (unilateral, bilateral, or both), and pushing and pulling (in-place or walking pushing and pulling against friction and inertia, plus the progressing of variable weights). Postures demonstrated by the client are recorded along with comments or responses to questions. These observations provide the information necessary to make recommendations on the need for body mechanics training. The results, along with heart rates, may also evidence a need for specific medical treatment or therapeutic exercise.

Posture and tolerance activities are sometimes assessed as independent components or included in a weighted materials handling activity. Many are covered in an instructed activity and checked for consistency in an uninstructed activity. Specific components include bending and stooping, squatting, multiple balance activities (toe walking, heel walking, braiding), kneeling, crawling, walking, standing tolerance, sitting tolerance, work hours per day tolerance, crouching, repetitive foot tolerance, reaching, climbing (ladders or stairs), and head and neck posture tolerances.

Tolerances are an area in which many assessment protocols are weak. This is especially true of the sitting and standing tolerances. In addition, there must be clear determinants for accuracy of all "occasional" and "frequent" activity categories. It must be remembered that tolerance categories need the same degree of accurate field testing that other FCA components require.

Upper extremity activities focus on assessing capabilities of clients with upper extremity injuries, especially those caused by repetitive motion. The components should include a variety of positions and relate to a basic category of work.

Measurements of an upper extremity assessment (UEA) should include most of the components previously identified in the categories of Weighted activities and Posture and tolerance. Those activities specific to upper extremities should also be assessed. Even if the upper extremity is the primary location of injury and activity, the rest of the body should also be assessed because it is important to know what the whole person can do. It is the whole body that returns to work.

The UEA should include circuit board and keyboard tolerances, small tool manipulation, normal tool manipulation, fine hand movements, and hand position tolerances. These tests are ideal for assessing skilled occupations requiring hand activities (Figure 13.7, *A, B, C*). Common occupations assessed include clerical and support staff, electrical and computer board assembly, dentistry, small parts assembly, and segments of the building trades industry.

Other measurements should be taken that assist in the determinations of tolerances, which can be used as consistency checks or input to the validity algorithms. These might include dynamometer readings[36,43,44,50,56] (resistance, grip, pinch), heart rates,[3,20,27,29,36,47] blood pressure, respiration rates,[25] oxygen consumption,[20,29,47] and other physiological signs (Figure 13.8).

Measurements Not To Include

Some measurements that are appropriate in a traditional clinical evaluation for an orthopedic case are not necessary, or applicable, to an FCA, which is work-related. Among these measurements are goniometric ROM and standard graded strength tests. This information is important in an FCA, and is measured differently—during functional components. In the FCA environment it is the work-related functional capabilities, not the clinical status, that is relevant. It would not be important that the arm cannot extend the full 180 degrees, missing 30° range, if the person is able to perform the required job functions.

The same principle applies for strength grades. It is necessary to test strength, but it is not necessary in an FCA to give specific muscle groups 3s, 4s, or 5s as grades. The muscle strength testing occurs in a functional measurement process. Weakened muscles will be expressed in terms of work-related functional limitations.

Some Therapists find it difficult to omit traditional range of motion and strength measurement techniques. It is important to remember that ROM and strength *are* being measured during the FCA, but from

FIGURE 13.6 A, B, C   The data collected during a Functional Capacity Assessment should reflect the primary work categories of weighted activities, postural categories and tolerances, and capabilities of the upper extremity injuries.

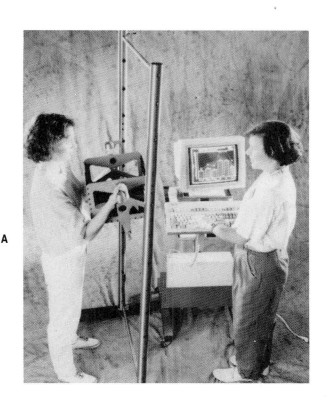

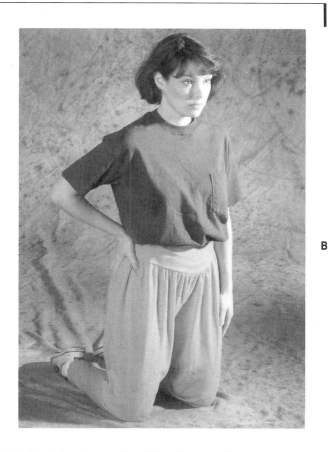

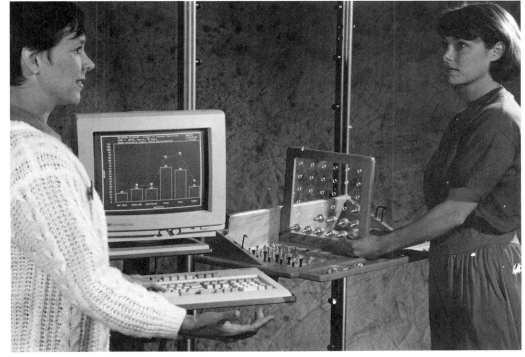

FIGURE 13.7 A, B, C   Upper extremity assessment tools enable determinations of capabilities and tolerances regarding skilled hand activities.

A

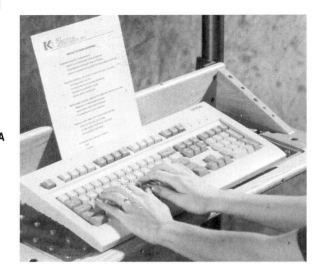

B

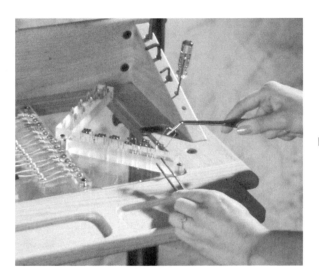

C

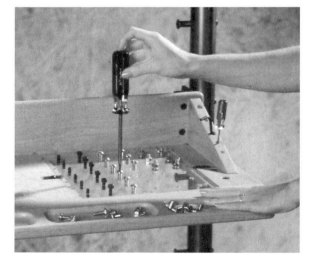

a dynamic, work-like, functional standpoint, rather than on a goniometric or individualized basis.

Including traditional clinical evaluations in the FCA process would in most cases constitute duplicating previous testing and measuring. This may be seen by paying parties as duplication of services. With the advent of EEOC and most recently the Americans with Disabilities Act, traditional ROM and strength tests in FCAs do not fulfill the functional requirements.[6,18,19,25,39,64]

Sequencing

It is important that the client be able to complete the entire assessment in the time frame designated. It is

also important to sequence activities allowing recovery from taxing movements, and ensure that fatigue does not artificially depress performance. Cardiovascular safety should be uppermost in the Therapist's mind at all times.

The Assessment Specialist should sequence the components based on the function being tested and the severity of injury. A taxing activity should be followed by another that is less taxing, this is called an interspacer. Interspacers are equally important parts of the Assessment and will allow a short relief period for the client. It is through this process that even though an individual may have only a two to three hour work day capacity, they will be able to complete the FCA.

FIGURE 13.8   Resistance, Grip, and Pinch Dynamometers enable additional measurements to be taken during an FCA to assist in tolerance and consistency determinations or as part of a validity algorithm.

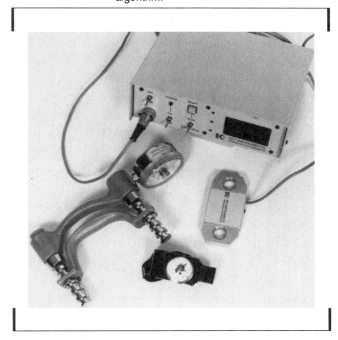

Reporting

FCA reports should clearly and concisely communicate important information to the users, including employers, insurance claims representatives, attorneys, judges, and vocational rehabilitation specialists. To accomplish this, reports should be written in users' language, with medical jargon minimized or eliminated.

Therapists must be mindful that many of the terms commonly used in therapy are not understood by FCA users. Such words as *pronation, supination, dorsiflexion, plantarflexion,* and anatomical terms such as *latissimus dorsi* should be expressed in lay person's terminology.

For example, rather than saying, "pronation," the report would say "palm down position." Unless comprehensible, important information in the report may be misinterpreted or misused, and the Therapist may have to spend an inordinate amount of time helping users interpret the report.

The Therapist or Assessment Specialist will have fewer depositions and court appearances if the readers can understand the report without interpretation by an expert witness.

Communication is also enhanced when the Assessment Specialist captures data that is a clear nonjudgmental portrayal of what occurred during the Assessment. This includes results of weighted activities, reports and behaviors during the progression up to and including termination. Without acute collection of data, accurate and appropriate reporting and recommendations cannot exist, and critical decisions will be difficult to make.

The Assessment Specialist must also remain objective in reporting results, taking care not to add their perceptions or subjective interpretations. The recorded statement "client rubbed low back because of pain," interjects the Therapist's conclusion as to why the rubbing took place. The Assessment findings should stand on their own without requiring subjective opinions.

It is helpful for all parties receiving the report, if there is a visual display of the major highlights of results. Figure 13.9 illustrates the most often requested information.[71]

Another way to present the results of an FCA for easy comprehension by industry is to match the categories in a table format as in Figure 13.10. This provides an immediate summary comparison of employee capabilities to job requirements.

It is common to report the candidate's results in terms of Physical Demand Levels (PDLs) specified by the U.S. Department of Labor. These results are often reported or described by statements such as "client's carrying capability measured to be 42 lbs, which is in the medium classification of the physical demand levels as published by the U.S. Department of Labor."

Completing The Visit

Upon completion of the assessment, if appropriate, the results should be briefly reviewed with the client. The importance of working on body mechanics may be discussed at this time. The client should also be reminded of who will be getting copies of the report and when.

It is protocol at the author's facility that clients are interviewed after the assessment and asked to sign a statement regarding whether they feel the weights achieved, repetitions, and other demands were at safe levels, unsafe levels, or "don't know."

Clients and referral sources should be asked to fill out a confidential customer satisfaction survey. It is important to become aware of any problems or potential problems so they can be addressed early and expeditiously.

STAFFING FOR FCAs

Staffing requirements to administer FCAs can be influenced by the protocols being used, the client mix, and the funds available for staffing.

FIGURE 13.9   Injured worker FCA results compared to job requirements relative to data bank norms.

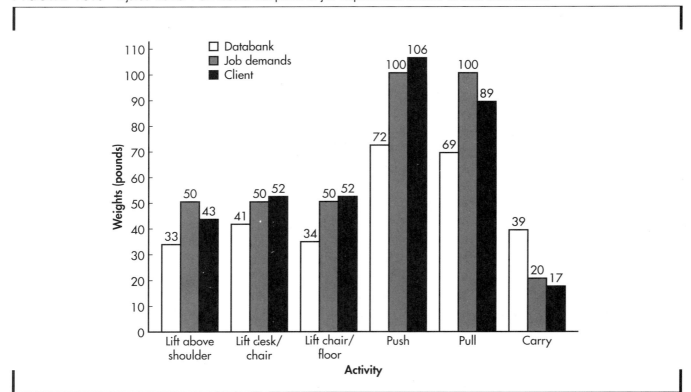

Protocol Considerations

Where protocols require the Assessment Specialist to make independent, clinically complex, kinesiological, and psychological decisions, a Physical Therapist or Occupational Therapist will be required to administer the assessment.

If the Assessment Specialist is not required to identify such detail as naming specific muscles involved, and if the Specialist has algorithms to assist in making final determinations, it is not necessary that a PT or OT administer the Assessment.

Occupational and Physical Therapist Assistants, Exercise Physiologists, Athletic Trainers and Kinesiologists can be trained as Assessment Specialists and fulfill all the requirements, assuming protocols are standardized and validated through outcome statistics.

Particularly unusual or atypical cases could be referred to experienced Therapists for assessment administration and consultation. Less experienced Assessment Specialists can be taught to recognize where postural issues require consultation with a more experienced Therapist. In such cases, the Therapist may determine that education or treatment should be initiated.

Although it is acceptable to have individuals who are not PTs or OTs being trained as Assessment Specialists, the final decision must be based on a number of additional considerations; such as reimbursement, state practice regulations, and the criteria required for credentialing.

Some Industrial Therapists are reluctant to have their assistants receive training or to bring others in to administer the assessments, because of fear of others infringing on the areas of care that "belong to Physical Therapy." Mitigating against this attitude is the fact that there is a shortage of Therapists and a growing number of needs that require the attention of experienced Therapists more so than FCAs.[13,42,48,49]

Combined with the continuing increase in salaries and the decrease in reimbursement, it behooves Therapists to organize the duties in the department to allow the lower salaried individuals to assume as much responsibility as is appropriate, and still maintain high quality, effective care. A note of caution, it is rare that someone calls themselves a Physical Therapist or Occupational Therapist when they are not actually credentialed. It is not so rare in some other fields of expertise. Verifying the accuracy of credentials is necessary.

FIGURE 13.10 Individual employee's capabilities compared to job requirements.

Essential functions & physical job requirements overview

Name: John E. Doe — Date of assessment: 03/14/94
Job title: Materials Packager — DOT code: 923
Validity determination: Valid — SIC code: 4783
Job information source: Risk Safety Manager
Referral source: Jane E. Smith, CRC

Activity	Client capabilities	Phys. job requirements
Work Day	8 hours	7 hours
Sit – (EF)	7 to 8 hours @ 60 minute durations, regular breaks	7 hours @ 60 minute durations, regular breaks
Stand – (EF)	5 hours @ 45 minute durations, regular breaks	5 hours @ 60 minute durations, regular breaks
Walk – (EF)	2 to 3 hours @ fequent, moderate distances	2 hours @ frequent, long distances

Activity	N	Occ	Freq	Cont	N/EF	Occ	Freq	Cont
Bend/stoop		X			N			
Squat			X		EF	X		
Stairs			X		EF		X	
Crawl		X			N			
Crouch		X			EF	X		
Kneel			X		EF	X		
Balance		X			EF	X		
Above shoulder – right								
Above shoulder – left								
Above shoulder – bilat.		43.4	34.6			50	25	
Desk / chair – right					EF			
Desk / chair – left					EF			
Desk / chair – bilat.		52.8	25.8		EF	50	25	
Chair / floor – right								
Chair / floor – left								
Chair / floor – bilat.		52.8	34.6			50	25	
Push		106.3	86.3		EF	100	50	
Pull		89.1	54.1		EF	100	50	
Carry – right		17.0	17.0		EF	20	10	
Carry – left		17.0	17.0		EF	20	10	
Foot – right			X		N			
Foot – left			X		N			
Hand – simp. grasp right		X			EF	X		
Hand – simp. grasp left			X		EF	X		
Hand – firm grasp right		X			EF	X		
Hand – firm grasp left			X		EF	X		
Hand – fine manip. right			X		N			
Hand – fine manip. left		X			N			
Head / neck - static		X			N			
Head / neck - flexion			X		N			
Head / neck - rotation			X		N			

OCC = 0 to 2.5 hrs. (1 – 33%)
Freq = 2.5 to 5.5 hrs. (34 – 66%)
Cont = over 5.5 hrs (67 – 100%)

'N' = Not at all
'EF' = Essential function
All weights listed are in pounds.

Client Mix

Another consideration in staffing for FCAs is what type of clients will be expected. If the referral base is such that many of the clients are in third and fourth surgeries and litigation is imminent, the selection of staff would be different from on-site Assessments for an industry that includes an operating therapy department.

This holds true in considering the employees' work history, style of person, and credentials.

ADDITIONAL CONSIDERATIONS

Treatment Pathways

The FCA results in conjunction with the Job Analysis can be used to establish the basis for the treatment plan. Using these inputs, a number of treatment pathways are possible. Some examples of options are as follows:

1. The person meets job requirements and returns to work.
2. The person meets job requirements but has capability levels considerably below average for the specific age and gender. Returns to work with recommendation to participate in a conditioning program to expand opportunities for the future.
3. The person does not meet job requirements. Poor posture is one of the major limiting issues. Individual is enrolled in body mechanics education, with the possible addition of Work Conditioning if body mechanics alone will not sufficiently raise capabilities to meet the job demands.
4. The person does not meet job requirements and tests out as Conditionally Valid on the Validity Index. The worker is underperforming, but not intentionally or consciously. The person is enrolled in Work Hardening with specific focus to changing the influences, psychosocial, or otherwise, that resulted in the Conditionally Valid on the Validity Index, while also increasing the physical capabilities.
5. The person does not meet job requirements and tests out as Invalid on the Validity Index. The person is called to a meeting where three options are offered:
   a. Client to undergo another FCA with instructions to show full effort this time.
   b. Employer to identify job options and offer job at levels of database averages for clients of similar age, gender, injury and occupation profile.
   c. Insurer to begin the process of reducing or terminating Workers' Compensation benefits.
6. The person does not meet job requirements and is significantly limited in some areas. The person is admitted to Work Conditioning. Simultaneously, job modification actions are initiated with employer.

These pathways are diagrammed in Figure 13.11. As can be seen by the options, the common factor is that FCA results are compared to the job requirements. The primary reason for administering an FCA is to identify capabilities for return to work. In order to do this, job requirements must be known. However, it is not necessary for the Assessment Specialist to know these requirements before administering the FCA. In many cases, the party requesting the FCA is thoroughly familiar with the job requirements and proficient in appropriately applying the FCA results.

There are situations in which a particular job has not been specified for the client. In such instances, the assessment is made to adjudicate insurance or legal issues, long term disability, and personal injury.

Cost of Offering FCAs

There are a number of factors that should be considered when reviewing the investment in providing FCAs. The initial consideration is the start-up cost of equipment, system components, and training. The second, which is of equal or greater importance, and is often overlooked in the purchase decision, is the ongoing cost of administering the FCAs.

The ongoing costs must be observed in combination with the start-up costs, to have a complete picture of the long term ramifications of each option. Many of these issues are illustrated in Table 13.1 on page 248.

Ongoing costs that are incurred, but sometimes overlooked when developing *pro forma* Return on Investment (ROI) calculations, may include annual license fees and maintenance, the length of time to perform the Assessment, and the length of time to prepare the report.

Excess hours that are not billable may be the most costly part of the total long term costs.

Assumptions included in Table 13.1 are as follows:

1. Assessments A and B require administration by PT or OT.
2. Assessment A's findings are not entered into the computer during the assessment, whereas B's and C's are.
3. Additional support staff time is required to prepare the report for assessment A, but for

FIGURE 13.11 Post FCA Pathways

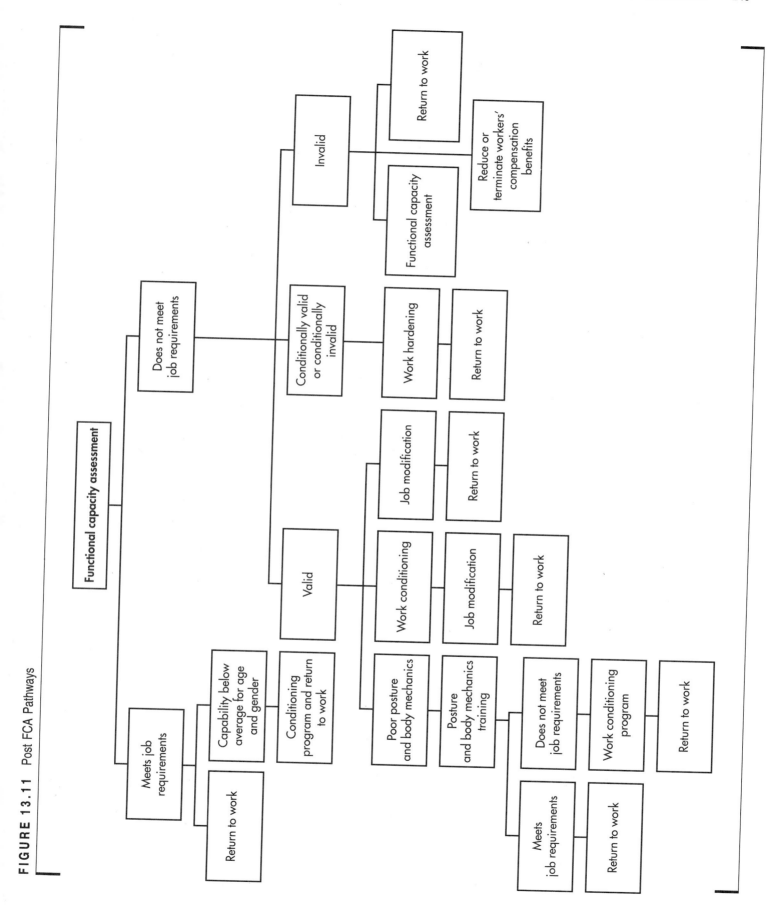

TABLE 13.1 Comparative Costs of Administering FCAs

	FCA System A	FCA System B	FCA System C

Point 1
Assessment hours:
  Therapist (PT or OT)
  Exercise physiologist
	5.00
	—
		4.00
		—
			—
			4.00

Point 2
Report and paperwork hours:
  Therapist (PT or OT)
  PTA, COTA, EP, ATC, or KIN
	2.00
	—
		.25
		—
			—
			.25

Point 3 Total hours:	7.00	4.25	4.25
Point 4 Assessment reimbursement:	$ 600	$ 600	$ 600
Point 5 Reimbursement per hour	$ 86	$ 141	$ 141
Point 6 Maximum number of assessments per month on one station	21	42	42

Point 7
Maximum revenue:
  Monthly
  Annually
	$ 12,600
	$ 151,000
		$ 25,200
		$ 302,400
			$ 25,200
			$ 302,400

Point 8
Salary plus 20% burden:
  Therapist
  Exercise Physiologist
	$ 54,000	$ 54,000	
			$ 30,000

Point 9
Average traditional
revenue per hour:
  Therapist
  PTA, COTA, EP, ATC, or KIN
	$ 100
	—
		$ 100
		—
			—
			$ 50

Point 10 Foregone treatment rev: (avg. rev. × total hrs.)	$(700)	$(425)	$(213)
Point 11 Gained (lost) revenue: (assess. rev.-treat. rev.)	$ (100)	$ 375	$ 587

ease of comparison, this extra time is not included.

4. Assessments B and C do not require additional support staff time to prepare their reports.

Calculating Therapist time requirements should include not only the length of the Assessment, but the entire process to administer it, analyze and write up the results, produce, and present the report (points 1,2, and 3 in Table 13.1). The salary overhead of the Assessment Specialist and support staff must be included (point 8 in Table 13.1).

The opportunity costs of the time the Therapist spends from preparation to completion must be considered. What fees would the Therapist have generated providing traditional services (points 9 and 10 in Table 13.1)? Moreover, what fees could be generated from additional assessments if the time required before and after the assessment could be condensed?

When considering the hours it takes to administer the assessment and produce the report, it is clear in reviewing points 3, 4, and 5 on Table 13.1, that the billing and reimbursement per hour is significantly different. Assessments B and C produce 64% greater revenue per hour than Assessment A.

In addition to the reimbursement, examine the availability of the equipment for full utilization. Points 6 and 7 illustrate that Assessments B and C have twice the full utilization revenue potential of Assessment A. Assessments that enable the use of qualified, well-trained staff at the PTA and COTA levels yield additional advantages in ROI, as illustrated by points 7 and 8.

> *The bottom line is that Assessment C, which can generate a $302,400 annual revenue with a $30,000 employee, nets $272,400. Assessment B nets $248,400 and Assessment A only $97,000.*

As the ROI considerations become more detailed, it is important to compare the assessment revenue with the revenue that the Therapist could have generated in traditional treatment. With reference to points 4, 9, 10, and 11, if the PT or OT can generate fees of $100 per hour in traditional treatment, the 7-hour Assessment A that pays $600 represents a $100 loss over traditional treatment earning potential. Assessment B, which takes less time, and Assessment C which saves both time and salary expense generate significant gains versus traditional services.

The point of this illustration is that FCA systems should be compared on the basis of total hours, not just assessment hours, and that the revenue the assessment personnel could generate in other activities should be calculated.

Other considerations in selecting an FCA system may include the level of support the manufacturer promises and their track record in providing it. Are they financially sound and sufficiently staffed to ensure long term support? Do they provide annual educational conferences to maintain state-of-the-art use of their product? Do they have the means to provide supporting data for litigation proceedings?

One of the most important components of support can be the library of outcome studies, and in some cases, the database maintained by the manufacturer. It is important to ascertain if these resources are available, and whether they are relevant for the purpose of recommendations, treatment, reimbursement, and marketing to new prospects.

The protocols and statistical disciplines need to be tight enough to render the information reliable. As employers, payors, and attorneys become increasingly FCA literate, proper science will provide market share and fee leverage.

Mobile FCAs

Mobility of assessments is becoming more important as the Industrial Therapist discovers the competitive

advantages of performing FCAs at locations convenient to the employer and client. Mobile equipment allows the Assessment Specialist to administer the FCA in the physician's office, the employer's office, the rehabilitation counselor's office, or even in the client's home. In addition to the convenience, mobile options offer immediate report generation that can be reviewed on-site for proper action (Figure 13.12).

Equipment that quickly assembles and disassembles is of critical importance. Portability in the trunk of an average sized car would be an additional plus, and assuring that all mobile units are built to the same dimensions as the stationary ones, with which the same database is shared.

Another alternative is to affix an Assessment Station to the inside of a van. This provides the mobility without requiring assembly and disassembly. This more convenient alternative is, of course, more expensive due to the cost of the van.

Reimbursement

Reimbursement is a major consideration. It is important to research the market to identify the going rates for FCAs. Fees generally range from $500 to $750 per

FIGURE 13.12 Mobile assessment equipment allows the Assessment Specialist to increase their service area and gain competitive advantages.

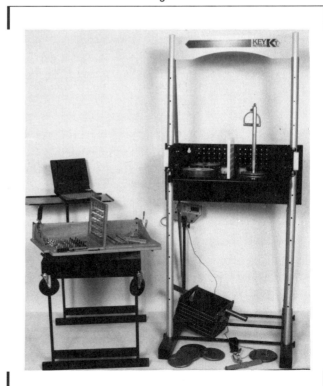

assessment, depending on the market, competitive climate, and nature of industries involved. FCAs may be included in a coding or fee schedule, supported by state regulations. Such schedules may, or may not, apply to self-insured businesses.

There are many levels of reimbursement that the creative therapist will consider and attempt to tap. If the published reimbursement is less than what is identified as fair and equitable, there are avenues for establishing special categories for a specific kind of assessment with separate reimbursement schedules.

Another significant trend is that more therapy organizations are generating business directly from industry, especially self-insured companies. As this continues, industry is becoming more educated as to quality differences that warrant commensurate fees. A factor in justifying value-added fees is the Therapist's ability to deliver measurable outcomes for the corporation or business.

Data Collection and Use

Given the increasing focus on outcomes to validate treatment procedures,[22,28,67,69] it is of growing necessity to build a database of FCA results. Reports can then be compiled from this database to support decisions to continue, discontinue, or modify treatment, particularly when decisions are being questioned. Data runs can also be beneficial in litigation cases and in marketing.

The benefits of data profiles and usages are illustrated in the following case histories.

Case A

A back injured male truck driver has demonstrated very little progress in Work Hardening for the past two weeks. FCA results identified client as a valid participator. Should treatment continue? Will this person actually get significantly better?

A data run was pulled to compare the client's attained capability levels with those of others of same age, gender, injury type, and occupation. In these comparisons, it was found that this client's rehabilitated capabilities far exceeded those of other rehabilitated workers with the same selection criteria. Rehabilitation, therefore, had reached a normatively acceptable level.

A data run of uninjured males in the same age group indicated that the client's capabilities were still below normative uninjured levels, but not significantly so. This uninjured profile became the goal of further conditioning efforts.

Based on this information, the client was given a home exercise program to follow for the residual progress. This was a cost-saving alternative to further treatment.

Without these data runs, Therapists may have continued expensive Work Hardening or closed the case without a return to work outcome. The use of data runs enabled Therapists to choose the most beneficial and reimbursable course of action for the client.

Case B

Another back injured client has met the job requirements, but is continuing to make progress in Work Hardening. FCA results identified client as a valid participator. Should this client's treatment continue?

A data run to compare this client with a similarly-profiled injured population indicated that although this client's rehabilitated capabilities met the job requirements, they were still below normative levels for injured workers. This information was used to demonstrate to the insurance company that there would be a good chance this worker could perform closer to norms, if rehabilitation or Work Hardening was continued for a specified period of time.

Without this data run, the worker may have been denied the opportunity to perform at higher levels, or the employer or insurer may have paid an early unnecessary settlement cost.

Case C

Therapists used analyses from a data base of FCA results to market injury prevention and other services to a large healthcare provider. The data runs served to focus the discussion on several areas in which the provider could see the benefits of the Therapists and their expertise.

A statistical analysis of 366 injured healthcare workers uncovered the fact that injuries in these occupations were more a function of years on the job than of age or gender.[38] Females, regardless of age, developed their injuries at an average of 8.2 years on the job, whereas males, also regardless of age, averaged 8.9 years. The provider instantly recognized the value of this information in ruling out age and gender as contributing factors to the incidence of injuries.

The provider was further enlightened by a breakout of 1,829 healthcare workers' validity of participation in FCAs as opposed to the general worker population (Figure 13.13).[71] This information reassured the provider that quite likely, only a small percentage of their injured workers were misrepresenting their condition or capabilities, and no more so than any other category of workers. It also demonstrated that they could expect about 25% of injury cases to be problematic.

The Therapists then presented a breakout of the typical healthcare workers' specific areas of injuries.

FIGURE 13.13   Validity of participation in FCAs.

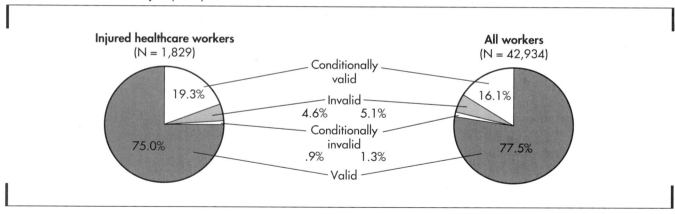

Injured healthcare workers
(N = 1,829)

19.3%

75.0%

Conditionally valid

Invalid
4.6%   5.1%

Conditionally invalid
.9%   1.3%

Valid

All workers
(N = 42,934)

16.1%

77.5%

Figure 13.14 indicates that 82% of healthcare worker injuries are spinal.[71] This established a base around which to discuss the provider's own injury and lost time history.

Figure 13.15 delves into the issue further by indicating the types of back injuries incurred by the sample of 1,829 healthcare workers.[71] The provider was eager to analyze this information based on injured employee experience, anticipating significant variances might lead to the discovery of causes.

Finally, the Therapists presented a comparison of uninjured and injured healthcare workers in terms of their assessed capabilities (Figure 13.16, page 252).[71] The uninjured workers underwent Job Placement Assessments and the injured workers were administered FCA's. These benchmarks provided a framework of comparison in discussing the provider's work force experience.

The preceding examples in Case C illustrate how the FCA data base can be used to initiate problem

FIGURE 13.14   Healthcare workers' injury profile.

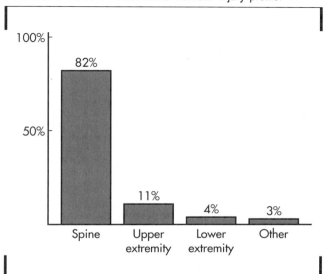

analysis discussions with companies in need of Industrial Therapy services. This is an effective first step in forming a consulting service relationship. Analyses from the data base serve to spark the prospect's interest, while enhancing the Therapist's recognized knowledge and credibility.

Case D

An injured worker was detected to be putting forth an invalid level of participation in an FCA. Data runs that compared this client's FCA results to norms for other injured workers and other invalid participators resulted in a negotiated settlement between the insurance company and worker that was 90% below the reserve that had been established.

To review, a determination of "invalid" participation is when the client has consciously demonstrated less than their full capability level. How much less is indicated in Figure 13.17 on page 252, which compares the client's results with norms of 1,372 injured healthcare workers found to be "valid" participators.[71] The comparison indicates the degree to which the client is underperforming relative to the norms.

The client's results were also compared to other invalid participators as displayed in Figure 13.18 on

FIGURE 13.15   Distribution of Healthcare Worker Back Injury Types.

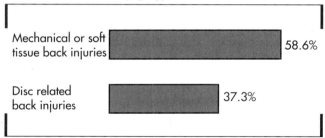

Mechanical or soft tissue back injuries   58.6%

Disc related back injuries   37.3%

FIGURE 13.16   Comparison of uninjured and injured healthcare workers in terms of their assessed capabilities.

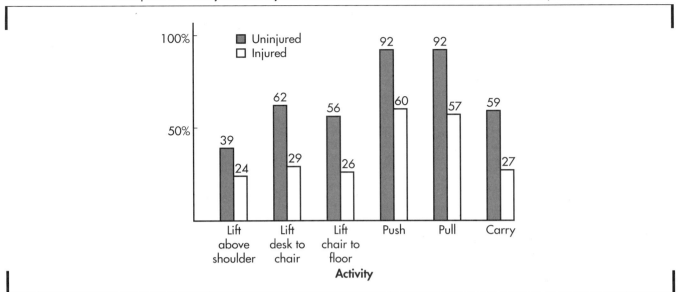

page 253.[71] The stark similarities were instrumental in arriving at a settlement that was 90% below the known reserve amount of $50,000. The client accepted and the case was closed.

This case accentuates the need for Therapists to expand their roles beyond simply delivering the assessment results, to becoming a problem solver. Particularly with the 25% of cases that are not valid participators,

FIGURE 13.17   Comparison of data bank norms of injured healthcare workers to client's results (invalid index rating).

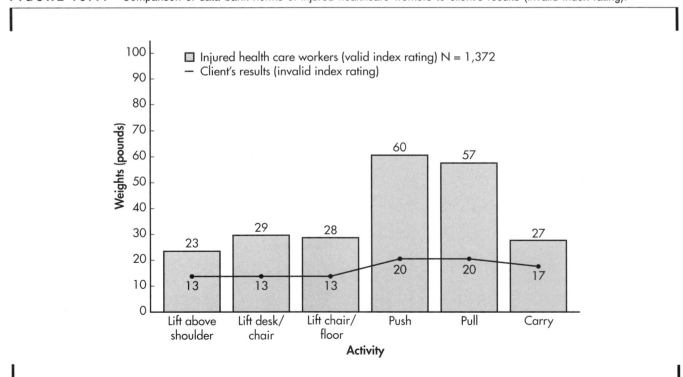

FIGURE 13.18 Comparison of injured healthcare workers (invalid rating) to client (invalid index rating).

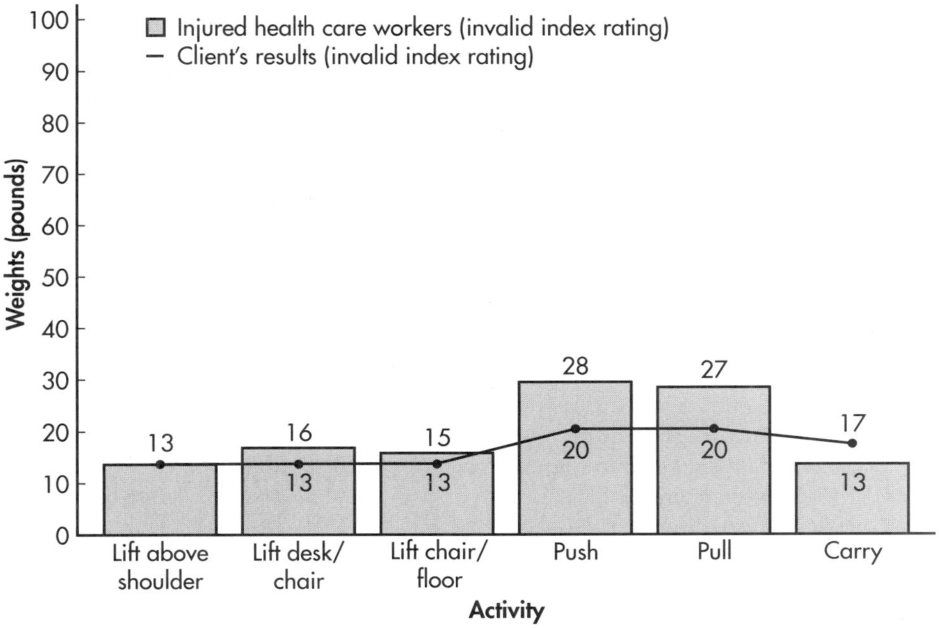

comparing these clients' results to normative data can be a key element in bringing about case closure at great savings to employers and payors.

Outcomes

Bringing about beneficial outcomes in industrial settings requires a shift in focus from "clinical advancement" goals in traditional therapy, to "return to work" and "injury prevention" goals in Industrial Therapy. It is no longer possible to simply provide the Assessment and abrogate accountability thereafter. Exposure continues throughout the rehabilitation phase and for many months after return to work.

The primary outcome sought in Industrial Therapy is defined in terms of the number of days at work without loss of work days. When establishing a system to track outcomes, the following information should be included:

1. Date of return to work.
2. Type of work resumed: same, modified or different job; same or different employer.
3. Elapsed time from date of injury to date of return to work.
4. Elapsed time from date of Assessment to date of return to work.
5. Elapsed time from return to work to date of follow-up.

6. Litigation status.
7. Loss of work days since return to work.

Follow-up for analysis of outcomes can be scheduled as often as possible. A minimum recommended frequency is at six months and 12 months, with six being the most important. If further follow-up is possible, it is usually at 24 months. These results may be used to support the continued use of FCAs, and in marketing to attract new accounts.

There is a wealth of other useful outcome information beyond the basic data discussed above. Waite studied the impact of FCAs on shortening the amount of time required for vocational evaluation of injured workers. The analysis indicated that clients undergoing a KEY Method FCA, required a median of 18 fewer days of vocational evaluations, translating to 18 fewer loss work days.[69] This kind of outcome information would be helpful in marketing FCAs to Vocational Rehabilitation Consultants, and to corporations that are increasingly focused on expeditious return to work.

SUMMARY

The role of Functional Capacity Assessment in Industrial Therapy has been growing in importance. The results are being used increasingly to assist job placement, to support the need for prevention programs, and to guide rehabilitation goal setting, design, planning, implementation, return to work, and outcome analysis.

FCAs are evolving to provide enhanced degrees of objectivity, validity, reliability, and predictability. These trends are being driven by the needs of Physicians, Employers, Vocational Rehabilitation Consultants, Attorneys, Insurance Companies, and Therapists. Out of this process, key principles are emerging to the effect that Therapists must be objective, equipment must be standardized, methodology must be consistent, and information processing and reporting, standardized.

In implementing FCAs, these emerging principles call for standard instructions, client-determined stopping points, minimized Therapist intervention or demonstration, algorithmic translation of results to recommendations, statistically determined validity of participation, and an increasing emphasis on outcomes to verify protocols and recommendations.

For Therapists contemplating adding FCAs to their services, or upgrading the current FCA system; key decision criteria are total long term costs (up front plus ongoing), the manufacturer's technical and upgrade support, reimbursement considerations, and the depth and breadth of database and outcome validations.

REFERENCES

1. Alexander RW, Maida AS, Walker RJ: The Validity of Preemployment Medical Evaluations, *J of Occup Med* 17:687-692, 1975.
2. AMA 1988 American Medical Association Guides to the Evaluation of Permanent Impairment, ed 3, Engleberg A editor, AMA Press, Chicago, 1988.
3. Astrand PO, Ryhming, I: A Nomogram for Calculation of Aerobic Capacity from Pulse Rate During Submaximal Work, *J of Applied Physiology* 7:218-221, 1954.
4. Ayoub MM, Mital A, Asfour SS, Bethea NJ: Review, Evaluation, and comparison of Models for Predicting Lifting Capacity, *Human Factors* 22:257-269, 1980.
5. Baran-Ettipio BJ, Centeno EJ: Early Return-To-Work Programs, *WORK*, 3(3), Summer, 1990.
6. Barlow WE, Hane EZ: A Practical Guide to the Americans with Disabilities Act, *Personnel J* June 1992.
7. Bechtol CO: The Use of A Dynamometer with Adjustable Handle Spacings, *J Bone and Joint Surgery* 36A(4): 820-832, July 1954.
8. Behan RJ: *Pain,* New York, 1914, D Appleton and Comp.
9. Bigos S, Spengler D, Martin N, et al: Back Injuries in Industry: a retrospective study III employee-related factors, *Spine* 11:252-256, 1986.
10. Bigos S, Spengler D, Martin N, et al: Back Injuries in Industry: a retrospective study-II, injury factors, *Spine* 11:246-251, 1986.
11. Blankenship K: Objectivity in Functional Capacity Eval-

uation, The American Physical Therapy Association Conference, Cincinnati, 1993.
12. Campion MA: Personnel Selection for Physically Demanding Jobs: review and recommendations, *Personnel Psych* 36:527-550, 1983.
13. Careers: need grows for physical therapists, *The New York Times,* March 3, 1988.
14. Chaffin DB: Ergonomics Guide for the Assessment of Human Static Strength, *Amer Ind Hyg Assoc J* 36:505-511, 1975.
15. Chaffin DB, Herrin GD, Keyserling WM, Garg A: A Method for Evaluating the Biomechanical Stresses Resulting from Manual Material Handling Jobs, *Am Ind Hyg Assoc J* 38:662-675, 1977.
16. Demers LM: Work Hardening: a practical guide, *Andover Medical,* 1992.
17. Deyo RA: Practice Variations, Treatment Fads, Rising Disability: do we need a new clinical research paradigm? *Spine* 18(15):2153-2162, 1993.
18. Equal Employment Opportunity Commission, Civil Service Commission, Department of Labor and Department of Justice. Adoption by four agencies of "Uniform Guidelines on Employee Selection Procedures," *Federal Register* 43:38290-38315, 1978.
19. Equal Employment Opportunity Commission: Technical Assistance manual for the Americans with Disabilities Act. IV-5 - IV-12.
20. Ergonomics Guide to Assessments of Metabolic and Cardiac Costs of Physical Work, *Amer Ind Hyg Assoc J* 32:560-564, 1971.
21. Fordyce W, Roberts A, Sternback R: The Behavioral management of chronic Pain: a response to critics, *Pain* 22:113-25, 1985.
22. Frymoyer JW: Quality: an international challenge to the diagnosis and treatment of disorders of the lumbar spine, *Spine* 18(15):2147-2152, 1993.
23. Graly J M, et al: Factors Influencing Return to Work for Clients in a Work-Hardening Center, *WORK,* 4(1), January 1994.
24. Greenberg SN, Bello RP: The Americans with Disabilities Act: what you don't know can hurt you, *Occup Health Forum* June 12, 1992.
25. Grossman P: Respiration, Stress, and Cardiovascular Function, *Psychophysiology* 20(3):284-300, 1983.
26. Hanson-Mayer TP: The Worker Disability Syndrome, *J of Rehab,* p. 50, July 1984.
27. Hastrup JL: Duration of Initial Heart Rate Assessment in Psychophysiology: current practices and implications, *Psychophysiology* 23(1): 15-18, Jan 1986.
28. Hazard RG: Functional Restoration Treatment Outcomes. Contemporary Conservative Care for Painful Spinal Disorders. 482-487:1991, Lea & Febiger.
29. Henschel A: Effects of Age on Work Capacity, *Amer Ind Hyg Assoc J* 31:430–436, 1970.
30. Herrin G, and Chaffin DB: Effectiveness of Strength Testing, *Professional Safety* 23(7): 39-43, 1978.
31. Holbrook T, Grazier K, Kelsey J, et al: The Frequency of Occurrence Impact and cost of Selected Musculoskeletal Conditions in the United States, *Am Acad Orth Surg* 27B, 1984.

32. Johnson & Higgins, subsidiary Foster Higgins: Survey on Workers' Compensation, 1992.
33. Kermond W, Gatchel RJ, Mayer TG: Functional Restoration Treatment for Chronic Spinal Disorder or Failed Back Surgery. In Mayer TG, et al, editors: *Contemporary Conservative Care for Painful Spinal Disorders*, Philadelphia, 1991, Lea & Febiger.
34. KEY Functional Assessments, Inc.: Follow-up Study on 100 Injured Workers, 1989.
35. Key GL: Key Functional Assessment Training and Resource Manual, 1984.
36. Key GL: Key Functional Assessment Policy and Procedure Manual, 1984.
37. Keyserling WM, Herrin GD, Chaffin DB: Isometric Strength Testing as a Means of Controlling Medical Incidents on Strenuous Jobs, *J Occup Med* 22:332-336, 1980.
38. Korthein TD, Gould JA, Key, G: Occupational Back Injury in the Health Care Employee Population, *Physical Therapy Today* 37-40, Summer 1993.
39. Lotito MJ, Allen JC: Legal Report: answers to commonly asked ADA questions, Human Resource Manag, Summer 1992.
40. Mahone DB: Job Redesign, Not 'Quick Fixes', Thwarts Many Back Injury Hazards, *Occup Health and Safety*, 63:51 Jan 1994.
41. Matheson LN: Effort Assessment During Functional Testing, Occupational Spinal Disorders Conference, Chicago, 1991.
42. Mathews, J: Physical Therapy: dramatic job increase, *Washington Post*, April 29, 1990.
43. Mathiowetz V, Weber K, Bolland G, Kashman N: Reliability and Validity of Grip and Pinch Strength Evaluations, *J of Hand Surg* 9A(2):222-226, March 1984.
44. Mathiowetz V, Kashman N, Bolland G, Weber K, Dowe M, Rogers S: Grip and Pinch Strength: normative data for adults, *Arch Phys Med Rehab* 66:69-74, February 1985.
45. Mayer T: The Shift from Passive Modalities to Reactivation from *Contemporary Conservative Care for Painful Spinal Disorders*, Philadelphia, 1988, Lea & Febiger.
46. Mayer T, Mooney V, Gatchel RJ: *Contemporary Conservative Care for Painful Spinal Disorders*, Philadelphia, 1988, Lea & Febiger.
47. Michael ED, Hutton KE, Horvath SM: Cardiorespiratory Responses During Prolonged Exercise, *J of Applied Physiology* 16:997-1000, 1961.
48. Medicine, *U S News & World Report*, April 25, 1988.
49. Morris M: 15 Fast-Track Careers, *Money Magazine* p 116 June 1990.
50. Nemethi CE: An Evaluation of Hand Grip in Industry, *Ind Med and Surg* 21:285-290, 1980.
51. Nordin M, Crites-Battié M, Pope MH, Snook S: Education and Training, In Pope MH, editor: *Occupational Low Back Pain: assessment, treatment and prevention.* St Louis, 1991, Mosby.
52. Osterweis M, Kleinman A, Mechanic D: Pain and Disability, Clinical, Behavioral, and Public Policy Perspectives, 1987, National Academy Press.
53. Park KS, Chaffin, DB: Prediction of Load-Lifting Limits for Manual Materials Handling, *Professional Safety* May 1975.
54. Personnel Decisions, Inc, Key Functional Assessment Preemployment Screening Battery as a Predictor of Job Related Injuries, Minneapolis, Minn, January 25, 1994.
55. Personnel Decisions, Inc: A Study of Statistical Relationships Among Physical Ability Measures on Injured Workers Undergoing KEY Functional Assessments, Minneapolis, 1986.
56. Petrofsky JS, William C, Kamen G, Lind AR: The Effect of Handgrip Span on Isometric Exercise Performance, *Ergonomics* 23(12):1129-1135, 1980.
57. Pope MH, Andersson BJ, Frymoyer JW, Chaffin DB: Occupational Low Back Pain: assessment, treatment, and prevention, 1991, St Louis, Mosby.
58. Powers, M: Psychocybernetics (Maxwell), N. Hollywood, Calif, 1960, Wilshire Book.
59. Quebec Task Force Study: Scientific Approach to the Assessment and Management of Activity Related Spinal Disorders, *Spine* 12:7S, 1987.
60. Salamy JG, Wolk DJ, Shucard DW: Psychophysiological Assessment of Statements About Pain, *Psychophysiology* 20(5):579-584, Sept 1983.
61. Saunders R, Industrial Rehabilitation: Functional Assessments and Work Hardening, The Missouri Physical Therapy Association, Osage Beach, 1993.
62. Schmidt RT, Toews JV: Grip Strength as Measured by the Jamar Dynamometer, *Arch of Phys Med and Rehab* 51:321-327, 1970.
63. Schwartz G: Healthcare Management and Physical Therapy: An Employer's Guide to Obtaining Physical Therapy Services: a study by the Washington Business Group on Health, commissioned by the Private Practice Section of the American Physical Therapy Association, Washington, DC, 1989.
64. Silvestri SM, Zimic DL: An Employer's Compliance Checklist, A Look at the Practical Aspects of Compliance with the ADA, *Federal Bar News & Journal* 39(1), January 1992.
65. Snook SH, Irvine CH: Maximum Acceptable Weight of Lift, *Amer Ind Hyg Assoc J* p 322-329, July 1967.
66. Snook SH: The Design of Manual Handling Tasks, *Ergonomics* 21(12):963-985, 1978.
67. Stewart DL, Abeln SH: *Documenting Functional Outcomes in Physical Therapy*, St Louis, 1993, Mosby.
68. US Department of Justice, Civil Rights Division: The Americans with Disabilities Act, Questions and Answers, Washington, D C, 1992, U S Government Printing Office.
69. Waite HD: Use of a New Physical Capacities Assessment Method to Assist in Vocational Rehabilitation of Injured Workers, 1987.
70. Webster's New World Dictionary, Third college Edition, 1988, Simon & Schuster.
71. Worker Data Bank, KEY Method, Minneapolis, 1994.

CHAPTER

14

Work Conditioning and Work Hardening

Glenda L. Key

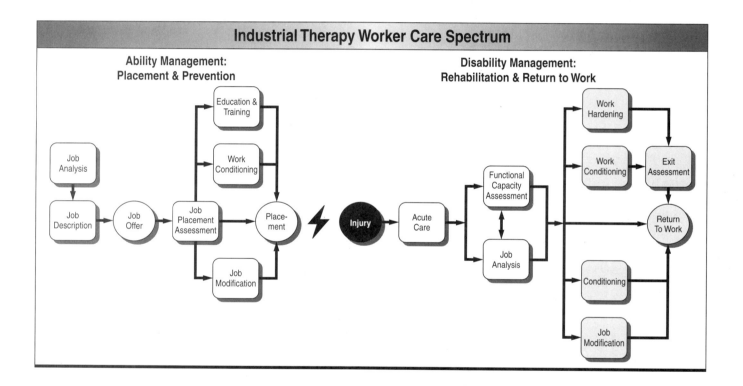

Work Conditioning and Work Hardening are rehabilitation systems, the individual components of which have evolved to address specific aspects of the return to work process. They have brought about increased success rates, accelerated time frames, increased restored function and productivity, reduced reinjury, and lower costs. In this chapter we will use the term "Work Retraining" as a more abbreviated and descriptive way to refer to either Work Hardening, Work Conditioning, or both.

Many of the Work Retraining components evolved independently, each in response to specific needs that were not being adequately addressed by traditional medical and therapeutic approaches. As more and more components accumulated, it became natural for people to begin grouping them. Since many of them addressed strengthening, conditioning, and preparation for the rigors of work, the terms "Work Conditioning" and "Work Hardening" were used regularly.

This chapter will review the emergence of Work Retraining to its present form and discuss issues influencing its growth and evolution. It will describe the basic hardware, staffing, organizational requirements, review an example process from beginning to end, and discuss the most important components of a good Work Retraining program.

FIGURE 14.1   Injury and capability status.

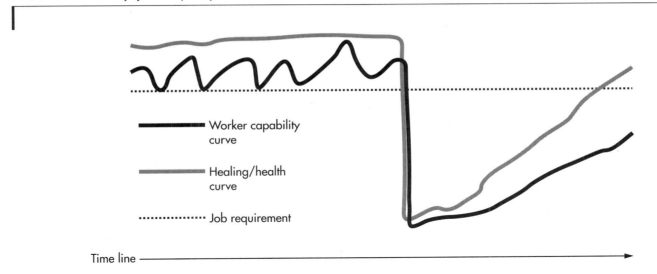

A. Pre-injury condition

1. Person's health/injury profile is not significant enough to cause problems fulfilling job requirements.

2. Person's capability is a range, generally covering the magnitude of the job requirements.

3. Job requirement is constant.

B. Injury phase

1. Person's health drops.

2. Person's capability drops.

3. Job requirement is constant.

C. Post-injury condition

1. Injured person is rehabilitated in stages.

2. Person's capability is initially greatly impaired and because injury recovery needs to precede capability recovery, the capability recovery comes later.

3. Job requirement is constant.

Why Work Retraining Has Emerged

Traditional medical methods of diagnosis and healing in the United States are at a level of quality unparalleled in the world. However, there are significant differences between a person who is medically healed, and a person who is prepared for return to work (RTW) at full job functions. The worker who is only medically healed has a number of deficiencies that need to be addressed:

1. The person's physical strength to perform the job has typically waned through inactivity
2. The individual's physiological resources such as energy level and endurance have often been depleted
3. The person's psychosocial equilibrium is often unsettled, with lingering fear of reinjury and other anxieties
4. The body part pronounced "healed" in medical terms may still be vulnerable to reinjury

when subjected to job demands

It is clear that a number of measures beyond healing are required in order to accomplish a safe and successful return to full productivity. There are a number of findings from the literature that suggest what these measures should be:

1. Physical strength needs to be built up and maintained by activity that puts "tension" on the musculoskeletal system
2. The injury or illness-induced physiological and chemical changes that impact energy levels and endurance must be reversed
3. The capability in strength and endurance depleted by inactivity must be restored[18,30,36,41,42]

Figure 14.1 summarizes the basic injury phases and capability status that characterize the traditional view of the injury cycle. The Work Retraining phase described in this chapter fills the gap between the last step in this traditional sequence and the resumption of work duties (Box 14.1).

BOX 14.1

Case Example
Social Versus Clinical
Responsibility[5]

Problem:

One of your therapists comes to you with Client A's file. Client A is in week four of Work Hardening with a diagnosis of degenerative disk disease. He reports pain symptoms at the end of the day. The Therapist reports that Client A's job requires daily heavy lifting. He is willing to work with some pain and it is the only kind of work he has ever had. He is married with two children in college. The Therapist reports, "I know his job is unsafe for him," and is requesting your help in telling the client.

Solution Options:

An ideal medical "best case scenario" might be to not return the employee to that job. But a socially responsible real life "best case scenario" might be to help get the client back to accommodated work and accommodated life style.

It may be important to take issue with the assumption that the job is unsafe for the client. Therapists may develop rigid views when it comes to "good" and "bad" posture, even though literature continues to support more than just one acceptable posture.

Some principles and actions to consider are:

- Review the FCA conducted prior to Work Hardening.
- If he cannot tolerate the job as is, the Therapist may need to make sure body mechanics training has included the various options of lifting, including bent back and straight legs.
- Consider ways to compensate for the deficits such as assistive devices or having coworkers assist with team or buddy lifts.
- Underscore the client's need to be very aware of and responsible for his continued fitness needs.
- In seeking accommodations, do not focus on what the person cannot do, but on what they can do.

The medical community's inattention to the returning worker's functional deficiencies was not a conscious oversight, but simply the result of the way health care has been structured. Physicians' education is in attending to anatomical and physiological aspects of the injury, with expertise in the medical management of the body and its parts. Since their education does not include RTW requirements or processes, Physicians have neither sought nor embraced involvement in it. They have willingly passed responsibility on to the Therapist.

Cost containment has also quickened the passage of RTW responsibility to Therapists. As doctors, hospitals, and private clinics have been required to limit the quantity and duration of interventions through DRGs (Diagnostic Related Groupings) and ICD 9s (International Classification of Diseases - 9th Revision), they have been effectively discouraged from expanding their spheres of involvement with each individual patient. It is no surprise, therefore, that Physicians and other providers have not attended to the RTW steps following their interventions (Figure 14.2).

Health Care and Employer Influences

Health care has been moving away from traditional approaches and facilities. With strict limitations on hospital inpatient medical care and growing restrictions on outpatient, new kinds of facilities and programs come into focus. Although hospitals could conceivably restructure services and facilities to serve

FIGURE 14.2   To ensure a safe, successful return to work, a worker needs the physical strength, flexibility, mobility, and endurance to perform the job functions.

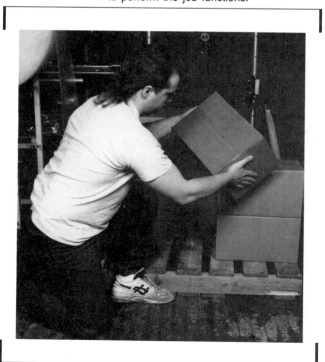

FIGURE 14.3   Direct working relationships between companies and providers has helped control health care costs while fostering innovation in planning and implementation.

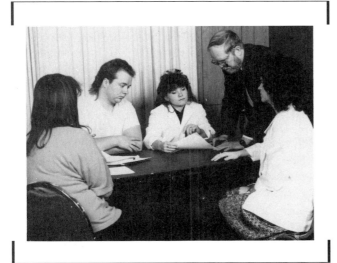

FIGURE 14.4   A Functional Capacity Assessment and Job Analysis are used to design individualized Work Hardening programs and to facilitate the consensus in planning and implementation that enables win-win outcomes.

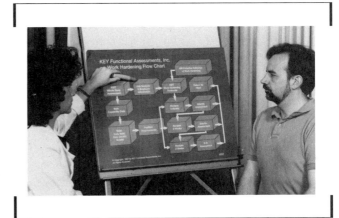

return to work needs, it appears that regulatory and perhaps cultural impediments have opened the door to new approaches, of which Work Retraining is one.

Employers have increasingly recognized the needs and benefits of taking control over health care costs, including those associated with Workers' Compensation (Figure 14.3).[6,9,15,24,33,36,40,43]

One avenue of better management has been to form more direct relationships with providers, and to participate in decisions with them in a partnership manner. These closer working relationships tend to more effectively intermingle medical and productivity considerations into rehabilitation planning and implementation. It is this blend of considerations that many innovative components of Work Retraining have addressed.

Another avenue of improved management is toward becoming self-insured.[33] In addition to saving money, breaking free from traditional insurance norms provides more opportunity to modify or eliminate procedures that do not fit the company's particular needs, and to test innovations that traditional insurers might not authorize. Self-insurance also enables more direct and precise analysis of costs and payback, with more relevance to the company's unique circumstances.

Work Retraining Benefits

Also fueling support for the systematic approaches of Work Retraining is the fact that everyone involved in the process benefits from the injured worker's expedi-

tious, safe, successful return to productivity. This engenders win-win outcomes (Figure 14.4).

The clients win because they are presented with clear realistic goals, and are imbued with the motivation and confidence required for success.

The physicians win because they know that their patients are in effective programs, and their return-to-work releases can be based on a comparison of Functional Assessment results and a Job Analysis, not just their own judgment call.

The employers win because the treatment approach focuses on restoring productivity to the worker and, hence, the company, while also lowering the risk of reinjury.

The vocational rehabilitation consultant, the insurance representative, Workers' Compensation case worker, and other involved parties win because they now have a formal system which facilitates gaining client cooperation, monitoring progress, making midcourse adjustments, and reaching more intelligent case closure.

The attorney who is truly looking out for the best interests of the client wins because the client wins. Supporting the RTW process may not yield the highest immediate financial gain, but serving the long term interests of the employer-employee is a wiser course over the long run.

Therapists win because Work Retraining is a conduit to additional services such as Job Analyses, Job Placement Assessments, employee fitness and ergonomics programs, and it also generates referrals from family members and friends of employees.

RTW REQUIREMENTS

With the increasing focus on workers' job-related functional capabilities, consensus continues to form as to what specifically is required. Figure 14.5 summarizes the capabilities necessary for successful RTW, and these are discussed in more detail on the following pages.

Physical Capabilities

The returning worker needs the physical wherewithal to perform the job functions, including physical strength, flexibility, mobility, and endurance.

Physical strength must be restored, specifically as it relates to required job functions such as lifting, pushing, pulling, and carrying.

Endurance must be rebuilt in order to tolerate full days of work activity, many days in a row, and long periods. The injured, nonworking individual usually does not have the desire nor the opportunity to assess these endurance needs themselves. They usually do not have the resources to set up an exercise or workout routine appropriate for rebuilding needed endurance.

Flexibility and mobility must be reestablished to enable the person to comfortably carry out daily home, social, and work activities.

FIGURE 14.5 Specific RTW requirements.

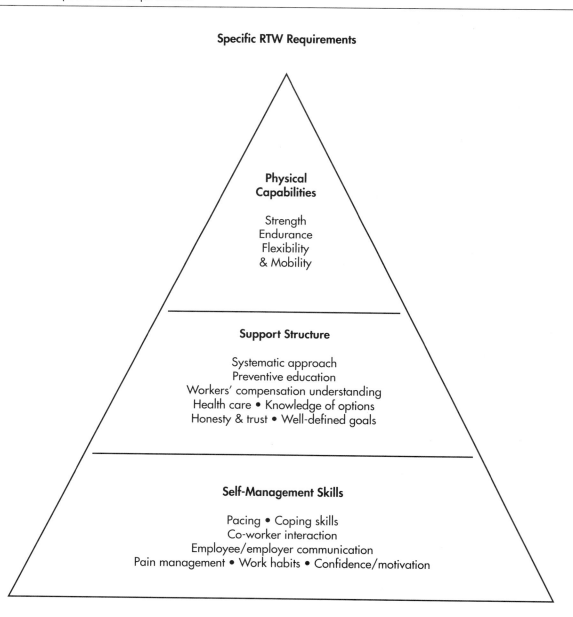

(Copyright KEY Method, 1994.)

Support Structure

The returning worker also needs a system that organizes and delivers needed resources and provides educational and psychosocial support to RTW efforts. The more important components of such a system are discussed below.

A Systematic Approach.   There must be an approach that incorporates full consideration of the functional components of the client's work world. Treatment must progress from general capabilities to the specific job demands, with consideration to the industrial and social context within which they must perform.

Prevention Education.   The client must understand what workstyles may have contributed to the injury, and what can be done, if anything, to increase safety.

Workers' Compensation.   Lack of confidence in the system can and does interfere with RTW progress. The client must feel they are receiving all due benefits in a timely manner. This is a complex system with multiple organizations and multiple players in each organization. Attempting to deal with this complexity can be a counterproductive distraction from the worker's necessary focus.

Proper Health Care.   Lack of confidence in the quality and duration of care being provided may hinder the worker's progress in other important areas of their rehabilitation. The client should have the impression that treatment consists of more than simply "try a bit of this, and if that doesn't work, try a bit of that."

Knowledge of Options.   The client is not usually aware of all the opportunities available to them, whether to return to their previous job, a modified job, a new job in the same field, or an entirely new field. A truck driver who can no longer drive may qualify for a job as a dispatcher (Figure 14.6). It is difficult for the injured worker to "buy in" to any program without a clear understanding of what can and cannot be achieved.

Honesty and Trust.   Members of the rehabilitation team—physicians, therapists, attorneys, counselors, employers, family members, peers, and others—must establish an atmosphere of honesty and trust in their dealings with each other and with the client. This is especially critical in cases of extended duration.

Well Defined Goals.   Ideally, all members of the rehabilitation team should be working in concert toward a shared set of goals. This is often not the reality. A player's individual goals, processes and time frames are often in conflict with those of other team members.

The physician's goal may be to speed up the medical process for RTW; the Vocational Counselor may want the individual to change jobs; the Attorney may want to perpetuate the status quo (no further medical recovery and permanent disability) in order to maximize the amount of settlement. In fact, in one instance a group of clients with attorneys had only a 9% return to work rate compared to a group without attorneys that achieved a 77% RTW rate.[15] An effective team rather than adversarial process serves to integrate and optimize everyone's goals and efforts.

Self Management Skills

Workers must also take an active role in their rehabilitation and RTW programs, and they can benefit from acquiring skills useful toward achieving the best possible outcome. The most beneficial skills are discussed below (Figure 14.7).

Pacing Mechanism.   Proper pacing regardless of weighted activity level is required in order to maintain safe cardiovascular and musculoskeletal integrity while being a productive, healthy employee.[9,30]

Coping Skills.   The injured worker needs to develop mental skills to cope with a number of psychosocial dislocations resulting from the injury. These include the loss of income; the necessity of the spouse to make up the difference; the loss of self respect associated with becoming a burden to loved ones; and the role reversal from primary breadwinner to responsibility for domestic activities and child care.

FIGURE 14.6   Vocational Rehabilitation Consultants are one resource in the RTW support structure that can facilitate the rehabilitation and reemployment process.

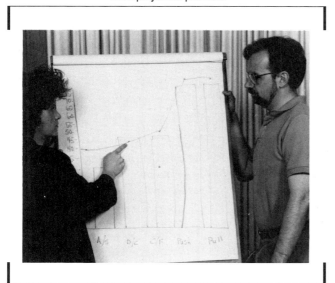

FIGURE 14.7 Work Retraining programs instill the self management skills of pacing, coping, coworker interaction, employer/employee communication, pain management, work habits, motivation, and confidence.

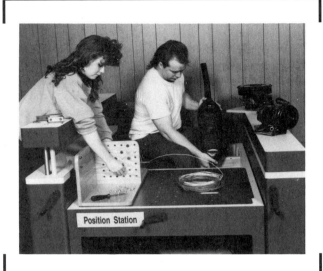

Position Station

If not addressed, this level of negative self reinforcement can lead to behavioral problems, or the use of alcohol or drugs, which further complicate an already complex situation.

Coworker Interaction. The injured worker needs a way to smoothly reintegrate with the peer group at work, which typically involves overcoming a number of fears such as, "Do they think I wasn't really hurt?," "Will they think I won't carry my own?," "Will they help me?," "Will they still like me?" Addressing these peer-related anxieties is an important component of successful RTW programs.

Employer/Employee Communication. It can be a powerful boost to morale and motivation if the injured worker knows that the employer is concerned about his or her health and return to work. Whatever level of communication that existed prior to injury is often discontinued once the injury occurs, and this breeds uncertainty. Good communication between the employer and the injured employee is as important for RTW as it is for the workplace in general (Box 14.2).[6]

Pain Management Skills. Injured workers can achieve a great deal more during rehabilitation and after RTW when they gain an understanding of the pain mechanisms and learn how to deal with each kind of pain they encounter. Pain that is the result of reinjury to soft tissue requires a change in workstyles

---

BOX 14.2

Case Example
Employer-Employee Relationship[5]

Problem:
A Work Conditioning client (Client B) reports to the Therapist that when he returns to work, he "knows" he will be laid off. That is what happened to all his peers when they returned to work.

Solution Options:
The overall challenge is to build or rebuild a constructive relationship between the employer and employee. Some principles and actions are:

- It is important not to assume the client's perception is correct or incorrect.
- Communicate the client's concerns to the Rehabilitation Counselor.
- Invite the employer to visit the Work Conditioning Center to see the employee at "work" in the clinic (not while receiving passive "pleasure" treatments like hot packs and massage). The employee also is encouraged by active employer involvement.
- If previous injured workers did not go through an extensive program, emphasize that difference to the employer.
- Consider moving the last week of the program to the job site to facilitate transition for both the employer and employee.
- Inform the employer of the Exit Assessment that will specify capabilities relative to job requirements. Everyone will see what can and cannot be done.
- Prepare the client for the worst case scenario—the employer does lay him off. Stress that he will have the benefit of knowing his capabilities in applying for new jobs.

---

or job functions, whereas pain that occurs when progressing exercise can be a positive sign of conditioning progress.[30] Without proper knowledge, the worker may interpret all pain as that which should be avoided, which would limit recovery and impair productivity.

Work Habits. An injured worker needs to regain any lost work habits that may have been second nature prior to the injury. These include arriving to work on time, properly attired; working at the job for sustained lengths of time; taking breaks only for lunch or other designated activities; communicating with coworkers to accomplish tasks; and leaving the work area orderly and clean at the end of the work day.

Injured workers must reestablish a positive attitude toward these disciplines, and reintegrate them into daily work routines.

Motivation and Confidence. Few injured workers can muster the necessary motivation and confidence to excel on their own. Motivation and confidence are strengthened by realistic goal setting, proper education, training, and positive support from employers, peers, and the family.

WORK RETRAINING OPERATIONS

Most of the necessary clinical skills are already a part of the Therapist's repertoire. Additional education and know-how as to organizing the program will be necessary to implement an effective one. A discussion of the basic components can begin that process.

Assessment and Evaluation

Just as in traditional medical care or any problem-solution discipline, the first step in a Work Retraining program is assessment and evaluation. This establishes the beginning status and provides a baseline of comparison for goal setting, planning, and progress monitoring.

Goal Setting

Once the current status and needs of the patient have been established, the next step is to set goals. In return-to-work treatment goals are determined by the rehabilitation team—employer, employee, peers, family, insurer, providers, and others—as contrasted to traditional care where goals are set by the Therapist alone.

The client is, of course, the focal point of goal setting, but each team member must translate the client's goals into specific objectives for their role in the RTW process. It must be decided where the team is going and what everyone's part is in getting there. Program goals for each client should be established upon entry to the program (Box 14.3).

Program Day Length

Determining program day length is dependent upon the treatment protocols. Previously, Therapists felt that it was necessary for clients to participate in Work Hardening for an entire eight hour day. As more clinics experimented with shorter day programs and demonstrated success in returning and keeping their clients on the job, six hour days came into practice.

The current trend is toward a four hour day program. Industrial Therapists have found that when treatment is highly programmed, truly focused, and well managed and supervised, the program can be condensed to four hours per day in most instances.[46] There are circumstances that require 6 to 8 hours per day. In fact, the Commission on Accreditation of Rehabilitation Facilities (CARF) requires that the facility be able to *accommodate* a full five day program if it is warranted, but accredits shorter programs in terms of hours per day and days per week.[10]

When a program has been successfully condensed to four hours per day, opportunities of time open up for other needs. Time can be used to accommodate more clients, administer assessments, implement marketing and selling activities, provide inservices, and conduct in-team updates, planning sessions, seminars, and conferences.

Program Duration

Once a philosophy on the length of the treatment day is established, it is important to determine how many weeks a program should last. Too often therapists have accepted clients into a Work Hardening or Work Conditioning program, with an open-ended plan of progressing the client until they can go no further. Without clear parameters, neither the therapist nor the client are committed to a completion point.

A frequent consequence is to extend programs up to as many as 12 weeks, resulting in excessive charges that can give a "bad rap" to all return to work programs.[4] Once an employer or claims representative has experienced such excessive charges without meeting return-to-work needs, they are much less likely to try another Work Retraining program—even from a different vendor. Referral sources do not simply stop referring to providers of below standard services, but to all providers of the service.

An accurately determined time frame enables all parties to plan more effectively. The insurance company and employer can be more comfortable authorizing a program with a well-defined time frame. The employer can also begin preparing the work environment, including any job modifications required.

In determining program duration it is important to apply standardized and useful protocols wherever possible. The question becomes, "What factors influence the amount of treatment a client will require to return to work?" The key variables this author considers in

---

BOX 14.3

Case Example
Goal Setting[5]

Problem:
Client C has been referred into Work Hardening by his spine surgeon—no surgery. His records show that he also sees a chiropractor, family doctor, and a Physical Therapist, each of which have given different Return to Work prognoses.

Solution Options:
This objective here is to generate positive action based on objective and accurate determinations of feasible goals and affordable treatment to achieve them. Principles and actions are:

- Before the client is considered for Work Hardening, a Functional Capacity Assessment should be administered and compared with the requirements of the job, to determine the following information:
    The client's functional capabilities
    The requirements of the job
    The feasibility of progressing the client to meet those requirements in an acceptable time frame
- If possible, the time frame should be determined quantitatively by factoring objective measures into a function such as the Predictive Index discussed later in the chapter. This will carry more weight than opinion, and will strengthen the recommendation to proceed.
- If the job requirements are deemed achievable, Work Hardening can proceed regardless of whether the conflicting medical opinions have been reconciled.
- If the job requirements are deemed unachievable, the employer should be notified, and the options of job modification or alternate employment discussed. At this point a VRC may be called in to coordinate the communication between the multiple medical providers involved.

---

this determination are diagramed in Figure 14.8 and include:

- Functional Capacity Assessment results
- Job analysis results
- Capability deficit of the worker relative to job requirements
- Validity determination
- Length of time out of work

- Status of litigation
- Compliance history

This author uses the term "Predictive Index" to denote the result of weighing these factors. This Index indicates whether the client requires a two week program (alpha), a four week program (beta), or a six week program (gamma). If the client does not meet the minimum requirements of the six week program, the client may qualify for Conditioning to prepare for subsequent Work Conditioning or Work Hardening.

Work Conditioning and Work Hardening programs generally vary in length from two to eight weeks, with the average being a four week duration. Programs lasting longer than six weeks should be reviewed for appropriateness of goals. Those lasting longer than eight weeks may represent abuse of the reimbursement system.

Functional Capacity Assessment results indicate the client's capabilities which, combined with *Job analysis results* enables determination of the *worker's capability deficit*. A deficit of 20% can usually be accomplished in a standard length program. A deficit of 50% or greater, however, may not be correctable through a standard program duration.[46]

The Validity Determination is an important input in governing program duration. An individual demonstrating "noncompliance" through an "invalid" rating in the FCA is unlikely to progress in the retraining program as quickly and successfully as "valid" participants.

Applying validity information may place the client outside the acceptable level for entry into the Work Hardening or Work Conditioning program.

The length of time out of work is well documented to correlate with a lower likelihood of returning to work.[2,7,14,16,24,31] In addition to the body becoming physically deconditioned, the individual may also become accustomed to a diminished level of responsibilities, deadlines, decisions, personal discipline, social, and family obligations.

Status of Litigation significantly affects the required duration of treatment. Although the literature is not clear about the cause and effect, it does confirm that cases in litigation extend longer, are less likely to return to work, and are therefore more costly.[15]

Compliance History from referrals, medical records, FCA findings, and past treatment experience affects program duration in that noncompliant clients tend to require more weeks of Work Retraining.

Program Planning

An accurately determined program duration provides clear direction for treatment content and progression, which is the next set of important decisions. For purposes of illustration, this author's approach to

FIGURE 14.8 Predictive index generation.

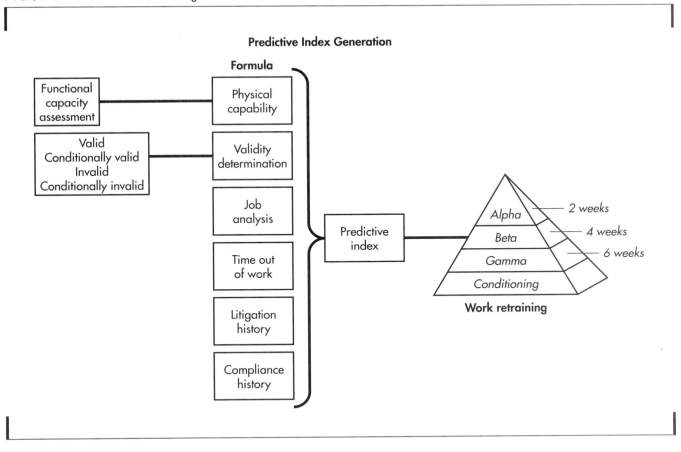

(Copyright KEY Method, June, 1992.)

selecting treatment components includes the following variables, some of which were applied to the determination of program duration:

1. The client's FCA results
2. The return to work job demands
3. The injury profile
4. The validity index scale results
5. Litigation status

The client's Functional Capacity Assessment results identify their present baseline physical job related capabilities against which to plan content and progression, and monitor progress.

The return to work job demands, accurately identified through a Functional Job Analysis, are the goals that drive the design and progression plan of Work Retraining. When a specific job has not been identified for the worker, job demands may be derived using the *Dictionary of Occupational Titles* in combination with information about the worker's previous employment.

Job demand levels may be modified upon communication with other parties of the team, but they serve as a starting point for program focus.

The injury profile classifies the client's injury ac-

cording to the occupation, the simulation stations that correspond to that occupation, the injured body part, and the specific activities that will be used to exercise that body part. This profile facilitates designing the program to address the relevant needs.

The Validity Index Scale results are important input to include in selecting treatment components. Although the percentages are lower than the perceptions, it is true that some injured workers misrepresent their injury and their capabilities, intentionally or unintentionally. Statistical methods exist that enable Therapists to detect such misrepresentation. This author compares the client's individual FCA tests for internal consistency, using an algorithm to derive a measurement of validity called the Participation Index. Box 14.4 describes four categories of FCA participation.[19,20,34,35] For a more detailed discussion of this derivation, see Chapter 13.

By following the Participation Index results from the FCA, the Industrial Therapist will be able to structure a program more appropriate for that individual. Examples of validity determinations and appropriate responses are discussed on the following pages.

BOX 14.4

Ratings of FCA Participation

1. Valid Participation: The individual demonstrated full effort, and the results reflect safe capability levels.
2. Invalid Participation: The individual consciously and intentionally demonstrated less than full effort, and the results reflect less than full, safe capability levels.
3. Conditionally Valid Participation: The individual unintentionally demonstrated less than full effort, and the results reflect less than full, safe capability levels. However, the results do reflect the client's own perception of capability limits.
4. Conditionally Invalid Participation: The individual demonstrated beyond what would be considered full, safe capability levels over long work periods, and the results reflect more than recommended safe levels.

A Valid Rating indicates the cooperative worker who is demonstrating full honest capability. It is legitimate and this designation must be remembered when evaluating problems that may arise. If a Valid Participator has difficulty in meeting the progression schedule, reports pain, or displays difficulty accommodating new posture techniques, chances are these are real concerns that require Therapist intervention. Similarly, the individual's Validity Designation should also govern the response to a person who shares personal information indicative of problem solving needs.

An Invalid Rating indicates an individual who does not show full effort, consciously demonstrating less than true capability level. In Work Retraining settings, this issue needs to be addressed prior to entry into the program. An individual who tests as Invalid in the FCA is likely to continue inconsistency of participation if not addressed. This will be manifested as tardiness, absenteeism, lack of cooperation, or disruptive behavior among other participants.

Although Invalid Participation is a burdensome problem, these individuals should not simply be ejected from the program. Industrial Therapists have the opportunity to turn this bad situation into a more desirable, if not good, outcome. To illustrate, one approach would be to offer a two step plan which if followed, would enable the individual to reenter the program:

Step 1: The issues of noncompliance and Invalid Participation are discussed directly with the client, offering the options of retaking the assessment, accepting one of several jobs offered by the employer, or participating in a Conditioning program as a prerequisite to Work Retraining.

Step 2: If the Conditioning program is chosen, the plan is laid out clearly including requirements of progress and compliance. After two weeks, if the client continues to choose to abuse the system, the client is discharged. If the requirements are met, the individual is admitted into the Work Retraining program. This approach rewards the individual for the decision to make positive and appropriate changes. It also provides a defined structure within which to make that change.

It is important for those in the medical profession to recognize and internalize that many injured individuals will not be returned to preinjury status. It is true that not everyone wants to be productive. It is also true that not everyone can be productive. To spend excessive amounts of time and money in Work Hardening or Work Conditioning may be a poor use of the medical and reimbursement systems. It would also unnecessarily hinder the success of the outcomes data for the program.

A Conditionally Valid Rating indicates one who is not putting forth full effort in demonstrating physical capabilities, but is not consciously trying to manipulate the results. The individual believes he or she is working at full capacity, and may be underperforming due to fear of reinjury. Whatever the reason, clients with this problem require a more tightly defined program plan and may warrant closer monitoring and staff involvement to reach their goals.

Although completely sincere, these individuals may present a variety of problems, such as extremely slow pacing, or over reacting and over reporting body responses. It is also not uncommon for them to become progressively more immobile, and to wonder why an injury that started out as a neck problem has spread to their back, hips, and arms. These clients will need more than average time in flexibility and mobility activities.

The challenge is to motivate the client to increase loads and body stretches beyond normal activity. Standard motivation approaches do not always work. One way to work toward increasing capability is to shift the focus away from the activity and toward the heart rate. This may require additional education for the client to understand the implications of the cardiovascular ranges and what constitutes an exercise level. Goals are expressed in heart rates, as are the tracking and monitoring. Once the client has been able to move forward, it is a little easier to use more traditional motivators and goals.

A Conditionally Invalid Rating indicates an overachieving person whose FCA results demonstrate that activities are not generally terminated as early as they should be.[8] Work Retraining treatments need to focus on pacing to prevent reinjury. Once the pacing problem is addressed effectively, increasing capabilities may be appropriate. This type of person often demonstrates an eagerness to participate, and tends to be very energetic, happy, and fun to be around. Although this may sound ideal for the Therapist, it is not easy to slow down the activity level and speed of these highly motivated individuals. For Therapists, it is critical not to mistake these people for just good, hard workers. As overachievers, they may be headed for further injury.

Telltale signs of conditionally invalid overachievers are:

1. Progressing themselves without consulting their Work Trainer or Therapist. They may not have completed the proper number of repetitions of a given weight or number of days at a given weight, but they increase the weights of the work simulation activity anyway.
2. Taking aerobic exercising to the next grade of difficulty before they should.
3. Paying little attention to body mechanics after the first few repetitions.

One strategy for advancing the program safely might include the use of biofeedback mechanisms with target heart rates, requiring the client to keep heart rate at or below a predetermined level. The author uses the term "Work Lightening" to describe this approach. It generally helps slow them down by providing a goal other than task completion. They may still have a tendency to speed at first, but the resultant "wasted" time waiting for their heart rate to recover is usually more of a bother than acquiescing to the slower pacing. The slower pacing also allows for time to incorporate improved postures. With Therapist reinforcement of positive changes, proper pacing is further reinforced (Box 14.5).

Litigation Status can significantly affect the success of Work Retraining. As mentioned earlier, cases in litigation are less likely to return to work.[15] It is important for Therapists to be cognizant of legal exposure and consequences, and to incorporate such considerations into the planning stage. Addressing these issues brings the team together in a problem solving mode in which major barriers to recovery may be addressed as early as possible in the goal setting and planning stages of the client's program (Box 14.6, page 268).

In summary, the individual client's own history extends far beyond medical or functional ability status. The variables that influence program content and progression are numerous and complex. Without standard protocols to assist in these determinations, it is difficult for an Industrial Therapy practice to offer

---

BOX 14.5

Case Example
Overworker[5]

Problem:
Client D has been in the Work Hardening Program for one week. He is unilaterally making modifications to his program progression, increasing weights and repetitions prior to scheduled progression. He reports increased pain at the end of the treatment day.

Solution Options:
It is this author's opinion that a determination should first be made as to whether the behavior is of a nature that could lead to injury, or whether it is simply an irritation to the Therapist. If the client's Validity Index rating was valid, and if he has only been in the program for one week, the Therapist should not be too quick to discount the client's belief that he can do more. The reports of pain should be investigated to determine whether it stems from discomfort normally associated with increased physical activity or from actual injurious tension to the musculoskeletal system. If it is due simply to conditioning, program modifications may be acceptable.

On the other hand, if his rating was conditionally invalid (an "overworker") and he is working into levels with risk of injury, this needs to be firmly addressed with him. He may not have a clear Point of Change (POC) reference system[8] and may need what was referred to earlier as Work Lightening—a process of lightening work response.[21] If not addressed, he may be at high risk for injury on the job. One of the rules that should be implemented is to require the client to have all changes or adaptations signed off by the Therapist prior to making them.

---

consistency from one clinician to another or from one facility to another.[25]

Protocol Guidelines

In the age of tracking and reimbursement based on outcomes, it is critical that Work Conditioning and Work Hardening programs strive for standardization. It is important that the program approach and results are consistent from one client to another and from one industrial customer to another.

Such consistency is not possible if the protocols within the provider facility are not standardized. Without standardization, each Therapist is responsible for

BOX 14.6

Case Example
Potential Plaintiff[5]

Problem:
Client E asks the Therapist if he thinks she should get a lawyer.

Solution Options:
Extreme caution is recommended. Although the Therapist would like to convince the client not to seek legal counsel, attempting such persuasion is not appropriate and may make things worse. Some principles and actions to follow are:

- A response that will not sway the client in one decision or another is best. The Therapist may ask, "What is your thinking on that?"
- Keep the conversations short and focused on gathering information required to prepare for the likelihood of legal intervention.
- Give State Workers' Compensation office telephone number as a resource for advice.
- Notify case manager and rehabilitation counselor.
- It is extremely important to document everything
- Issues to consider:
  Is litigation feasible?
  If so, how will it affect the client's treatment, progress, and return to work possibilities?

BOX 14.7

Case Example
Alcohol Detected On Breath[5]

Problem:
Coworkers and other clients report that Client F's breath smells of alcohol.

Solutions Options:
The critical first step in this kind of situation is to gather information before taking any action:

- Medical records—It is possible that chemical responses of the body in certain diagnoses (diabetes) and in certain medications can cause a person's breath to mimic that of alcohol even when none has been consumed
- Attendance record
- Program progress toward goals

The result of this information gathering should be documented. Depending on the determination, some principles and actions that typically apply are as follows:

- It is extremely important to document everything.
- If alcohol is involved, notify the physician.
- Make staff and other clients' safety the top priority.
- Consider bringing in a Vocational Counselor or Psychologist.
- Review with the client the agreement they signed upon entry into the program, underscoring that it is a potential basis for termination
- Consider moving the client from the afternoon to the morning program, if the consumption appears to start during lunch.

inventing the approach, without benefiting from the lessons of others. As a result, there may be little consistency between programs, and even less as employees leave and take continuity with them.

Protocols in Work Hardening and Work Conditioning are quite extensive. They must address requirements from intake to discharge and weave together many disciplines and processes. They must allow flexibility to treat each client as an individual, with a program designed to meet the specific needs. This individual tailoring can be accomplished while still working within standard parameters for all participants (Box 14.7).

Simulation Guidelines

Contrary to earlier philosophies, the prevailing belief today is that the program does not have to *exactly* *duplicate* the real world. It needs only to *simulate*

relevant portions of it. It is not necessary to create a real fire in order to build ladder climbing and hose carrying capabilities in fire fighters. Aspects of simulation that are superfluous to Work Retraining goals, such as using the exact technical skills or producing actual products, may interfere with the rehabilitation progress.

The differences between job duplication and job simulation may be subtle, but they are important when establishing the intended scope of the program offered by the facility. Most rehabilitation programs have expanded to include job simulation, but have not included the complexity of job duplication (Figure 14.9, *A, B*).

1 4 . 9 A, B   Simulation need not duplicate the actual job—only the dynamic body mechanics and resistances involved.

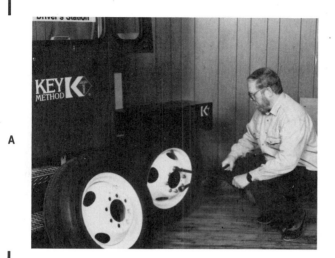
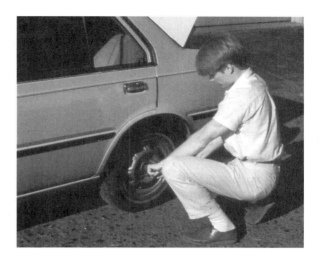

Client Progress Reviews

Client progress reviews, often called "Staffings" are weekly meetings of the clients' in-house rehabilitation team. The purpose of this meeting is to provide a vehicle for multi or interdisciplinary case management. Client progress monitoring should be scheduled at given intervals, with success based on achieving the predetermined RTW goals. A significant difference between Traditional Therapy and Industrial Therapy is that in IT, success is not defined as the completion of the program, but rather, as the successful return to work.

During Staffings, all members of the team are expected to have input on clients' progress reports and to provide direction for the next step in each client's program (Figure 14.10).

The team includes those directly and indirectly involved in the case; the Industrial Therapist who manages the case and the Work Trainer who has the day-to-day tracking and monitoring responsibilities. Where psychology and vocational rehabilitation components are offered from in-house staff, they may also be in attendance. If they are not in attendance, their progress notes should be available and reviewed prior to the Staffing.

It is common practice that this meeting be held every week with the Program Manager presiding. CARF mandates this meeting no less often than every other week.[10] These should be only summary review meetings that take no more than five to ten minutes for each client. All weekly summary information should be prepared for presentation prior to the meeting.

In the Staffing, the Work Trainer reports on the client's progress including the areas of:

1. Attendance and compliance with other policies
2. Body mechanics progress
3. Weighted activity progress
4. Communication
5. Relationships with coworkers
6. Safety practices
7. Compliance with policies
8. Interim assessment results

FIGURE 14.10   Weekly staff meetings involving the in-house rehabilitation team members are held to review client progress, discuss problems, and provide direction for next steps.

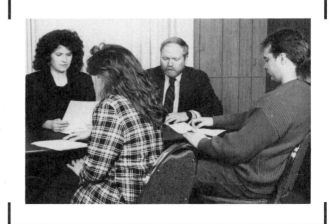

Where goals are not being met or change is required, the team discusses options and chooses the appropriate approach to take. This is an opportunity to benefit from the expertise of others.

The documentation and results of these meetings should be sent with every progress report and invoice that is generated.

WORK RETRAINING STRUCTURE

Space Requirements

The amount of the space required will depend, to an extent, upon the length of the program. If the policies and procedures dictate a program length of four hours per day, the space will be able to accommodate more clients (assuming two shifts) than with a six or eight hour standard protocol (Figure 14.11).

Space is also dictated by the amount and size of equipment specified in the program. This, in turn, is dependent upon the population to be served. If the primary customer is a railroad company, it may be worth the extra cost to bring in rail car mechanisms. This may also dictate the required height of the room.

If the population is primarily heavy labor, equipment that simulates manual labor situations would be appropriate. Examples would be a simulated factory conveyor, or shipping area involving materials handling, a simulated construction site with cement blocks and other building materials, or a simulated truck driver's cab.

Although there are many different equipment mixes based on the surrounding client base, the average size space for a Work Conditioning or Work Hardening Center is 2,500 square feet.[18,21] For CARF accreditation, this space must be a designated area specifically for Work Hardening. The space must also approximate a real working environment.[10]

In a four hour per day program (assuming two shifts) up to 30 or 40 participants can be treated each day. If the center is expected to do more volume than that, the space may have to be expanded. Another alternative is to have certain aspects of the program, such as the FCA's, administered off-site.

Equipment Requirements

The equipment purchase can be the largest single capital outlay next to the building itself. The three primary determinants of equipment requirements are; the type of work the surrounding population performs, the number of clients and types of injuries expected each month, and the specific Work Conditioning or Work Hardening protocols (Figure 14.12).

FIGURE 14.11 The equipment mix and space requirements of a Work Hardening Center are determined by the surrounding industrial base.

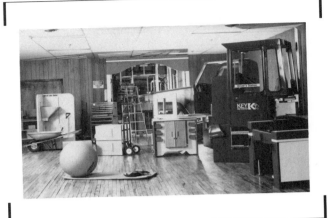

In some instances, it may be necessary to have duplicate pieces of equipment at the facility. If the location and population served is predominantly small manufacturing, with high incidence of upper extremity injuries, it might make sense to have two or three small assembly simulation stations instead of truck cab simulators.

Regarding protocols, depending on what beginning postures and weights are called for, a "position

FIGURE 14.12 Equipment requirements determination.

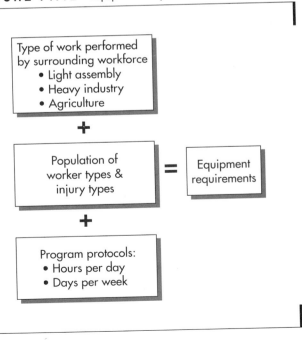

station" that requires holding various body positions will help build static posture capabilities. A "sorting station" that requires handling small parts may also be helpful if protocols call for high repetition activities. Small parts manipulation simulation is also used to build posture capabilities, through the process of getting the body comfortable with the extremes and practicing postural progression in nonloaded activities.

Equipment Selection Criteria

An overall set of guidelines to help when selecting equipment is that it should be:

a. Functional—to simulate real job activities.
b. Manufacturer warranted—generally one year parts and labor is standard.
c. Multi-user capable—to accommodate multiple users simultaneously on each piece of equipment and get the most from invested space and capital.
d. Multi-occupation flexible—to simulate a variety of occupational needs with each piece of equipment and get the most from invested space and capital. Separate stations for

each specific kind of work can be cost prohibitive. The governing philosophy is to simulate the job, not duplicate it (Figure 14.13, A, B).

e. Durable—for heavy-duty activities from treadmills and exercycles to building trades and materials handling stations. The users of this equipment are often accustomed to forceful activity levels, and many are overweight.
f. Space efficient—this is part of the reason for purchasing multi-user, multi-occupation stations. The height of the equipment in relationship to the room is also an important consideration.
g. Client friendly—to feel and look somewhat like work, avoiding the "sterile" medical look and minimizing computer interaction if any.
h. Therapist friendly—easy to operate, requiring little or no knowledge of the real world equipment. Real equipment or real work should not be used if its complexity adds unnecessary time or burden to the Therapist's treatment processes.
i. Reversible assembly—finished product from simulated manufacture or construction can be

FIGURE 14.13 A, B   Work Retraining equipment that accommodates multiple users and multiple tasks economizes on equipment expense and space.

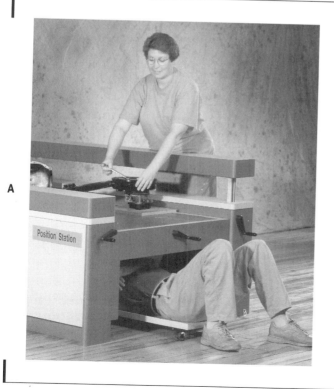
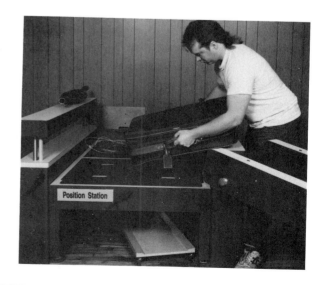

taken apart so that components do not have to be replenished, saving time and money.

j. Non-trendy design—so that the equipment design or color combination does not look "dated" in too short a time period.

A Therapist is more likely to feel fulfilled as a treating Therapist in a setting when most of their time is spent focusing on the progress, postures, and education of clients. The equipment must simulate real world postures and dynamic functions, but it need not replicate the actual production of real finished products.

If real equipment is used, it should not require the Therapist to be an expert in its operation, or to monitor an actual industrial process. This would take unnecessary time and energy away from monitoring and facilitating the client's physical progress. It is important to Industrial Therapists to still practice as Therapists, not industrial process technicians. Attention to this distinction will impact staff enthusiasm and retention.

Location Selection

In Work Retraining, facility location is an important consideration. Referral sources prefer nearby locations, and clients' travel distances affect compliance with attendance requirements once in the program. Since referrals impact revenue and poor attendance cuts return to work success rates, facility location should be evaluated carefully. Accordingly, the facility should be easily accessible from major highways, and within a 30 minute drive of those it is intended to serve.

Space Selection

Warehouse buildings were once thought to be not only ideal, but the only way to go. Now they are recognized as being one of the many options available and only ideal if the population it serves works in similar environments and are located nearby. An advantage of warehouse space is that it is usually less expensive to rent or purchase. It is also common to find previously used space in medical buildings. Changes in reimbursement as well as mergers and acquisitions have resulted in not only vacant rooms, but the availability of entire wings or floors. In any case, the space must be accessible and meet ADA requirements for accommodation.

Patient Mix

It is important that the location does not require the mixing of the worker with the more acute patients. Some view such a mix as a motivator to both populations. That is, the severely impaired may be motivated by seeing a later stage of recovery and would get encouragement from being around those who are making progress. And the Work Retraining client with a back injury may be more inclined to feel fortunate in having avoided a more serious injury, and as a result, may have a more positive attitude toward moving forward. Although there is some logic to these views, it has become generally regarded as a "downer" for the healthy but injured clients to be mixed with acute care patients.[46]

Many clinics create separated spaces within the same building, or use separate buildings next to each other. In this way, the return-to-work program can still be an incentive and motivator for the acute care patient. It is also a practical solution for scheduling staff, especially if employees rotate through different programs.

Staffing

The number of people needed at each level of credentialing depends primarily upon the client caseload and the protocols used. An operation can begin with a single Physical Therapist or Occupational Therapist designated as the Program Director. This person is initially responsible for every aspect of the program's daily operations, including planning, patient or client treatment, monitoring, reporting, and making any adjustments that are indicated.

As the staff grows, the Program Director assumes a more managerial role involving program management of each client and specific clinical management of their postures and progress. The Program Director supervises the other Therapists and employees, and presides over staff meetings regarding program design, planning, and progress reporting.

As the caseload increases, a Work Trainer would be the next staffing addition. This individual might be an Exercise Physiologist, an Athletic Trainer, a Physical or Occupational Therapist Assistant, or a Kinesiologist. This individual would assume responsibility for the daily monitoring of progressions of weights, repetitions, and clients' compliance with program policies and procedures. The Work Trainer contributes to the weekly progress report and provides input and recommendations regarding the week's plan.

Regarding the number of staff, if the program begins with fewer than 10 new clients per month, it is relatively easy for a single Therapist to manage a four week, four hours per day general treatment approach. Assessments, reports, and meetings can take place in the afternoons. More staff may be required if the protocol is a six or eight hour program per person every day.

Above 10 new clients per month, the Work Trainer

should be added and the staff of two can manage up to 20 new clients per month, assuming the four week, four hours per day protocol. This size population can also still be housed in the initial 2,500-3,000 square foot space. There may be a need for some support staff, part time or full time, for scheduling, accounting, and possibly marketing.

ADMINISTERING WORK RETRAINING TO CLIENTS

In administering Work Conditioning or Work Hardening, it is important to follow a structured, step-by-step process, governed by consistent standards and tailored to each client's needs wherever possible. Each Industrial Therapy practice may devise their own unique variations and touches, but a general outline is presented in Box 14.8, some of which are discussed in more detail.

Of course, the first steps of contact with the client are vital to the success of the program in terms of establishing a comfort level, initiating the building of trust and confidence, and generally setting the proper tone for the relationship.

Thereafter, the critical elements of Work Retraining are to:

- Restore dynamic function to the highest achievable levels within the reimbursable time frames and treatment procedures.
- Address the needs of the whole person—the psychosocial needs as well as the physiological.
- Organize treatment professionals and other stakeholders and participants into a team which includes the client as the center of the team's focus.
- Involve the client in understanding the current needs, goal setting, planning, monitoring progress, and making adjustments as progress proceeds.

To better understand the elements within each client's program, it is important to clearly define the difference between the terms Work Hardening, Work Conditioning, and Conditioning. Figure 14.14 illustrates the difference in relationship to the ten elements of consideration. All ten elements will be described briefly here. They are also covered in other chapters in greater detail.

Assessments

There are three types of assessments that are important to provide in Work Conditioning or Work Hardening programs. The FCA, covered in Chapter 13, is the preprogram assessment. Interim Assessments are performed at regular intervals during treatment. The Exit

---

BOX 14.8

Work Conditioning & Work Hardening Program Implementation Outline

A. Scheduling
1. Take the referral
2. Set up the file
3. Schedule the client

B. Intake
1. Intake Interview
2. Orientation to and signing of facility policies
3. Authorization for release of information
4. Client's rights lists
5. Job Analysis or Work Information review

C. Establishing the plan
1. Administer Functional Capacity Assessment (FCA)
2. Review medical history
3. Compare results of FCA with job requirements
4. Develop exit goal
5. Identify length of program
6. Confirm probability of reaching job requirements level
7. If numbers indicate low probability rating, select plan for job modification in those areas
8. Identify starting point
9. Identify weekly progression check
10. Identify body mechanics adaptations needed
11. Identify educational needs
12. Identify exercise needs
13. Plan job simulation activities
14. Identify need for outside services

D. Implementing the plan—key elements
1. Assessments
2. Flexibility/mobility
3. Strengthening
4. Conditioning
5. Job simulation
6. Functional circuit
7. Education—group and individual
8. Vocational rehab (Work Hardening)
9. Psychosocial (Work Hardening)
10. Outcomes

Assessment offers a posttreatment measurement of progress.

Functional Capacity Assessment is an entry point

FIGURE 14.14   Comparison of the terms Work Hardening, Work Conditioning, and Conditioning.

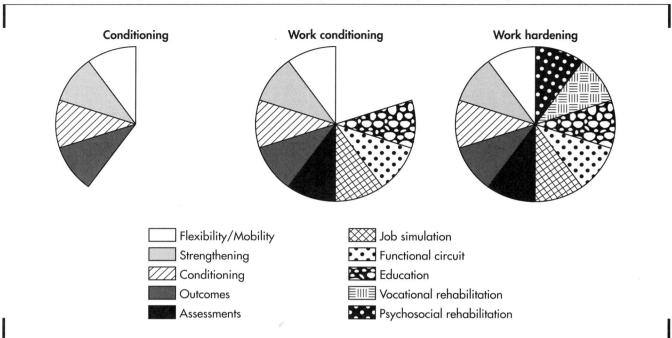

assessment. The results of this assessment are used as a base of data from which treatment plan decisions are made. The results of the FCA include physical capability levels and information specific to the client's validity of participation. Both of these factors are necessary in determining the future management of the plan. Possible uses of the results are enumerated in Figures 14.15 and 14.16.

Figure 14.15 lists options that are likely to result from an assessment that was referred into the clinic as a stand-alone referral. This contrasts with Figure 14.16 which represents recommendations from an FCA that is an integral first step in a Work Retraining program.

An analogy of the use of the FCA in Work Retraining programs can be drawn with the use of an x-ray, in the acute care of a patient. Just as a physician

FIGURE 14.15   Options following a stand-alone Functional Capacity Assessment.

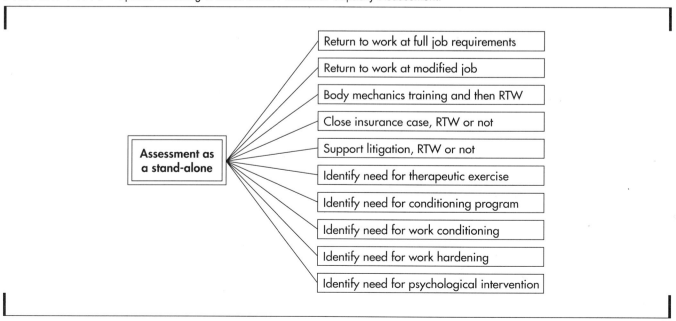

FIGURE 14.16 Uses of a Functional Capacity Assessment in the design and planning of work retraining programs.

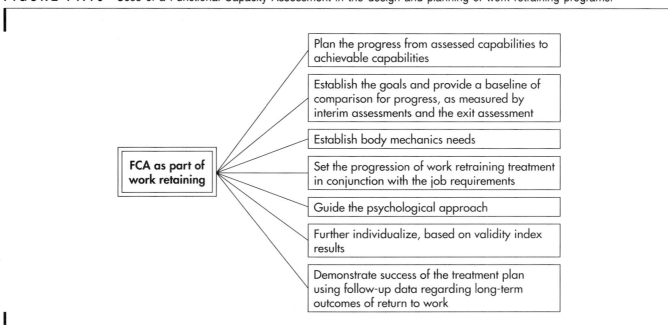

FCA as part of work retaining

- Plan the progress from assessed capabilities to achievable capabilities
- Establish the goals and provide a baseline of comparison for progress, as measured by interim assessments and the exit assessment
- Establish body mechanics needs
- Set the progression of work retraining treatment in conjunction with the job requirements
- Guide the psychological approach
- Further individualize, based on validity index results
- Demonstrate success of the treatment plan using follow-up data regarding long-term outcomes of return to work

is not likely to set a bone until they have a clear picture of its condition, Industrial Therapists do not initiate rehabilitation without a clear picture of the client's initial status and how far they have to go to meet job requirements. This is also consistent with therapists' traditional approach to treatment—evaluate the patient's status prior to treatment.

Interim Assessments are used to objectively monitor progress in the program. In combination with daily documentation, Interim Assessments compare attainment with the baseline data from the initial FCA.

General guidelines for content of each component included is that they must be:[3,21,22]

1. Well structured—Clear policies and procedures consistent with the entry FCA must be followed in order for the results to be valid and reliable.
2. Job related—The physical tasks required must simulate the dynamic functional activities found on the job. It must be possible to measure increases in weighted capabilities, changes in tolerances, posture improvements, and changes in cardiovascular responses. The Assessment must have a direct relationship to the entry FCA and to the job requirements. As it provides capability, tolerance, postural, and cardiovascular measurement results, program plans and goals can be modified if necessary.
3. Easily reproducible—The results should be the same regardless of the Assessment Specialist administering the Assessment.

4. Safe—The procedure must be safe and pose no hazard to the client.
5. Cost effective—As this is performed with each individual every two weeks of the program, one must keep the length of time to a minimum—no more than ten minutes per client is recommended. It is unlikely that a separate billing will be possible. This Assessment must therefore be covered in the standard Work Retraining billing.
6. Ease of documentation—The documentation and reporting of the information should be quick. Also, if it is information that will be distributed, it must be easy to read and understand by those receiving the report.

The Interim Assessment allows the Work Retraining Specialist to indirectly assess pacing skills, flexibility and mobility, postural adaptability, and physical compensation patterns. The cardiovascular response is monitored to assess physical exertion levels at increased capability levels. This provides a ratio on a cardiovascular stress index.[21,23,41]

The Industrial Therapist may also identify efficiencies and inefficiencies of movement, transferability, concentration, memory, follow-through, consistencies of pain reports and behaviors, and patterns of neuromuscular recruitment.

Interim Assessments should be a standard part of any Work Retraining protocols.

Exit Assessments are performed at the conclusion of the Work Conditioning or Work Hardening program, just prior to discharge. This should be the same as, or part of what was used for the entry FCA. Exit Assessments are generally 1½ hours in length. The results should be reported in an overview format, providing a complete picture of initial status, job demands, intervals of progress, and exit status.

Flexibility and Mobility

All participants in both Work Conditioning and Work Hardening will be scheduled for activities of flexibility and mobility. The purpose of these activities is to improve the client's postural adaptability for performance of functional and work related tasks.

These activities are designed to improve circulation, reduce neuromuscular inhibition, provide carryover into functional activities, and improve confidence in the ability to safely move into postures.[48] This is especially important when many postures have not been used for quite some time because of their painful nature. A list of Level 1 flexibility and mobility exercises is presented in Box 14.9. Flexibility and mobility are covered in greater detail in Chapter 15.

Activities are selected on the basis of the client's area of injury, the diagnosis, job requirements, and medical status limitations. These exercises are usually carried out as part of the warm-up and cool-down periods. It is from these exercises that those included in a client's home program will be selected. The home program occurs during the Work Retraining program and continues after completion of the program.

Strengthening

All participants in both the Work Conditioning and Work Hardening programs will be scheduled for strengthening activities specific to their individual needs. The selection of the exercises is based on the results of the Functional Capacity Assessment, the job requirements, and the specific body part that is injured. As with the flexibility and mobility exercises, the Industrial Therapist must consider any medical diagnosis and limitations. Strengthening is covered in greater detail in Chapter 15.

The objectives of the strengthening component are to:
- Develop strength in select areas of the body.
- Work through specific areas of deficits.
- Support general improvement within the program.
- Improve the client's ability to perform the job simulation activities.
- Strengthen body parts to accommodate mechanical stresses that will eventually be placed on the body.

BOX 14.9

Level 1 Flexibility/Mobility Exercises

Common cervical ROM and stretch exercises include:

> Flexion, extension, retraction, rotation, lateral flexion, and upper trapezius stretch.

Common shoulder ROM and stretch exercises include:

> External and internal rotation, horizontal abduction and adduction, extension, Codman's pendulum, and caudal glide

Common back ROM and stretch exercises include:

> Pelvic tilt, single knee to chest stretch, prone on elbows, standing foot on chair low back stretch, and prone back extension.

Common hip and knee ROM and stretch exercises include:

> Inner thigh and groin stretch, seated or supine hamstring stretch, quadriceps stretch, hip flexor stretch, and piriformis stretch.

- Increased localized strength for maintaining static postures necessary for the job.

Strengthening exercises may be carried out using any variety of combination of equipment. Common examples include Universal, Nautilus, Hydrafitness, Keiser, Cybex, and Kincom.

Some strengthening exercises will be taxing to the injured part of the body. Others will not. As a result, it is important to space them out, allowing ample rest and recovery between exercises, especially early in the program.[15,21,42] Once the client has adapted to the activity, and it is not as taxing to the injured body part, the Industrial Therapist is able to include more taxing activities sequencing them more closely together. The sequencing should also progress toward levels similar to the job.

Strengthening exercises should be part of each day of treatment. They should be mixed in with other Work Conditioning and Work Hardening components, such as job simulation, education, functional circuit, and aerobic conditioning activities. Box 14.10 lists the most common strengthening exercise recommended for Work Hardening and Work Conditioning programs.

BOX 14.10

Level 1 Strengthening Exercises

Common cervical strengthening exercises include:

AROM, isometrics, and stabilization exercises.

Common shoulder strengthening exercises include:

AROM, PRE's, plate, hydraulic, pneumatic and isokinetic exercises involving external and internal rotators, supraspinatus, flexion, abduction, biceps, triceps, and rhomboids

Common back strengthening include:

ROM, stabilization, and equipment-specific back extensions, gluteals, and abdominals

Common hip and knee strengthening exercise include:

Quads, hamstrings, abductors, adductors, gastroc, and gluteals

FIGURE 14.17 Work stations that simulate dynamic job functions should be matched to the individual based on job classification, postural treatment needs, and the body part that has been injured.

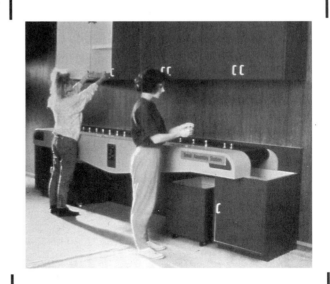

Job Simulation

All participants in both Work Hardening and Work Conditioning programs should be scheduled for job simulation activities.

To identify the specific job tasks to simulate, the Industrial Therapist can use the Job Analysis, a job description, the client's description of the job, or the DOT (Dictionary of Occupational Titles). It is important to *focus only on those capabilities demonstrated by the FCA results to be insufficient relative to the job requirements.*

Work stations that simulate dynamic job functions should be matched to the individual based on:

1. Job classification
2. Postural treatment needs
3. Body part injured (Figure 14.17)

The particular equipment chosen does not have to duplicate the exact job, as long as it includes the relevant postures and motions involved in the job. The goals can be met by using many combinations and varieties of equipment. General types of work stations used in a RTW program are illustrated in Figures 14.18 through 14.26 and include:

Materials Handling. (Figure 14.18) Function: To simulate lifting, manipulating, and moving containers of different sizes and weights to different heights and distances.

OCCUPATIONS:
- Production and stock clerks
- Motor freight
- Transportation
- Packaging and material handling
- Food and beverage preparation
- Museum, library, and archival sciences

COMPONENTS:
- Upright section
- Reversible power conveyor
- Reversible inclined power conveyor
- Adjustable height off-load roller section
- Ten pound weights
- Transition tables
- Roller conveyor
- Tote containers
- Under cabinet lower shelf
- Ladder

Driving simulator. (Figure 14.19) Function: To simulate entry, exit, driving, use of foot pedals, trailer hook-up, and tire repair.

OCCUPATIONS:
- Transportation
- Protective service (police, security guards, fire fighters, etc)
- Mechanics and machinery repair
- Amusement and recreation services

FIGURE 14.18 Materials handling station.

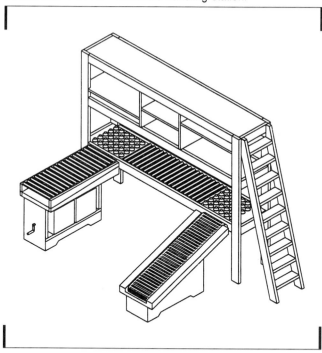

(Copyright KEY Method, April, 1994.)

FIGURE 14.19 Driving simulator.

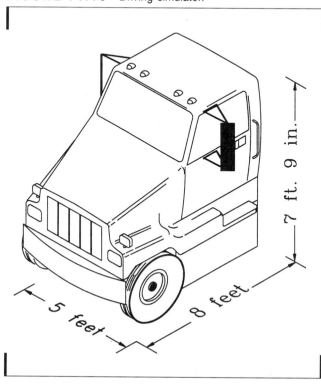

(Copyright KEY Method, April 1994.)

- Excavating, grading, and paving
- Motor freight
- Animal farming
- Forestry
- Route sales and delivery
- Construction
- Plant farming

COMPONENTS:
- Driver station cab
- Trailer dolly crank
- Lug wrench
- Removable weighted tires
- Scissors jack with handle
- Cleaning kit

Building Trades. (Figure 14.20) Function: To simulate working with a broad range of building trades tools and materials using a variety of postures.
OCCUPATIONS:
- Construction
   Carpentry
   Electricians
   Plumbers
   Ductwork installation and cleaning
- Structure work
   Assembly and repair of equipment

COMPONENTS:
- Stud walls and ceiling joists
- Step ladder
- Reusable attachment blocks
- Plumbing activity materials

FIGURE 14.20 Building trades station.

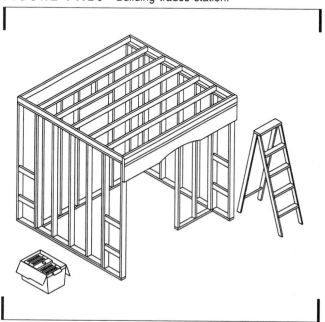

(Copyright KEY Method, April, 1994.)

- Carpentry, electrical, plumbing, and heating tools
- Electrical activity materials

Sorting Station. (Figure 14.21)   Function: To simulate reaching, bending, and stooping forward and manipulating small items using a variety of postures.
OCCUPATIONS:
- Architecture, engineering, and surveying
- Medicine and health
- Clerical, accounting, recording, and computing
- Building and related service occupations
- Machine trade occupations
- Bench-work occupations
- Structural work occupations
- Transportation
COMPONENTS:
- Pigeon hole units with bin drawers
- Time clock with time card racks
- Filing drawers with removable letter and legal size bins

- Weighted flats
- Start-up kit (tube set, small box set, envelope set, hanging file folders, small hardware package, ball set, and time cards)
- Ball sorting station
- Mail cart
- Interchangeable vertical and horizontal sorting slots
- Peg board section with hooks

Position Station. (Figure 14:22)   Function: To simulate manipulating tools and materials using a variety of static and repetitive postures involving upper extremities, spine, and lower extremities.
OCCUPATIONS:
- Mechanics and machinery repair
- Construction
- Patient care workers
- Transportation
- Fishing and related occupations
- Assembly line workers
COMPONENTS:
- Large center table with adjustable height

FIGURE 14.21   Sorting station.

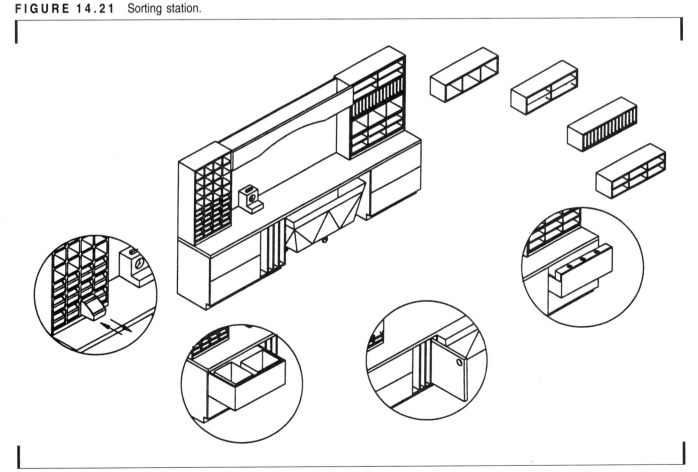

- Movable and interchangeable center flats
- Height adjustable side tables
- Hydraulic adjustment
- Accessory mounting available on flats
- Creeper
- Accessory storage
- Flats interchange with Building Trades Station.

Manual Labor Station. (Figure 14.23) Function: To simulate digging, shoveling, lifting and moving materials using a variety of weights, heights, and postures.

OCCUPATIONS:
- Building and related service occupations
- Structural work
- Packaging occupations
- Material handling occupations
- Excavating and grading occupations
- Ore refining and foundry
- Ambulance drivers
- Feed mill workers
- Construction
- Plant farming
- Animal farming
- Forestry
- Paving and related occupations
- Landscaping and lawn service
- Cemetery workers
- Snow shoveler

COMPONENTS:
- Open base bin
- Adjustable elevated materials bin
- Platform base bin
- Gravel, sand, or rock
- Broom and shovel
- Wheelbarrow

Small Assembly Station. (Figure 14.24) Function: To simulate repetitive assembly of small components using a variety of standing, sitting, and upper extremity postures

OCCUPATIONS:
- Packaging and material handling
- Fabrication, assembly, and repair of products
- Processing food, tobacco, and related products
- Fabrication and repair of products made from assorted materials
- Processing paper and related materials
- Assembly and repair of electrical equipment
- Electrical assembling, installing, and repairing

COMPONENTS:
- Reversible, variable speed conveyor
- Shelving and cabinets
- Safety switches
- Catch bins
- Ring pins
- Small assembly components

FIGURE 14.22   Position station.

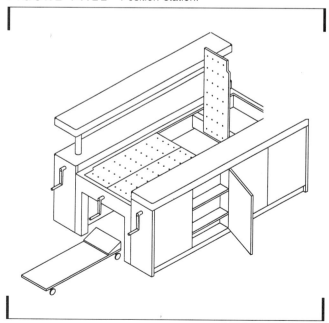

FIGURE 14.23   Manual labor station.

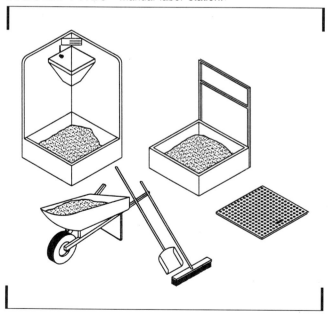

FIGURE 14.24   Small assembly station.

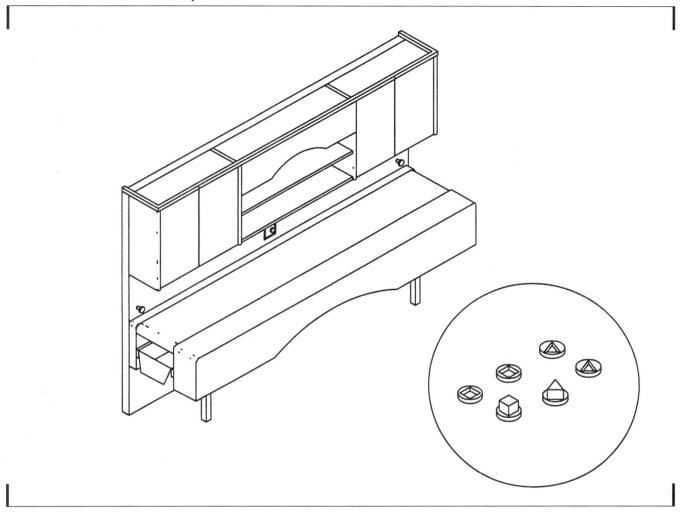

(Copyright KEY Method, April 1994.)

Patient Room Station. (Figure 14.25)   Function: To simulate healthcare and domestic occupations involving beds and other furnishings in a variety of tasks and postures.
OCCUPATIONS:
- Medicine and health
- Emergency services
- Domestic fields (home/hotel/motel)

COMPONENTS:
- Patient room surround
- Patient bed
- Child size mannequin
- Adult size mannequin
- Rolling cabinets
- IV pole
- Stretcher
- Wheel chair
- Curtains
- Bed linen
- Wash basin
- Vest for varying weight of mannequin

Work Table Assembly Station. (Figure 14.26)   Function: To simulate finger, wrist, full upper extremity, back, and lower extremity activities using a variety of body mechanics, heights, and postures.
OCCUPATIONS:
- All bench work occupations
- Electrical assembling, installing, and repairing
- Plant farming
- Animal farming
- Data entry
- Mechanics and machinery repairs
- Packaging and material handling

FIGURE 14.25 Patient room station.

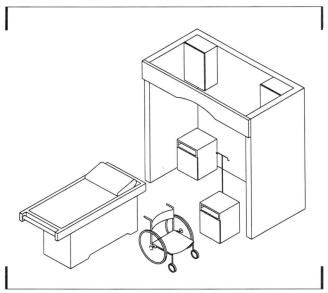

(Copyright KEY Method, April 1994.)

COMPONENTS:

- Table components for assembly
- Storage work cart with top
- Brackets, connectors, nuts, and bolts for assembly
- Multiple option tools for assembly

FIGURE 14.26 Work table assembly station.

As a rule of thumb, a 2,500 square foot facility usually begins with four to five stations that are versatile enough to meet the needs of a number of industry populations (Figure 14.27, *A, B, C*). These are typically augmented by smaller items that also help restore dynamic function, such as gym balls, theraband, theratubing, and sports cords.

The purpose of the job simulation component is to build capabilities of all the musculoskeletal body parts and postures involved in the dynamic functions of the job. If only some of the muscles or joints are strengthened while others remain weak, the returning worker is at risk of reinjury.

As with strengthening exercises, it is important to interspace simulation activities, so the injured body parts are not overtaxed. The progression should be designed to gradually incorporate the job tasks in sequence, while closely simulating the actual sequence and pacing on the job. Job Simulation is covered in greater detail in Chapter 16.

Functional Circuit

The activities included in a Functional Circuit are meant to be a distraction from pain while the individual is carrying out increased levels of postural complexities. To accomplish this purpose, the activities need to be short in duration (about three minutes each). In addition to motivating participation, activities with a

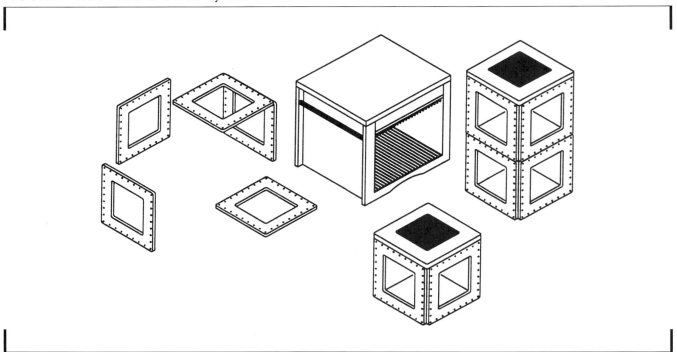

(Copyright KEY Method, April 1994.)

FIGURE 14.27 A, B, C   Rehabilitation goals can be achieved using a variety of equipment, as long as it replicates the relevant postures and motions used in the job.

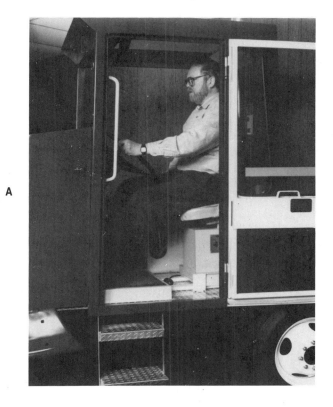

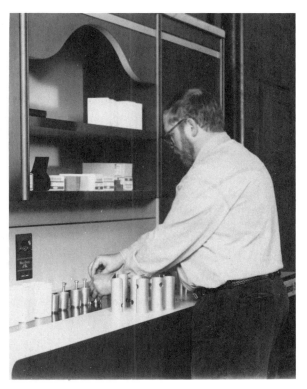

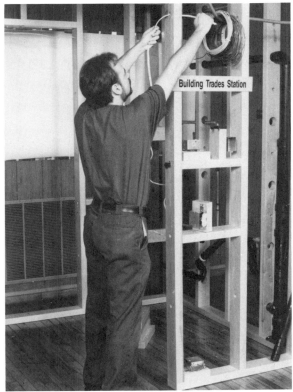

certain amount of enjoyment, contribute to the positive attitude that should be encouraged and nurtured at the center. The total time each day devoted to these activities should be approximately 30 minutes (Figure 14.28, *A, B*).

Functional circuit activities should be based on the SAID principle—Specific Adaptation to Imposed Demands.[41] Activities should be structured to require postures and movements that are in need of rehabilitating and strengthening. One client may be asked to shoot a basketball into the sand bin of a manual labor station, while another client retrieves the ball for the shooter. The shooter is required to reach up and out, bending slightly while the rebounder will have to bend and stoop, reach into the bin with both arms, grasp with both hands, stand up, pivot, and throw.

Such activities provide ample opportunity to carry out instructed postures, or demonstrate that these learned postures are not a part of daily activity yet, and may only be a part of the structured environment.

In monitoring functional circuit activities, the focus for the Industrial Therapist falls into two categories: the direct observations that will also be somewhat obvious to the participants; and the indirect observations, which are more subtle, but just as important.

Direct observation includes the following:

1. The activities included in a standard FCA such as kneeling, crawling, bending, stooping, squatting, reaching, and grasping.

2. Eye-hand coordination
3. Mobility
4. Reports and behaviors
5. Hearing and seeing

Indirect observation includes the following:

1. Pacing
2. Sequencing
3. Ability to follow multiple instructions
4. Safety practices
5. Partner and group responsiveness
6. Guarding
7. Segmental abilities and limitations
8. Motivation and cooperation
9. Consistency

Two examples that illustrate activities, their purpose and possible results are as follows:

Activity A

Two people (one sitting on a creeper and the other standing) toss a small gym ball to each other, attempting to toss within the reach of the receiving person. The standing client may be required to bend and stoop, or reach very high or out to the side. The seated client will be more limited in movement, but will be required to use considerable upper body control.

Activity B

One person rolls or "bowls" a small gym ball

FIGURE 14.28 A, B   Functional circuit activities should be fun while rehabilitating and strengthening relevant postures and movements.

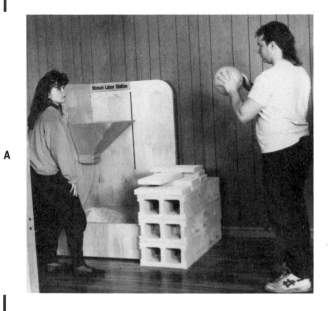

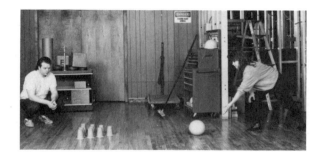

to knock down paper cups. The second person is responsible for retrieving the ball and re-setting up the cups. As one might imagine, this allows the Industrial Therapist to see how both, especially the pick-up person, use their body in bending, stooping, and squatting activities. By adhering to a short time allotted for each person (three minutes), they try to get as many throws in as possible to win the game.

Functional circuit activities are rapid-paced, so clients are more likely to carry out postures that are natural at the time. It can be a humbling experience for the Therapist if the client has been carrying out excellent modified and improved posture during the rest of the program, but when put in a "fun" environment, they do not carry out the new behaviors.

Functional circuits are also a good opportunity to develop client's adaptations to immediate demands. While a client may have been hesitant during work type activities to assume certain postures, the functional circuit activity may bring out the postural goal quite easily, proving to themselves that they are able to do it without the previously feared consequences.

All clients should participate in functional circuit activities, rotating from station to station, as set up by the Therapist or Work Trainer. Activities are usually organized so that the starting point each day is at a different station. With this schedule, all participants perform each activity over a few days time. This is a very active, busy part of the program. Once organized, it is very informative for the therapy staff and enjoyable for the clients and staff.

Education

The needs of a client as he or she progresses through a return-to-work program are numerous and vary with each individual. The client may need to learn basic body mechanics training, as lack of knowledge may have contributed to the injury. The client may need to learn how to perform a job that has been significantly modified to eliminate risk factors. Whatever the individual needs, the overall objective is to educate clients on the proper use of their body to perform jobs comfortably, and to prevent reinjury. Education programs are valuable for personal health, job performance, and long term employment security.

Although the range of education topics is dependent upon the market being served, some topics are felt to be important for safe job performance and functional independence regardless of the category of workers involved. For the purposes of this chapter, these topics will be referred to as "primary topics."

"Secondary topics" are those that may be important to some clients and not others. Many secondary topics may arguably qualify as important enough to be primary, but because of restrictions of staff time and natural restrictions of client availability, triaging is required to focus time on the areas that can have the most impact for the most people.

Primary Topics include Back Education, Upper Extremity Education, and Stress Management.

Back Education is intended primarily to teach proper lifting techniques for prevention of any recurring or potential back injury.

Upper Extremity Education teaches proper use of the upper extremities and prevention of cumulative trauma disorders, of which the most widely known is carpal tunnel syndrome. With the increased movement away from the heavy job categories, more people will be involved in increased use of their wrists and hands. As a result, many practitioners include this as a primary topic, even for those who do not have upper extremity injury (see Figures 14.29, *A, B, C*).

Stress Management is a topic which can take many forms in this setting. The focus may relate to pain control, teaching clients the different techniques of recognizing and managing the stress brought about by physical pain. This can be of significant importance during the work retraining program. It can also provide them with coping skills to properly handle the possible recurrence of pain once they leave the structured program environment.

Stress Management may also encompass the broader area of helping participants deal with overall stresses in their lives. A frequent focus is on the stress brought about by the injury itself. It can be stressful to deal with the complexities of the health care and Workers' Compensation system, or the impact on the family's financial and emotional stability. Stress in one form or another is shared by all participants, and hence is a primary topic of educational programs.

Secondary Topic subject matter is dictated by the needs of the individual clients and the expertise available to the center. Common programs include family relationships postinjury, getting and keeping a job, how to interview, nutrition, drug and alcohol counseling, low impact aerobics, exercise at home and work, weight gain and loss, heart care, understanding the Workers' Compensation system, what to do about pain, and safe work habits. Typically covered in smaller groups and sometimes one-on-one, these secondary topics provide an opportunity for clients to focus on their more individualized and unique needs. These topics provide perspective and guidance that can enhance their lifestyles on and off the job.

It is beneficial to schedule one group education session each week, alternating between primary and

F I G U R E   1 4 . 2 9   A , B , C   Educational programs should incorporate large group sessions emphasizing primary topics and small group or individual sessions focusing on secondary topics.

A

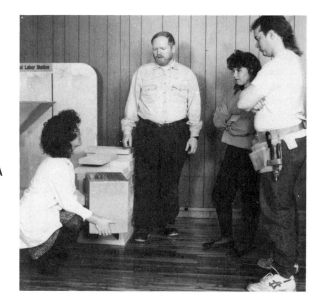

B

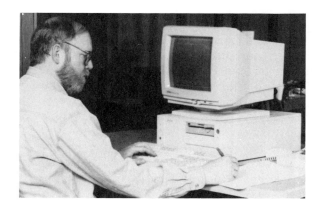

C

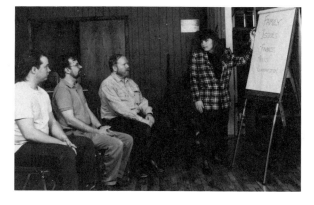

secondary topics every other week. This ensures that in a six week program, each client is exposed to all three primary topics, providing a good base of posture education and coping skills.

The individual study time, defined clearly in the schedule for the client, should be assigned according to the very specific needs of that individual. Video tapes, computer programs, reading materials, and worksheets should be made available wherever possible to facilitate the learning process.

In individual sessions, material from the group sessions may be reviewed where special emphasis is warranted. An individual session may also focus on an exercise or topic that is hard for a particular client to master.

It is important to consider the different learning styles of clients when structuring the programs, to permit the highest possible transfer of usable information to them. The daily individual education sessions are most commonly scheduled following a more strenuous, physically taxing activity. They occur when other clients can be kept busy in group activities. Education is covered in more detail in Chapter 17.

The Vocational Rehabilitation Consultant

It is important that the Industrial Therapist understand the role of the Vocational Rehabilitation Consultant (VRC). There are many titles this person may have; Rehabilitation Coordinator, Case Manager, Vocational

Rehabilitation Counselor, Vocational Expert, Rehabilitation Specialist. The responsibilities may vary minimally or greatly. It is necessary to take them on a case-by-case basis.

For the purpose of this chapter, this area of specialization will be called Vocational Rehabilitation Consultant (VRC) and a broad spectrum of responsibilities is assumed.

The VRC may be a self-employed practitioner having contracts with a variety of entities. Clients may be industry, insurance carriers, other rehabilitation firms, case management organizations, attorneys, third party administrators, or the State Workers' Compensation Fund. The VRC could also be a direct employee of any of the above.

The role of the VRC specific to Work Conditioning and Work Hardening programs can be organized into five major categories.

1. Referral source
2. Communication and information facilitator between parties
3. Source for specialty testing and needs
4. Guidance and advisory
5. Facilitator for processing of paperwork, billings, and payment

As a *referral source* the VRC's focus is to facilitate the return-to-work process for their client. This includes recommending providers for assessments and programs of treatment. Counselors have many options available to them on where to refer clients. It is up to the therapist to assure that vocational counselors are aware of services and quality outcomes.

As a *communication and information facilitator*, the VRC may be involved in fulfilling the considerable information and communication needs of all parties involved. This can be one of the overwhelming challenges in a return-to-work program. In this role the VRC offers a welcome, competent reprieve for the Therapist. It is this author's experience that VRC's are very effective in handling sensitive issues between the employee and the employer, like when an employee may be afraid of a particular job, or the employer may not want the employee back.

The barriers to reentry to work take many forms. If the client is experiencing complications in receiving Workers' Compensation benefits on a timely manner, the VRC can be instrumental in correcting the problem. If the client has transportation issues, either in getting to treatment or to work, the VRC often has knowledge of resources to overcome that. When job modification is found to be helpful or necessary, the VRC may be the person most effective in bringing about the necessary changes. This is also true if the Therapist is

recommending job rotations and transfers within a company or department. When new employment is required, it is often the VRC who has current information on job availability within the company, industry, or other sources for employment (Figure 14.30).

Another very important contribution the VRC often makes is in accessing needed records. Due to the relationship with all parties involved, VRC's can be very resourceful in gathering and compiling medical records, job descriptions, job matching needs, availability of job retraining, compliance history, and vocational and psychological testing results.

Finally, the VRC is a clearing house and communicator of issues and problems arising from all parties involved in the client's rehabilitation. This function facilitates goal congruence and coordination among the rehabilitation team members. In this role, the VRC should participate and provide input in the staffing meetings on each client. The VRC can provide valuable information regarding case management and resolution as well as coordinate services with other specialties.

As a *source for specialty testing and needs,* the VRC is a key referral source for the Industrial Therapist's Functional Capacity Assessment services.[47] Such referrals arise from the VRC's need for information specific to the client's capabilities, in order to support case resolution.

In addition to referrals into the program, they will be identifying mental and emotional capabilities to

FIGURE 14.30 The Vocational Rehabilitation Consultant can be a valuable resource to the Industrial Therapist in providing referrals, assisting in specialty testing, and facilitating communication and coordination with other parties.

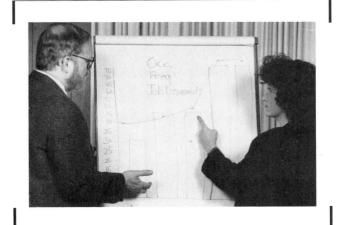

facilitate return to the competitive work environment for the client. This may include medical tests such as MRIs, EMGs, and x-rays. It may also include standard capability tests such as Purdue Pegboard, Minnesota Rate of Manipulation, or Functional Capacity Assessments. Interest, aptitude, and IQ testing may unveil the need for psychological testing recommendations.

The VRC is a good resource for the Industrial Therapist when there are complicating factors interfering with a treatment program. The expertise that both parties bring to problem solving is exceeded only by their mutual commitment to the client.

As a provider of *guidance and advisory*, VRC's are able to leverage their relationships with all parties involved to assist with consultation. These include the cost and productivity concerns of the industry, the fiscal responsibility of the insurance company, the legal rights of all parties involved, and the best interest of the client.

VRC's can be especially assistive in working with clients who are embroiled in compliance issues. Even well motivated clients can be hampered by home and family complications. Some case problems can be resolved with the intervention of the VRC alone. Where psychological intervention is warranted, the VRC will be able to advise accordingly.

The legal rights of the client are closely safeguarded by the VRC. In light of this, relevant legal questions that the Industrial Therapist may have can be directed to the VRC.

As a *paperwork and payment facilitator* it is not uncommon for the VRC, as liaison for all parties, to be asked to intervene on behalf of the client for expediting necessary paperwork, including the processing of bills. VRCs recognize the importance of treating providers with fairness, to maintain a positive atmosphere that maximizes the clients chances for success.

There may be situations in which the role of the VRC overlaps with that of the Claims Adjuster or other rehabilitation specialists. It is important to clarify the roles in each case, to assure goal congruence and optimum orchestration of all parties involved.

Working With The VRC. The VRC can be so instrumental as a referral source in bringing clients and problem solving, during case progression, that meeting the VRC's needs should be high on the Therapist's priority list. In handling VRC referrals, therefore, the Industrial Therapist should seek to ensure:

1. Prompt admission into FCA and the return-to-work program
2. Prompt reporting—verbal and written
3. Clear reporting—easy to read and explain
4. Responsive reporting—answers the specific questions that have been asked
5. Clear recommendations with sufficient supporting documentation
6. Goal setting congruent with the case plan
7. Clear delineation of time frames
8. Solution-oriented approach to problems
9. Defensible assessment and treatment protocols
10. Standardization and consistency of approach and outcomes
11. Flexibility to accommodate unique needs of each client

Each member of the rehabilitation team is in a position to positively impact the efforts of other team members, and the client's prospects for an expeditious and safe return to work. Helping VRCs perform their facilitating functions, and reinforcing the appropriateness of their referrals, can be important ingredients in the Industrial Therapist's success. Vocational Rehabilitation from a VRC's perspective is covered in detail in Chapter 19.

Psychosocial Factors

Psychosocial considerations are important for a well rounded Work Hardening program. In fact, the psychological component is one of the primary defining differences between Work Hardening and Work Conditioning. As defined by CARF and APTA, Work Hardening includes addressing the psychological issues as an integral but independent element of the Work Hardening treatment program.[1,10] Work Conditioning does not include this focus (Box 14.11).

Work Hardening is designed to return the injured person to work level capability. It is important to recognize that physical impairment is often only one of the deterrents for return to work, and that psychosocial factors are almost always present.[5,11,21,26,27,28,29,32]

One of the important issues for the Industrial Therapist to remember is that the Psychologist is there to further the return-to-work progress. It is the responsibility of the Program Director to select the appropriate professionals and practitioners who are interested and willing to become members of the client's Rehabilitation Team.

The Psychologist will be responsible for selected group meetings, individual counseling when appropriate, and will have input into the initial program plan, weekly reviews, and the continuum of care for specific clients, and for all program clients in general.

Triggers that indicate a potential need for psychosocial intervention regarding a specific client include:

CARF Work Hardening Definition:

Work Hardening is a highly structured, goal-oriented, individualized treatment program designed to maximize the person's ability to return to work. Work Hardening Programs are interdisciplinary in nature with a capability of addressing the functional, physical, behavioral, and vocational needs of the person served. Work Hardening provides a transition between the initial injury management and return to work, while addressing the issues of productivity, safety, physical tolerances, and work behaviors. Work Hardening Programs use real or simulated work activities in a relevant work environment in conjunction with physical conditioning tasks. These activities are used to progressively improve the biomechanical, neuromuscular, cardiovascular/metabolic, behavioral, attitudinal, and vocational function of the person served.

APTA Work Conditioning Definition:

Work Conditioning is a work related, intensive, goal-oriented treatment program specifically designed to restore an individual's systemic, neuro-musculo-skeletal (strength, endurance, movement, flexibility, and motor control), and cardiopulmonary functions. The objective of the Work Conditioning program is to restore the client's physical capacity and function so the client can return to work.

APTA Work Hardening Definition:

Work Hardening is a highly structured, goal-oriented, individualized treatment program designed to return the person to work. Work Hardening programs, which are interdisciplinary in nature, use real or simulated work activities designed to restore physical, behavioral, and vocational functions. Work Hardening addresses the issues of productivity, safety, physical tolerances, and worker behaviors.

1. A conditionally valid or invalid determination on the Validity Index of FCA results
2. Indications of little or no communication with coworkers or the employer since injury
3. Compliance issues such as tardiness or not showing up at all for daily scheduled activities
4. Being disruptive in either the group sessions or as a coworker with other clients
5. Revealing thoughts or actions related to suicide or other violence against self or others
6. Demonstrating good progress until shortly before discharge, at which time old pains or problems reappear
7. Demonstrating inability to work with equipment that simulates the equipment the client was using upon injury

It can be seen from these examples that the level of intervention required can range from telephoning the employer to reestablish communication and involvement, to bringing in a psychologist to deal with a potentially life threatening situation.

The Therapist must develop the knowledge and ability to identify not only when outside experts are warranted, but also what kind of expertise is needed. Issues of immobilizing fear and severe anger may need to be addressed by a person credentialed for those issues. For each issue that may arise, there is an outside professional or consultant with sufficient expertise to handle it. These experts can also be instrumental in program planning to address the particular needs involved.

It is this author's experience and recommendation that it is important to bring on professionals, whether independent or a group practice, who are interested and willing to become part of the Work Retraining Team. All team members must understand the unique return-to-work process from medical, legal, insurance, and social viewpoints.

The psychosocial specialist should have experience in subject matter that includes:

1. Pain management—distraction techniques, relaxation and imagery, and medication
2. Dependencies
3. Fear of return-to-work
4. Employee/employer relationship issues
5. Managing family and work issues
6. Pain and cultural belief systems
7. Coworker issues
8. Anxiety and stress management techniques
9. The "injured" self image syndrome

These are the topics that psychologists must be prepared to address with clients. It is important that professionals recognize their role in supporting the return-to-work focus of the program. This will be monitored by the Industrial Therapist in connection with progress and goal setting.

Recognizing the need to rehabilitate the whole person, psychosocial factors—present to some degree in every case—must be understood and covered in treatment planning. With attention to signals that indicate the severity of need, Therapists may opt to include a professional psychologist or counselor on the client's rehabilitation team. At all times, the focus is on furthering return-to-work progress. Psychological aspects of rehabilitation are covered in more detail in Chapter 18.

Outcomes

Pressure to increase productivity and reduce costs has focused a great deal of scrutiny on Industrial Therapy programs and procedures. As a result, there is growing demand for outcome studies that enable quantified cost-payout analysis.[17,26,38] This is particularly important with newer treatment approaches.[37] The complexity of Work Hardening complicates the communication and decision process. Outcome studies that address bottom line results define what is really important to prospects.

A study by Sachs et al. found that 45 clients with spinal dysfunction benefited significantly from Work Retraining.[38] Compared to 33 similarly impaired clients who did not participate, the Work Retraining participants had higher employment rates at six months (73% versus 38%).

A study by Mayer found that 116 chronic low back pain clients who participated in Work Retraining had higher return to work rates than 72 nonparticipants (85% versus 39%).[26] In the first year after the program, participants also had lower incidences of additional surgery (4% versus 12%) and lower incidences of doctor visits (33% versus 75%).

There are a limited number of published outcome studies that serve to substantiate the benefits of Work Hardening. Therapists should develop their own outcome tracking program. With it they can better tailor treatment to a specific client base, improve assessment and treatment procedures overall, support treatment and reimbursement, and market Industrial Therapy services to new prospects.

There are three categories of outcomes that should be measured to fully evaluate Work Retraining programs:

1. Clinical solutions—Return to work and reinjury percentages
2. Satisfaction surveys—Client and Referral Source
3. Follow-up client reports—Six and 12 months post RTW

Specific measures worth including are:

- Length of time between injury and start of Work Retraining
- Length of time between start of Work Retraining and RTW
- Program components administered
- Return to work status:
    Same employer/same job
    Same employer/modified job
    Same employer/different job
    Different employer/same job
    Different employer/modified job
    Different employer/different job
    Not reemployed

- Reinjury rates

Further insight and analysis is gained by comparing these measures to the following:

- Attendance record
- Days in the program
- Having reached or not reached goal
- Litigation status present and at time of treatment
- Having completed or not completed program
- Reason for discharge
- Time interval from discharge to date of work
- Date of injury to date of admission into program

By monitoring clients on these measures, results can be tracked to assess whether the Work Retraining programs yielded the prevention, return-to-work, or productivity outcomes that were sought. In some instances, outcome studies may indicate shortcomings in Work Retraining procedures that the Therapist may have been using for years. In such instances, paradigms may have to be broken.

Sachs et al. report their results of adding the B-200 Isostation (isometric strength testing, ROM measurement, and velocity of motion monitoring) to a work tolerance rehabilitation program. They found no statistical difference in the improvement of the patients' functional capabilities with the additional exercise routine.[39] Often, it is as important to find out what does not make a difference, as it is to confirm what does.

With the growing presence of reimbursement caps, there is increasing pressure to reduce treatment procedures to the lowest common denominator at the expense of quality. Outcome studies can be used to relieve these sources of pressure—to defend against further cuts in cost or quality, or to support that reductions can be achieved without adverse consequences.

KEY ISSUES AND STRATEGIES IN WORK RETRAINING

Some critical issues in Work Hardening and Work Conditioning deserve special focus because of their impact on the success of the client and on the industrial therapy practice itself.

Pain Issues

It is important that pain does not play a major role in Work Retraining. Goals within a program should provide strategies for management of pain, but only inasmuch as they support the central, RTW focus. The emphasis is on function, not pain.

An Industrial Therapist might instruct a client to stop when the heart rate elevates to 130 bpm. This differs from a traditional therapeutic program where the Therapist might have the client go to the point of pain.

An Industrial Therapist is less likely to start out the day with questions like, "How are you today?," so as not to focus on pain but redirect attention toward abilities. The traditional Therapist, however, would purposely ask a pain question to obtain guidance on the changing location, character, and intensity of the pain itself.

It is the responsibility of the Industrial Therapist to develop strategies to assist in clinical management of an individual's pain. This begins with a determination as to whether the pain is simply discomfort from exertion or actual damage to the muscle tissues. Remedies may include individual educational sessions, deemphasis on pain drawings and pain scales, creation of partner or "buddy activities," and possibly psychologist intervention in one of the monthly meetings.

In attempting pain management strategies, there are many variables that influence the client's response to pain:

1. *The extent or severity of pain.* Is it a mild dull ache or the intensity of a stab wound or heart attack?
2. *The duration of the pain.* Does it come and go, and do only certain activities trigger it, or relieve it?
3. *The genesis of the pain.* A person's response to pain from a severed limb would be quite different from their response to a gradually developed musculoskeletal injury.
4. *The current stage of the pain.* How long the pain condition has existed and how it is handled by the medical community has an influence on the impact it has on the client.
5. *The client's cultural background.* Some ethnicities have religious or cultural responses to pain that affect their response. It may be considered proper penance for sins to bear the pain or an admirable act of bravery to ignore it. It is important for Industrial Therapists to become knowledgeable about such beliefs.
6. *Fear and anxiety levels.* These vary from individual to individual and can be responsible for differences in the perception of pain. They can also produce cardiovascular and physiological changes that will modify the response to pain. Neural mechanisms can be effected which modulate transmission in primary pathways or modify emotional reaction.
7. *Psychosocial influences.* These can be one of the hardest hurdles because of the multiple and ever changing variables involved. For ex-

ample, family issues such as severe role modifications, loss of breadwinner status, financial hardships, and loss of influence in decisions. Even the inability to attend children's sports activities can significantly exacerbate response to pain. Similarly, loss of camaraderie due to the inability to participate in extracurricular activities can also influence the client's perception of and response to pain.

8. *Monetary award.* It is becoming all too well known that exaggerating the severity of pain, perhaps even unknowingly, can yield significant monetary settlements.

The Industrial Therapist must understand the above influences on pain response. The Therapist must be able to manage the program to extinguish negative, unproductive behavior and foster self-management of pain to control and change its influence on progress. Some strategies to accomplish this include:

- Identify consistencies and inconsistencies with performance; activity to activity, day to day, and week to week
- Monitor changes in the location, character, and intensity of the pain
- Request assistance at Staffings
- Make appropriate changes in the treatment program
- Educate for adaptive postures
- Educate for proper understanding of acceptable and unacceptable types of pain
- Prepare for initial increase discomfort level with an increase in difficulty in the program
- Make appropriate referrals when necessary to group sessions, psychologist, physicians, and therapists

Pain can and does have an influence on an individual's safe physical functional capabilities and tolerances. It may be a protective agent, preventing reinjury, or a barrier to recovery. The Industrial Therapist must establish a structured program that assists in the tracking and management of this influential variable.

Clinical and Physical Issues

Often during the course of a Client's program, issues regarding clinical or physical phenomena arise that require careful consideration and creativity. Some of the more common ones are as follows:

Issue. The Client is pacing self too fast.
Strategy. The Therapist should confirm the determination and help the client develop safer pacing, using additional reference points such as heart rate. Otherwise, the client may be at risk upon RTW.

Issue. The Client is quitting activities prematurely while demonstrating consistent but questionable workstyles and postures.

Strategy. The Therapist or Work Trainer should teach proper methods while also modifying weights and activities temporarily until learning takes place.

Issue. Inexperience with equipment or an exercise is inhibiting performance.

Strategy. The Therapist or Work Trainer must give accurate instruction, provide encouragement and support, then observe and address any incorrect techniques.

Issue. The Client experiences increased pain while performing an exercise.

Strategy. The Therapist must help client differentiate between tissue damage pain and conditioning discomfort, then address each separately and accordingly.

Issue. The Client reports discomfort.

Strategy. The Therapist should use accurate judgment on whether to respond, so as not to either encourage indiscriminate reports of unimportant episodes, or ignore important ones.

Issue. The Client displays anxiety progressing to more demanding activities.

Strategy. The Therapist must educate the Client as to the physiological dynamics and benefits involved in transitioning to more demanding levels.

Motivational and Mental Issues

Emotions and psychosocial factors are important influences as mentioned a number of times in this chapter. Although it is impossible to anticipate every situation, some of the more common ones can be mentioned:

Issue. The Client is not adhering to the program rules to which agreed at the beginning of the program.

Strategy. The Therapist or Work Trainer must initiate communication to examine the possible causes, then work with the Client, possibly with the help of other peers and providers, to renew commitment and abide by it.

Issue. The Client perceives, accurately or not, a lack of employer support for return to work.

Strategy. The Therapist must help reestablish communication between the Client and employer, and draw the employer into closer involvement with the program. The employer could be invited to visit the center for a one-on-one review of the program and the employee's progress.

Issue. The Client is encountering problems at home.

Strategy. The Therapist must initiate communication to examine the possible causes, then enlist appropriate educational or professional resources to help overcome this barrier to recovery.

Issue. The Client exhibits depression.

Strategy. The Therapist must thoroughly document observations, report to the physician and other team members, possibly followed by professional consultation.

Issue. The Client questions other program participants about the timeliness of Workers' Compensation checks.

Strategy. The Therapist should initiate a one-on-one with the Client to ascertain any problems and initiate corrective action, while emphasizing the importance of not discussing this topic with other clients.

Issue. The Client is working too slowly.

Strategy. The Therapist should confirm the determination and help the client meet the weight, endurance, and output requirements. This involves alleviating barriers, building motivation, rewarding progress, and instilling confidence. Additional reference points such as heart rate may also be used. If the pace is not increased, the client may not be reemployable.

Issue. The Client is quitting activities prematurely for no apparent reason.

Strategy. The Therapist or Work Trainer should observe and accurately document the pattern, then initiate communication to examine the possible causes and discuss the consequences, including possible termination from the program.

Issue. The Client does not trust that the medical system or the program staff is providing proper care or prognosis as to program completion dates and return to work options.

Strategy. The Therapist must communicate clearly with the Client, employ objective methods of predicting completion dates, and enlist the Client's participation and consensus in setting realistic treatment goals and plans.

Issue. The Client demonstrates inconsistent capabilities from station to station.

Strategy. The Therapist or Work Trainer should accurately document the observations, discuss them with the Client, and gain agreement on corrective measures.

Issue. The Client reports that prior experience with exercise has been ineffective.

Strategy. The Therapist or Work Trainer should explain to the Client the work-related reasons for and science behind the exercise, using outcome studies for support where available.

Issue. The Client inappropriately schedules outside appointments such as dentist or eye doctor appointments that conflict with treatment times.

Strategy. The Therapist must reiterate to the Client the importance of adhering to the program schedules in order to successfully meet the return to work goals. If necessary, the Therapist might enlist the help of other peers and rehabilitation team members to reinforce and support the Client's recommitment to the rules.

Issue. The Client offers a negative verbal response to virtually every aspect of program activities or instruction.

Strategy. One remedy would be to persuade this Client to commit every reaction to writing, and to make declining written reports an important program goal. The Client should also be made aware that this pattern may delay or prevent their return to work.

Issue. The Client assigns blame to the Therapist or Work Trainer for consequences they anticipate or experience. "If I can't sleep tonight because of this exercise, it's your fault."

Strategy. The Therapist or Work Trainer should help the Client realize that he or she is the beneficiary of the program, not a victim.

Combination Clinical and Motivational Issues

Often, issues are a combination of both clinical and motivational factors. The more commonly recurring ones are as follows:

Issue. Client reports a minor injury from the previous day.

Strategy. The Therapist and Work Trainer must establish at the beginning of the program, and reinforce where necessary throughout, that all injuries, however minor, must be documented when they occur. The general rule is, "If it isn't documented, it did not happen."

Issue. The Client evidences fear of reinjury.

Strategy. The Therapist or Work Trainer should accurately document the observations and discuss the issue with the Client. They may then educate the Client as to the physiological dynamics and benefits involved in progressing to more demanding levels, so that knowledge can overcome fear of the unknown.

Issue. The Client does not take some of the activities seriously.

Strategy. The Therapist or Work Trainer must reit-

erate that certain activities are interim steps in the "part to whole" progression toward dynamic work functions.

Issue. The Client does not follow instructions, either on purpose, through forgetfulness, or inability.

Strategy. The Therapist or Work Trainer must ensure that instruction, demonstration, and coaching are practical and understandable. Where Clients still fail to follow instructions, staff must emphasize the importance of safety and meeting RTW goals in predicted time frames (Box 14.12).

The Dictionary of Occupational Titles

It is difficult to get an accurate understanding of the requirements of a job without the benefit of a well written job description. There are times, when an accurate job description is not available and it is not an

---

BOX 14.12

Case Example
Union Issues[5]

Problem:
Client G works at his job four hours per day and spends two hours in Work Conditioning. Employer would take him back at six hours per day. Union contract requires he go back at either four or eight hours per day.

Solution Options:
Client G must first have a Functional Capacity Assessment. With a formula process, an accurate work day tolerance is established. From here, the options are dependent on the Functional Capacity Assessment results.

- If the results are eight hours or more, client can return to work at full eight hours per day.
- If the results are less than eight hours, have a joint meeting with employer, client, and union representative to persuade them to heed the FCA results, primarily for reasons of safety.
- Explain to all parties that the employee can return at six hours per day and progress to eight over a few months time.
- Start with four hours on the job and build the additional four hours of capability in the Work Hardening Center.

option for the therapist to perform a Job Analysis. It is in this circumstance that the Dictionary of Occupational Titles (DOT) becomes a valuable resource.[13]

An Industrial Therapist should know how this resource works. These job classifications, as defined by the Department of Labor cover nine primary categories, including a "Miscellaneous" category. In the most current edition, 1991, the Physical Demand Level (sedentary, light, medium, heavy, very heavy) is indicated for each job.

The complete code for each job classification contains nine digits. The first number represents the primary classification. As numbers are added, they represent a finer designation of the requirements or makeup of that job. The third, fourth, and fifth digits represent the responsibility and judgment required of the worker in areas of data, people, and things.

Insurance companies, industry, and rehabilitation counselors classify occupations using the DOT. It may not cover all jobs, and many jobs do not fit the precise description. It is however, the most comprehensive listing that presently exists and is used as a standard.

All clients' and patients' files should be designed to capture this code. Most Industrial Therapists' record only the first three digits of the code. Without it, it is unlikely that the therapist or facility is gathering data by occupational groupings.

The description of a particular job, as found in the DOT, can be included as part of the correspondence in cases where the Industrial Therapist does not have access to a job description. In such instances, reference and comparisons can be made to the job description as found in the DOT.

Another example of use is when a Work Retraining client has no specific job in which to return, and hence, no specific job description. If it can be assumed that the injured worker will most likely return to similar types of work, the DOT description will provide overall information that can be used to help identify work related goals.

The categorization of work demands is very broad, ranging from sedentary to very heavy. The DOT does not provide specific "pound" weighted requirements. It will not classify a job as requiring sixty pounds of lifting. It will instead, identify the job as having a "heavy" Physical Demand Level (PDL).

SIC Codes

Another classification that Industrial Therapists are using more often is the Standard Industrial Classification or SIC code.[44] These are employer industry classifications. Using the SIC code in combination with the DOT code further refines the segmentation of job types. Truck drivers in the agriculture industry have different demands and risks than those in manufacturing. This distinction becomes more meaningful with more discriminating use of database contents.

SUMMARY

The many components of Work Conditioning and Work Hardening have evolved because they address injured workers' needs between acute care and return to work. After acute care, the injured body part may be healed but not ready for an eight hour workday; other muscles and limbs may have been deconditioned; psychosocial problems may be hampering progress; and the worker needs help in preventing reinjury. Programs and procedures that address these needs, while benefiting the bottom line, have gained growing acceptance among health care professionals, insurers, and employers.

Physical and Occupational Therapists have traditionally treated patients after acute care and have been the natural recipients of return-to-work business. To serve this market, Industrial Therapists are offering programs in specially equipped centers, on-site, or both.

In most programs, practitioners have also adopted the team concept in which a multiplicity of professionals and disciplines are coordinated around the worker as focal point. The worker's employer, family, and peers are often brought into involvement.

A central focus of Work Conditioning and Work Hardening has been to simulate dynamic job functions and weights. The purpose is to ensure that the relevant musculoskeletal capabilities are properly developed to meet job demands. In designing simulation stations, it is not necessary to exactly duplicate the work station or equipment, only the components required to condition the relevant body parts.

Functional Capacity Assessment at intake, interim points, and exit have been instrumental in goal setting, planning, monitoring progress, and delineating safe performance levels on the job. FCAs can help determine the required length of the program, and whether the client is participating validly.

Since Work Retraining involves increasing innovation and complexity, numerous issues arise, answers which cannot be found in manuals or journals. For this reason, it is important for practitioners to be open to continued learning, flexible, and resourceful enough to improvise where the knowledge or resources may not yet exist.

In all, Work Conditioning and Work Hardening have brought about increased RTW rates, accelerated time frames, increased restored function and productivity, reduced reinjury, and lower costs.

REFERENCES

1. American Physical Therapy Association, 1101 17th Street Northwest Suite 1000, Washington, DC 20036

2. Andersson GBJ, Pope MH, Frymoyer JW, Snook S: Epidemiology and Cost, *Occupational Low Back Pain: Assessment, Treatment & Prevention*. St Louis 1991 Mosby.

3. Andersson GBJ, Duncan J, Troup G: Worker Selection, In *Occupational Low Back Pain: Assessment, Treatment & Prevention*. St Louis, 1991 Mosby.

4. Baran-Ettipio BJ, Centeno EJ: Early Return-to-Work Programs, *WORK* 3(3), 1993.

5. Baum B et al: Clinical Problem Solving: Working with Industrial Clients, Minn Industrial PT Study Group, a symposium, Minnesota APTA Spring Conference, April 22, 1994.

6. Bigos et al: Back Injuries In Industry: A Retrospective Study. III. Employee-related Factors, *Spine* 3(3), 1986.

7. Bigos SJ, Spengler DM, Martin NA, Zeh J, Fisher L, Nachemson A, Wang MH: Back Injuries in Industry: a Retrospective study, II Injury Factors, *Spine* 2(3), 1986.

8. Campion MA: Personnel Selection for Physically Demanding Jobs: review and recommendations, *Personnel Psych* 36:527–550, 1983.

9. Certo CME: Enhancing Cardiopulmonary Function, In Scully RM, Barnes MR: *Physical Therapy* by Scully, Philadelphia, 1989 JB Lippincott.

10. Commission on Accreditation of Rehabilitation Facilities (CARF), *Standards Manual for Organizations Serving People with Disabilities.* Tucson, Arizona, 1992.

11. Demers L: *Work Hardening, A Practical Guide,* 1992 Andover Medical Publishers.

12. Doherty C: Beyond Work Hardening 101, WORK 1(1), Fall 1990.

13. *Dictionary of Occupational Titles,* U.S. Department of Labor Employment and Training Administration 1991, Vol. II, ed 4, Rev. 1991.

14. Frymoyer JW, Andersson GBJ: Clinical Classification, *Occupational Low Back Pain: Assessment, Treatment & Prevention,* St Louis 1991 Mosby.

15. Frymoyer JW, Haldetman S, Andersson GBJ: Impairment Rating—The United States Perspective, in *Occupational Low Back Pain: Assessment, Treatment & Prevention.* St Louis 1991 Mosby.

16. Graly JM, Yi S, Jensen GM, Gibson M, Laborde T: Factors Influencing Return to Work for Clients in a Work Hardening Center, *WORK* 4(1) 1994.

17. Hazard RG, Fenwick JW, Kalisch SM, et al: Functional Restoration with Behavioral Support: a one year prospective study of patients with low-back pain, *Spine* 14:157–161, 1989.

18. Hazard RG, Matheson LN, Lehmann TR, Frymoyer JW: Rehabilitation of the Patient with Chronic Low Back Pain, *Occupational Low Back Pain: Assessment, Treatment & Prevention.* St Louis 1991 Mosby.

19. Key GL: *Key Functional Assessment Leaders Guide: Training and Resource Manual,* 1984.

20. Key GL: *Key Functional Assessment Policy and Procedure Manual,* 1984.

21. Key GL: *Key Work Retraining Operating Systems Manual,* 1992.

22. Keyserling WM, Herrin GD, Chaffin DB: "Isometric Strength Testing as a Means of Controlling Medical Incidents on Strenuous Jobs, *J Occup Medicine* 22:332-336, 1980.

23. Mangine R, Heckman TP, Eldridge VL: Improving Strength, Endurance, & Power, *Physical Therapy,* 1989.

24. Masset D, Malchaire J: Low Back Pain. Epidemiologic Aspects and Work Related Factors in the Steel Industry. *Spine* 19(2), 1994.

25. Matheson LN, Mooney V, et al: Effect of Instructions on Isokinetic Trunk Strength Testing Variability, Reliability, Absolute Value, and Predictive Validity, *Spine* 17(8), Aug 1992.

26. Mayer TG, et al: A Prospective Two Year Study of Functional Restoration in Industrial Low Back Injury, *JAMA,* 258, Oct 1987.

27. Mayer TG, Gatchel RJ, Kishino N et al: Objective Assessment of Spine Function Following Industrial Injury. A Prospective Study with Comparison Group and One-Year Follow-up, *Spine* 10(6), 1985.

28. Mayer TG, Mooney J, Gatchel RJ: *Contemporary Conservative Care for Painful Spinal Disorders,* Philadelphia, 1991 Lea & Febiger.

29. Menard MR, Hoens AM: Objective Evaluation of Functional Capacity: Medical, Occupational, & Legal Settings, *JOSPT* 19(5), May 1994.

30. Moffroid MT, Aja D, Laflin K, Haugh LD, Henry S: Efficacy of a Part-time Work Hardening Program for Persons with Low Back Pain, *WORK* 3(3), 1993.

31. Moffroid MT, Zimny N: Musculoskeletal Causes, In Scully RM, Barnes MR *Physical Therapy.* Philadelphia, 1989, JB Lippincott.

32. Morrison MH: Rehabilitation and Return to Work. Do Other Countries Succeed?, *WORK* 3(1), 1993.

33. Nelson WJ: Workers' Compensation: Coverage, Benefits and Costs, 1990-91, *Social Security Bulletin*, Social Security Administration, Office of Research and Statistics, 56(3), Fall, 1993.

34. Personnel Decisions, Inc., A Study of Statistical Relationships Among Physical Ability Measures on Injured Workers Undergoing KEY Functional Assessments, Minneapolis, 1986.

35. Personnel Decisions, Inc., KEY Functional Assessment Preemployment Screening Battery as a Predictor of Job Related Injuries, Minneapolis, Jan 1994.

36. Pope MH, Andersson GBJ, Frymoyer JW, Chaffin DE: *Occupational Low Back Pain: Assessment Treatment and Prevention,* St Louis 1991 Mosby.

37. Rothstein JM: Introduction to Outcomes Research, American Physical Therapy Association: Combined Sections Meeting, Feb 1994.

38. Sachs BL, David JF, et.al: Spinal Rehabilitation by Work Tolerance Based on Objective Physical Capacity Assessment of Dysfunction: a prospective study with control

subjects and twelve-month review, *Spine* 15:1325-1332, 1990.

39. Sachs BL, et al: Objective Assessment for Exercise Treatment on the B-200 Isostation as Part of Work Tolerance Rehabilitation, *Spine* 19(1), 1994.

40. Schwartz G, Galvin D, Watson S, Dickinson S: Healthcare Management and Physical Therapy: An Employer's Guide to Obtaining Physical Therapy Services, a study by the Washington Business Group on Health, commissioned by the Private Practice Section of the American Physical Therapy Association, Washington, DC, 1989.

41. Scully RM, Barnes MR: *Physical Therapy*, Philadelphia 1989 JB Lippincott.

42. Sharp MA, Harman EA, Boutilier BE, Bovee MW, Kraemer WJ: Progressive Resistance Training Program for Improving Manual Materials Handling Performance, *WORK* 3(3), 1993.

43. Spengler et al: Back Injuries In Industry: A Retrospective Study I, Overview & Cost Analysis, *Spine* 3(3), 1986.

44. *Standard Industrial Classification System.* U.S. Office of Management and Budget, U.S. Government, 1987.

45. Steward DL, Abeln SH: *Documenting Functional Outcomes in Physical Therapy*, St Louis, 1993, Mosby.

46. Carlson L. et al: Work Hardening Think Tank: A Private Practitioners' Symposium, Minneapolis, 1991 (unpublished).

47. Worker Data Bank, KEY Method, Minneapolis 1994.

48. Zachazewski JE: Improving Flexibility, In Scully RM, Barnes MR: *Physical Therapy* Philadelphia, 1989, JB Lippincott.

CHAPTER

15

Flexibility, Mobility, Strength, and Aerobic Conditioning

John Hilson
Stephanie Hatlestad

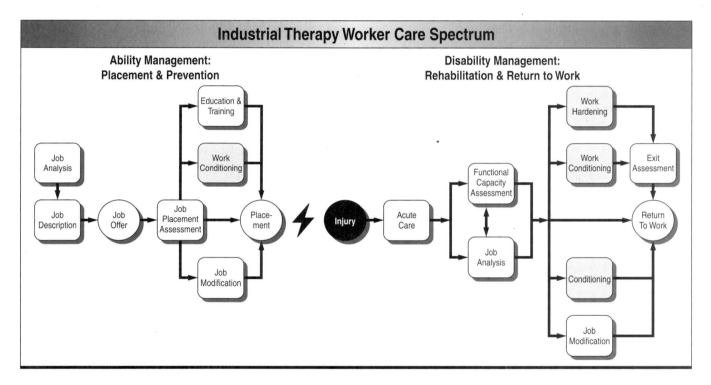

Industrial Therapy programs can be as diverse as the clients and jobs from which they come. While each program may be highly individualized and tailored to the specific needs of each client and their work situation, there are basic components that will be fundamental to any program. Enhancing flexibility, mobility, strength, and aerobic conditioning are basic components that should be part of any program, regardless of occupation or the type of injury the worker has sustained.

Many clients entering a Work Hardening or Work Conditioning program will have a specific weakness or tightness that is present as a result of injury. Generalized loss of strength or flexibility is usually present as a result of a decrease in activity level, stemming either from the injury or possibly from a sedentary lifestyle. Accompanying this deficit is usually a low level of aerobic fitness, which further complicates the person's rehabilitation and return to work.[2,4,11,18] By addressing these deficiencies in the Industrial Therapy program, the client is better prepared for job simulation and ultimately a successful return to work.

The activities discussed in this chapter are to be used individually or in combination, to enhance job simulation capabilities. Just as an athlete would participate in an exercise program to improve flexibility, strength, endurance, coordination, and other skills required by the sport, the worker must develop sufficient flexibility, mobility, strength, and aerobic conditioning to be able to perform the job as required. Without adequate physical preparation, safe performance of the job cannot be expected (Figure 15.1).

STRENGTH TRAINING

Strength training is a process in which a series of progressive exercises or work is used to attain strength, speed, and endurance. Work is defined as applying a force to an object and moving the object through a distance (w = f × d).[16,17] Greater strength, or the ability to generate greater forces, will allow for more work to be done. Further, if a muscle or muscle group is stronger and capable of generating greater forces, it does not have to work as hard to perform submaximal levels of work. As the muscle group is not strained to perform the task, it has a greater tolerance to performing work, and risk of injury is reduced.[16]

Physiological Changes

Strength training produces a number of physiological changes in the muscle tissue. The three major categories of tissue change that occur are aerobic changes, anaerobic changes, and slow and fast twitch muscle fiber changes.

The aerobic changes that occur in skeletal muscle are:
1. *Increased myoglobin* content which aids in the delivery of oxygen from the cell membrane to the mitochondria.
2. *Increased oxidation* of carbohydrates (glycogen) which increases the muscles capacity to generate energy.
3. *Increased size and number of mitochondria* along with a higher concentration of enzymes that are involved in the Kreb's cycle. Thus, the muscle can store more glycogen.
4. *Increased oxidation of fat* through submaximal endurance activities resulting in less lactic acid buildup and less fatigue.

The anaerobic changes are an increase in the muscle's capacity to store adenosine triphosphate-phosphocreatine (ATP-PC) along with key enzymes that break down the PC. This system allows a fast release of energy by the muscle cells for short bouts of activity.

The fast and slow twitch muscle fibers increase their aerobic potential equally with aerobic training. The fast twitch fibers, however, have a greater glycolytic capacity due to the increased number of mitochondria. Hypertrophy is selective to both groups being dependent on the specificity of the exercise.

These physiological changes demonstrate that the body will adapt to the specific demands imposed upon it (SAID Principle).[16] Physiological changes will occur with any type of training program. It must be remembered that training effects are specific to the type of exercise performed. Consequently, the Industrial Therapist must design a specifically-targeted strength training program that incorporates diagnosis, healing constraints, orthopedic evaluation, Functional Capacity Assessment results, psychological status, patient tolerance, body involvement, job analysis, and other medical concerns.

Postural Changes

Strength training also involves a variety of postures categorized as open chain, close chain, and sustained positions.

An open chain position (Figure 15.2, A) is when the proximal aspect of the muscle is fixed and the distal end moves through a range of motion. An example of an open chain exercise of the quadriceps would be a long arc quad.

A close chain position (Figure 15.2, B), conversely, is when the distal aspect of the muscle is fixed and the proximal end moves through a range of motion. An example of a close chain exercise of the quadriceps would be a partial squat.

Sustained positions (Figure 15.2, C) are when opposing muscle groups are contracted to maintain a particular static position. For example, static standing requires the cocontraction of the back extensors as well as the abdominals. Work activities requiring constant postures can be facilitated by strengthening the opposing muscle groups. By providing greater muscular endurance and strength, training will make it less strenuous to maintain the specific posture over time.

The type of exercises chosen for the individual can

FIGURE 15.1 Flexibility, mobility, strength training, and aerobic conditioning used individually or in combination can enhance the physical performance of a worker.

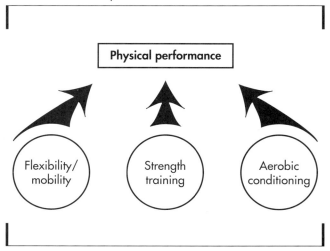

include all three postures, but emphasis should be placed on the exercises that are functional and can be translated into work simulation and enhancement activities.[7,12]

Part/Whole Concept

The Part/Whole concept involves working on individual muscles first, before commencing strengthening activities that involve muscular groups. In this manner, the program includes strengthening exercises for specific individual muscles, general muscle groups, as well as job simulation activities.[7,12]

A worker with a rotator cuff injury will require specific exercises of the rotator cuff musculature, in addition to general strengthening such as lifting a box off the floor, or a sustained activity such as reaching.

The Part/Whole concept can be taken one step farther to prepare for job simulation. A job simulation activity can be broken down into parts that can be practiced individually (Figures 15.3, *A, B*). Once the worker masters each activity, these activities can be combined to simulate the job to which the worker is returning. (Figure 15.3, *C*)

To illustrate this sequence, suppose the worker is a car mechanic who has sustained a rotator cuff injury. The job requires lifting through a variety of ranges, performing sustained reaching, and using tools that vibrate. Initially, exercises to strengthen individual rotator cuff muscles are executed. Then the client progresses to general strengthening of lifting boxes, working with arms overhead, working with arms reaching out in front, and holding onto a vibrating tool. Once these activities are mastered, the worker can combine them through job simulation of working on a car in preparation for return to work.

The Part/Whole concept is supported through findings in a study by Kahanovitz et al. in which a strength assessment of trunk musculature, after lumbar discectomy, was found to demonstrate diminished trunk flexion and extension strength and endurance, with persistent decrease in extension strength noted after long term follow-up, averaging seventeen months.[10] Weakness following injury can persist for an extended length of time, unless specifically addressed.

Muscular strain occurs when stresses placed on the muscle exceed the strength or endurance of the muscle, becoming chronic if sustained over time. If the original injury was related to the muscle-tendon unit, return to work will not be possible unless specific measures are taken to return the appropriate muscle groups to sufficient strength. It is also conceivable that new injuries could result after a worker, either a new hire or previously injured, is placed in a job that exceeds their strength capabilities.

Program Goals

With the above information in mind, the goals of the strengthening program would be to:
- Improve the capability to handle or apply force to weighted objects
- Improve the endurance to sustain an activity

Through specificity training and using the Part/Whole concept, the Industrial Therapist can improve the workers' neuromuscular recruitment patterns, providing greater coordination and agility.[12] All persons in the Industrial Therapy program, Work Hardening, or Work Conditioning, would be expected to participate, because this is the foundation upon which work simulation is built.

Assessment

Typically, 20 to 30 minutes of time would be spent in strengthening activities each day. Prior to designing the program and establishing the specific exercises to be performed, an assessment of the individual's strengths and weaknesses should be performed. The Therapist can use the results of the Functional Capacity Assessment and orthopedic evaluation to identify specific muscle and muscle group weaknesses and strengths. A program can then be developed that will address these issues as they relate to the injury and job requirements. Severe deconditioning may have occurred in those persons with chronic injuries, requiring an extensive strengthening program.

Equipment and Exercise Selection

Isometric and active exercises are the most gentle variety, yet they still provide for strengthening. These exercises can be easily instructed, require no equipment, and are ideal for use in a home exercise program prescribed for additional activity outside the therapy center. Isometrics are very useful in the cervical area, an area where it is difficult to specifically exercise on gym equipment. This form of exercise is not intimidating and allows the client greater control over the intensity of exertion (Figure 15.4).

Free weights, dumbbells, and cuff weights, are beneficial not only to exercise a specific muscle, but also to strengthen the muscles stabilizing the joint being moved. Caution must be used in this type of exercise. Injuries may occur if the movement of the weight is not carefully controlled, or the amount of weight is not carefully controlled or appropriately selected (Figure 15.4, *C*).[7]

Resisted exercise machines may also play a role in strengthening programs. The exercise movement is

FIGURE 15.2 A, B, C The types of exercises chosen for the individual can include open chain **(A)**, close chain **(B)**, or sustained positions **(C)** with the emphasis on the exercises that are functional and can be translated into work simulation activities.

A

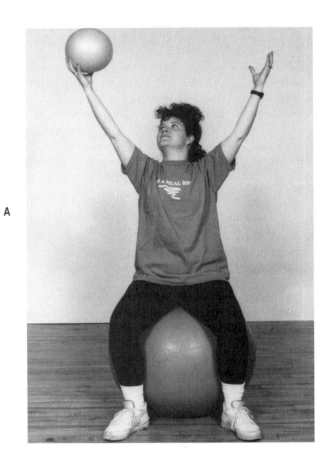

B

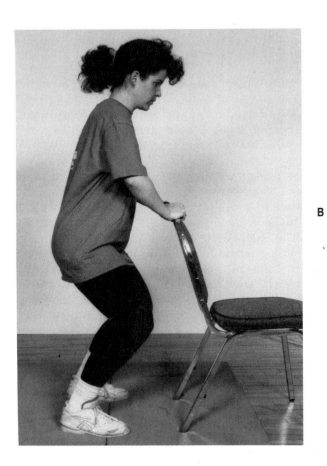

C

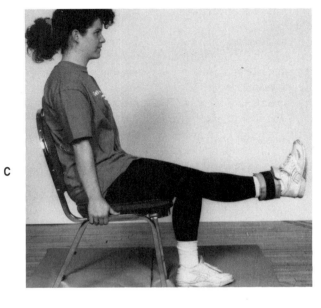

FIGURE 15.3 A, B, C   A strengthening program should use the Part/Whole concept of working on specific muscles individually prior to strengthening activities that require a muscle group or the whole body.

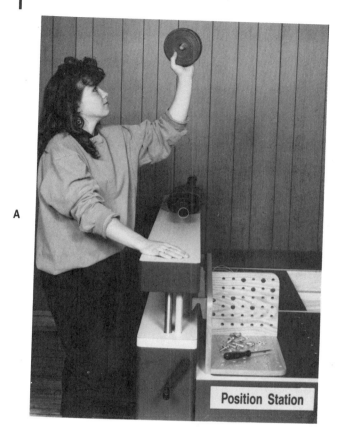

A

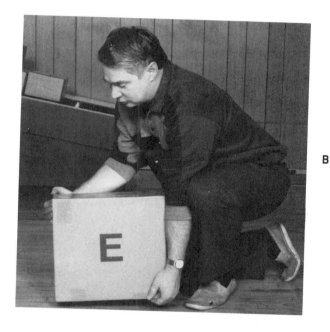

B

Position Station

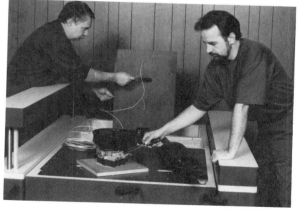

C

controlled by the machine, with less chance of injury due to loss of control of the weight by the user. Many types of resistance are available, from more traditional plate loaded machines (Universal, Nautilus) to hydraulic (Hydrafitness) or pneumatic (Keiser). As with the selection of weight in free weights, care must be used in selecting the amount of resistance to be used so the muscle group to be exercised is not overloaded (Figure 15.5, *A*).

With hydraulic resistance, the force generated by the machine is dependent on the force applied by the individual using the machine. In other words, the harder the client pushes, the harder the resistance will be because the machine works at a constant speed. This can be very beneficial to the injured. If the person exercising stops at some point during the range of motion, there is no resistance remaining. This provides a measure of safety and comfort to the individual using

FIGURE 15.4 Isometrics **(A)** are the gentlest form of strengthening followed by active range of motion **(B)** and free weights **(C)**.

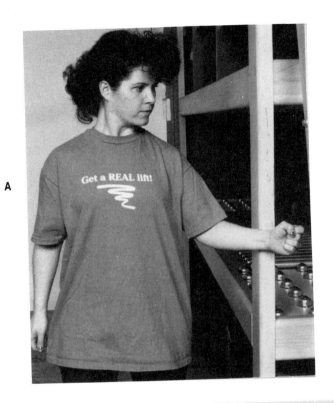

A

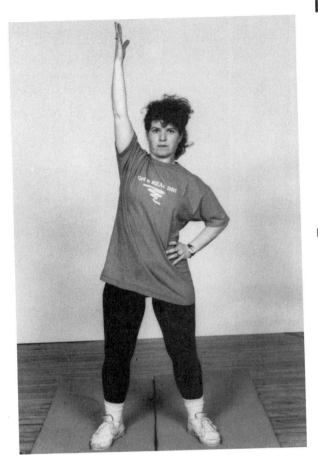

B

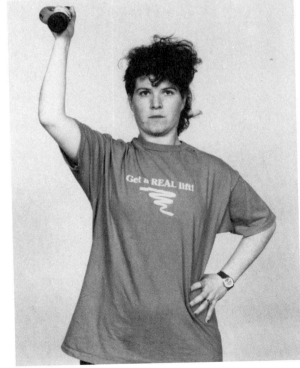

C

FIGURE 15.5   Plate **(A)**, hydraulic **(B)**, pneumatic, and isokinetic **(C)** equipment provide a variety of strengthening alternatives.

A

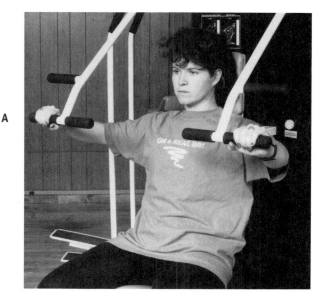

B

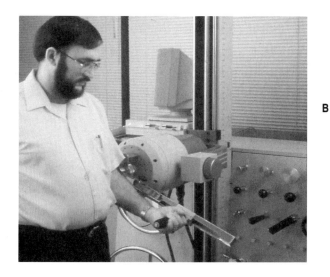

C

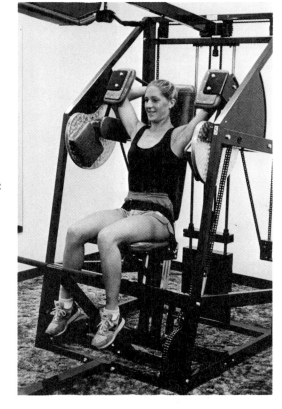

15.5, **C** (From Gould, Orthopedic and Sports Physical Therapy, ed 2, St Louis, 1990, Mosby.)

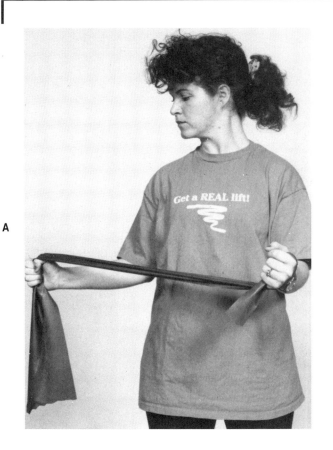

A

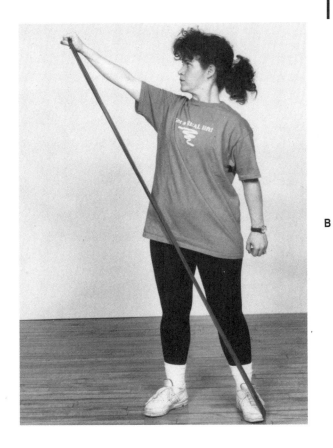

B

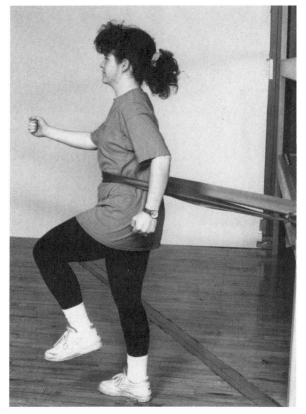

C

the equipment, who may be at risk for reinjury (Figure 15.5, *B*).

Isokinetic equipment (Cybex, Kincom, etc.) may also be used for strength training. Similar to hydraulic resistance, a speed of movement is selected and resistance is variable depending on the input of force from the client. Both hydraulic and isokinetic devices eliminate the eccentric portion of the muscle contraction. Instead they exercise opposing muscle groups on one machine in a concentric-concentric fashion. This can significantly reduce muscle soreness as the eccentric portion of the contraction is eliminated (Figure 15.5, *C*).[7]

While free weights and resisted exercise equipment may first come to mind in a strengthening program, there are several other ways this may be accomplished.

Theraband, theratubing, and sports cords are becoming increasingly popular and are available to most clinicians (Figure 15.6). Several grades of resistance are available, and its use is restricted only by the imagination of the Therapist. It is useful not only in the therapy setting, but may also be dispensed to the client to provide resistance in exercises that are prescribed as a home program.

Gymnastic balls are also useful in the Industrial Therapy setting (Figures 15.7, *A, B, C, D*). Using the ball in conjunction with a strengthening program will serve to improve coordination and proprioception, as well as to strengthen. Lumbar stabilization programs rely heavily on the use of a gymnastic ball in the rehabilitation of low back injuries.[13,14]

Work Hardening and Work Conditioning equipment itself is also valuable to the strengthening program. The lifting, carrying, pushing, pulling, and other activities that are done with resistance will serve to strengthen and may provide job simulation for some clients (Figure 15.8).

Session Guidelines

As previously noted, at least twenty to thirty minutes should be spent in the strengthening portion of the program each time the client attends. It is appropriate to stagger exercises, alternating upper and lower body exercises to allow for a brief rest of the particular part and sufficient recovery from earlier bouts of exercise.

In the Industrial Therapy setting, exercises are generally completed in sets of ten. The client will progress from one set of ten to three sets of ten as strength and tolerance of the activity increases. Once three sets of ten can be completed, the resistance should be increased to the next level.

Planning

Before beginning the strengthening portion of the program, the progression plan should be discussed with the client. First, the individual should understand that by increasing strength, greater forces can be generated and work can be more easily tolerated. It is easy for the client to comprehend why these exercises are part of a Work Conditioning and Work Hardening program even though the activities are very different from those done on the job.

Second, the client should be educated on the program's starting point which should also include a discussion of the job demands and weekly goals. The client can provide valuable insight on how the job is performed and this information can be incorporated into the exercise selection process. Besides exercises targeted at weaknesses, it is important to identify areas of strength, so that exercises can be selected that will reinforce the client's abilities and improve confidence.

Progress and goals should be reviewed weekly with the client in order to incorporate exercise modifications. Involving the client in the treatment plan shows great concern, clarifies expectations and responsibility, and allows the client to become comfortable with the plan.

Monitoring

The client should also be instructed to monitor symptoms during the exercise. While it is expected that sensations of stress, fatigue, or even muscular pain may accompany this type of exercise, care must be taken so the symptoms, related to the injury for which the client is off work, do not increase. The client must be able to differentiate this "Point of Change" where symptoms related to exercise begin to include an increase in pain. By observing this, it is possible to exercise without exacerbating symptoms. It also makes the client responsible for increases in symptoms.

The principle of delayed onset muscle soreness should also be explained.[8,16,17] The soreness accompanying strengthening exercises is normal and expected, and should not be a cause for alarm to the client. An easy way to explain this to a client is to talk about a familiar home activity that has caused soreness the next day. Raking leaves is an activity that is done only once or twice a year. Most people are sore the next day because their muscles have not been used in the activity for some time. Strength exercises follow the same principles because the exercises will be new to the muscles. If these symptoms become problematic, measures can be taken to minimize them, such as icing or stretching following the exercise session.

It is important for the Industrial Therapist and client to communicate to determine whether the level of treatment is acceptable or not. The client is responsible for monitoring the "Point of Change" when exercising and notifying the Therapist of any difficulties. The Therapist is responsible for educating and

FIGURE 15.7   Gymnastic balls are used to improve coordination, proprioception and strength. **A,** Initially, the patient learns to maintain trunk position while using gentle weight shifting; **B,** Trunk stability is advanced through removing leg stability and relying on the trunk musculature to maintain the position; **C,** The addition of free weights requires the trunk to tolerate greater loads; and, **D,** Dynamic activities require the patient's trunk to adapt quickly, similar to daily activities.

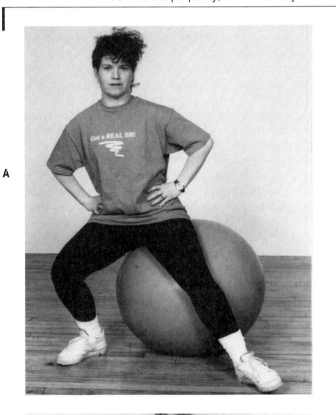

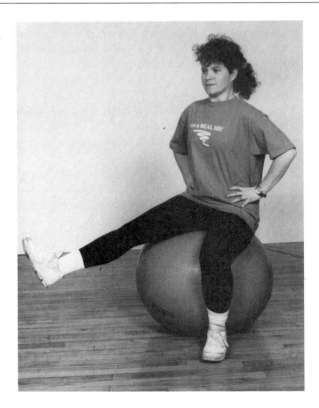

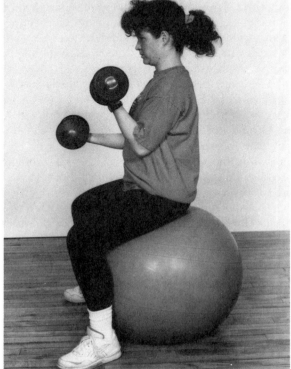

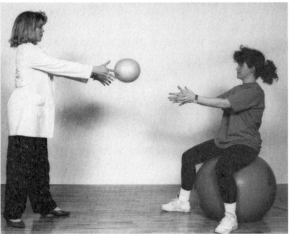

FIGURE 15.8   Job simulation in Work Hardening **(A)** or Work Conditioning **(B)** provides another environment to work on strengthening as well as flexibility and conditioning.

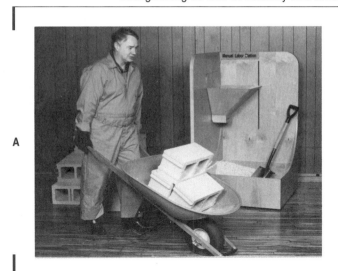

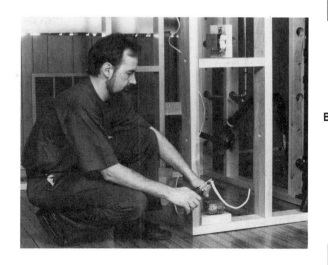

reinforcing the "Point of Change" principle as well as modifying the exercises when needed. Modalities should be kept to a minimum with ice being the only alternative. This reinforces client responsibility for the strengthening program in addition to independence from modality treatment. Figure 15.9 illustrates sample strengthening exercises.

FLEXIBILITY AND MOBILITY

The Industrial Therapy program must also include exercises that will restore the flexibility and mobility of the joints and soft tissues that have been reduced by the injury. If the injury has become chronic, or there has been a long lapse from the time of injury to the time of entering the Industrial Therapy program, it can also be reasonably assumed that inactivity is a secondary contributor to the loss of flexibility and mobility.[2,4,11,18]

Loss of flexibility could have been a cause of the injury in the first place. It was found that a reduction in lumbar extension was predictive of low back trouble by Burton et al.[5] The study indicated that maintaining lumbar extension is important in both sexes to reduce the risk of low back trouble.

It is, therefore, important to observe the worker for functional limitations in joint range of motion and loss of soft tissue mobility, whether in a preemployment assessment for a new hire, or in a Functional Capacity Assessment post-injury. For those individuals entering a Work Hardening or Work Conditioning program, a more specific assessment of mobility can be made through neck, trunk, upper, and lower extremity range of motion testing. It is important that these results are

compared to the dynamic movements performed in the Functional Capacity Assessment.

Exercise Selection

Passive stretching can be effective in increasing muscle and tendon length, while improving the flexibility of the tissues being stretched. If there has been a soft tissue injury resulting in scar tissue formation, stretching can help to make the scar tissue more flexible and more functional. Improvement in local circulation is another possible benefit. Confidence and tolerance to activity can also be anticipated.

Specific tightness and general flexibility must be considered when selecting exercises. Tightness in the area of injury must be addressed, perhaps with multiple exercises to assure a thorough stretch of the part and return of functional range of motion. Knowledge of the type of work done by the client is another consideration in designing the stretching program. A heavy laborer may need attention to trunk and lower extremity flexibility, while a typist's stretching program might center around flexibility of the upper extremities and cervical spine. Figure 15.10 illustrates sample stretching exercises.

Session Guidelines

Flexibility exercises can be integrated into the strengthening and conditioning section of the Industrial Therapy program. They can be used both in warming up prior to strengthening and cooling down upon completion. All clients who participate should be involved in

FIGURE 15.9 Examples of strengthening exercises that can be used in a work hardening or work conditioning program.

Shoulder external rotation

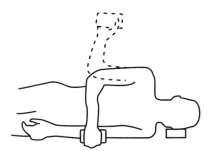

Raise arm up toward ceiling. Keep elbow bent and in at side.

Shoulder internal rotation

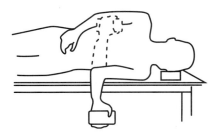

Bring arm up toward body. Keep elbow bent and in at side.

Shoulder abduction

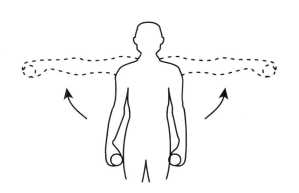

Raise arms out from body.

Shoulder: Supraspinatus strengthening

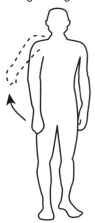

Bring arm up and forward about 30 degrees from side. Keep elbow straight, thumb pointing down.

Shoulder flexion

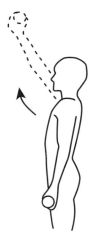

Raise arm out in front of body and lift toward ceiling. Keep elbow straight.

FIGURE 15.9 *Cont'd*

Trunk stability
Hook-lying bent leg lift

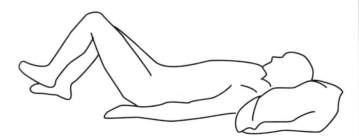

Flatten stomach muscles to keep trunk rigid and slowly raise leg three to four inches from floor.

Trunk stability
Bridging

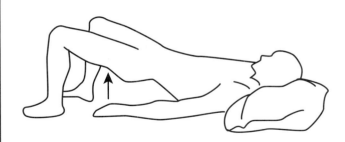

Slowly raise buttocks from floor, keeping stomach tight.

Back
Diagonal curl-up

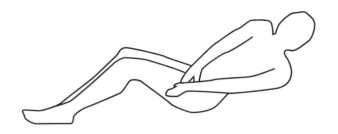

With arms at sides, tilt pelvis to flatten back. Raise head and shoulders, rotating to one side as shoulder blades clear floor.

Back
Alternate arm and leg lift

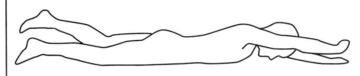

Keep knee locked and lift leg eight to ten inches from floor, along with opposite arm.

Back
Curl-up (phase 2)

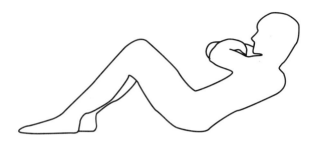

Keeping arms folded across chest, tilt pelvis to flatten back. Raise head and shoulders from floor.

FIGURE 15.10 Example of stretching exercises that can be used in a work hardening or work conditioning program.

Cervical Spine
Levator scapula stretch

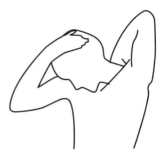

Place hand on same side shoulder blade. With other hand gently stretch head down and away.

Cervical Spine
Flexibility: corner stretch

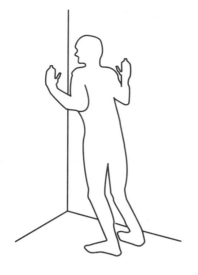

Standing in corner with hands at shoulder level and feet two to three feet from corner, lean forward until a comfortable stretch is felt across chest.

Back
Press-up

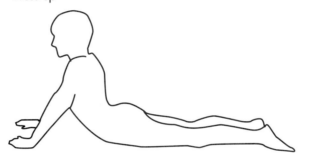

Press upper body upward into position shown, keeping hips in contact with floor. Keep low back and buttocks relaxed.

Back
Single knee to chest stretch

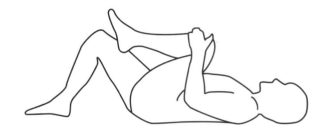

Pull one knee in to chest until a comfortable stretch is felt in the lower back and buttocks. Repeat with opposite knee.

Back
Angry cat stretch

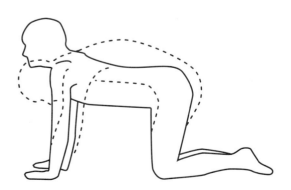

Tuck chin and tighten stomach, arching back.

Back
Mid back stretch

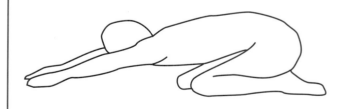

Push chest toward floor, reaching forward as far as you can.

FIGURE 15.10   *Cont'd*

Hip and knee Gastroc stretch

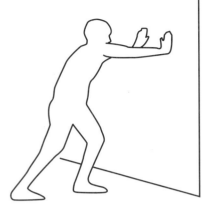

Back leg kept straight, heel on floor and turned outward, lean slightly until stretch is felt in the calf.

Hip and knee Supina piriformis stretch

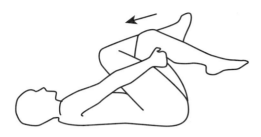

Cross legs with one leg on top. Slowly pull opposite knee toward chest until a comfortable stretch is felt in the buttock/hip area.

Hip and knee Inner thigh/groin stretch

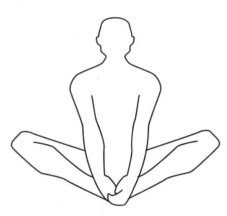

With heels together, pull toward groin until stretch is felt in groin and inner thigh.

Hip and knee hamstring wall stretch

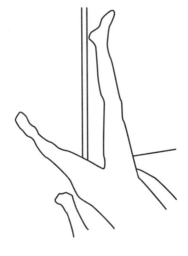

Lying on floor with one leg on wall and other leg through doorway, move closer to wall until a stretch is felt in back of thigh. As leg relaxes, move closer to wall.

stretching, whether in a conditioning program or in Work Hardening. The flexibility exercises can be particularly useful in the more severely debilitated client, as stretching can be easily controlled by the individual and enables new movement without fear of reinjury.

Consideration can be made for a group stretch, selecting an assortment of general exercises in which all clients could participate. Afterward small groups could perform more specific exercises. Some clients may find this approach encouraging, allowing them to see others with similar problems. It also helps the director of the program to monitor an individual's progress with regard to flexibility, and the client's socialization skills.

The specifics of stretching exercises vary among practitioners, client populations, and types of injuries. In the Industrial Therapy program the client will have a variety of activities to complete, stretching being just one. For each exercise, it is suggested that the stretch is held for five seconds and repeated five times. This allows for a simple program that is effective but not too time consuming. It would be expected that stretching exercises are done at each session of therapy.

Monitoring

It is important for the client to work until the first sign of tightness, pulling, or slight pain, then stop the movement, and return to the resting or starting position. If the client works within comfortable ranges, they will be able to progress. If they do not, discomfort will persist. Once again the "Point of Change" principle should be emphasized.

As soft tissues are viscoelastic in nature, the amount of deformation a structure can tolerate is dependent on the length of its elastic components, while the maximal rate of deformation depends on the viscosity of its fluid.[17] A prolonged load causes stretching as desired, but can also cause deformation or even breakage of the tissue being loaded. Thus, the client should understand that there is a certain amount of uncomfortable sensation that may accompany a stretching exercise, but these exercises should not exacerbate symptoms.

The client should be instructed to stretch slowly and avoid ballistic stretches. Any problems should be reported to the Therapist supervising the program. This helps to relieve any anxiety the client may have that the exercises may hurt, and allows some responsibility for avoiding increases in symptoms.

AEROBIC CONDITIONING

Aerobic conditioning involves overloading the aerobic system, stressing it beyond its current limits, to gain improvement in aerobic capability.

Benefits

Aerobic conditioning can yield a number of benefits. First and foremost, endurance is improved. Tolerance for work activity is also improved, particularly for those most deconditioned. A successful return to work can only be anticipated if the individual has the endurance or tolerance for the work day, whether part time, modified job, or full time employment.

Second, cardiovascular efficiency is improved, allowing more blood to be circulated with less demand on the heart. This result is a function of reduced heart rate and increased stroke volume.[6]

Stroke volume is defined as the volume of blood ejected from the heart per beat. The increased stroke volume can be a result of either intermittent exercise or continuous exercise. With intermittent exercise, the stroke volume is higher during the immediate recovery than during the activity. Since intermittent programs contain numerous recovery periods, the stroke volume increase is an adaptation.

Continuous exercise, on the other hand, only entails one recovery period, and requires the same energy expenditure and oxygen use, so the mechanism

for the lower heart rate is an increased stroke volume.[6] This improvement in cardiopulmonary function can also facilitate the tissue healing process, through improved oxygen delivery and removal of carbon dioxide and metabolites.[17]

A third benefit of an aerobic conditioning program is weight loss. Aerobic training provides a greater ability to mobilize and oxidize fat.[8] While the Industrial Therapy program is not designed to be a weight loss program, obesity can certainly be an obstacle to rehabilitation, and may be a factor in work injuries. Deyo and Bass found that there was an increase in back pain prevalence with increasing obesity.[6]

An individual's level of cardiovascular fitness may also affect the response to an episode of back pain, suggesting that with a lower level of cardiovascular fitness, a higher response of disability may be observed. There is also evidence that aerobic training in clients with back problems can be beneficial in reducing chances for developing chronic back pain disability. Individuals with higher fitness levels had less costly claims and fewer recurrences.[3,6]

A fourth benefit of aerobic conditioning is the release of endorphins whose effect resembles that of certain opiates.[14] They serve to reduce pain and enhance a feeling of well being. The increased release of endorphins during exercise may partially explain the feeling of well being commonly experienced at the end of a training session.

For these and other reasons, participation in aerobic conditioning may motivate the client to develop a long term involvement in this form of exercise.

Program Guidelines

There are three variables to consider in an aerobic conditioning program, the intensity, frequency, and duration of the exercise.[9]

Intensity of the exercise is generally governed by the individual's age and pulse rate. There are a few basic methods for determining intensity. If the individual has had a stress test, the physician interpreting the results of the test should be able to give a range of pulse rates for exercise. If this information is not available, exercise pulse rates may be easily calculated.

Maximum pulse rate is determined by subtracting the client's age from 220 and multiplying by 60 to 80 percent. (In some cases a level of intensity below 60% may be required). If the client is 50 years old, the calculation is 220 minus 50 equals a maximum heart rate of 170, multiplied by 60% and 80% yields a range of 102 to 136 beats per minute.

For individuals with very low resting pulse rates, or possibly those on medications altering the resting pulse, the Karvonen formula may be helpful.[8] This is determined as follows:

EHR = RHR + X(MHR−RHR)
EHR is exercise heart rate
RHR is resting heart rate
MHR is maximum heart rate
X is the percentage of maximum heart rate desired (the 60 to 80% used above).

This formula allows for a more specific determination of the exercise heart rate.

Determining frequency and duration of the conditioning program is a simpler matter. It would be expected that the client participates in this type of exercise each time he or she attends. Depending on the program, this is usually three to five times per week. In order to achieve the beneficial effects of the exercise, the conditioning program must be completed a minimum of three times a week. Aerobic exercise can be done on a daily basis and the Therapist might encourage the participant to continue on days off as part of a home program.

Duration of the exercise is variable and can be suited to some extent to the type of industrial program in place. A minimum of 15 minutes of continuous activity is suggested. This allows for the pulse rate to rise to the desired level, and be held for a sufficient length of time. Depending on the time available for aerobic conditioning in the program, this exercise may be continued for 30 minutes or longer.

Tolerance and condition of the patient are also factors in determining exercise duration. A severely deconditioned client, or individual with significant pain, may be able to only tolerate five minutes of exercise. It may be possible to allow some rest between bouts of exercise by using two or three five minute sessions interspersed in the program. As tolerance of the exercise, as well as endurance, improve, longer durations can be used.

Setting specific goals is recommended and will help the participant increase duration of the activity, particularly if pain tolerance or motivation are factors to be considered. A program could be designed to start with five minutes of activity and increase one minute every other day. In three to four weeks (depending on the client's program attendance), 15 minutes of activity would be tolerated.

Monitoring

Pulses can be monitored on electronic pulse monitors. If one is not available, manual monitoring of pulses must be done, using either the radial or carotid pulses. The client should be instructed in the method of pulse rate monitoring. If possible, exercise should be continued while checking the pulse rate to avoid an inaccurate count due to slowing of the pulse while the activity is stopped.

If exercise must be stopped while counting, the pulse should be taken over a 15 second period and multiplied by four. Pulses taken over longer periods may be inaccurate as the heart may begin to slow when activity is stopped to take the pulse.

It is important to consider the Point of Change principle, where the client understands that some discomfort may be experienced with the exercise, and that the intensity or duration of the exercise should not cause an exacerbation of symptoms. This concept is important throughout the activities of the Industrial Therapy program.

One last consideration in determining intensity is that at no time should the client be out of breath while performing an aerobic exercise. This suggests the demand for oxygen is greater than what the body is able to supply, thus the exercise is no longer aerobic and is not providing the desired benefit. It may be comforting for the client to know that aerobic conditioning will be comfortable and regulated, not an uncontrolled exercise that becomes uncomfortable.

Exercise Selection

To be aerobic an exercise must use large muscle groups, be repetitive in nature, and maintained over a period of time.[9] There are many aerobic exercises available that are very functional, yet inexpensive to provide. Walking, running, biking, rowing, cross country skiing (simulated on a machine), stepping, or swimming are activities that are perhaps most well known.

Walking can be performed on a treadmill, or in larger facilities a walking circuit can be laid out. Clients could work at different walking stations for three minutes and then switch to another station, (five stations would add up to 15 minutes of aerobic activity). Station possibilities could include; treadmill, walking on a beam on the floor, carrying a box, pushing a broom, and walking a fixed floor pattern (Figure 15.11).

Biking can be done on any type of exercise bike. Biking alternatives include airdynes which use both upper and lower extremities at the same time and stationary bikes which use only the lower extremities.

Stepping can be done on a machine if available, or on a flight of stairs. When using stairs, the client should climb five steps, then turn and come back down the steps. By doing this, pulse rates become steady. If an individual uses a flight of stairs at a time, pulses increase while going up, and can decline as they come

FIGURE 15.11 A–E   A walking circuit is a creative way to combine aerobic conditioning, coordination, flexibility, and strength training.

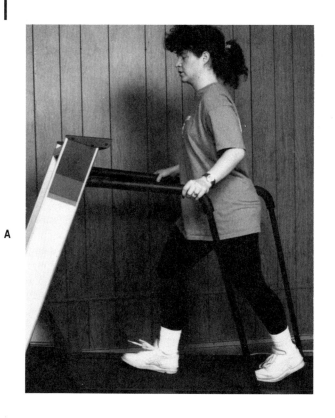

A

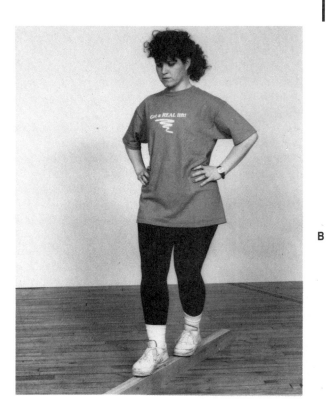

B

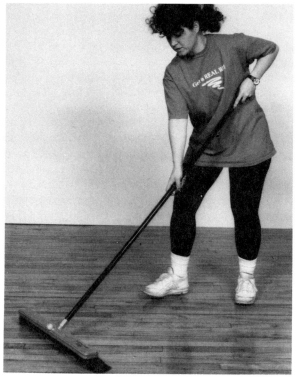

C

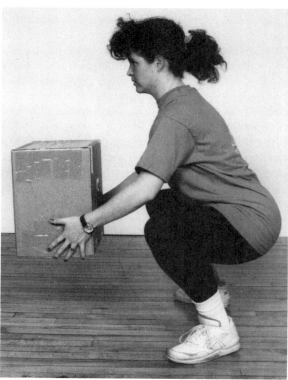

D

FIGURE 15.11   *Cont'd.*

E

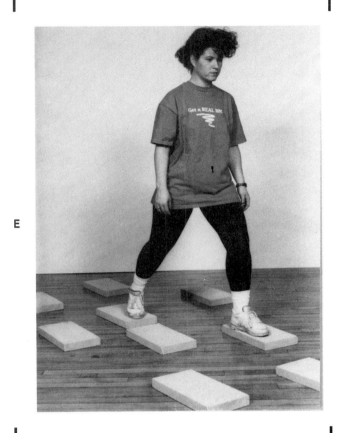

back down, never staying consistently in the targeted range.

Rowers are found in many clinics, and have the added benefit of using the upper and lower extremities. Caution must be used due to the posture used on this exercise, as it may prove problematic for those with low back or other injuries.

If a pool is available, swimming, walking in the water, or even a supervised water aerobics program can be pursued. As long as the exercise fits the requirements noted above for aerobic exercise, and is tolerated well by the client, it may be used in the Industrial Therapy program.

Upper body ergometers may also play a role in the conditioning part of the program, smaller muscle groups are used, it is repetitive, and is maintained over a period of time. This form of exercise may also benefit those clients with upper extremity injuries, or those persons having limited tolerance for use of the lower extremities.

Safety Considerations

Aerobic exercise may pose risks for some clients, particularly those that are obese, severely deconditioned, or with a history of cardiac problems. If a person participates in a sudden, vigorous, and unaccustomed exercise, there is a five to tenfold increase in the chances of cardiac death while the activity is continuing.[19] The risk is much less when the exercise is well matched to the clients physical condition. However, any type of exercise leads to some statistical increase of acute cardiac risk.[19] It is important that the staff be trained in CPR techniques should the need for this arise.

Equipment used in aerobic conditioning may also pose some risk if used improperly. Equipment should be inspected weekly and an equipment safety sheet signed by the Therapist who performed the inspection. The equipment used should be well maintained, and the staff should be well instructed in its proper use. The client must also understand thoroughly how to use specific pieces of equipment and appropriate supervision must be provided.

SUMMARY

The addition of these flexibility, mobility, strengthening, and aerobic conditioning exercises are essentially the foundation upon which the Industrial Therapy program is built. It is not difficult to develop this aspect of the program, and the Therapist should already have the knowledge to comfortably develop these components in the overall program. This is one aspect of the program that will demonstrate consistency in benefits for each client.

REFERENCES

1. Astrand P, Rodahl K: *Textbook of Work Physiology*, New York, 1986, McGraw-Hill.
2. Akeson W, Amiel D, Woo S: Immobility Effects on Synovial Joints: the pathomechanics of joint contracture, *Biorheology* 17:95–100, 1980.
3. Battie et al: A Prospective Study in the Role of Cardiovascular Risk Factors and Fitness in Industrial Back Pain Complaints, *Spine* 14(2).
4. Bortz W: The Disuse Syndrome (commentary), *West J Med* 141:691–694, 1984.
5. Burton et al: Prediction of Low-Back Trouble Frequency in a Working Population, *Spine* 14(9).
6. Cady I, Bischoff DP, O'Connell ER, Thomas RC, Allan JH: Strength and Fitness and Subsequent Back Injuries in Firefighters, *J Occup Med* 21:269–272, 1979.

7. Deyo, Bass: Lifestyle and Low-Back Pain: the influence of Smoking and Obesity, *Spine* 14(5).

8. Gatchel, RJ: *Early Development of Physical and Mental Deconditioning in Painful Spinal Disorders, Contemporary Conservative Care for Painful Spinal Disorders*, Philadelphia, 1991, Lea & Febiger.

9. Gould J, Davies G: *Orthopedic and Sports Physical Therapy*, St Louis, 1985, Mosby.

10. Hanson P: *Clinical Exercise Testing. Resource Manual for Guidelines for Exercise Testing and Prescription*, Philadelphia, 1988, Lea & Febiger.

11. Kahanovitz et al: Long-term Strength Assessment of Postoperative Discectomy Patients, *Spine* 14(4).

12. Mayer TG et al: Comparison of CT Scan Muscle Measurements and Isokinetic Trunk Strength in Postoperative Patients, *Spine* 14:33–36, 1989.

13. Mayer TG, Gatchel RJ: *Functional Restoration for Spinal Disorders: the sports medicine approach*, Philadelphia, 1988, Lea & Febiger.

14. Nutter P: Aerobic Exercise in the Treatment and Prevention of Low Backpain, *Spine* 2(1): 137–145, 1987.

15. Morgan D: Concepts in Functional Training and Postural Stabilization for the Low-Back-Injured, *Top Acute Care Trauma Rehabil* 2(4):8–17, 1988.

16. Saal JA, Saal JS: Nonoperative Treatment of Herniated Lumbar Intervertebral Disc with Radiculopathy, *Spine* 14(4):431–437, 1989.

17. Saunders R, Anderson M: Early Treatment Intervention. In Isernhagen S editor: Orthopedic Physical Therapy Clinics, *Ind Physical Ther* 1(1).

18. Scully RM, Barnes MR: *Physical Therapy*, Philadelphia, 1989, JB Lippincott.

19. Torg J, Welsh P, Shephard R: *Current Therapy in Sports Medicine*, ed 2, 1990, BC Decker.

20. Woo S, Buckwalter J: Injury and Repair of the Musculoskeletal Soft Tissues. Park Ridge, Il, AAOS Symposium. 1988.

16

Job Simulation

Anne K. Tramposh

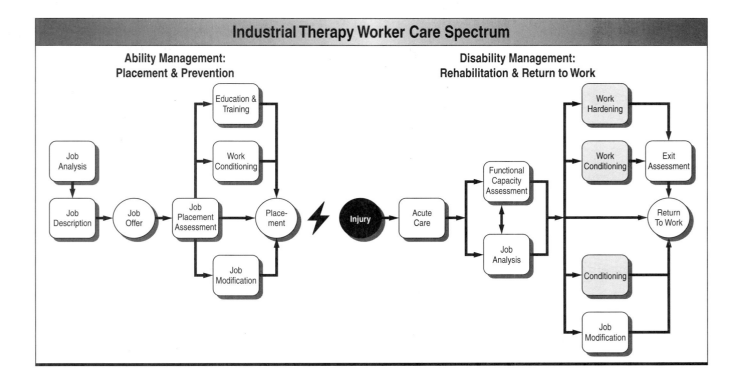

Job simulation can be defined as putting a worker in a similar or mock situation that closely resembles the task or tasks that the worker performs on the job. Job simulation is an essential component of an effective Work Hardening or Work Conditioning program. It enables and requires the worker to simulate the tasks which are involved in a given job.

Through analysis of the worker's performance and with appropriate education, the worker can experiment and practice different techniques, increase loads and learn the safest and most energy efficient way to complete job tasks. The worker can then refine the techniques and "muscle memory" can be trained in a safe, low pressure environment (Figure 16.1, *A*). This will increase the likelihood of success upon actual return to the job. (Figure 16.1, *B*)

Education, progressive increase of weighted activities, and practice in a safe environment can be the primary purposes of job simulation. There are other purposes for performing job simulation. These include reducing workers' fear of return to work by gradually increasing successes in the performance of job tasks or modifying the job to make tasks safer for the worker.

Job simulation is, in essence, the use of work related activities to increase strength, endurance, coordination, and range of motion. Use of work related activities serves to reduce preoccupation with symptoms and reinforces well behaviors.

HISTORY OF JOB SIMULATION

The use of work as a therapeutic medium is not a recent development. It has been the focal point in the fields of Occupational Therapy and Vocational Rehabili-

FIGURE 16.1   Progressing to safe and efficient workstyles in job simulation **(A)** ensures a more successful return to the real job **(B)**.

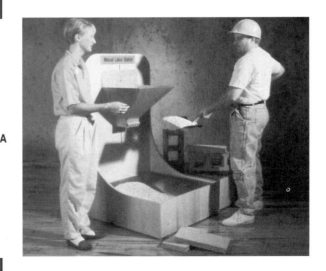

A

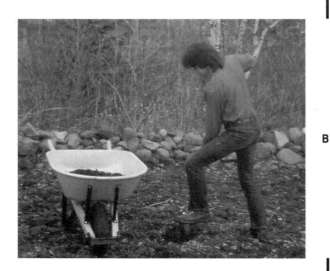

B

tation. Many people have benefited from this type of therapy over the years, including victims of war, heart attacks, strokes, amputees, the mentally ill, the congenitally handicapped, the blind, and elderly.[18]

In the late 1970's and early 1980's, the use of work related rehabilitation became more prevalent in Industrial Therapy. Early pioneers in job simulation in Work Hardening include Len Matheson, Keith Blankenship, KEY Method (formerly KEY Functional Assessments), Polinsky Medical Rehabilitation Center, and Wx: Work Capacities.

> *Len Matheson is credited with defining Work Hardening as "a work oriented treatment program that has outcome which is measured in terms of improvement of the client's productivity. This is achieved through increased work tolerances, improved work rate, mastery of pain (through the effective use of symptom control techniques), increased confidence, and proficiency with work adaptations or assistive devices. Work Hardening involves the client in highly structured, simulated work tasks in an environment where expectations for basic worker behaviors, (timeliness, attendance, and dress) are in keeping with work place standards."[19]*

Matheson's work included the use of the WEST equipment to quantify a worker's functional abilities and to simulate the work environment. Matheson replaced the use of the overused term malingering with the more appropriate terminology symptom magnification.[20] Matheson continues to be a major contributor to the field of Industrial Therapy and job simulation.

Keith Blankenship began his work in Industrial Therapy with David Apts, founder of the American

Back School. His work in the area of Functional Capacity Assessments (FCAs) included the use of easily obtainable materials to simulate physical demands of a worker's job.[5] His company, American Therapeutics is responsible for training thousands of Therapists in techniques of Functional Assessment, Job Simulation, Work Hardening, and Work Conditioning. His company has also made Job Simulation equipment readily available to rehabilitation centers that provide industrial services.

KEY Method is responsible for developing a standardized system of Functional Capacity Assessment using standard equipment. Beginning in the early eighties, Key also developed a system of train-the-trainer classes in the field of Carpal Tunnel Syndrome and other upper extremity Cumulative Trauma Disorders.

The founder of KEY Method, Glenda Key describes the Worker Care Spectrum as a framework of Industrial Therapy. It includes the point of hire through job placement, prevention, injury, acute care, rehabilitation, and return to work. Her continuing contributions in the areas of Work Hardening, Work Conditioning, and Functional Assessment have also enabled thousands of Industrial Therapy facilities to offer comprehensive effective services to the industries they serve.[17]

Polinsky Medical Rehabilitation Center developed a standardized Functional Capacity Assessment system in the early 1980's. This assessment utilized commonly available equipment in a standardized manner, to evaluate an individual's capabilities with regard to work requirements. The primary developers of the Polinsky FCA, Sue Isernhagen and Margot Miller continue to contribute to the field of Industrial Therapy through continuing education courses, research, development, and contributions to the Industrial Therapy literature.[14,23]

Wx: Work Capacities similarly contributed to the field in the early 1980's with the introduction of a job related, functional evaluation, that utilized standard components which matched the worker's capabilities with the worker's job requirements.[18]

This method of functional evaluation also included a psychosocial evaluation that screened for appropriateness of a candidate for a rehabilitation program.[13] The founders of Wx: Work Capacities, Suzanne Tate Henderson, Carol Lett, and this author also continue to contribute to the field of Industrial Therapy in the areas of prevention of injury and early return-to-work programs in industry.

In the past decade, there have been literally hundreds of contributions to the field of Industrial Therapy. The art and science of job simulation has been refined and improved through its application in many different industries and work settings. Job simulation is now used in virtually any type of injury or illness where returning or staying at work is an issue.

Job simulation became a critical component in Industrial Therapy in view of rising Workers' Compensation costs in industry.[24,31] In the management of a Workers' Compensation case, the primary goal is case resolution. This means, the worker will be provided with the medical and rehabilitation services that will most efficiently and effectively achieve maximum medical improvement (MMI). Where traditional methods of therapy failed to produce successful return to work outcomes, programs with job simulation were able to successfully move cases toward resolution.[22]

Case resolution, using job simulation, works efficiently for a number of reasons, depending on the specific situation. Job simulation can force the injured worker to face the issues and discover whether or not they are physically capable of performing a given job. Job simulation also decreases fear and increases worker self-confidence.[30] Often this has become then catalyst for successful return to work.

Successful or earlier case resolution using job simulation as a part of rehabilitation efforts has literally produced an entire new industry in the field of rehabilitation. In 1980 there were only a handful of U.S. rehabilitation facilities offering varying degrees of job simulation activities. In the past decade Industrial Therapy has become a well accepted model.[15]

While job simulation in Work Hardening programs has been used primarily in Industrial Therapy, rehabilitation intervention has gained popularity in other patient populations. Rehabilitation in sports related injuries has paralleled Industrial Therapy in simulating activities required by a given sport.[4] Cardiac

---

> ### BOX 16.1
>
> ## Job Simulation Fields of Applications
>
> 1. Industrial Therapy
> 2. Sports Medicine Therapy
> 3. Cardiac Therapy
> 4. Auto and Personal Injury

---

rehabilitation has used job simulation as a treatment modality.[32] Victims of automobile and other personal injury cases have also benefited from job simulation and simulation of other activities of daily life.[28]

Simulating physical demands for the purpose of evaluating an individual's capabilities is increasingly used in disability determinations for personal injury, product liability, social security disability, and long term disability cases.[28]

As programs using job simulation have demonstrated themselves as cost effective mechanisms for returning injured workers to work, programs have become increasingly more popular in the workplace itself.[31] Innovative Therapists have instituted Work Hardening programs in employer facilities which emphasize a combination of actual work duties, education, exercise modalities, and simulated job activities to improve workers' abilities to perform physical demands.

Job simulation is not new as a therapeutic modality, but its use has increased dramatically in the past decade. While the increase has primarily occurred in the field of Industrial Therapy, job simulation in various forms is also being used in other specialty areas and general rehabilitation. The effectiveness of job simulation as a treatment modality will unquestionably cause it to continue to grow in scope and use in rehabilitation practice.

JOB SIMULATION CONSIDERATIONS

In theory, the best way to simulate a job would be to actually perform it (Figure 16.2). There are a number of situations discussed below in which on-the-job simulation is not possible. However, when a worker can remain "on the clock" at work, it is usually preferred to Work Hardening off the job. The primary reasons are to avoid secondary gain and to keep the individual on normal work routine.[8]

FIGURE 16.2 Job simulation in the workplace is sometimes the ideal approach, but is not always possible.

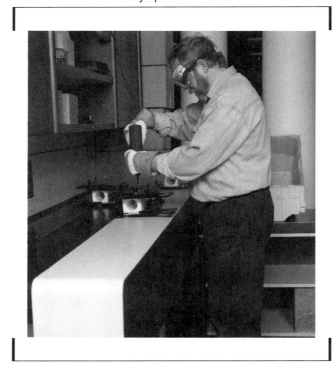

Human resources managers know that once a case involves lost time, the problems associated with the case multiply. Accordingly, it is preferable if an individual can be kept working, even on restricted duty, with progression and appropriate rehabilitation and education.

Safety Considerations

Safety is a primary reason why actual performance of the job is not appropriate rehabilitation after injury. It may not be safe for the worker to simultaneously perform all of the motions required by the job. It becomes necessary to break tasks into independent

---

BOX 16.2

Benefits of Job Simulation

1. Case resolution and return to work
2. Reduces fear of reinjury
3. Improves confidence in performing tasks
4. Determines client's job task capabilities
5. Provides a safe, controlled environment

---

components in order to learn to perform them in a safe manner before combining them again. Thus, from the standpoint of worker education and prevention of reinjury, safety is one reason why rehabilitation on the job may not be the best approach.

One example of the safety issue would be a delivery truck driver with a back injury. Drivers often handle loads at all heights and weights. They must also carry these loads on level surfaces, up and down stairs and ramps, and at times in adverse weather conditions.[2] Some of the independent components in this job would be the following:

- Lifting at waist level
- Lifting from floor to waist level
- Lifting from waist level to overhead
- Carrying on level surfaces
- Carrying on uneven surfaces
- Carrying up and down a ramp
- Carrying up and down stairs
- Carrying on potentially slippery surfaces

When workers are first injured, they may be able to handle the maximum amount of weight required by the job, but only at waist level. If rehabilitation occurred on the job, the conditions could not necessarily be controlled so that the worker would be able to lift only at waist level.

In the controlled, Work Hardening or Work Conditioning environment, the injured employee can begin handling the maximum load at waist level, then lesser loads from the floor and overhead. The worker could build endurance for carrying on level surfaces, and practice climbing stairs, ramps, and uneven and slippery surfaces with no load.

As the worker progresses in the program, physical demands can be combined. The individual can begin to carry light loads on stairs and ramps, and progress to heavier loads, then carrying on uneven or slippery surfaces. This controlled environment is a safe and preferred alternative to rehabilitation on the job in this case (Figure 16.3).

Fear Considerations

Another primary reason for job simulation off the job is to break down the barrier of fear.[26,29,30] If a worker was injured on a given job, there can be considerable fear of the tasks that caused the injury. In this case, breaking tasks into independent components makes them less recognizable to the worker as tasks that caused the injury.

It is quite common for workers entering a rehabilitation program to suffer from fear of reinjury. Efforts at rehabilitation will fail unless the issue of fear is addressed. In this instance, the worker is gradually improving and has just one more doctor's appointment before returning to work. Suddenly, the worker experi-

FIGURE 16.3 Job simulation starts with lower weights and demands (empty crates versus full crates) and safely progresses the worker to actual job demands.

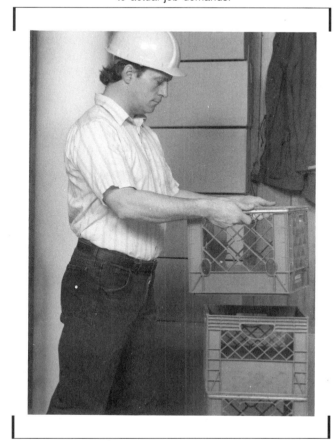

ences a relapse of the symptoms, and the Therapist (and Physician) are baffled. The action taken, generally, is to administer more therapy . . . and the pattern repeats itself. Without confronting the real issue, the patient may be perceived as a "gameplayer" who is exploiting the situation for secondary gain.

The injured worker does not necessarily recognize that fear is an issue. In fact, if asked, the individual would typically deny it. If rehabilitation includes job simulation, the worker can gradually overcome the fear motion-by-motion, task-by-task through the process of job simulation. Often job simulation itself will create avenues that will begin the process of working through the fear. As the job simulation becomes more like the job the worker must perform, small successes will help overcome the fear and will enhance the ability to face the actual situations that are perceived to have caused the injury.

A Case History—Fear of Reinjury[2]

In the author's experience with individuals having

a "fear problem," the injured worker who stands out in my mind was responsible for working on billboards on the highway. The worker had injured his back when he stepped too far backwards and fell off of the platform that supported him. He was approximately 50 feet off the ground. His safety belt caught him, but he hung there for a while before help arrived. This author was personally very concerned about the prospect of putting him back in that position; how frightening it must have been for him!

This gentleman had been sent for rehabilitation to a number of different Therapy centers. In each program, he had progressed well until it was time to return to the job. He would suddenly have a relapse just before it was time to return. His insurance company was certain that he was manipulating the system.

When he entered our Work Hardening program, he was able to perform all of the physical demands of his job individually. He did have minimal symptoms when lifting and had some difficulty lifting properly. We accepted him in the program; primarily for instruction in proper techniques, especially given the situations in which he was required to lift. He was a model patient during the educational sessions and early job simulation.

As we began simulating his job demands more specifically by combining lifting and climbing in confined spaces, he began to be more symptomatic. The Therapist working with him had noted that he would literally break into a cold sweat when working on one particular job simulation activity that had been designed specifically for his job. As the Therapist worked with him, he confided that he "just couldn't figure out why it was so scary" to climb with a load and work in a confined space. As they discussed the situation, it became evident that fear of falling was the primary issue.

Certainly he had good reason to be afraid. His coworkers and all of the Therapists working with him acknowledged that they would be afraid too. This seemed to be what he needed to face the fear. When he realized that it was all right (and normal) to be afraid, he was able to face it head-on and overcome it. Until he recognized the fear, he could not work through it. Job simulation, beginning with individual components of his job and working toward more specific and combined components of the job helped him gradually face the fear and move beyond it. He returned to work and is one of the center's chief cheerleaders.

Other Considerations

There are also other reasons to not undergo rehabilitation on the job. These include cases where there are uncooperative employers; where the injuries are too severe to even consider the approach; or where the workers have been off of the job and have already exhibited difficulty returning.

Many employers are unwilling to make accommodations for light duty to accommodate an injured worker. Although medical personnel may view such employers as uncooperative, there are often very good reasons for this reluctance.

Many employers have felt that they have been "burned" by temporary light duty becoming permanent. Medical personnel must remember that employers have to produce a product in order to stay in business.

In other cases, employers must deal with seniority issues, particularly if there is a union. Workers who cannot return to their former job often cause morale problems with other workers, even if they are not playing games.

The employer may be uncooperative simply because it is difficult to overcome these workplace issues. In such instances, off-site job simulation is an effective alternative. Work Hardening including job simulation is like the real workplace in important ways. It requires the worker to report for duty and spend a considerable portion of the day at the work center. And it incorporates the social aspects of being on the job, which minimizes the development of secondary issues. Therefore, off-site job simulation in a Work Hardening program has many of the same benefits that "staying on the clock" has, in instances of uncooperative employers (Figure 16.4).

There are workers who are already off work or have injuries too severe to consider rehabilitation on the job. Job simulation in these cases serves to condition the employee back to the workplace in a controlled, well supervised manner.

In summary, when rehabilitation on the job is not possible, job simulation is an effective alternative. It is often safer to break job tasks into small segments that can be eventually combined to resemble the actual job. It can address a worker's fear of reinjury, and benefit employees whose employers cannot accommodate them in the workplace.

General to Specific Job Simulation

Due to the needs to break up job tasks in a rehabilitation setting, one option is to begin with "generic" or "general" simulation and progress to "specific" simulation.[1]

JOB SIMULATION APPROACHES

General Simulation

General job simulation tends to work on a part of the body or part of a task. Specific job simulation involves

FIGURE 16.5   Job simulation starts with parts of the job and parts of the body, and progresses to whole job and whole body functionality.

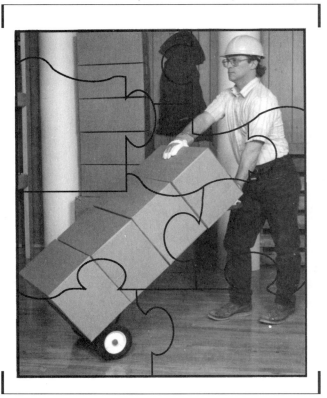

FIGURE 16.4   Work Hardening and Work Conditioning simulate a "real" work day down to the detail of punching in and out on a time clock.

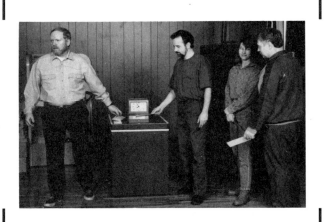

the whole body or a whole task. In general job simulation of lifting, the task can be structured so that the worker is lifting low weights only at waist level. This may initially involve primarily the arms, and may only be a portion of the actual lifting the worker must do on the job. In specific job simulation, the worker may be required to use the entire body including the back, legs, and arms when performing the entire task (Figure 16.5).

General simulation uses simulated physical demands (as opposed to actual job tasks). The physical demand of overhead reaching can be initially simulated by having a worker work with a bolt box on a high shelf. This may not be exactly like the actual task that a worker has to perform on the job.

In the case of an automobile mechanic, in order to install a muffler on a car, the worker may have to reach overhead. Working with the bolt box overhead will increase the worker's ability to install the muffler, by increasing the individual's tolerance for performing any type of activity in an overhead position (Figure 16.6).

General job simulation is used as a bridge between education, specific exercise techniques, and specific job simulation activities. In education sessions, workers learn appropriate techniques for lifting. They are also instructed in stabilization techniques, and strengthening exercises are performed to support and protect the injured body part. Following this education, general

lifting is a means of allowing the worker to apply the information learned and to practice stabilization techniques in a job related activity (lifting). A mirror can assist the individuals in self correcting as they practice. General lifting can be progressed in force, repetitions, and range, and the worker can eventually progress to specific simulation closer resembles the actual job.

Specific Simulation

After improving the worker's ability to perform the general physical demands of a task, the worker is ready for more specific simulation. Injured workers can begin accomplishing the actual task or a simulation of the actual task, simultaneously performing more than one of the physical demands. This is termed specific job simulation; that is, the task the worker is asked to perform is the actual task or a task that resembles the actual task in the combination of physical demands required.[1]

In specific job simulation, the individual is working at or near the required heights. The individual may also be working with the required weights, depending upon the objects the worker must handle. Specific simulation can also be progressed in the amount of time that is required of the worker and in the speed at which the worker performs the task.

One approach to job simulation begins with gener-

FIGURE 16.6 A, B   General simulation can be used as a bridge between education, specific exercise techniques, and specific job simulation activities.

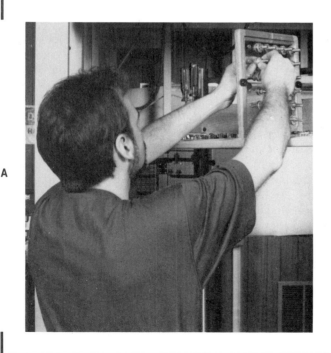

A

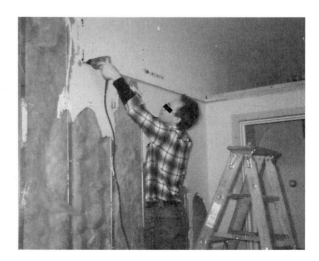

B

al simulation of physical demands and progresses to specific simulation. Specific simulation can then be progressed in time, speed, and loads. General job simulation works primarily on one physical demand at a time, which may be a part of an actual task a worker is required to perform. General job simulation also tends to involve only one body part at a time. On the other hand, specific job simulation tends to involve multiple physical demands simultaneously, an entire job task and the entire body.

Progressing from general to specific job simulation in a setting other than the actual worksite is appropriate for three major reasons—1) to more effectively overcome fear, 2) to provide more comprehensive education, and 3) to avoid risk where the injury poses a hazard to the employee or other workers.

GENERAL JOB SIMULATION

Equipment Selection—Considerations

As discussed previously, general simulation is typically used before specific simulation to build tolerance to job related activities and to break down a worker's fear of a task.

A wide variety of equipment can be used for general activities that build tolerance to physical demands. These include everything from home built equipment and common materials to purchased equipment.

In determining what type of equipment and materials to use for general job simulation activities, it

---

BOX 16.3

Equipment Needs Checklist

1. Equipment already owned?
2. Equipment used for FCAs?
3. Target industries and clientele?
4. Safety and liability issues?
5. Methods of documenting activity progression?
6. Cost and benefit of the equipment?
7. User friendliness?
8. Staffing, supervisory, and new hire requirements?
9. Space requirements?
10. Program capacity?
11. Program length? (Determines variety needs)

---

is helpful if an individual clinic considers a number of issues (Box 16.3). These include the following
- Equipment already owned by the clinic
- Equipment the clinic uses or is considering for Functional Capacity Assessments
- Types of industries from which the practice will attract its clientele
- Safety and product liability issues
- Ability to measure and document progress with the activity
- Cost benefit of the equipment to the clinic's potential other uses of the equipment
- User friendliness of the equipment
- Space availability in the clinic
- Staffing requirements needed to supervise activity on the equipment compared to staff availability in the clinic
- Number of workers in a program at a given time
- Hours per day workers are typically in the program (longer time requires more variety in activities and requisite equipment)

Since there are a number of issues to consider in choosing specific activities, no two clinics will approach job simulation equipment in exactly the same manner. The two primary issues to consider in choosing equipment are safety and the clientele the clinic will attract.

Safety Considerations

The importance of safety is easily seen. A Therapist does not want to injure an individual during an evaluation or in a rehabilitation program. In recent years, there have been several instances where rehabilitation centers and Therapists have been sued for injuries that allegedly occurred while using job simulation equipment.[3] In some of these cases, the equipment itself failed. The equipment must be sturdy and dependable. When considering the purchase of equipment, clinic personnel should investigate the track record of each piece under consideration. The following questions in Box 16.4 should be asked of the manufacturer.

Additionally, clinic personnel should think about what could potentially happen with the equipment. If you are thinking about a piece of equipment that has free weights, the following scenarios might be considered:
- How are the weights stored on the equipment? Could they easily fall or accidentally slip?
- How is the weight increased or decreased? If the client must lift it, could that alone cause an injury?
- Can the weight suddenly slip or fall off of the equipment once it is placed on the equipment?
- Can the weight shift around in or on the equip-

BOX 16.4

Equipment Manufacturer Safety Issues

1. Have there been any equipment incidents that have been reported to the manufacturer? If so, what happened and what was the outcome?

2. What type of product liability does the manufacturer have in case of equipment failure?

3. Does the equipment need periodic inspections or calibration? If so, how often? Who should do it? What does it entail?

4. Does the manufacturer have protocols for the proper and safe use of the equipment?

ment causing a sudden jolting or jerking force on the client?

Protocols for proper and safe use of the equipment should be readily available from the manufacturer or should be developed by the clinic.

In the case of home built simulation equipment, the same safety issues apply. At a minimum, if home built equipment is considered, the following questions should be asked:

- Does the clinic have adequate liability insurance in the event that the equipment fails?
- Will the equipment withstand the amount of force or weight that will be used with it? For example, if shelving units are to be built, how much weight is the maximum that should be placed on it and will more than that be required? Has it been tolerance tested?
- What protocols will be used? How will the protocols for the equipment be developed? Is it important to have these protocols tested prior to using them in the clinic setting?

Safety is a primary concern. It should be kept in mind that the clientele in an Industrial Therapy setting are already disabled. The risk of injury may actually be higher than for a more general population. Considering that there may be a greater propensity for litigation with this type of population, you cannot be too careful when selecting equipment.

Clientele Considerations

In addition to safety, the specific clientele of the clinic should be carefully considered in selecting equipment

for general job simulation. A clinic with a clientele of primarily white collar injured workers or light manufacturing industries will have different needs than clinics with a primarily heavy industry clientele. Clinics with a high percentage of hand injury patients will have different needs than those with primarily back injury patients.

A clinic with patients primarily in the railroad, trucking, and lumber industries will want to provide a number of different general lifting activities including stations with large and awkward loads. On the other hand, a clinic that works primarily with light manufacturing companies will tend to have lifting stations with more compact and lighter loads.

Clinics working with the construction trades may want to have a small house inside their clinic with electrical, plumbing, framing, drywall, painting, cabinetry, and other such activities that require stooping, squatting, and kneeling.

Rehabilitation centers working with large numbers of mechanics have been known to put actual trucks and car engine assemblies inside their clinics to simulate both general and specific job simulation activities.[10] Those working with the barge industries have been known to install lashing posts either inside or outside their clinics.[11]

Those working with primarily hand patients will tend to have activities that involve gross manipulation, fine manipulation and dexterity. They may use the BTE[e] or similar general simulation equipment which enable them to concentrate on activities specific to rehabilitating hand injury patients.

Simulating Physical Demands

Based on safety and clientele issues as previously discussed above, a clinic should choose activities and equipment for each physical demand that they wish to simulate. The following list of general physical demands, equipment, and activity suggestions should provide ideas for a clinic interested in adding general simulation workstations.

Some of these ideas can be suggested as home activities as well. It is important to keep in mind that you are billing for Work Hardening time. Activities that could be performed by the client at home should be performed at home. Often the group atmosphere of a Work Hardening program will provide motivation for the client to initially perform a given activity.[18] Later, the client can be expected to perform the activity at home.

Lifting and Carrying. All commercial functional evaluation systems provide some method of evaluating lifting and carrying. Many of these can be effectively used in Work Conditioning and Work Hardening for general lifting and carrying activities.

When choosing lifting activities for a given individual, one should begin with small, compact loads lifted close to the body and between waist and shoulder level (ideal lifting). As the individual progresses, the load is increased and the heights can be adjusted (to above and below the waist to shoulder range). The size of the load and where it is carried (relative to the body) can be progressed.

When moving from compact loads in the ideal lifting ranges, the Therapist should help the individual retain the body posturing and stabilization techniques that have been learned. The type of progression will depend upon the type of lifting and carrying that is required by the job. If the individual does not lift above shoulder level on the job (or in home or recreational activities) then simulating them in Work Hardening or Work Conditioning is not necessary or helpful.

General lifting and carrying activities can include the following:

- Any type and size of container and weights (Bricks can serve as weights - new bricks generally weigh five pounds. As they wear however, the weight decreases.)
- Commercially available lifting boxes[d,f]
- Heavy duty plastic bags filled with sand
- Lumber
- Concrete blocks (Figure 16.7)
- Buckets
- Burlap bags with gravel
- Lifting and stacking stations and various heights of shelving[d,f,n]
- Work Simulator equipment[e,p]
- Commercially available lifting evaluation stations[a,b,c,d,i,j,m,n,p,q,s,t,u]
- Commercially available materials handling stations (Figure 16.8)[f,n,r]
- Bags of cement or other substance (wrap them in plastic with duct tape to prevent leakage)

Stationary Standing. An upper extremity activity can be used as a standing activity if it can be used in a standing position. It is important to vary the activities to avoid boredom. Examples of activities which can be used while working on stationary standing include:

- Functional assessment upper extremity work sample equipment[n]
- Circuit board[n]
- Small assembly (Figure 16.9, A)[n]
- Nailboard and wallboard activities[f,n,o]
- Small bird cage assembly activity[f,o]
- The Work Cube[d]
- Building trades equipment (i.e. plumbing, electrical and carpentry equipment)[h,k,n,o]
- Pipe tree[f,n]

FIGURE 16.7 Concrete blocks are used to reinforce general lifting techniques. This is later incorporated into a work site task.

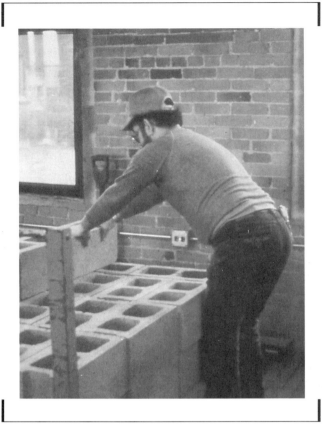

- Bolt box[e,n,t]
- Assembly tree[n]
- Office and factory modules[f,n]
- Component work samples (i.e. Valpar, Singer, WEST etc.)[r,t,u]
- Brick stacking on various heights of shelves
- Work simulator activities (Figure 16.9, A, B)[e,p]
- Macrame
- Electronic hobby kits[1]
- Woodworking kits[1]

Standing and Walking Combination or Walking. Program features can be alternated with activities that involve walking or moving from one activity to another to simulate standing and walking combinations. Other specific methods of simulation of a standing and walking combination include the following:

- Collating, filing, and copying (clerical type duties that require standing and walking)
- Alternating between two standing activities with a timed pattern which simulates the work situation
- Light carrying or pushing and pulling can be considered walking activity

FIGURE 16.8   A materials handling station can be used for general lifting as well as job task simulation.

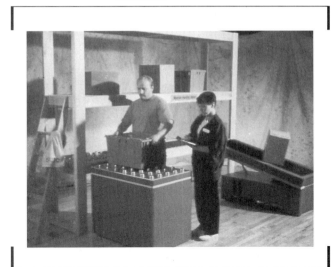

- Actual walking with a group (the companionship and semi-competitive atmosphere of a group is more motivating than simply walking at home. Additionally, walking just after a lunch break is an excellent way to begin a lifelong habit for the injured worker and provides a good warmup for afternoon activities.)
- Treadmill
- Cross country skiing type device
- Swimming with a flutter kick (this activity in-

volves many of the same muscles groups as walking but is unloaded).
- Stationary bicycle (seat should be such that pedals can just barely be reached to most closely approximate a walking type position for the spine).

Sitting.   Many of the same activities as listed under standing are also appropriate for sitting. As in walking, the group therapy aspects of doing activities with other people can be as beneficial as the actual simulation. Additional activities to consider while sitting might include the following:
- Typing
- Sewing
- Driving simulation[e,n,p] (Figure 16.10)
- Puzzles
- Stuffing envelopes
- Small assembly projects
- Knitting, crocheting, and needlework projects
- Other therapeutic activity projects such as those that are at times used in Occupational Therapy or Recreational Therapy departments.

Pushing and Pulling.   Pushing and pulling can be either static or dynamic, or a combination of both. Many Work Simulator pieces of equipment have some form of static and dynamic pushing and pulling activities. Some are isokinetic activities in which the speed is controlled, and the resistance is variable. These are least like actual dynamic pushing and pulling situations but can be considered safer due to the variable resistance.[12]

FIGURE 16.9   A small assembly station **(A)** or a variety of commercial equipment **(B)** provide the opportunity to work on stationary standing while utilizing the upper extremities.

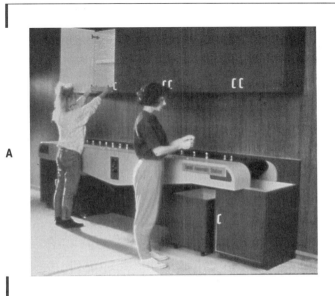
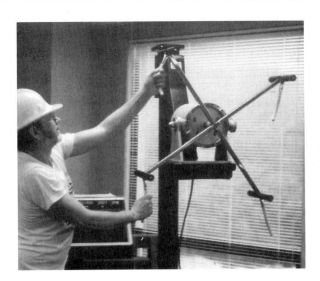

FIGURE 16.10   A driver's station provides a sitting environment with activities for the upper and lower extremities.

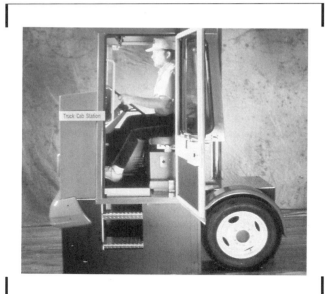

FIGURE 16.11   Push/pull activities can be simulated through the use of isokinetic equipment due to its safe and variable resistance. The patient can then progress to actual, dynamic push/pull situations.

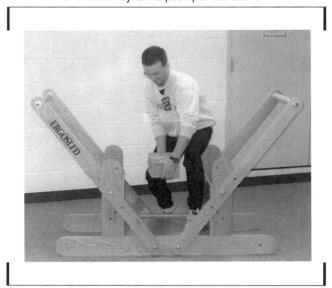

Pushing and pulling can be highly repetitive such as using a paint-roller, or more sustained such as pushing a cart. When simulating pushing and pulling, the direction of the pushing and pulling should match the actual job task the individual performs. The height of the pushing and pulling should also be similar.

It is important to know the amount of force that is used on the job and the amount of force that an individual is capable of exerting. The resistance should be adjusted to the level of resistance required by the job, as the individual progresses.

Examples of general pushing and pulling activities (Figure 16.11) include the following:
- Work simulator equipment (variety of push and pull situations can generally be simulated)[e,n,p]
- Shoveling
- Two wheel hand truck (the type of apparatus that is used to move a refrigerator)
- Four wheel cart
- Wheelbarrow
- Pushing and pulling object(s) on a dolly (a dolly is a platform with wheels on it).
- Paint roller (without paint is preferred)
- Push and pull sled[d]
- Sanding a board
- Many woodworking activities
- A pulley type apparatus
- Overhead pulley[n]

Repetitive Reaching.   Repetitive reaching can be forward, backward, sideways, or overhead. General simu-

lation of repetitive reaching requires activities where the individual alternatively moves the arms back and forth from a neutral position to a position over the head, or backward, sideways, or forward. This is unlike sustained overhead backward, sideways, or forward reaching which requires individuals to maintain their arms in the position. Repetitive reaching can be weighted or unweighted by virtue of the activity itself or by placing weights on the individual's arms.

Examples of repetitive reaching activities and equipment include the following:
- Work simulator equipment[e,p]
- Brick stacking on various levels of shelving with bricks placed based on the specific type of reaching to be performed
- Nail boards or pegboards where the individual inserts nails or pegs into a board at a height or distance that simulates the specific type of reaching to be performed on the job[f,n,o]
- Assembly activities where the individual must reach overhead, forward, sideways, or backward for short durations
- Electrician or plumbing type activities where the individual must reach overhead, forward, sideways, or backward for short durations[h,k,n,o]
- The West VII Bus Bench[u] on a shelf that requires reaching to and occasionally above shoulder level
- Paint rolling
- Macrame projects hung from the ceiling can be worked on in a sustained overhead reaching position

- Upper extremity coordination activities where the individual works on a variety of activities at a height or distance that simulate the specific type of reaching to be performed on the job (Figure 16.12), See standing and extremity coordination sections for specific activities to be performed.

Sustained Reaching. General simulation of sustained reaching can use many of the same activities as repetitive reaching. In this instance however, the individual must perform the activity for longer durations while maintaining the position. For example, the same nail or pegboard can be used, but the individual must move the nails or pegs from one slot to another at the given height, rather than from a waist level position to an overhead position.

Kneeling and Sustained Squatting. Kneeling or sustained squatting can be simulated by having the individual perform any of the activities that might be performed in a standing or sitting position. Many of the previously mentioned activities may be performed while an individual is kneeling or squatting. A brick stack can be used with the individual placing bricks from one low shelf to another.

Other activities that can also be performed in a kneeling or squatting position include the following:
- Paint rolling along a baseboard
- Electrician or plumbing type activities where the individual must kneel or squat[n,o]
- Assembly activities placed so that the individual must kneel or squat[n,r,t,u]

Climbing. The following can be used as climbing activities or to work on the motions used in climbing:
- Stairs
- Stationary vertical ladder
- Stepladder
- Portable stairs
- Stepper type exercise machines[d]
- Bicycle or stationary bicycle

Balancing. Balance activities can be performed alone or with other physical demands. Climbing a ladder can be a balance activity. The following activities can be used to work on balance:
- Balance beam
- Various types of ladders
- Sloped surface such as a ramp, or a simulated roof (Figure 16.13)
- Walking on uneven terrain
- Walking in a long narrow sand lot

Repetitive Stooping and Squatting. Repetitive stooping or squatting is differentiated from sustained

FIGURE 16.12   A position station allows the patient to work within their reaching capabilities and advance their reaching capabilities through incremental height and width adaptations.

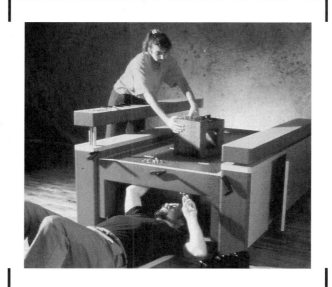

stooping or squatting in that the individual moves back and forth from a normal upright position as opposed to maintaining that position for long durations. Repetitive stooping can be performed while standing or while sitting. Simulating repetitive stooping or squatting can be done by using upper extremity coordination activities such as repetitive assembly tasks that require the worker to stoop or squat to perform them.

The following activities can be used to work on repetitive stooping and squatting:
- Brick stacking from a waist level shelf to a lower shelf
- Woodworking activities (larger objects that require stooping over or squatting to reach part of the object)[n]
- Paint rolling along a low surface
- Electrician or plumbing type activities where the individual must bend forward at the waist[n]
- Assembly activities placed so that the individual must bend forward at the waist[n,r,t,u]
- Work table assembly[n]
- Position station[n]

Dexterity and Upper Extremity Coordination. There are numerous methods on the market to measure upper extremity coordination and dexterity (Figures 16.14, *A, B*). Such tests are all useful as mentioned in previous sections as activities to perform while simulating other physical demands (such as kneeling, squatting, sitting, or standing).

FIGURE 16.13 Uneven surfaces allow the patient to work on balance and can be incorporated with other physical demands to work on a job task.

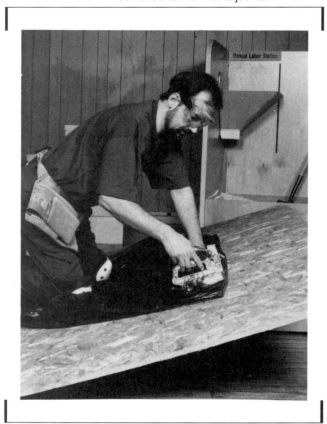

The following are examples of some of the upper extremity coordination activities available:

- Circuit board[n]
- Keyboard keystrokes[n]
- Valpar I and IV[t]
- Minnesota Rate of Manipulation[d]
- Crawford Small Parts[d]
- West II Brief Tool[u]
- Macrame activities
- Woodworking activities[l]
- Work simulators[e,p]

A clinic has many options when selecting general simulation activities. There are a number of issues to consider when selecting equipment and activities, but the two primary concerns are safety and job activities of the clinic clientele.

SPECIFIC JOB SIMULATION

As an individual increases in ability to perform general physical demands of a given job, simulation should become increasingly specific to the tasks which the worker will have to perform on the actual job. In moving from general to specific job simulation, an individual is progressing from the part to the whole. This progression occurs both from part of the body to the whole body, and from part of a task to the whole task.

FIGURE 16.14 The Minnesota Rate of Manipulation **(A)** and the O'Connor Finger Dexterity **(B)** are upper extremity coordination and dexterity testing methods that can be used as activities while simulating other physical demands.

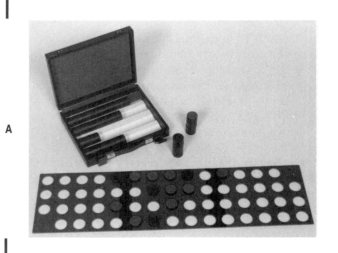

A

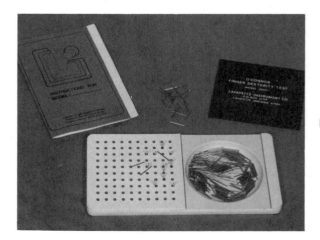

B

In many instances it is not necessary to specifically simulate every task the individual will perform on the job, nor is it always necessary to simulate the whole body motion that the individual is required to do. The Therapist must determine from the general simulation process which demands or tasks the individual will find difficult. These are the demands or tasks for which a specific simulation should be designed and implemented.

In the case of a railroad worker with a back injury, the individual must regain the ability to jump on the stationary vertical ladder of a moving train.[2] After the individual has practiced and demonstrated the ability to perform generic stationary vertical ladder climbing and running, it is likely that the individual will still have difficulty jumping the moving train. This is an instance where specific simulation is necessary.

Equipment Considerations

In determining how specific job simulation will be done, a great deal of creativity is often necessary. Equipment such as the BTE Work Simulator,[e] the Lido Work Simulator[P] and the KEY Position Station[n] are generally helpful in simulating some specific activities.

In the case of an automobile mechanic that must work under a car, the individual can lie on their back and use a screwdriver or other tool simulation attachment. This provides a reasonable simulation of the tasks that automobile mechanics must perform. There are many other examples however, where equipment from the workplace will be more helpful.

Installing Actual Equipment

In cases where a given clinic provides service to a specific industry in great numbers, it is always helpful to obtain equipment or props from companies with which the clinic works. Companies are generally more than willing to assist in actually installing such equipment in a clinic that will be seeing a number of their employees. Examples have been numerous, including the following:
- Railroads have installed switches and have donated railroad ties to clinics that work with large numbers of their employees[10]
- A utility has installed a telephone pole and telephone cable for use in one clinic setting[2]
- A barge company has installed lashing posts and ropes outside one clinic[11]
- Local post offices have provided mail sorting bins and mail carts for a number of clinics working with their employees[2]
- Grocery warehouses have provided groceries for a number of clinics[2]

In working with a company with high numbers of employees that are being seen in a given clinic, such options for a specific job simulation should be explored.

Equipment On Loan

In cases where an individual worker is actually being seen in a clinic and there is no special equipment already available, it is often possible to borrow equipment or supplies for specific job simulation. Involving the injured worker in the process of obtaining such equipment or supplies is actually good therapy in itself.[29,30]

If an injured employee has been off the job, there may be barriers to returning to work other than the injury itself.[29,30] Often, the worker and employer may be "out of sight, out of mind" in each other's minds. This may not necessarily be at a conscious level, but nevertheless, it may exist. The employer may have found a way to work around the fact that the employee is missing, and the employee has gotten used to not working.

The process of the employee participating in obtaining job simulation equipment forces the individual to establish contact with the employer. If there are communication problems between the employee and employer, this process will often begin to establish improved communication. The worker will have an opportunity to observe the employer being helpful and taking an active role in the rehabilitation process.

In addition, the employer will see the worker's active participation in a realistic and functional rehabilitation process. Improving communication in Workers' Compensation cases is always good therapy. This chapter discusses examples of equipment provided on loan in a clinic setting.

> A roofer fell from a roof and sustained a mild head injury, fractures in the right humerus, radius, and ulna and a severe cervical and lumbar strain. The employer provided the center with rolls of roofing materials, shingles, and a tool belt. These were used in conjunction with balance activities to simulate the more specific situation while working on a roof. In this case, the fear of falling and a mild balance deficit were problematic. Simulating the actual activities the worker performed enabled the individual to face the situation in a controlled environment.

In this case, it was determined that working on high sloped roofs was not appropriate for this individual. However, he had no difficulty with flatter surfaces. The individual had worked for the company for a long time and was considered by his employer to be a valuable employee. His employer decided to promote him to a supervisory position in which he would be better able to control his individual work situation.[2]

An individual working for an automobile assembly plant was provided a bumper by the employer. In this situation, the worker was status-post lumbar discectomy. The main problem for the worker was not the amount of weight that he had to lift, but the position in which he had to lift and hold it. The job involved lifting a bumper that was $4.5' \times .5' \times .5'$ and weighed 65 pounds. He had to lift every other bumper, pass it across a pit (for workers working under the car) to another individual and the two of them hooked it onto brackets on the car. At the next station on the assembly line, the bumper was actually adjusted and secured to the car.

Hooks were placed on a standard shelving unit at the proper height and the individual, with the assistance of a center employee was able to simulate lifting and passing the bumper over the pit. Boards were placed on the floor to indicate the placement of the pit that runs under the car so that the worker would appropriately learn placement of his feet while installing the bumper.[2]

A circuit board assembler who was status-post Carpal Tunnel Release was provided with actual circuit boards and the components to work on the specific activities on which she had experienced difficulty. This involved positioning the board with her unaffected hand and attaching small parts using a pair of tweezers with her affected hand. Additionally, the individual had difficulty with testing the circuit boards. This involved clipping wires which connected the boards to a piece of testing equipment. Opening the clips that attached to the circuit board required 11 pounds of pinch force in a lateral pinching position.

While working on the specific simulation, it was determined that exerting the 11 pounds of pinch force to open the clips was problematic. In researching the possibilities for modifications, it was found that there was an alternative clip that could be used that only required two pounds of pinch force. This modification was made to the workstation which enabled the employee to return to work. Without trying the simulation in the clinic, the individual would probably have returned to work and failed. With the simulation, the problems could be explored and modified. Thus, the worker returned to the job confident in her ability to perform her job.[2]

A retail clothing store stocker with a lumbar strain was provided with clothing samples and a clothing rack to work on the specific lifting requirements of her job. This job involved lifting up to 35 pounds of clothing on hangers, and placing them onto a rack which was above shoulder level. On the general lifting stations, the worker had demonstrated the ability to lift up to 40 pounds from waist to overhead. The individual was somewhat leery however, of her ability to lift the actual clothing, as it was awkward and the load would often shift.

After obtaining the bundles of clothing samples and the racks, the individual found specific techniques to stabilize the load while lifting, which gave her confidence in her ability to perform the job. She was able to return to work with no modifications to her job.[2]

A waitress was able to obtain a tray, a bus tub, dishes, and a server stand to work on the specific requirements of her job. This individual had sustained a lumbar and cervical strain when involved in an automobile accident while catering an off-site function. The restaurant was no longer involved in catering and the employee would be returning to a normal waitress job.

The employee had demonstrated the ability to manage the weights required by the job (lifting up to 40 pounds from waist to shoulder levels), but was unsure of her ability to reach forward and sideways to serve customers that were on the inside of a booth. She feared situations where she had to work quickly (during peak hours) and felt that she would be unable to balance a loaded tray and reach forward to serve someone at the same time. By simulating her specific work situation, she was able to practice and gain the confidence she needed to return to work.[2]

If it is not possible to obtain specific equipment, a little creativity between the clinic and the injured worker will often produce a simulation idea that will work. Getting the worker involved is important. Specific examples of creativity that have been applied toward simulating specific demands include the following:

It was determined that the primary difficulty with one individual's job involved the vibration of a tool that was used in the process. The worker needed to find appropriate protective equipment that would protect her hands from the vibration. The Therapist determined that the vibration from a hand sander was similar in frequency to the tool she used. The hand sander was used to assist in problem-solving the best combination of protective equipment to use.[2]

One worker had to perform certain tasks in assembly of a light fixture. Component parts were made available by the employer, but fixtures to hold the components were not available. An industrial specialist on the staff of the clinic designed and built holders for the components to enable the employee to simulate her job activities.[2]

One clinic designed a moving ladder on a wall that could simulate the vertical ladder from which a railroad employee had to jump while the train was moving.[10]

A clinic that had a contract with the local police and fire department designed and built an obstacle course that included climbing, crawling, and other activities to simulate rescuing people from burning buildings while carrying simulated bodies (burlap bags filled with gravel).[2] Rescue Randy mannequins are commercially available for this purpose.

When progressing individuals from general simulation activities to specific simulation activities, the following should be kept in mind:

- Not all job activities need to be simulated in every case. Therapists should determine which activities are critical to the job and which activities are problematic for the worker based on the results of general simulation.
- Specific equipment can and should be obtained from the employer where possible. Involving the injured worker in obtaining materials is often therapeutic in that the injured worker begins to accept responsibility through the rehabilitation process.
- Creativity is often a key component in designing specific job simulation. Brainstorming with the injured worker is a good way to generate ideas for simulation of specific tasks.
- Safety must always be a concern in specific job simulation. Since the individual is beginning to work on whole tasks and is using the whole body, specific simulation activities lend themselves to less of a controlled environment than general job simulation activities. Therefore,

Therapists should closely supervise individuals working on specific simulation activities.

Worksite Simulation

If the individual has already demonstrated the ability to handle the amounts of weight and the ranges of lifting required by the job, specific job simulation can also be done at the worksite by having the individual work at slower speeds or for shorter durations. This is a good way for the employee to make the transition from Work Hardening to the job. Once an individual has begun specific job simulation, return to work or case closure should be imminent.

PROGRESSION FROM GENERAL TO SPECIFIC SIMULATION

Job simulation is naturally only a part of work oriented rehabilitation. As an individual progresses in the program, more time should be spent performing general and eventually specific simulation activities. Commensurately, less time is spent on education, pain and stress management, and other components of the program.

This progression and application of general to specific approach to job simulation is demonstrated in the following case study.

General to Specific Job Simulation[2]

Linda is a 36 year old employee of a light paperboard products company. Linda worked as a scrapper for this company for seven years before she sustained a back injury that required a lumbar discectomy.

The scrapper is responsible for removing the excess scrap from a pallet-load of die-cut paper. This is done by using a jackhammer-type tool that is suspended from the ceiling. The tool is outfitted with a vibration-dampening device that minimizes the whole-body and hand vibration to the worker. The scrapper also is responsible for clearing the scrap that is generated, and moving the product to and from the workstation.

Job Analysis

The following physical demands are required in this operation: (Note—for the purposes of this illustration, only the physical demands that apply to the specific injury of the employee will be discussed. For purposes of understanding the job, the physical demand information from the job analysis is presented in narrative format.)

Lifting and Carrying. Twenty repetitions per day moving empty pallets approximately 15 feet. Lifting can occur from floor to shoulder level if one person handles and actually lifts the pallet. The actual weight of this company's pallets is approximately 75 pounds. However, the employee typically lifts just one end of the pallet (maximum force of 30 pounds to lift one end) and drags it (see pulling) approximately ten feet before dropping it.

The employee lifts (and carries approximately three feet) completed stacks of the product from one pallet to another. Product varies in dimensions; the smallest being 8½ inches wide by 11 inches long, and the largest being 45 inches wide by 45 inches long. The number of sheets per stack is determined by the individual employee.

Employees are free to move less than a one inch stack or more than a thirty inch stack, depending on how much they want to move at a time and how many trips they want to make. The lifting range is from 8–60 inches off the floor. The frequency is determined by the size of the stack the employee chooses to lift at one time. Employees average 20 pallets per day. The minimum frequency of lifting observed per pallet was 15 and the maximum was 28 (range of 300 to 560 lifts per day).

Pushing and Pulling. The individual tends to lift and pull the empty pallet approximately ten feet. Pulling force (at approximately waist height) varies from 20 to 50 pounds, depending on the surface and the condition of the pallet.

The employee also sustains a pulling force from shoulder to waist level (pulling downward) on the jack-hammer that is suspended from the ceiling while scrapping. The force varies from 10 to 20 pounds, and is maintained for an average of three minutes, six times per pallet, 20 pallets per day (120 repetitions maintained for three minutes each per day).

Additional pushing and pulling involves using a manual pallet jack. Force required is 15 pounds at waist level while employee maneuvers pallet jack into position (sustained for 1.5 minutes on the average). This occurs ten times per day on the average.

Stooping. (Forward bending at the waist). The employee begins using the jackhammer at a position just below shoulder level (the employee is standing upright at this point) and then gradually bends until the employee is in a fully stooped position. This is done 120 times per day with the stooped position occurring for an average of 1.5 minutes per repetition. The employee has control over whether or not this is accomplished by squatting, stooping, or other alternative positions, but all employees observed used stooping.

Squatting. No employees were observed using this position, but it is an alternative.

Standing and Walking. Employees are on their feet for eight hours per day. Most of this time they are stationary as they perform the scrapping operation described above. Short distance walking is required as they perform the cleanup operation and move products.

Physical Examination and History

The following is a summary of the findings from Linda's initial evaluation:

- Linda is status-post L4/L5 micro-discectomy—30 days.
- Linda had been off work with this injury a total of 75 days. Conservative treatment had been attempted, but with continued pressure on the nerve root as evidenced by increasing neurological signs; surgery had been recommended and performed.
- Linda had no prior history of back injury. She stated that she was just "doing her job one day" when she felt "something just give-way" in her back. She said she had continued working, but that night and the next day the pain became severe and was "from my back all the way down my right leg to my big toe."
- Linda attempted to return to work three weeks post surgery but was only able to complete one half day on the job. She stated "it was the bending and the lifting" that caused an increase in her symptoms.
- Current symptoms are a dull ache in the L4/L5 region of the low back with radiation into her right leg to the knee. She also reports "shooting pains" in the same area (and occasionally to the foot) when bending, and occasionally when lifting.
- Linda expressed considerable anxiety about not being able to return to work. She stated that she makes $12 per hour on her job and needs the money to support her daughter. She said "Workers' Compensation pay just doesn't cut it." She also told the evaluator "I probably pushed the doctor to let me go back to work sooner than I was ready . . . but I needed the money."
- Musculoskeletal evaluation indicated the following findings:
    Flat back posture with a mild lateral shift (posterior view—upper body shifted to the left, hips shifted to the right).
    Severe restriction in lumbar extension (low back did not move at all when attempting this motion)

Guarded lumbar flexion with patient using her knees as support. Range of motion was severely limited and not measured due to severe guarding by the patient. Linda refused to perform side bending and lateral shifting motions—she stated she was "afraid of hurting something." No neurological deficits were noted.

- Evaluations indicated the following maximum capabilities: (Note: for the purposes of this illustration, only the capabilities that apply to the specific injury of the employee will be discussed.)

  Lifting and Carrying—repetitive—25 pounds at waist level; unable to perform repetitive lifting other than at waist level.

  Lifting and Carrying—one time maximum—15 pounds floor to waist; ten pounds waist to shoulder and 40 pounds at waist level.

  Pushing and Pulling—Static maximum at waist level—42 pounds; static maximum pulling from shoulder height—31 pounds.

  Stooping—Unable (Linda self limited this test and stated she was "afraid she'd hurt something.")

  Squatting—Unable (Linda self limited this test and stated she was "afraid she'd hurt something.")

  Standing and Walking—Longest single duration on her feet during the functional evaluation was 45 minutes. Total time observed—90 minutes. Linda paced the floor as a form of pain relief.

Work Hardening

Linda was admitted to a full day (6½ hours/day) Work Hardening program. She completed the program in four weeks and was discharged and returned to work with restrictions. The following is a summary of her activities in the program.

Week 1

The focus this week was on orientation to the program, education, symptom control and instruction, and practicing exercises involving stabilization and postural correction. General job simulation activities were initiated which stressed application of the principles learned in the education and individual exercise sessions.

These simulation activities involved parts of the types of tasks she had to do at work, and parts of the body required to perform the tasks.

Linda completed three hours per day (a total of 15 hours for the week) of educational classes on back care, pain and stress management.

Linda worked in the gym for 90 minutes per day (a total of 7½ hours for the week) on her individualized exercise program which included correction of the lateral shift, extension exercises, and stabilization and postural correction techniques.

Linda worked in the general job simulation area for two hours per day (total of ten hours for the week) working on the following activities (grouped by physical demand):

Lifting and Carrying

- Lifting station waist level (with mirror)—20 pounds; 5 sets of 15.
- Lifting station knee to waist level (with mirror)—5 pounds; 5 sets of 5.
- Lifting station shoulder to waist level (with mirror)—5 pounds; 5 sets of 5.
- Carrying (small box)—20 pounds; 20 repetitions of 15 feet.

Standing and Walking

- Brick stacks—10 minutes—2 times—waist level move bricks from front to back of shelf (also mild stooping).
- Goal—Work on all other activities as assigned; increase total on-feet time to 2 hours; longest on-feet duration to 1 hour by the end of the first week.

Pushing and Pulling.   Push cart—(waist level—static force required to push—30 pounds)—1 minute durations; 10 repetitions.

Stooping.   Work on bolt box—just below waist level (requiring a minimal sustained stoop) 30 second durations; back bends in between each repetition, 20 repetitions—spread throughout job simulation time frame.

Squatting.   Work in sustained squat position 30 second durations on wall board; 10 repetitions—spread throughout job simulation time frame.

As expected, Linda was extremely sore after the first two days of the program and continued to be sore throughout the rest of the first week. She did note, however, that her pain was now confined mostly to her back; and did not involve the right leg as much.

The Therapist noted reduction of the lateral shift following the second day and the beginning of improved lumbar flexion and extension mobility. By the end of the week Linda was able to reduce her leg symptoms by doing lateral shift correction and extension exercises.

Week 2

The focus this week was on increasing the general job simulation activities and maintaining control of her leg symptoms throughout the activities, by using her stabilization and postural correction exercises. Thus, parts of tasks and parts of the body were still the emphasis this week.

All frequencies were increased by 100% on Monday. All weights were increased by 10 pounds on Wednesday. Brick stacking from waist to shoulder and from waist to knee level were also added to increase her tolerance to postures required by her job. Total time in general job simulation activities was now 3½ hours per day; individual exercise program, two hours per day and instructional sessions with practice of body mechanics and stabilization techniques, one hour per day.

By the end of the second week, Linda was reporting periods of time when her back "just hurt a little." She stated that for the most part she was "now feeling much better about being able to control her symptoms." She stated that she was not really having much leg pain anymore; "sometimes just a little at night." She did complain of being "sore all over from the exercises." She reported still being "a little leery about using the jackhammer."

The Therapist noted that range of motion was approaching normal in all spinal movements and was able to progress her stabilization activities against gravity. The Therapist stated "the client's overall excellent conditioning and flexibility has allowed Linda to progress quickly in the stabilization protocols."

Week 3

In this week, the goal was to begin introducing specific job simulation activities and increase the total on-feet time. For this purpose, the employer was contacted, and stacks of product of differing sizes were provided. The rehabilitation center had pallets that were similar in design and nature to the pallets used in the workplace. An old jackhammer assembly was obtained and hung from the ceiling. The jackhammer was not operational, but did provide the aspects of pulling and positioning needed to simulate the scrapper job.

In the general simulation activities, Linda had achieved good symptom control and had learned to stabilize her spine in all positions. All activities were increased to match the heights and weights of the job.

Repetitions were not increased, and no further general activities were added. Specific simulation activities were introduced to begin to focus more on whole tasks, and to integrate the parts of the tasks that had been introduced previously. Rather than working

on parts of the body individually, the focus shifted to a whole body approach with specific job simulation. The following specific job simulation activities were added:

Lifting and Carrying.
- Ten repetitions per day of moving empty pallets approximately 15 feet. (Linda was instructed to perform this activity in front of the mirror to ensure that she used good stabilization techniques).
- One hundred repetitions of lifting and carrying stacks of product, range from 8 to 60 inches. (Linda had to determine an appropriate weight for each product and keep track of the approximate stack height for each size of product represented. This was done so that the total repetitions per day could be determined based on her comfort level with the weight).

Pushing and Pulling.   (See lifting pallets above for simulation of push and pull associated with lifting pallets on the job.)

Scrapping Simulation.   Using the jackhammer suspended from the ceiling in the clinic, Linda was instructed to perform 50 repetitions per day of simulated scrapping (using the stabilization techniques she had been taught and varying her postures from stooping to squatting). She was instructed to maintain the force and postures for 1.5 minutes each repetition.

Stooping.   Forward bending at the waist—(See scrapping simulation above for stooping.)

Squatting.   (See scrapping simulation above for squatting.)

Week 4

Linda stated she was feeling good about her ability to return to the job. The Therapist contacted the employer at the end of week three and asked if Linda could work on the job for three hours and complete the day in Work Hardening as a transition to returning to the job. The employer was cooperative and Linda decided to work in the morning and go to Work Hardening in the afternoon.

In the afternoons during the fourth week, the Therapist worked with Linda to refine her postural techniques with the scrapping simulation. The Therapist worked with Linda to find the ideal balance between the weight and repetitions of lifting the product. Symptom control exercises and activities were also reviewed as Linda prepared to return to work full time.

Linda was released to return to full duty with a restriction regarding overtime. The employer agreed to allow Linda to work overtime only when absolutely necessary, and when she was working overtime, she would perform jobs that did not require her to lift or stoop.

Progressing Job Simulation Activities

As was demonstrated in Linda's case, activities should be progressed from general to specific; part of the body to the whole body; part of the task to the whole task. Progressing job simulation activities becomes the key to moving cases toward resolution. The ultimate customer, the employer, and the insurance company that represents the employer look favorably on programs that can progress injured workers quickly.[21]

It is important to know when and how to progress job simulation activities. While each case is certainly different, the following guidelines are useful in progression of activities (Box 16.5, page 336).

- Activities should be progressed twice per week in a full day program and weekly in a program less than a full day.
- The Therapist should work with the injured worker in progressing the activities. This gives the individual a feeling of control, ownership, and participation in the rehabilitation program.
- If the program is predicted to last four weeks, the progress should equal approximately one quarter of the total goal each week. For instance, if the individual initially can lift 20 pounds and must ultimately lift 60 pounds, the individual must progress by approximately 10 pounds per week. On the other hand, if the program is scheduled to last two weeks, the same individual will have to progress by 20 pounds per week to reach the goal. Repetitions, durations, and frequencies must also increase proportionately to the length of the program. Progressing by more than 10 pounds per week is probably unrealistic for most patients.[2] Likewise, increasing beyond doubling the frequency, repetitions, and range each week is probably also unrealistic.[2]
- Increasing frequency and duration is generally easier than increasing ranges and loads. If activities are increased twice per week, increase the frequencies and durations the first time then loads and ranges the second time.
- Individuals vary greatly in their capacities to increase weight, frequencies, durations, and ranges depending on the type of injury, age, and general fitness level. This is why it is

important to work with the individual in determining what is appropriate. As in general rehabilitation, the Therapist must balance pushing the injured worker with sensitivity, empathy for pain, and other symptoms the individual is experiencing.
- Motivation is an important factor. Generally, other clients in the program will provide motivation for the individual. The Therapist can assist this process by encouraging a first week client to talk to a motivated fourth week client who is making good progress. Likewise, the Therapist must keep in mind the opposite effect of one bad apple in the program demotivating the rest of the client population.
- If the individual is reluctant to increase activities, the Therapist must assist in viewing the big picture. Finding motivation for the employee and keeping that in focus will help the employee work beyond the symptoms.
- Since most patients will have sore muscles, especially the first week in a program, it is helpful to prepare the client for that eventuality. Some have said that this might be a self-fulfilling prophecy. Experience indicates that if they are not warned, they may become afraid and not come back. Counteract the self-fulfilling prophecy by letting them know that they will begin to feel better by the second week. Letting them know that they will be sore, but only temporarily, is preferred to their being surprised by the pain.

The ability to progress in job simulation activities varies from individual to individual. One must also keep in mind the above guidelines and consider the total length of the program in progressing activities.

Program Length

Over the past decade, as more facilities have become involved in work oriented rehabilitation, there has been a wide range of appropriate program lengths. Programs have averaged from several weeks to several months in duration.[9] Naturally, appropriate durations will vary depending upon the client base of the clinic.

Clinics with high populations of lighter industry may be expected to have shorter lengths than clinics with high populations of heavier industry. Further, clinics that specialize in difficult clients can expect longer average durations than those that see primarily acute clients. Clinicians have been known to keep injured workers too long. There are two primary reasons why this occurs:
- The program is progressed too slowly
- The client is inappropriate for the program

BOX 16.5

Guidelines for Progressing Job Simulation Activities

1. Activities progressed twice per week in a full day and weekly in a half day program.
2. Therapist and worker should work together in progressing activities because each worker has different capacities.
3. Program length should be determined by weight, frequencies, repetitions, and range. General rules to follow are 10#/week and doubling the frequency, repetitions, and range per week.
4. Increasing frequency and durations is easier than increasing ranges and loads.
5. Determine workers' motivation and use it to advance activities.
6. Inform the worker about the general discomfort they will develop as a result of increasing their activity.

Program Progression

Full day programs, by definition, are predicated on the worker being off work. However, the trend is away from full day programs for a number of reasons— 1) to condition the worker more slowly, 2) to incorporate some on-the-job rehabilitation, 3) to allow for vocational activities, and 4) to reduce costs.

Less than full day programs are particularly effective in more acute situations where individuals can only work part of the day. Whether running a full day or partial day program, a number of guidelines have proven beneficial.

Clients should be progressed at a pace that provides a sense of daily progress and minimizes boredom. No matter how many activities a clinic has, the clients may at some time become bored. At a glance, this phenomenon may be difficult to understand. After all, jobs that Work Hardening clients do are often repetitive and appear boring. The difference is, on the job, the worker is producing something of value. In a Work Hardening program, while the worker may be gaining in strength and endurance, there is no tangible evidence that they have produced anything of value.

Producing something of value is a critical factor in maintaining motivation.[21] It is advantageous to return the worker to the job as soon as they are able to handle a job-level pace, usually by the fourth week as dis-

cussed below. Returning to the job instead of two additional weeks of Work Hardening represents tangible progress that maintains motivation. If the worker must repeat the same things another week, despite a possible increase in strength and endurance, motivation suffers.

It is important to begin Work Hardening or Work Conditioning activities as early as possible post-injury. In the early days of work oriented rehabilitation, it was thought that an individual must be completely stable before beginning job simulation activities. Today, earlier work-related intervention is becoming preferred. It has been shown that programs instituted quickly will prevent many of the secondary issues that plague lost time Workers' Compensation cases.[7,8]

Initially in a program, there is a considerable amount of education that must take place. The first week of a full or partial day program may involve only five to ten hours of job simulation activities and exercise. This amount can be spread throughout the week, interspersed with education classes, pain and stress management classes, self management teaching, and individual and group counseling sessions.

The second week in the program, the individual will begin to tolerate more hours of job simulation activities and exercise and fewer hours of education.

The third week, as the individual has completed education sessions, most of the time will be devoted to job simulation activities.

Work Hardening on the job can begin, in many cases, by the fourth week, or at the point in time when a client is able to perform five days of work. Naturally this takes considerable coordination with the employer. The employer must be willing to work with the injured worker and the clinic to make the transition. This ideal situation is not always present with a given injured worker. But clinics do not always persue these options with their clients' employers.

The above schedule may not be appropriate for all workers. Some workers simply need a heavy dose of education and can return to work after one or two weeks. Others may not be able to return for four to five weeks.

When looking at cases in which clients were kept for one to two weeks after they were able to tolerate job-level activity, they actually regressed in Work Hardening.[2] In interviewing these clients, it became apparent that the primary problem was boredom.

Screening, Admission, and Continuation in the Program

In its early development, Work Hardening was considered a last resort for many clients. There were no known factors which would assist a Work Hardening or Work Conditioning clinic in knowing whether or not a program would be successful. After more than a decade of experience with these programs, it is much easier to determine who is appropriate and who is not.[6] The following general guidelines apply:

- If the barrier (reason the individual is unable to do their job) is purely physical, a single discipline Work Conditioning program, with or without job simulation is generally appropriate.[26,27,29,30]
- If the barrier involves secondary issues other than physical, a multidisciplinary full day program with job simulation is generally indicated.[27,29]
- If the worker must progress in the ability to lift more than 30 to 40 pounds, the goal is probably unattainable.[2]

Vocational rehabilitation or case settlement is generally indicated. A major exception to this guideline is an individual demonstrating extremely unsafe lifting, due primarily to a lack of understanding of how to lift safely. This individual may only be able to lift 10 to 20 pounds on an initial evaluation but with education in appropriate lifting techniques will quickly be able to lift 40 to 50 pounds. If the job requires lifting of 70 pounds, this goal may be attainable.[2]

If after the first five to seven days of a program, the individual's symptoms do not change, the individual is not a good candidate for continuing in the program. It is expected that the client will be sore or will get a little worse the first few days. However, the worker should begin to improve at least by the middle of the second week. If the individual continues to worsen, they may be too unstable and may require additional medical intervention (potentially surgical intervention).

Alternatively, the client may have other issues that are not being resolved in the program. The program should be altered at this point to address the appropriate issues. This may include exploration of whether or not the worker truly wants to return to work, or more emphasis placed on pain management, vocational intervention, or other nonphysical types of intervention.[6,7] If these types of services are not available to the center, the client should be discharged or referred to a center that can manage the nonphysical issues.[6,7] Continuing the program without progress is not appropriate and may actually harm the reputation of the rehabilitation center.[9]

If the client demonstrates progress until the day of, or just before the next physician's appointment, it is a good bet that the barrier is not purely physical.[7,8,26,30] It could be that the true barrier is fear of returning to work, or some family issue that the client is having difficulty facing. In these cases, the real issue must be discovered and addressed for the individual to return to work.

No amount of additional conditioning and job simulation will help this patient without additionally addressing the real issue. Many times this can be managed very simply by talking with the client, along the lines of the following. . . . "I'm a little puzzled . . . you were making such good progress . . . and now you seem to be losing ground. You know, if I were in your shoes, I might be a little afraid that I'd hurt myself if I went back to that job. I wonder . . . are you feeling a little bit that way?" Often by initiating this type of conversation, and then by listening to the client's response, the real issue will surface.[2]

Beyond this form of intervention, clinics unable to solve particular problems should establish a referral policy to transfer these patients to clinics or other settings that can manage these cases. The clinic will enjoy a much improved success rate if that policy is followed.[27,29]

In summary, the work schedule should be progressed aggressively beginning with the first week. The program can and should be instituted immediately, particularly for individuals that are not working. The program should begin with heavy emphasis on educational components and five to ten hours of activity in the first week.

In the second week, job-related activity should be increased and educational activity reduced. In the third week, devoting most of the time to job simulation is appropriate. If possible, the fourth week should be Work Hardening on the job.

If clients are not able to progress at this rate, it is probable that there are other issues that should be addressed if a successful outcome is to be achieved. A clinic must alter it's program to discover and address the issues or should refer the individual to another clinic that can address the problems.

Determination of the Job Modifications Required

Job simulation is an excellent means of determining what modifications can and should be made to a given job. There are three primary types of job modifications or controls. These are worker controls, administrative controls, and engineering controls[25] (Figure 16.15, *A*, *B*, *C*).

Worker controls are Changes or modifications that employees can make themselves.[1]

Examples of worker controls include:

- Proper use of tools and equipment
- Changes in the technique or the way the job is performed including adjustments in posture.

FIGURE 16.15 *A, B, C* Job simulation can help determine worker, administrative, and engineering modifications for a given job.

A

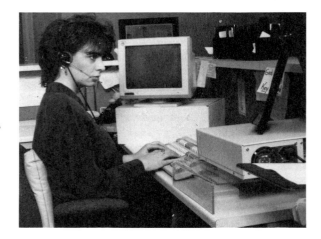

B

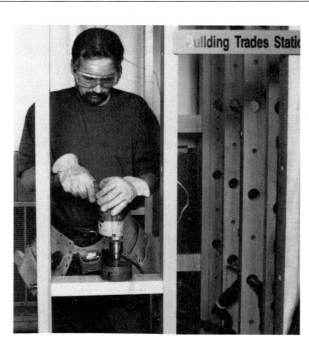

C

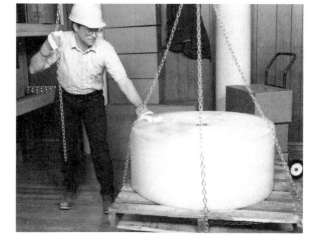

- Adjustment of the height or orientation of the workstation.
- Rearrangement of where things are placed.[1]

Administrative controls are changes or modifications that are generally under the control of management. This type of control may involve changes in policies and procedures.[1,25]

Examples of administrative controls include:

- Protective equipment for employees, such as vibration-absorbing gloves or rubber mats
- Rotating workers from one job to another to provide time for relief from certain risk factors
- Matching workers to jobs based on job requirements and worker capabilities
- Providing training programs in safe work methods
- Enforcing safety practices
- Changing pay practices to encourage appropriate rest breaks
- Scheduling exercise and stretch breaks
- Arranging work to interrupt static postures[1]

Engineering controls are changes that eliminate or limit the exposure of risk factors to workers by redesigning the methods, equipment and environment.[1,25] Examples of engineering controls include:

- Additional equipment, such as mechanical lifting devices, rotating storage bins, adjustable chairs, adjustable workstations etc.
- Modifying existing equipment, including adjustability, reorientation of work surfaces, provision of jigs or static holding devices, and counterbalancing existing tools
- Providing redesigned or automated tools, such as curved handled knives, scissors, and tools or electric drills, wire strippers, and cutters
- Redesigning to include increased automation in areas of material handling and where there are repetitive or forceful motions

Implementing Modifications

Worker controls are the easiest for a clinic and an injured worker to implement because they do not involve changes in the workplace itself. One does not need the cooperation of the employer to implement worker controls; only the cooperation of the employee. According to OSHA, worker controls are the least reliable means of ensuring safety and least desirable form of job modification.[25] This is because the worker will not always follow through. Sometimes they will forget and do it the unsafe way. Or, the effects of training may wear off and the worker may slip into old patterns.

Even with the best technique, a worker can still be hurt on a poorly engineered workstation. Engineering controls, therefore, are cited by OSHA as the first and preferred method of job modification, followed by administrative controls.

Where worker controls are not enough or are not preferred, clinics should interface with company personnel in determining administrative and engineering modifications that would enhance the employee's ability to safely return to work. Administrative controls can often be suggested, particularly the easier ones, such as providing personal protective equipment. Simple engineering controls can be fairly easy to institute in the case of an injured worker.

Industrial Therapists have often been frustrated in attempting to work with employers in the area of job modification. There are a number of reasons employers are unable or unwilling to work with medical personnel in modifying jobs or making other accommodations in the workplace. Those reasons include the following:

Rigid union seniority rules. If there is a union representing the employees, the employer must work under the seniority rules established by the union contract. An injured worker cannot have administrative or engineering controls that may be perceived as special privileges that are not available to all workers.[26,31]

Stereotypes regarding injured workers. Many employers believe that all injured workers are taking advantage of the system. As a result, they are not necessarily open to accommodating an injured employee's return to the job. They often consider injured workers troublemakers, and may prefer to get rid of them, rather than see them return to work.[26,31]

Medical personnel's suggestions may be naive or inappropriate. Many employers have had medical personnel make suggestions as to how to avoid injuries. The intention on the medical person's part is generally noble, but may not be fully understood. For instance, it's not necessarily easy to simply ''raise the conveyor belt'' or ''tilt the workstation.'' Raising the conveyor belt may cause problems in another work area. Tilting the workstation may cause productivity problems. Medical personnel have excellent ideas. Without a team approach to problem-solving at a given workstation, suggestions will often not be feasible or well designed.

Lack of availability of jobs that an injured worker can do. Generally, most companies operate on fairly thin profit margins with the work force as lean as possible. There are no extra jobs that an injured worker can occupy. Every job has to contribute to the bottom line in order for the company to remain in business. Keeping people around that are a drain on profitability is not feasible.

Production demands. The company is in business to produce products or services required by customers. If job modification is perceived to reduce productivity, it will be seen to undermine the company's ability to deliver its products or services to customers, thus threatening survival of the business. While companies should care about safety and injured workers, they must be concerned about production.

Cost of implementing the modifications is too great. Companies generally have limited funds. Just as rehabilitation clinics have capital equipment budgets, so do companies. Job modifications may save money in the long run by reducing injuries, but the funds to finance them may not be available.

Fear of reprisals from other workers if favoritism is perceived. If an injured worker is given special treatment, all workers will want special treatment. Companies have experienced the "domino effect" of one employee's injury turning into a number of employees reporting injuries. Once this phenomenon has been experienced by a company, there will be a resistance to any modifications that may be perceived as special treatment.

Lack of understanding of the need for modification. A fellow worker might have the attitude, "I've done this job myself . . . Mr. Injured Worker is just a pansy." Often supervisors have been promoted through the ranks. They may have done the injured employee's job. A supervisor may figure that if they could do the job, then so can the injured worker.[26]

SUMMARY

As costs of Workers' Compensation have risen and the Americans with Disabilities Act has become more understood, employers are rethinking their strategies in dealing with return-to-work issues. Companies that previously would not have considered modified or restricted duty are now implementing programs of their own to keep workers on the job.[16]

Industrial Therapists can serve as valuable resources in the implementation of these programs. With knowledge of job simulation techniques, creativity, and a willingness to work with employers and injured workers, the prospects of improving an injured worker's chance of success upon return to work is increasing. Understanding and implementing job simulation is a key component to the ultimate success of a Work Hardening program.

REFERENCES

1. Advantage Health Systems, Inc., *Training Materials* 1991 –1993 920 Main Street, Suite 700, Kansas City, MO, 64105.
2. Author's personal experience; Except where otherwise noted, all examples of specific job simulations, case histories, and program length data has been taken from author's actual experience at Wx: Work Capacities, Inc., 8000 Reeder Road, Lenexa, KS. Specific patient data is confidential. All names and other identifying information have been changed to protect patient confidentiality.
3. Author's personal experience in expert witness testimony in malpractice cases against Therapists in Industrial Therapy.
4. Bandy W: Functional Rehabilitation of the Athlete; in Timm K editor: *Orthopaedic Physical Therapy Clinics, Exercise Technologies* 1(2) Oct 1992.
5. Blankenship K: *Work Capacity Evaluation: industrial consultation* American Therapeutics, 1984.
6. Commission on Accreditation of Rehabilitation Facilities: *1990 Standards Manual for Organizations Serving People with Disabilities*; Tuscon, Az, 1990.
7. Darphin LE, Smith RL, Green EJ: Work Conditioning and Work Hardening in Isernhagen, S editor, *Orthopaedic Physical Therapy Clinics, Industrial Physical Therapy*; 1(1) July 1992.
8. Derebery VJ, Tullis WH: Delayed recovery in the patient with a work Compensible Injury, *Journal of Occupational Medicine* vol 25: 1983.
9. Goldberg S: Workers' Compensation Reimbursement: What's happening across the nation, What does the future have in store?, *Journal of Hand Therapy* April, 1990.
10. Healthline Work Hardening Center, St Louis.
11. HealthSouth Cole Center for Work Hardening, St Louis.
12. Hislop HJ, Perrine JJ: The isokinetic concept of exercise, *Physical Therapy* vol 47, 1967.
13. Hudson: *The Clinical Measurement Package, A Field Manual*, Homewood, Il, 1982, The Dorsey Press.
14. Isernhagen Susan: Functional Capacity Evaluation in Isernhagen S editor, *Work Injury: management and prevention*, Aspen, 1988.
15. Isernhagen S: Past and Present of Industrial Physical Therapy in the Work Injury Management Spectrum in Isernhagen, S editor, *Orthopaedic Physical Therapy Clinics, Industrial Physical Therapy*, 1(1) July 1992.
16. Isernhagen Susan: Return to Work Testing in Isernhagen, S editor, *Orthopaedic Physical Therapy Clinics, Industrial Physical Therapy*, 1(1) July 1992.
17. Key Glenda: *Key Method of Functional Capacity Evaluation*, Key Method, 1010 Park Avenue, Minneapolis, Minn, 55404.
18. Lett McCabe, Tramposh, Henderson: Work Hardening in Isernhagen, S editor, *Work Injury Management and Prevention*, Aspen, 1988
19. Matheson LN, Ogden LD, Violette K, et al: Work Hardening: occupational therapy in industrial rehabilitation, *Amer J Occup Therapy* vol 39: 1985.
20. Matheson LN: *Work Capacity Evaluation*, Trabuco Canyon, Calif, Rehabilitation Institute of Southern California, 1982.
21. Matkin RE: *Insurance Rehabilitation* Pro-Ed, 1985.
22. Mayer TG, Gatchel RJ, Kishino N, et al: Objective Assessment of Spine Function Following Industrial Injury: A Prospective Study with Comparison Group and One Year Follow-Up, *Spine* vol 10, 1985.
23. Miller M: Cost Savings in Four Cases in Isernhagen, S editor, *Work Injury: management and prevention*, Aspen, 1988.
24. National Commission on Compensation Insurance, *Workers' Compensation Cost Data, Annual Reports*, 1980–1993.
25. OSHA, *Management Guidelines for the Meatpacking Industry*, 1989.
26. Tramposh: *Avoiding the Cracks: a guide to the Workers' Compensation System*, Praeger, 1991.
27. Tramposh: *Correlation of Subjective vs. Objective Functional Capacities in Workers' Compensation Patients.* non published, 1989.

28. Tramposh: The Functional Capacity Evaluation, Measuring Maximal Work Abilities, *Spine, Sept 1991.*
29. Tramposh: The Work Injury System in Orthopedic Physical Therapy Clinics, *Ind Physical Therapy,* July 1992.
30. Tramposh: Work Related Therapy for the Injured Reduces Return to Work Barriers, *Occup Health and Safety,* April 1988.
31. Welch EM, editor: *Workers' Compensation: Lowering Costs and Reducing Workers' Suffering,* LRP, Fort Washington, Penn, 1989.
32. Wilke NA, Sheldahl LM: Use of Simulated Work Testing in Cardiac Rehabilitation: a case report, *Amer J Occup Therapy,* vol 39, 1985.

EQUIPMENT REFERENCES

a. ARCON: ARCON, Inc 2 McLaren, Suite D, Irvine, CA 92718
b. B-200: Isotechnologies, Inc, PO Box 1239, Elizabeth Brady Road, Hillsborough, NC 27278
c. Biodex: Biodex Corporation, PO Box 703, Shirley, NY 11967
d. Blankenship: American Therapeutics, PO Box 5084, Macon, GA 31208
e. BTE: Baltimore Therapeutic Equipment, 7455-L New Ridge Road, Hanover, MD 21076
f. Creative Specialists, PO Box 213, Cloquet, MN. 55720.
g. Cybex: 2100 Smithtown Avenue, PO Box 9003, Ronkonkoma, NY 11779.
h. Easy Street Environments, Health Services Marketing, LTd., 6908 East Thomas Road, m Suite 201, Scottsdale, AZ 85251.
i. ERGOS: Work Recovery Systems Inc., 1141 N. El Dorado Place, Suite 332, Tucson, AZ 85715.
j. Functional Capacity Assessment, Polinsky: Subs of KEY Method, 1010 Park Avenue, Minneapolis, MN 55404.
k. FFFWA: Wx: Work Capacities Inc, 8000 Reeder Rd, Lenexa, KS 66111.
l. Greymark International Inc, PO Box 5020, Santa Ana, CA 92704.
m. Isernhagen: Isernhagen and Associates, 2202 Water Street, Duluth, MN 55812
n. Key: KEY Method, 1010 Park Avenue, Minneapolis, MN 55404.
o. Lett McCabe, Tramposh and Henderson, Equipment drawings in Work Hardening in Isernhagen, Susan editor *Work Injury Management and Prevention,* Aspen, 1988.
p. LIDO: Loredan Biomedical Inc, 1632 DaVinci Court, PO Box 1154, Davis, CA 95617.
q. LiftTrak: Motion Analysis Corporation, 3650 Laughlin Road, Santa Rosa, CA 95403
r. Singer: New Concepts Corporation, 1141 N El Dorado Place, Suite 332, Tucson, AZ 85715.
s. SWEAT: Bi-State Medical, 7110 Wyandotte, Suite B, Kansas City, MO 64114.
t. Valpar International Corporation, PO Box 5767, Tucson, AZ 85703.
u. Work Evaluation Systems Technology, 1950 Freeman, Long Beach, CA 90804.

CHAPTER
17
Educating the Worker for Maximum Productivity

Olivier Corbeel

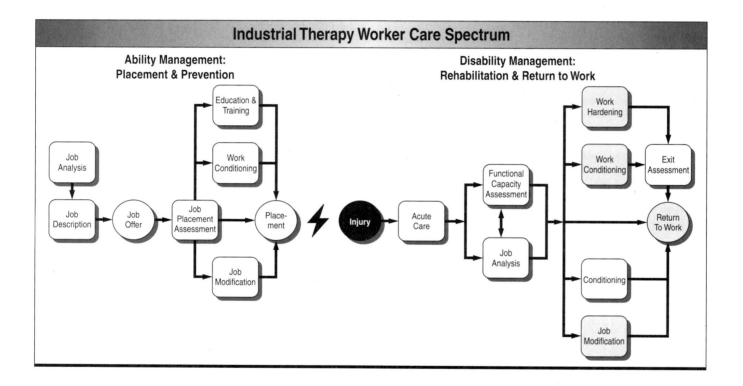

Industrial Therapy Worker Care Spectrum

Ability Management: Placement & Prevention

Disability Management: Rehabilitation & Return to Work

Education has long been recognized as a major factor in the success of modern medicine.[19,32] Its usefulness in all types of prophylactic and therapeutic endeavors accounts for it being one of the valued components of a successful return-to-work program.

Education's role in rehabilitating injured workers began initially in the form of injury prevention classes in the 1960's. Since then, it has evolved to include much more than simply basic concepts in anatomy and physiology. Educational components within a Work Hardening program have now been expanded to address numerous physical, psychosocial, and environmental factors involved in the return-to-work process (Box 17.1).

In this context, education's role extends beyond providing information and instruction. Its positive impact in the psychosocial aspects of rehabilitation has gained growing recognition. It is well documented that most of the clients seen in a Work Hardening program exhibit some degree of psychological distress.[20]

Research has demonstrated that psychological behavior, after a work related injury is an important factor in predicting the success potential of various therapeutic treatments and the possibilities for returning to work.[35] By helping the worker understand the nature of the injury, its causes, and techniques for avoiding recurrence, education can relieve anxiety and contribute to building confidence in the rehabilitation process.

Recognition of these effects on the outcome of rehabilitation explains the increasing emphasis placed on a well-structured educational program. To examine the role of education in rehabilitation, this chapter will first define its basic function, then describe the various aspects and how it is integrated into a Work Conditioning or Hardening program.

THE FUNCTION

Educating the injured worker means providing the information needed to understand the injury and how to cope with the many-faceted problems that arise from it, both before and after return to work. The new knowledge helps the worker gain more control, both physically and emotionally, over the symptoms of the injury and determine how to safely perform the job without being reinjured. As a safe level of performance is established, the participant's confidence in being able to overcome the injury increases, and productivity improves. With effective education, the participant becomes more actively involved in, and committed to, the rehabilitation process.

As an example for illustration, a mechanic is being admitted to a Work Hardening program after sustaining a back injury. Initially, this participant might not attempt to lift anything out of fear of reinjury, and may experience anxiety or depression, knowing that this disability makes it impossible to reassume the former job. By learning lifting techniques in back

school, this worker would learn the possibility of lifting a certain amount of weight without increasing back pain.

With fear reduced and progress experienced, the participant is encouraged to focus on achieving higher levels of performance. Eventually, the client should be able to confidently lift heavier weights without exacerbating symptoms (Figure 17.1).

It is in the worker's best interest to regain the highest possible productivity level, since this directly affects the individual's potential for returning to work. The key objective of the education program, is to change the injured worker's focus from pain and pain limitation, to achieving functional goals and returning to maximum productivity.[38]

COMPONENTS OF AN EDUCATIONAL PROGRAM

The components of an educational program can be divided into *primary* and *secondary* topics.[13]

Primary topics are the most important and of greatest need to all participants in the Work Retraining program. Primary topics like "Coping With Pain" are generally covered during group sessions.

Secondary topics have value for everyone, but are more relevant to some of the participants. Topics such as "Overcoming Chemical Dependencies," are covered during small groups or individual sessions.

FIGURE 17.1   How education enhances rehabilitation.

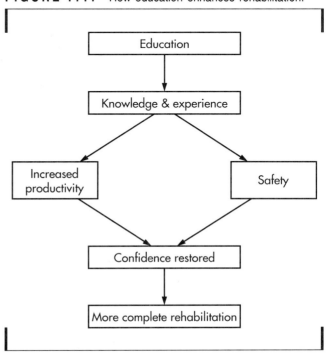

BOX 17.2

Primary Topics

- The injury (back, neck, upper extremities)
- Prevention
- Pain management
- Stress management

Secondary Topics

- Dependencies
- Nutrition
- Fitness
- Getting and keeping a Job
- Pain and interpersonal relationships
- Other

BOX 17.3

Injury Topics To Be Covered

- Basic anatomy of the body areas involved
- Description of the injury and related physiopathology
- Explanation of clinical test results: EMG, MRI, CT Scans
- Explanation of the treatment options: medications, surgery, rehabilitation

---

Box 17.2 contains a list of topics most commonly covered in a typical Work Retraining program. Additional topics can be added depending on the needs of the participants.

INJURY

The worker's need for information after an injury is extremely important. The amount of information retained can be significantly correlated with the worker's perception of improvement.[12,1]

A worker's dissatisfaction can sometimes arise from a misconception of the cause of injury.[7] There can be a lack of information about the diagnosis, the the severity, options, duration, and expected outcome.

A correct diagnosis or explanation may be given in medical terminology, which can be difficult for a worker to understand. A statement of the clinical findings does not always communicate the severity of the symptoms, and leaves the worker in need of further explanation about the condition.

Injuries most commonly referred to a Work Retraining program are back, neck, and upper extremities. Different program content is required to cover different conditions, although back and neck programs can be very similar. Information describing and defining the injury should be provided to participants early in the Work Retraining program. The majority of questions concern the nature and scope of the injury and the treatment. The information provided to clients should be as clear as possible, in nonmedical terms. Box 17.3 outlines the topics that a typical session on the injury should cover.

To build confidence among clients and the reha-

bilitation staff, educational information should be consistent and on-going throughout the course of treatment. This information must be well-grounded in thorough knowledge of the participant's diagnosis and medical condition, based on the results of clinical evaluations and the physician's analysis and recommendations.

PREVENTION

There must be a balance between information about the injury and information on how to prevent recurrence. Dwelling on the injury, in too much detail, can cause the worker to perceive greater severity than is warranted, or to imagine symptoms that do not actually exist. A balance of symptoms with key elements of prevention to answer the question, "How can I prevent this from happening again?" is outlined in Figure 17.2.

Identifying the Risk Factors

Prevention of reoccurrence begins with education. The worker needs to learn the elements involved in causing the injury. Injuries are seldom the result of an isolated accident or event. Recognizing and identifying the many contributing events and risk factors is the first step in prevention. Box 17.4 summarizes the major

FIGURE 17.2 Prevention of reoccurrence or aggravation.

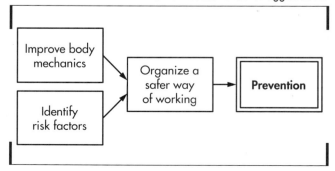

Personal Risk Factors:
- Posture and pattern of motion
- Fitness, personal health habits, dependencies, hobbies
- Lack of observance of the safety rules
- Inappropriate use of equipment

Environmental Risk Factors:
- Type of industry
- Type of work performed
- External events (accident)

personal and environmental risk factors that might be covered in a prevention education program.

As they learn about personal risk factors, participants begin to understand the extent of their personal responsibility for the injury. This realization causes them to become more involved in the prevention process.[31] It makes them aware that safety is not only the employer's responsibility, but theirs as well.

Improving the Body Mechanics

This topic covers controlling the affects of mechanical forces on the human body and reducing the stress on various body parts, by developing a safer and more efficient scheme of motion, to perform a given task. It includes static and dynamic positioning of the body and postural control.[30] Improving body mechanics is a valuable way the client can safely improve the level of function in the Work Retraining program.

Often, the corrected position or pattern of motion does not feel natural to the injured worker because of bad habits, or some segments of the body are too weak to accommodate the new dynamics. Repetition and practice are the only ways to change habits or strengthen a capability. Instructive supervision of the injured worker plays a major role in ensuring that a better and safer motion replaces the old pattern.

Improving body mechanics must be addressed early in the program because of its safety aspect. A single presentation is not enough.

Guidance and feedback are extremely important to successfully correct bad habits. It helps to demonstrate both the correct and the incorrect motion. Video taping the participant or use of a mirror can provide additional feedback for improved results.

In some cases optimal posture or motion cannot be

realized due to physical impairment, functional weakness, improper diagnosis or treatment of injury, or external factors present in the job or the work station. The contribution of the educational program in such instances will encourage individuals to think in terms of alternative postures or adaptations. Functions to be performed should become the focus, not limitations.

It is necessary that the design of the program is flexible enough to allow for individual modifications in performing the task, as long as safety and efficiency rules are observed.

If the client cannot bend at the waist to load a weight into a bin, correct placement of the knee on the edge of the bin to safely maintain the proper center of gravity should be taught. The employer of a participant in a Work Conditioning program might ask the employee to perform somewhat different tasks on the job immediately upon return to work. It is therefore important for the worker to learn alternative positions and movements that can be used to safely perform a variety of tasks (Figure 17.3, *A, B*).

Organizing a Safer Way of Working

Proper mental preparation before beginning a task is important for improved safety and comfort. Accordingly, the educational component of a Work Retraining program instills a "Think First" problem solving approach. This entails instructing the participant to mentally feel and visualize the task to be performed before doing it (Figure 17.4). As a result, the effort required will not be unexpected, and more optimal use is made of the equipment.

Proper pacing is an additional factor that enhances comfort, safety, and performance. During the Work Retraining program, the participant is trained to schedule work activities and resting periods, thus pacing themselves through the program, so the level of function continues to progress.

Ergonomic instruction in basic work place rules enables the worker to make modifications that will render the work environment more productive and possibly safer.[28,22,11] The educational program should stress the need for a proper sitting and standing position, and how to best work with the equipment already in place.

The best designed seat will not be of any help if the individual keeps slouching, or does not know how to use any available adjustment settings. Ergonomic education focuses more on the adaptations of existing conditions at home and at work (like adjusting the height of a computer screen to ease a cervical discomfort). Improved ergonomic awareness and knowledge means improved safety and productivity.

FIGURE 17.3   Sometimes the "correct way" (A) has to be modified (temporarily or permanently) due to a weakness or impairment (B).

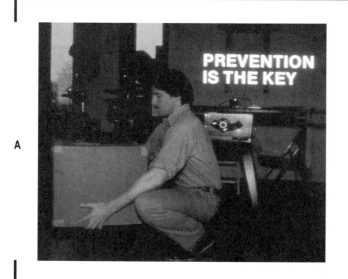
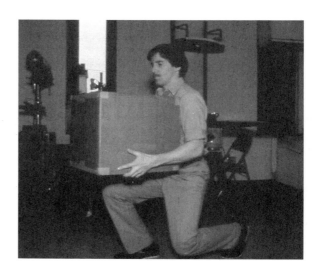

A   B

Program Content Resources

There are a number of existing resources to draw upon in developing a prevention educational program:

- Information about various injuries and their prevention can easily be found in medical literature and professional publications for rehabilitation specialists.
- Some excellent programs for back school, neck school, or upper extremity cumulative traumatic disease prevention are available in the market.

Commonly audio and video aids are used to clarify the presentation. It is a good idea to view several programs to select the one best suited to the specific needs.

- Community physicians will often provide more specific and detailed medical information about certain injuries when it is needed, such as in the case of an uncommon surgical procedure.
- The safety department of a large facility such as a hospital is also a valuable source of information.

FIGURE 17.4   Visualizing the task in advance helps to ensure safe and proper performance.

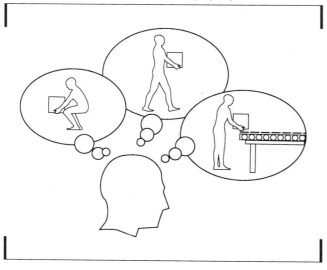

PSYCHOLOGY

The psychological well-being of the participant in a Work Retraining program has an influence on the outcome. Psychological support is provided within this program to favorably influence the outcome. This does not replace professional intervention when it is needed, but intends to respond to the needs of the majority of the participants.

During the evaluation at the onset of the program, a baseline assessment should be performed to identify the needs for psychological support, the potential problems, and coping skills of the client.

Several facilities in the US use a battery of tests, including the Pain Questionnaire and the Minnesota Multiphasic Personality Inventory, to define the worker's psychological profile and identify the worker's needs.[16] It is recommended that the utilization and interpretation of these tests is performed by someone with a thorough knowledge of the matter, especially if the facility does not have a psychologist or similar professional on staff.

When professional psychological evaluation cannot be obtained, an individual interview will be utilized to outline the problem areas to be addressed by the education program.

PAIN MANAGEMENT

Pain can be a distressing presence in an injury, bringing with it many negative emotions such as fear, anxiety, and depression. These emotional states can divert attention from the rehabilitation process. The participant must be taught how to get beyond pain and focus energies on regaining function and returning to work.

Understanding the Mechanism

The first step in helping clients manage pain is to give them an understanding of its mechanism. The anatomical and physiological information that the participant is given at the beginning of the educational program, provides insight into the nature of the pain. This alleviates some fear of the unknown and replaces it with objective information that the participant can use in planning and visualizing the recovery process.

Identifying Contributing Factors

Once the mechanism is understood, the next step is to help clients identify the factors and circumstances that positively or negatively influence the degree of discomfort.

The initial evaluation *identifies the different factors* and circumstances that positively or negatively influence the level of discomfort. Some of the issues to explore include:

- Does the pain increase as the activity is prolonged? Does it decrease when the activity is stopped?
- Does a specific motion or position increase or decrease the discomfort? (Driving, standing).
- What type of action relieves the pain?

During the evaluation or the first treatments, a careful observation helps to recognize additional factors. The participant should be aware that pain perception varies from one individual to another, according to the person's mental and physical status.

Establishing Guidelines

Using that knowledge, the client is advised on what to do (or to avoid) in order to reduce discomfort. A set of general and individual *guidelines* for the participant is then established. General and individual guidelines are outlined in Box 17.5. Individual guidelines are further detailed with each client after an evaluation.

The following case is an illustration of applying individual guidelines. During the Functional Capacity Assessment at the start of a Work Retraining program, a 45 year old cook with a diagnosis of degenerative disc disease reports that he does not tolerate prolonged standing and sitting. Results of the FCA verify limited sitting and standing tolerance. An additional finding is that lumbar extension produces pain. Accordingly, the educational program will teach the participant:

- How to organize his activities in the program to, at least initially, avoid a succession of standing or sitting activities.
- How to position his spine in order to prevent the lumbar extension while performing the task required in the program. (This is presented as a coping technique, not a treatment method.)

The participant is responsible for following the guidelines and reporting the results, and takes a more active role in the Work Retraining program.

BOX 17.5

Guidelines For Pain Management Instruction

General

- Document the discomfort and its interference with the task to be performed in the Work Retraining program[24,13]
- Distinguish between the soreness associated with the practice of a physical activity and a true aggravation of the injury symptoms
- Report change or appearance of the symptoms
- Work within comfortable tolerance and stop the activity if the symptoms increase
- Analyze the reasons for a pain increase, if an activity not related to the Work Retraining program is responsible for the pain increase, discuss the findings
- The body will adapt to the specific demands imposed upon it.
- Pace yourself.

Individual

- Listen to your body and recognize the clues that precede a flare-up
- Use your personal most comfortable, safe position
- Avoid the position and motion that increases your discomfort[16]

Relaxation

The practice of relaxation techniques is a must in any serious educational program.[25] The client learns about basics in mental and physical relaxation including:

- Breathing control and diaphragmatic respiration
- Mental distraction and focusing
- Contraction and relaxation techniques and reestablishment of body tone
- Stretching techniques appropriate to the injury

Instructions are also given to the client so relaxation techniques can be applied at home and at work. During the program the client is taught by example how to isolate a specific muscle group to perform the work while adjusting the rest of the body and relaxing unnecessary muscle contractions and tensions.

It must be realized that teaching a given relaxation method takes a great deal of time, and in some cases years of practice to realize the benefits. Since Work Retraining programs do not cover such long time frames, it is practical to teach only the basic relaxation techniques and hope that participants will practice what they have been taught. To ensure thorough instruction, relaxation techniques are taught in small groups.

The instructors should also make sure that a quiet place is available for the group to practice and that no one disturbs the session (Figure 17.5).

Some clients, will require a "one on one" approach to ensure the topic is thoroughly covered. During an individual session, practicing relaxation can also be part of the daily Work Hardening routine.

Distraction

Distraction from the pain is often an effective way to cope with the discomfort.[2] Distraction involves focusing on something other than the task at hand, or the pain, so that better performance is possible. The effort to avoid pain seems lighter when the mind is not focused on it. This skill is definitely helpful in the Work Retraining process as it breaks the "pain thinking" pattern and fosters progress. Distraction, however, should not interfere with the safety of the worker or the productivity.

There are two types of distraction: *active* and *passive*.

- *Active* distraction is used when the mind is kept focused on something different than the effort. Example: A group of participants in the Work Retraining program plays cards while working on improving their sitting tolerance.
- *Passive* distraction is illustrated when someone is using a "Walkman" and is listening to some music while exercising. The music helps the mind to be distracted from the effort.

These techniques should be used in a well con-

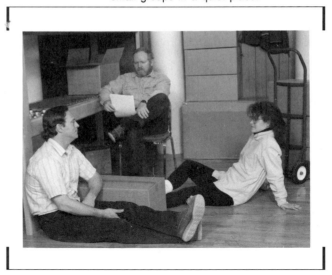

FIGURE 17.5 Relaxation techniques should be taught in small groups in a quiet place.

trolled environment. When distraction is used, clients should understand that the goal is to help them improve tolerance and enhance performance. They should not perceive that the staff is trying to "trick" them. Indeed, they should learn to use these techniques both at work and home.

Medications

Since most of the clients seen in a Work Hardening program use some prescribed medication, this topic is presented during the group sessions as a part of pain management.

Here, the participant is educated about the various types of medications prescribed for a given injury with the action and possible side effects. Instruction should simply relay the information given by the physician and help the client to understand medication's use and effects, and to follow the directions for prescription. The information content can be easily reviewed by a physician or a nurse.

Individual problems and discussions should always be reported to the treating physician. The participant may report some symptoms or side effects from the medication that may interfere with the ability to safely perform the task required in the Work Hardening program. The staff should be knowledgeable of the effects of the most commonly prescribed medications, and should be on the lookout for tell-tale problems during the Work Hardening program (pain killers, muscle relaxers, etc.).

Some Work Hardening centers want their clients to be medication-free. This may not be wise considering that if the medication is still prescribed, it might be necessary and helpful to the participant. Once again, this has to be discussed with the physician.

Drug abuse is a complex problem and should be addressed by a professional. The client's behavior during the conditioning program supplies good indications about a potential problem and in that case, further investigation and treatment is required.

Physical Agents

Physical agents include hot packs, cold packs, TENS units, etc. The participant is educated in the Work Hardening program on the usage of agents to manage discomfort at home and at the center. The use of a physical therapeutic technique or modality during the program consumes valuable time and should be as limited as possible. Often only cold pack application is used to limit inflammation and discomfort.

STRESS MANAGEMENT

The education program must explain the role of stress in exacerbating pain, and then identify stressful factors for the client at home and at work. It is not possible to address all the specific situations faced by participants, so the format is to teach them a problem solving approach that can be used to address whatever circumstances that may arise (Figure 17.6).

FIGURE 17.6   Meeting everyday obligations can become a stressful problem and impede progress.

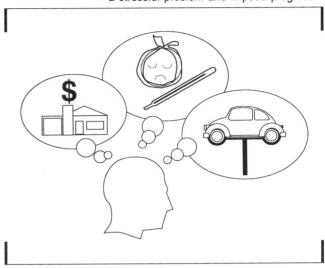

Work Related Stress

Box 17.6 lists some of the sources of work-related stress and the explanations and answers given in the educational program.[33]

As the client realizes progress, stress associated with returning to work should decrease as the goal gets

---

BOX 17.6

Work Related Stress

Source of stress	Educational approach and explanation
• Fear of reinjury	The worker has to know that a reinjury is always possible, although applying the different techniques taught during the Work Retraining program will notably reduce that risk.[30]
• Lack of confidence in one's physical capabilities • Anxiety regarding the quality, cadence, quantity of the work • Apprehension about tolerance for aspects of the job	The final Functional Capacity Assessment performed at the end of the program will help determine the worker's new, safe functional level as well as postural tolerances. The participant in the program should be evaluated regularly and apprised of their current level of function as compared to their initial status and how far they stand from the goals set for the program.[34,18,13]
• Need for job modification	The observation of the participant's performance in the program and the results of the final FCA will help to document the need for a modification.
• Lack of relationship with the employer or the insurance company[36]	A therapist can initiate contact with the employer by requesting a copy of the client's job description. Following that, the employer or insurance company may be invited in to learn more about the treatment process. Ideally, the employer would agree to bring in tools or equipment and receive a demonstration of rehabilitation programs.
• Fear of the future relationship with the supervisor or coworkers	Reassure the client: the restored self confidence and the involvement with a group of people facing similar problems has a positive influence on their interpersonal skills.

closer. Stress may increase shortly before discharge from the program, usually evident in increased reports of pain, or a "new injury" appearing just before the discharge. The best strategy throughout the educational program is to keep the focus on the performance, the progress accomplished and the final result.

Personal and Family-Related Stress

This type of stress arises from the frustrations that injury can cause in someone's life away from work. This topic should be covered in general during a group session in pain and stress management, but specific cases are more effectively treated during individual sessions, preferably with a psychologist, or a specialized counselor. In some cases, the participant may prefer to discuss the subject with another staff person, rather than a psychologist.

It is important to recognize that some personal or family-related problems are preexistent to the injury and are out of the field of treatment in Work Hardening.

In dealing with problems attributable to the injury, the educational approach is to focus on simple practical solutions to individual problem areas, rather than trying to solve the problem in totality. Needless worry has to be identified and replaced by a more optimistic outlook. Sometimes, as a way to ease family problems or questions, family members can be invited to one of the educational sessions, or they can visit the center when it is convenient (Figure 17.7).

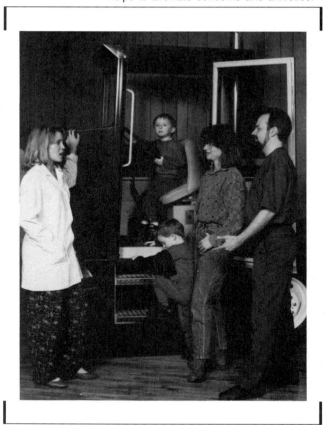

FIGURE 17.7   Many times a family visit to the center helps to alleviate concerns and anxieties.

Program Content Resources

There are a number of existing resources to draw upon in developing educational programs for pain and stress management:

- Documentation on pain management, stress control, relaxation, and distraction can be found in medical literature.
- A public library generally has a wealth of information on relaxation and distraction issues.
- Videotapes on specific techniques (like Yoga) are readily accessible on the market.
- In general, psychologists are knowledgeable in these topics and typically have a great deal of references and documentation.

DEPENDENCIES

The educational program should address dependency problems by focusing on the effects of such dependencies on the pain, job performance and safety at work.[5]

The influence of alcohol or drugs in the ability to operate a machine is well known. Few people are aware, however, of the possible impact of cigarette smoking on the recovery from low back pain.[4,5,8]

When a substance abuse problem is suspected, the participant's physician should be notified. Referral for further investigation and eventual treatment should be sought in agreement with the physician, especially if professional help is not available in the facility.

In Work Retraining, alcohol and street drugs should be prohibited on the premises as well as indoor smoking. This should be stated clearly to the client as part of the program's policies. If applicable, the participant should be given the local address and phone number for AA, drug counseling, and smoking cessation programs.

NUTRITION

Eating habits have an impact on a person's physical performance and health in general. Nutritional education sessions can be prepared with consultation from a dietitian and should include the following information:

- The need for and benefits of a balanced diet for general good health and physical performance.
- A description of the different food groups and their nutritional effect (qualitative and quantitative).
- The detriments of excess weight on the recovery from some injuries encountered in the Work Retraining program (incidence of the weight on spinal loading).[10]
- The determination of an individual's ideal weight.
- A brief description of the most common diet programs and their potential dangers, stressing the advantage of discussing alternatives with a specialist.

This information should be given during a special group session. Individual problems requiring more attention should be referred to a specialist. A close relative or spouse of the participant can also be invited to attend the class, which gets the family involved positively in the educational process and leads to more material being retained from the class.

Healthy eating habits can also be encouraged in the Work Retraining program by monitoring the client's weight. Weight control is not a primary goal of the Work Retraining program, but it can be addressed as an overall issue.

Program Content Resources

Documentation and didactic materials on the topic of nutrition are available at the Red Cross, The American Heart Association, The Cancer Society, and the Diabetes Foundation.

FITNESS

Aerobic conditioning is an essential element of the Work Retraining program. The participant has to be educated in the importance of whole body fitness, how to successfully recover from an injury, and how to achieve optimal work performance. Even clerical occupations will benefit from the aerobic conditioning that increase postural tolerance and improve muscle tone.

Participation in the conditioning aspect of Work Retraining requires medical clearance for physical activities, and the staff should be aware of the client's medical condition. Most injured workers have deconditioned since their injury because they have not kept their cardiovascular or motor functions up to their preinjury status. In addition, some worker capabilities are found to have been below the job's fitness and force requirements prior to the injury.[26]

Although it has never been clearly demonstrated,

some authors attribute the higher frequency of back related injuries to inadequate physical education and information in school.[21,37] In other cases, the pre-existing low fitness level could have played a role in the injury.

In addition to the aforementioned factors, the worker should know:

How to accurately take the pulse
This can be easily taught in group sessions—taking pulse on themselves and fellow participants—before and after the completion of aerobic activities, such as the treadmill or group exercise, etc.

How to interpret their heart rate
The value of measuring their heart rate, the importance of reaching their target rate, and when the rate indicates a too intense or too light effort during an aerobic exercise.

For more information on employee fitness programs and aerobic conditioning, see Chapters 11 and 15.

Program Content Resources

The American Heart Association has a wealth of information on cardiovascular issues. The YMCA currently publishes a number of brochures and there are videotapes and magazines that illustrate aerobic exercises and provide good documentation.

GETTING AND KEEPING A JOB

For many participants, their former job is no longer available and they will have to look for another job on completion of the program. In some cases they are required to do a job search by the insurance company.

Often, a Vocational Rehabilitation Consultant is brought in to identify and address problems. Individuals may also be referred to State vocational rehabilitation programs. This process can be initiated through contacting the Rehabilitation Nurse or case manager of the client. For more information on the role and involvement of a Vocational Rehabilitation Consultant, see Chapter 19.

In the educational program, the accent is placed on the qualities needed to get and keep a job: presentation, punctuality, honesty, quality, and consistency of the work. Problems can be identified and addressed even by a nonspecialist. If a participant consistently shows up late for the Work Retraining program or misses treatment without a valid reason, it is likely there will be a similar pattern at work.

PAIN AND INTERPERSONAL RELATIONSHIPS

An individual session on this topic is scheduled only if a real problem is identified that interferes with performance, or negatively affects the other participants in the Work Retraining program.

Most of the participants in a Work Retraining program experience some form of frustration attributable to the injury. Through our individual experience, it is known that chronic pain sometimes affects behavior and relationships. Participants in a Work Retraining program are no different. In most cases, these problems can be handled in informal conversations with the staff, or as part of a stress management session. If an individual session is needed, a psychologist should become involved, if at all possible.

The therapist can initiate the contacts and facilitate coordination between the client, the insurance company, the physician, and the attorney to alleviate the frustration and maintain an optimal communication among the different persons involved.

INTEGRATING EDUCATION INTO WORK RETRAINING

Having determined the educational needs, topics, and content guidelines, the remaining challenge is how to integrate all of this into the Work Retraining program. In this connection, the major issues are:
1. Who should educate the worker?
2. How should the program be organized?
    a. Description and guidelines for the educational sessions
    b. Scheduling the sessions
       - Primary topics
       - Secondary topics
       - Group sessions
       - Individual sessions
       - Home study

Who Should Educate the Worker

Most Work Hardening or Work Conditioning programs are organized in a multidisciplinary fashion to respond better to the variety of needs required in the treatment. The effectiveness of the educational program is the responsibility of all staff members and the participant.

Staff's Role

All staff members are responsible for helping the client put into practice the information given during the educational session. They also uphold the standards of consistency and continuity. Weekly staffings should include discussion of the educational programs with regard to:
   - The primary topics for the week
   - Individual sessions to be scheduled
   - Educational focuses for certain participants

The staff should consistently apply the rules and concepts taught to the clients, especially regarding the postural correction and the use of proper body mechanics. The participant will always observe the way staff members act and move, therefore setting a good example is important in the educational process.

Participant's Role

Clients in the program can also become role models for each other. For that purpose, it is sometimes beneficial to pair a new client with a more advanced participant who can serve as a mentor. Seeing that someone has overcome the same type of injury is valuable for the newcomer and being an example reinforces the confidence of the advanced client.

Specific Responsibilities

In general, the Retraining program director is responsible for the conception and organization of the educational program. Box 17.7 provides a list of the professional specialties commonly involved in a Work Retraining program and their strength in teaching specific topics. This list is certainly not all inclusive or limiting.

Depending upon the organization of the staff, the billing process, the reimbursement system, the expertise and the philosophy of the facility, the contribution to the educational program from various professionals can be quite different.[15] Some specific problems encountered with a client have to be managed by a specialist.

Description Of A Session[13, 14]

Educational sessions in the Work Retraining program should be conducted in small groups, in order to make them highly participatory and interactive. Illustrating material such as videotapes, interactive programs, or slides are a plus but cannot replace an active, personalized demonstration containing humor and originality.

Knowledge of the clients' background helps in adapting the content to the audience. For instance, in explaining body mechanics to a group of construction workers, the therapist might use actual concrete blocks

---

BOX 17.7

Typical Educational Responsibilities of the Work Retraining Team Members

The injury's treatment and prevention.	Occupational or Physical Therapist, Chiropractor; Nurse. Occupational therapists have in general an excellent knowledge of the upper extremity injuries and of the daily living applications. Physical therapists are more comfortable with the spinal problems and body mechanics.
Pain and stress management	Psychologist; Occupational or Physical Therapist. Group sessions can certainly be handled by a physical or occupational therapist. Sometimes they have a certification or specialization in relaxation or psychology. Individual sessions are scheduled with a Psychologist.
Fitness and Healthy living	Exercise Physiologist; Athletic Trainer; Physical Therapist
Nutrition	Dietitian.
Medications, Dependencies, drug abuse (individual problems)	Physician; Psychologist;
Getting and keeping a job	Vocational Rehab Counselor.
Interpersonal and personal problems (individual sessions)	Psychologist; Family Counselor.

BOX 17.8

Guidelines For Educational Sessions

- Avoid large medical words. Use plain language.
- Keep the subject to 3 or 4 points you want the participant to remember.
- Distribute handouts illustrating the points presented.
- Do demonstrations, give examples, illustrate.
- Ask questions and invite the clients to share experiences and opinions.
- Do not embarrass anyone in front of an audience. People learn better when they feel an atmosphere of confidence and acceptance.[3]
- Promote self discovery by encouraging questions and interactions between clients.
- Do not fake an answer. If you do not know the answer, tell them that you will get the answer later.

to demonstrate proper lifting techniques (Figure 17.8, *A, B*).

Instructors should follow guidelines that will make the session more stimulating and constructive for the participants. Box 17.8 provides some of these guidelines, but each Work Retraining program will discover additional ones as they gain experience over time.

Scheduling Of the Sessions

Primary topics are presented during group sessions and scheduled in a fashion to ensure that all the participants in the Work Retraining program will attend all the primary topic sessions.

A six week Work Hardening program might select three primary topics such as Back Education, Upper Extremity, and Stress Management and rotate these topics every other week. In this way, no matter when a client enters the program, they would be exposed to all three primary topics over the six week stay.

Secondary topics are rotated in a fashion similar to primary topics described above and indicated in Box 17.9. They are interspersed with primary topics so that every week has either a primary or secondary topic group session.

Sometimes, a secondary topic can be an "in depth"

FIGURE 17.8 A, B   Making demonstrations as realistic as possible facilitates the learning process.

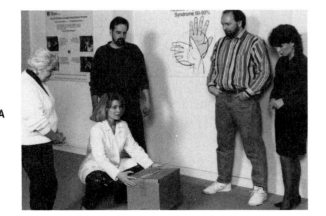

A

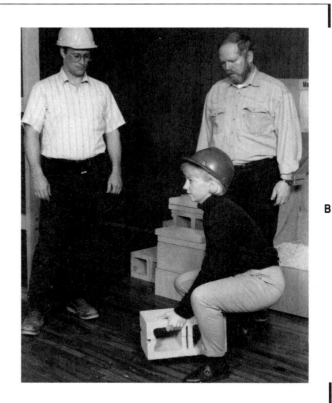

B

review of some aspect of a primary topic, participants can be scheduled for a special session in body mechanics or stress control, to reinforce the material already presented in a primary topic session.

Group Sessions

Group sessions are organized for the primary and secondary topics that are of importance to all partici-

---

BOX 17.9

Scheduling Group Education Sessions

	Primary Topic	Secondary Topic		Primary Topic	Secondary Topic
Week 1	Back education		Week 8		Workers' Compensation system
Week 2		Employee-employer relations	Week 9	Upper extremity	
Week 3	Upper extremity		Week 10		Dependencies
Week 4		Relaxation techniques	Week 11	Stress management	
Week 5	Stress management		Week 12		Nutrition
Week 6		Family issues	Week 13	Back education	
Week 7	Back education				

pants. As indicated in Box 17.2, the primary topics are Back Education, Upper Extremity, and Stress Management. As to secondary topics, in addition those indicated in Box 17.2, others might be:
- Workers' Compensation
- Coworker issues
- Recreation and hobbies
- Pain and belief systems

These Group Sessions should be about 60 minutes in duration.

Individual Sessions

This is the time to give each participant a chance to address certain issues related to the specific injury, and to address more personal or private issues, either through "one-on-ones" or self study (Figure 17.9). Some of these topics may have been covered in group sessions as well. In individual sessions topics can be customized to the client's needs.

> *The dietitian can review several eating habits and help to establish a more targeted and balanced diet for the days to come.*
>
> *The therapist can help the client to adjust a car seat and steering wheel to decrease back discomfort while driving.*
>
> *A therapist can practice a golf swing with a participant using an alternative type of motion to help the client to get back to a favorite hobby (Figure 17.10).*

In addition to addressing the worker's specific injury, the individual session can also be an informal discussion to make sure that all the problems are being addressed and the client feels comfortable with the program.

Home Study

To complement the material of the educational sessions, the client also can have articles or abstracts to read on a specific topic. For that purpose, it is practical to set up a small library of easy-to-read references on the topics presented. The content of the home study can also be reviewed during the individual or group session. Home study can prepare participants for upcoming sessions. All the resources cited earlier can be explored to provide some material for home study. The client can be issued a type of folder to gather the educational information for review at home.

SUMMARY

Education is an important part of a Work Retraining program. It requires skilled professionals to provide education to break the treatment dependency chain and progress toward recovery and functional independence.

FIGURE 17.10   Showing clients that they can resume recreational activities (sometimes modified) can be an important motivator.

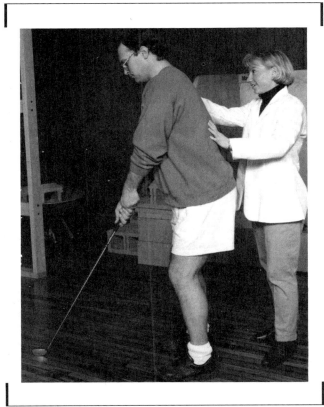

FIGURE 17.9   A variety of self study resources enables clients to delve into selected topics more intensely.

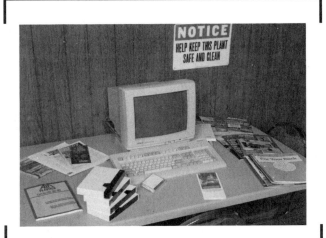

For the staff of the Work Retraining program, it is a rewarding and challenging experience. It takes time, patience, and dedication to teach something to someone. An efficient program is one that helps the worker to translate the theory into practical application at home and in the workplace.

Focusing on maximum productivity is the best way to ensure the effectiveness of treatment because it is the only approach that takes into consideration the worker's need for returning to work and the requirements of an industry that has to face a more competitive environment each year.

REFERENCES

1. Anderson L: Educational approaches to management of low back pain, *Orthopedic Nursing* 8(1):43–6, Jan 1989.
2. Arntz A, Dreessen L, Merckelback, H: Attention, not anxiety, influences pain, *Behavior Research & Therapy* 29(1):41–50, 1991.
3. Bates RE: Professional selling skills I, Key Functional Assessments, Inc, Marketing Course unpublished, 1988.
4. Boshuizen H C, Verbeek J H, Broersen J P, Weel A N: Do smokers get more back pain?, *Spine* 18(1):35–40 Jan 1993.
5. Deyo R A: Lifestyle and low-back pain: the influence of smoking and obesity, *Spine* 14(5):501–6 May 1989.
6. Deyo R A: Nonsurgical care of low back pain, *Neurosurgery Clinics of North America* 2(4):851–62, Oct 1991.
7. Deyo R A, Diehl A K: Patient satisfaction with medical care for low-back pain, *Spine* (1):28–30, 1986.
8. Dewey M E, Dickenson C E, Foreman T K, Troup J D: Back pain, ventilatory function, chest symptoms, and smoking, *J Spinal Disorders* 2(4):241–8, Dec 1989.
9. Galka M L: Back injury prevention program on a spinal cord injury unit, *Sci Nursing* 8(2):48–51, June 1991.
10. Garrett B, Singiser D, Banks S M: Back injuries among nursing personnel: the relationship of personal characteristics, risk factors, and nursing practices, *Aaohn Journal* 40(11):510–6, Nov 1992.
11. Grandfram: *Fitting the task to the man—A textbook of occupational ergonomics*, New York 1988, Taylor and Francis.
12. Hall H, Iceton J: Back school clinical orthopedics and related research 179(10):10–14, 1983.
13. Key G: The Key Method of Functional Work Hardening (unpublished) Key Functional Assessments Inc, 1992.
14. Key G: Industrial Physical Therapy: an Introduction. In Gould JA, editor: Orthopedic and Sport Physical Therapy, St. Louis 1990, Mosby.
15. King P M: Profiling the work-hardening therapist: education and experience, *Amer J Occ Ther* 46(9):847–9, 1992.
16. Kinney R K: The SCL-9OR evaluated as an alternative to the MMPI for psychological screening of chronic low-back pain patients, *Spine* 16(8):940–2, Aug 1991.
17. Kohles S, Barnes D, Gatchel R J, Mayer, T G: Improved physical performance outcomes after functional restoration treatment in patients with chronic low-back pain. Early versus recent training results, *Spine* 15(12): 1321–4, Dec 1990.
18. Lepping V: Work Hardening: A valuable resource for the occupational health nurse, *Aaohn Journal* 38(7): 313–7 Jul 1990.
19. Mackenback J P: Socioeconomic health differences in the Netherlands: a review of recent empirical findings *Social Science & Medicine* 34(3): 213–226, Feb 1992.
20. Main CJ, Wood PL, Hollis S, Spanswick CC, Waddell G: The Distress and Risk Assessment Method: A simple patient classification to identify distress and evaluate the risk of poor outcome, *Spine* 17(1):42–52, Jan 1992.
21. McKenzie R: *Treat your own back,* Spinal Publication, Ed 4, 1988.
22. McElligott J, Miscovich S J, Fielding L P: Low back Injury in Industry: the value of a recovery program, *Conn Med* 53(12):711–715, Dec 1989.
23. Miller RJ, Hafner RJ: Medical visits and psychological disturbance in chronic low back pain: a study of a back education class, *Psychosomatics* 32(3):309–316, Summer 1991.
24. Nicholas MK, Wilson PH, Goyen J: Comparison of cognitive-behavioral group treatment and an alternative non-psychological treatment for chronic low back pain, *Pain* 48(3):339–47, Mar 1992.
25. Nicolas MK, Wilson PH, Goyen J: Operant-behavioral and cognitive-behavioral treatment for chronic low back pain, *Behaviour Research & Therapy* 29(3):225–238, 1991.
26. Pederson DM, Clark JA, Johns RE, White GL, Hoffman, S: Quantitative muscle strength testing: a comparison of job strength requirements and actual worker strength among military technicians, *Military Med* 154(1):14–8, Jan 1989.
27. Peters P: Successful return to work following a musculoskeletal injury, *Aaohn Journal* 38(6):264–70, 1990.
28. Pinkham J: Carpal tunnel syndrome sufferers find relief with ergonomic designs, *Occ Health & Safety* 49–53, Aug 1988.
29. Rakowski W, Wells BL, Lasater TM, Carleton RA: Correlates of expected success at health habit change and its role as a predictor in health behavior, *Amer J Preventive Med* 7(2):89–94, Mar 1991.
30. Saal JA: Dynamic muscular stabilization in the nonoperative treatment of lumbar pain syndromes, *Orth Review* 19(8):691–700, Aug 1990.
31. Selby NC: Developing and implementing a back injury prevention program in small companies, *Occup Med* 7(1):167–71, 1992.
32. Simons-Morton DG, Mullen PD, Mains DA, et al: Characteristics of controlled studies of patient education and counseling for preventive health behaviors, *Patient Education & Counseling* 19(2):175–204, Apr 1992.
33. Svensson H, Anderson GBJ: The relationship of low back pain, work history, work environment and stress: a retrospective cross sectional study of 38 to 64 year old women, *Spine* 14:517–522, 1989.
34. Taylor ME: Return to work following back surgery: a review, *Amer J Ind Med* 16(1): 79–88, 1989.
35. Taylor RS, Bonfiglio RP: Industrial rehabilitation medi-

cine: Assessment of the outcome of treatment in industrial medicine, program development, documentation, and testimony, *Arch Phys Med & Rehab* 73(5): S369–373, May 1992.

36. Tramposh AK: Work-related therapy for the injured reduces return-to-work barriers, *Occ Health & Safety* 57(4): 55–6, 82, 1988.

37. Vicus-Kunse P: Educating our children: the pilot school program, *Occ Med* 7(1): 173–7, 1992.
38. Waddell GA: A new clinical model for treatment of low back pain, *Spine* 12: 632–644, 1987.
39. White AH: The back school of the future, *Occ Med* 7(1): 179–182, 1992.

18

Rehabilitation of the Injured Worker from a Psychological Perspective

Robert L. Karol

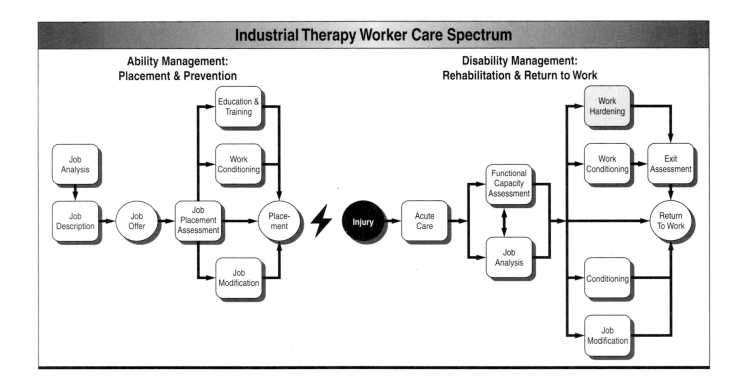

Therapists must attend to alteration in function and pain to achieve successful rehabilitation. In some cases, altered or lost function dictates the outcome, whereas in others pain is the predominant hindrance to return to productivity. In either situation, inattention to psychological considerations is likely to result in failure.

Loss of Function

When loss of function is the primary variable under consideration in rehabilitation, Therapists must weigh psychological variables. Therapists must attend to patients' strengths and shortcomings in coping with the life impact of altered physical ability. Patients must cope with the challenge of handling social, recreational, marital, financial, and vocational changes. If patients cope poorly, anger, frustration, guilt, and depression result.

The emotional responses of patients to injury often determine how well they apply their abilities in the real world. Therapists help patients make better advancements in treatment when they understand the psychological adjustments made by injured workers. Ignorance of how patients respond to injury consigns Therapists to suboptimal results. Hence, psychological factors help determine the degree of loss of function.

Pain

Often, pain plays a primary role in the determination of rehabilitation outcome. Pain is an internal psychological event which can be precisely known only by the individual. Pain is multidimensional. It varies in intensity and location, and it may have diverse sensory and affective elements. It may change with body posture, activity level, and emotional status and may have acute and chronic elements.

Some people may experience the full "richness" of pain: it is multifaceted, with subtleties and variations. To these people, pain exists in a context of emotions, thoughts, and behaviors. To other people, pain is undifferentiated, experienced without much reflection. They tend to see pain relatively concretely as a "thing." Their psychological state is as much a part of their pain as it is for the first group of individuals, but they may be less aware of their psychological state and less likely to acknowledge it.

There is a continuum ranging from experiencing the multifaceted nature of pain, with a concomitant acknowledgement of psychological variables to something without differentiation. Most people apply the same level of analysis to their pain that they apply to other life challenges. The emotional, cognitive, and behavioral resources they use in life are the same resources they use to understand and cope with pain.

The availability and sophistication of patients' resources determines how they approach pain, treatment, rehabilitation, and return to work. It is incumbent upon Therapists to evaluate and utilize patients' psychological abilities to maximize intervention outcome. A mismatch between patients' experience of pain and Therapists' approach is likely to lead to unsuccessful treatment. An appreciation of patient psychology is essential.

Role of Psychology

Psychological considerations can be crucial throughout the treatment and rehabilitation of injured workers. Health care professionals, who take a psychological perspective are more likely to succeed in their therapeutic efforts, from medication management or surgery, to manual manipulation or rehabilitation programs, such as Work Hardening. This chapter will primarily consider how the incorporation of a psychological perspective can benefit patient care in Work Hardening programs, though those in other settings should be able to apply similar principles.

THE STRUCTURE OF REHABILITATION

The Psychological Nature of Rehabilitation

Rehabilitation follows psychological principles of intervention. Work Hardening program Therapists who best understand the inherent psychological nature of rehabilitation, are most likely to succeed in treating injured workers and returning them to work.

Taber's Cyclopedic Medical Dictionary[38] defines rehabilitation as follows:

> *The processes of treatment and education that lead the disabled individual to attainment of maximum function, a sense of well-being, and a personally satisfying level of independence. The need for rehabilitation may be due to any disease that causes the person to be impaired either mentally or physically. The post-coronary patient, the post-trauma patient, and the post-surgical patient all need and can benefit from rehabilitation efforts. The individual who is recovering from a mental disorder is also in need of rehabilitative support. The combined efforts of the individual, family, friends, medical, nursing, allied health personnel, and community resources are essential in order to make rehabilitation possible.*

This comprehensive definition bears close attention to appreciate the psychological character of rehabilitation. First, rehabilitation is a process, not an event. There is a fundamental difference between an isolated treatment which ameliorates pain, damage, or cures illness, and the sequential, interactive rehabilitation dynamic. The whole is different from the sum of the parts.

Isolated treatment is done to a passive patient-bystander. Through rehabilitation people grow, change, and adapt. Psychologists recognize that treatment changes people beyond the specific care that Therapists provide. Successful programs understand how intervention broadly effects patients, also.

Psychologist-Patient Relationship

In rehabilitation, the broad impact Work Hardening programs have on patients is partially a function of the psychological relationship Therapists build with patients. Table 18.1 summarizes the relationships between patients and professionals in different situations.

In some areas of health care, professionals act on passive patients. Success is a function of the professionals' skill. There are numerous examples in health care: setting a broken bone, performing surgery, or responding to a heart attack in the emergency room. Much like parents caring for infants, professionals care for patients.

TABLE 18.1 The relationships of patients and professionals

Professional	Patient	Model	Example
Acts	Passive	Parent to infant	Surgery
Directs	Obeys	Parent to child	Office visit
Advises	Consults	Adult to adult	Rehabilitation

In other cases, traditional health care involves directive providers, prescribing the actions of patients who obey. When patients follow the instructions, they get better. Providers are governing the behavior of the patients, just as parents govern children. When patients take medication to cure illness, they are following the dictate of the professionals.

Rehabilitation, however, requires a different model.[14,16] When patients are passive or merely following directions, rehabilitation programs, such as Work Hardening, will fail. Patients must be active partners in the treatment endeavor, and providers must be flexible. Patients' input and compromise by providers are crucial. Intervention is a function of adults bringing their skills and knowledge together to achieve an agreed upon goal. If providers do not adapt to patients or patients do not follow through, success is difficult to achieve.

Education

In examining the definition of rehabilitation, it is apparent that education is part of rehabilitation. Notwithstanding some reimbursement policies which view education as a nonreimbursable activity because they deem it distinct from reimbursable "treatment," patient-participants should be more knowledgeable when they leave the program.

Future behavior ought to be different because of enhanced patient understanding. Psychologists have long recognized that behavior change must originate with the patient; the professional is a guide and teacher, but is unable to impose change. In contrast to Therapist-conducted manipulation or Physician-provided surgery, the Work Hardening Therapist is an instructor and the patient is a learner.

Goals

The goals of rehabilitation are multifaceted. Rehabilitation strives for increased function, well-being, and independence. Psychological status is essential to these ends. Moreover, rehabilitation does not strive to cure. This bodes well for the application of rehabilitation in Work Hardening programs to the recalcitrant injuries that plague patients, insurers, employers, and providers. Such injuries are chronic, not acute in nature, and lend themselves poorly to curative efforts.

Disciplines

Rehabilitation requires a combined effort of patients, health care providers, and others affected by the patients' limitations. A coordinated team approach is crucial.

Successful programs must consider all of the factors which interfere with the desired outcome. Poor body mechanics, depressed patient mood, a frustrated employer, or an apprehensive insurer can ruin the chance of a positive result. The weakest link left unaddressed is likely to cause failure. Oftentimes, this is the psychological status of the patient and the psychological orientation of the employer.

Programs should be ready to facilitate intervention wherever and with whomever is necessary to achieve a successful outcome. While not everyone requires help with everything, programs should address everything with which patients require help, if it interferes with the rehabilitation process.

Intervention Points

Artificial boundaries regarding where to intervene diminish outcome. In general, programs can change patients or environmental influences on patients. Interventions targeting patients' attitudes, emotional status, or coping skills are important, but it is a mistake for professionals to restrict themselves to only changing patients.

It is overly restrictive to omit intervention with those whom patients interact from the professionals' armamentarium. Furthermore, prevention and avoidance of reinjury is best accomplished through a broad approach that includes environmental and systems changes.[41]

At times, programs can be more effective with intervention elsewhere than with patients. The attitude, position, and behavior of insurers, lawyers, employers, and coworkers can unintentionally undermine rehabilitation. A patient may present as depressed and anxious. Despite physical therapy and individual psychological counseling, the patient remains depressed because of legal wrangling about the case. Both lawyers agree that the patient is depressed (though they may disagree over financial responsibility for its treatment). Prescribing speedy legal resolution, as a treatment for depression, recognizes that the behavior of players, other than the patient may have a greater impact on the patient than Therapists can overcome with traditional treatment.

Other examples could be drawn citing the importance of other players. At times, the primary focus of intervention needs to be through families, employers, insurers, or lawyers; as they can be most helpful. Programs have more leverage when they are willing to help orchestrate everyone's impact. The Therapist's own treatment modalities are often not powerful enough to overcome all of the forces acting on patients.

Psychologists generally realize that it is often impossible to achieve and maintain behavior change by just working with patients. Outside influences which reward, punish, or put pressure on patients can easily degrade therapeutic progress. There must be outside intervention where patients must apply their newly acquired abilities.

Broad-based intervention is hard. Most Therapists are trained to provide their therapy, be it manual manipulation or psychotherapy, with patients in their office or clinic. Going on-site or calling a meeting of the other players requires effort and Therapists must innovate. Despite these obstacles, the improvements in patient outcome make the effort worthwhile.

Team Models

Conducting rehabilitation in this comprehensive fashion requires teamwork. Individual practitioners usually are incapable of successfully managing such a broad-based approach. Work Hardening teams permit a wider effort and insure that treatment addresses psychological issues.

The Multidisciplinary Model.   The Therapists own treatment modalities are often not powerful enough to overcome all of the forces on patients This is the most rudimentary team model. As shown graphically in Figure 18.1, *A,* a group of professionals in different disciplines work separately within their own traditional fields of expertise. Each slice of the pie represents a distinct discipline and patient problem. Each Therapist treats a part of the patient's problem. There is little communication between disciplines since each has a fairly independent set of problems with which to deal.[7]

Team meetings usually consist of reports by different Therapists on the problems their discipline treats. Each sits silently as the other disciplines report on other problems. Often a team leader listens to everyone's report and gives directions to each Therapist.

There are a number of assumptions in this model. First, this model assumes that the areas of treatment each discipline feels responsible for derive from a sensible division of expertise. Rather, it is likely that historical, political, economic, and social forces also helped shape the development of health care professions.[21] There was no blueprint. Even today, battles

wage within legislatures over licensing, independent practice, and reimbursement for various disciplines.

Second, this model suggests that rehabilitation requires little cross-discipline communication. It is as if Therapists think that there is truly little overlap between their efforts. Yet, no one really believes that the brain belongs to the psychologist, the upper extremities to the Occupational Therapist, the lower extremities to the Physical Therapist, the heart to the physiologist, the bones to the orthopedist, the nerves to the Neurologist, the muscles to the Physiatrist, the domicile to the Social Worker, and the job to the Vocational Counselor.

It should become obvious that when patients are able to move with no pain, their mood is affected, a good mood affects attention to body mechanics, and body mechanics affect their job, etc. Nevertheless, this model would have one believe that the efforts of Physical Therapists, Psychologists, and vocational placement experts, can be conducted independently. In reality the success of one Therapist affects everyone else's treatment planning. Since treatment rates vary across disciplines and diagnostic problems, this model falls short of the ideal rehabilitation team model. Moreover, this model is the one least likely to permit effective psychological care.

The Interdisciplinary Model.   This team represents a somewhat better model. As shown in Figure 18.1, *B,* Therapists working within this model acknowledge that there is overlap in the problems they address and the treaments they provide.[21] Communication between disciplines becomes more important. Therapists no longer work in isolation. The information one Therapist provides in the team meeting is important to the other Therapists.

Communication occurs among Therapists, not just through a central team leader. Nevertheless, in this model there are core areas reserved to each Therapist that do not cross disciplinary boundaries.

The Supradisciplinary Model.   This team optimizes the rehabilitation outcome.[17] This label represents treatment organized around patient problems, not Therapists' disciplines, and it is the model most likely to incorporate consideration of patients' psychological functioning into all aspects of the Work Hardening program.

In Figure 18.1, *C,* each ring represents patients' problems. Disciplines contribute to the amelioration of problems from each discipline's perspective and knowledge base simultaneously. The team develops a hierarchy of problems, including psychological issues, identifying the sequence in which problems require treatment. The problems are defined narrowly enough to suggest intervention strategies.

FIGURE 18.1   A graphic representation of three types of team models. **A**, In the multidisciplinary team model, a group of professionals in different disciplines work separately within their own traditional fields of expertise; **B**, With an interdisciplinary team model, Therapists acknowledge that there is overlap in the problems they address and the treatments they provide; and, **C**, With a superdisciplinary team, treatment is based around the patient's problems, not the Therapists' disciplines.

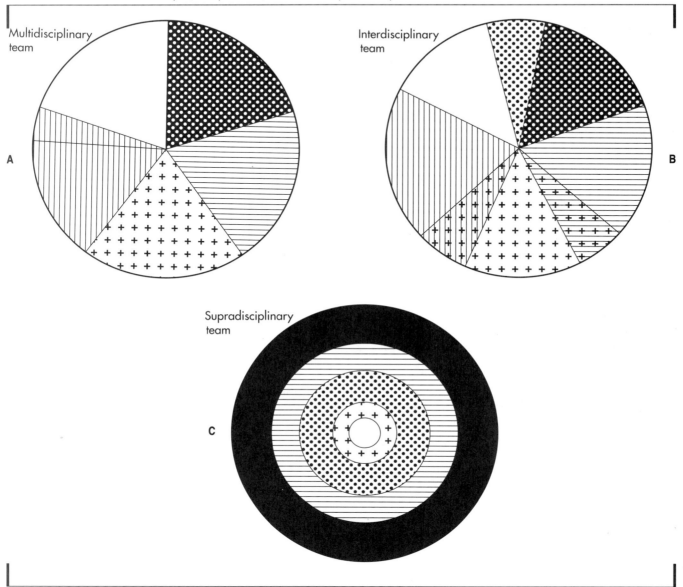

Note. From Karol RL: Dealing with Mental Health Issues After Brain Injury: A User's Guide to Approaches Real and Imagined, 1991, Paper presented at Mental Health Issues of Adults With Brain Injury. Copyright 1986 by Robert L. Karol. Reprinted by permission.

Therapists can simultaneously address multiple problems, but some situations may require them to address a specific problem first. Some problems may require the full team, while others may require only one or two Therapists or disciplines.

In training body mechanics, the Physical Therapist and psychologist might both intervene. The psychologist might first conduct a group of patients encouraging them to identify challenges at the work site. The psychologist might show how thinking, "X interferes.

How do I do X?" encourages problem solving, whereas thinking, "I can't do X" generally insures that no attempt will be made. The former leads patients to seek advice, whereas the latter leads to withdrawal and failure.

With the psychologist's help, the group conducts an exercise in generating a possible list of solutions. The psychologist instructs the patients to tell the Physical Therapist what is on the list. The psychologist then checks patients' compliance with the Physical

Therapist, regarding whether the patients informed the Therapist about the problem solving exercise, in which the patients developed the list.

The Physical Therapist working separately shows the patients how to refine the solutions and put them into practice. The Physical Therapist might work with the job placement counselor to see how the employer will respond to the solutions. In follow-up, the psychologist motivates the patients to try the activities in the real world, and the Physical Therapist monitors their recall of proper body mechanics over time.

Meanwhile, the psychologist could begin to tackle patient perceptions of the Workers' Compensation system that might hold up placement efforts. The psychologist might bring into play the insurance adjuster and patient lawyer as team members.

Therapists in a supradisciplinary model address problems regardless of discipline, and tackle problems in a sensible sequence. When psychologists observe poor body mechanics, they should be free to join the Physical Therapists.

If Physical Therapists can help motivate patients, they should join the psychologists. It is advantageous to use everyone's skills, including psychologists, physicians, physical therapists, occupational therapists, exercise physiologists, lawyers, case managers, claims adjusters, vocational counselors, or placement experts, to their utmost with few professional turf issues. This does, of course, require confident, secure professionals.

PSYCHOLOGICAL EVALUATION

Regardless of how Therapists structure care, the psychological status of patients is crucial. Without appropriate psychological assessment, intervention is going to be less efficacious. A thorough psychological assessment includes both psychometric and clinical evaluation. Total reliance on either component of a full evaluation limits the extent and quality of the information available on which to base care. While it may be unreasonable to expect that Therapists alone will be able to gather complete information on patients' psychological functioning, Therapists can be excellent sources of crucial data and insights.

Therapists need to understand the nature of psychological assessment to best incorporate psychological findings into their treatment efforts. In addition, some Therapists may have access to psychologists only as consultants. In such cases, Therapists ought to appreciate the types of issues psychologists can assess and treat, to know when to refer a patient to a psychologist.

Psychometric Assessment

Psychometric assessment can provide insight into patient functioning beyond that which is easily obtainable in a diagnostic interview. This is particularly true if programs want recommendations in a timely fashion. Therefore, it is advantageous to select psychometric tests to cover a wide domain of possible areas concerning the injured worker patient population. There are numerous articles on individual tests[5,8,10,22,24,25,28,29,30,32,34] and reviews that summarize the field.[1,4,27,39]

It is beyond the scope of this chapter to catalog these tests. However, it is important for programs to understand the domain that psychologists ought to sample using psychometric instruments.

Emotions. Tests should assess patients' emotional status. Emotions influence how patients perceive messages from health care providers. Feelings also affect patient behavior. Mood strongly influences how well patients can rally their coping mechanisms in response to health problems. Patients experiencing negative emotions are less likely to avail themselves of all of their resources.

Assessment of emotional status is important, too, because the patients mood is a worthy target for intervention. Patients' feelings deserve attention regardless of their impact on other health care problems. Physical rehabilitation and return to work that leaves patients depressed, is incomplete intervention. Too often, Therapists, insurers, and employers view rehabilitation as complete when they resolve the vocational impact of an injury, while they ignore the emotional fallout of the disability or off-work experience. Even with return to vocational success, the disability experience may change patients in detrimental ways. There can be residual changes in self image, trust, sense of security, or family relationships.

Perceived Capabilities. Psychometric assessment should include a measure of patients' self report of their activity capability. It is important to know what patients see as their functional ability. Their concept of their own walking, sleeping, driving, sitting, and sexual activity tolerance is important. The outcome of treatment on concepts of their own abilities may be more important for a successful result than any actual change in their abilities, such as the amount of weight they can lift.

Pain Beliefs. Testing ought to include a measure of pain beliefs, pain fear and anxiety, or pain cognition. These terms refer to how patients think about pain and injury. Patients evaluate their lives in light of their pain and limitations. It is important to know what judgments patients make regarding pain, disability, self-worth, and the future. Change is difficult to achieve without knowing about patients' expectations for their roles in life. How patients view their injury is crucial.

Pain Assessment.   A test battery should assess pain. Too often professionals apply sophisticated techniques for the assessment of organic damage (Magnetic Resonance Imaging), physical abilities (Functional Capacity Evaluation), psychological functioning (Minnesota Multiphasic Personality Inventory), and then simply ask the patient "How much does it hurt?"

Pain is a complex, multi-dimensional, multi-determined phenomena. It is inadequate to assess it by only asking how it rates "on a scale from one to ten." It is important to choose an assessment instrument that evaluates the diversity and richness of the pain experience. An appreciation of various pain elements can lead Therapists to greater comprehension of the patients' condition.

Coping Skills.   A comprehensive assessment ought to measure coping skills and broad patterns of adjustment. Personality provides the foundation upon which patients formulate their response to pain and injury. It is essential that Therapists be aware of behavioral tendencies, attitudes, or even psychopathology. These may affect the nature of patients' symptom presentation and may have large implications for case management.

Diagnostic Interview

Face to face patient evaluation can be essential. Psychometric assessment is necessary, but not sufficient, for a comprehensive determination of patients' psychological status. Too often Work Hardening programs may include a few psychological tests as part of an evaluation of the patients' condition without including a good psychological interview. This is unfortunate because testing can generate hypotheses to pursue in clinical examination, or it can confirm findings from clinical examination, but tests usually work best in conjunction with a diagnostic interview. Excellent patient care requires confirmation of clinical tests.

A diagnostic interview of injured workers ought to include questions in special areas of inquiry pertinent to injured workers. Box 18.1 provides a sample format for such an interview. Psychologists might expand on various sections during the interview based on the information the patients provide and the test results. If possible, it is helpful to have the test results available prior to the interview so they can guide interview inquiry.

BOX 18.1

Problem-Oriented Diagnostic Interview

Evaluation purpose
Why were you referred?

Onset
How were you injured?
When?

Vocational status
What was your job?
Did you like it?
What was your relationship with your employer?
Supervisor?
Is your old job being held for you?
If you must change employers or fields, what would you like to do?
What was the last grade of school you completed?
   If less than 12, did you get a GED?
    Why did you leave school early?
      Were you ever in any special education classes?
      Any diagnoses of learning disability?

Were you ever in trouble in school?
How well do you read?

Financial status
What was your salary prior to your injury?
Are you receiving workers' compensation?
   How much?
   Is it on time?
   Do you have financial troubles?
     Have you had to sell things?
     Declare bankruptcy?
   Do you have any private disability insurance?
   Do you have another source of income?

Workers' Compensation
Do you have a case manager?
What is your relationship with your case manager?
What is your relationship with your insurance carrier?

continued

B O X   1 8 . 1 — *c o n t ' d*

Marital history

Are you single, married, divorced?

If married:

How long?

Children? Ages?

Spouse's occupation?

How is spouse coping?

How is the relationship?

Were you ever married before?

If single:

Are you in a relationship?

How long?

How serious?

Significant Other's occupation?

How is the relationship?

Were you ever married before?

If divorced:

How many times?

When?

How long were you married?

Any children? Ages?

Whose idea was it to divorce?

Reasons?

Emotional status

Are you depressed?

Do you have increased irritability?

If yes, do you leave, yell, throw things, hit people?

Have you ever contemplated suicide?

Chemicals

What medications do you take?

What is each for?

How much caffeine do you drink each day (coffee, tea, soda)?

Do you smoke? How much?

If you quit, when? How much before quitting?

Do you drink alcohol? How much?

Have you used more in the past? When? How much?

Any past or current street drug use? When? What?

Any history of DWI? When?

Any history of chemical dependency treatment? When?

Legal

Any lawsuits pending?

Any run-ins with the law in the past?

When? What for? What happened?

Abuse

Have you ever been a victim of physical, sexual, or emotional abuse?

Have you ever perpetrated physical, sexual, emotional abuse? When? Whom?

Past psychological history

Have you been seen by a psychologist, psychiatrist, or counselor in the past? When? For how long? Why? Who?

Were you an inpatient or outpatient?

Were you prescribed any medications? What?

Basic Functions

How is your sleep?

Trouble with falling asleep?

Trouble staying asleep?

How is your appetite?

Have you gained or lost weight? How much?

Has there been a change in your interest in sex?

Does pain interfere?

For men, any trouble getting or keeping an erection?

Activity

If you are off work, how do you spend your time now?

What leisure time activities did you pursue before onset?

Are you bored?

Goals

Is your primary goal pain relief or increase in function?

If pain relief, how much relief would be the minimum that would be acceptable?

What specific activities do you want to be able to do?

PSYCHOLOGICAL RECOMMENDATIONS

Psychometric and clinical evaluation ought to lead to concrete recommendations. Psychologists ought to record recommendations in terms clear to those who will use the findings. Psychologists might hope that the crucial nature of subtle psychological variables were more obvious. Unless one presents psychological findings succinctly, the import may be lost.

Patient Categorization

Many times, psychologists can best present recommendations regarding patients' psychological status using a method of categorization. Table 18.2 outlines such a system.

These four categories summarize recommendations in an easily understandable format. Psychologists may use this system to categorize patients from a

TABLE 18.2 Psychological Evaluation Recommendations

Good	Handle care in standard fashion
	Proceed with intervention
Fair	Handle care with attention to specific patient needs
	Proceed with care
Uncertain	Care likely to present case management problems
	Proceed with caution
Poor	Care presents clear problems
	Recommend defer planned intervention

(Adapted from Karol RL: Presurgical Psychological Evaluation Results, unpublished, 1990.)

psychological perspective in a number of cases: Work Hardening program participant, returning employee, or even surgical candidate. Psychologists could use this system to rate how they expect a patient to do in treatment.

Good Candidate. The first of the four categories is a "good candidate." A good candidate requires little special attention. There are few, if any, psychological variables that might adversely effect outcome. As issues arise, Therapists should handle them with little difficulty.

Fair Candidate. This patient might need Therapists to pay attention to specific patient needs. There might be a particular way that communication works best, a particular issue that is especially difficult for the patient to handle, or a well-defined concern about something in the patient's care. Nevertheless, Therapists, in consultation with the psychologist, ought to be able to adapt intervention to meet the patient's needs.

Uncertain Candidate. This patient raises more concern and it is questionable whether the patient will do well. Issues of the patient's ability to cope loom sufficiently large, and there are doubts about outcome. It is possible that the challenges in the case may be too great to overcome. This may not preclude proceeding with the proposed plan, but Therapists should be very aware of the challenges and should anticipate the possibility of less than optimum success. The psychologist might not be able to provide sufficient help.

Poor Candidate. This candidate shows signs of problems. It is likely that the intervention or plan will fail. This may be due to active chemical abuse, significant depression, extreme hostility, poor comprehension, or compensation manipulation agendas. Therapists should recommend prerequisite treatment to the

care plan or even an alternative, more appropriate, course of action.

Clinical professionals often have a difficult time saying "no." Many Work Hardening programs and chronic pain programs take all patients referred to them. They sometimes believe that poor candidates may surprise them and do better than Therapists expect. If the program is the last resort, Therapists may hesitate to turn patients away, believing that whatever they can achieve, is worth attaining.

Poorly empowered, nonmedical professionals may hesitate to refuse a Physician's referral. They may anticipate loss of future referrals and money. Interestingly, surgeons also, wrestle with this problem. Surgeons can find it very difficult to withhold treatment from poor surgical candidates when confronted with patients in pain who are desperate.

Nevertheless, Therapists ought to carefully select intervention, ranging from individual outpatient treatment to Work Hardening programs, or chronic pain programs to surgery. Poorly selected intervention is poor care. It wastes insurance money and Therapists' resources. Poor candidates can be a detrimental influence on other participants, whether they are Work Hardening program participants or patients on a surgical floor.

Furthermore, patients do get hurt in conservative care programs, and invasive procedures carry risk. Patient selection is crucial to balance cost and risk with likelihood for desirable outcome.

Recommendations from a psychological perspective should concretely contribute to clinical decision making. Psychological information is most helpful when Therapists can use it to help clarify treatment planning.

In addition to concise recommendations, psychological assessment ought to explain the reasons for the recommendations. These should include how the psychologist reached the conclusions and what support the psychologist attached to particular variables. The factors which are intuitively obvious to a psychologist may fail to be apparent to other health care providers. Caution must be taken that discussion of the findings does not obscure the clearness of the recommendations.

Discussion of the recommendations can have a broad range. A psychologist may report on case management issues and delineate how to handle them. The discussion may propose particular types of programs or individual approaches. Then, suggestions may include advice on adjunctive, but often essential, treatment intervention for issues having psychological impact, such as physical, sexual, or emotional abuse;[2,18,20] financial status; chemical dependency; etc.

Finally, in a setting using invasive techniques,

psychological information can facilitate making a determination as to whether to proceed.[3]

TREATMENT FROM A PSYCHOLOGICAL PERSPECTIVE

Psychological Orientation

Individual and programmatic treatment have "psychological footprints," a term that describes the cumulative psychological atmosphere surrounding intervention. The first factor that contributes to the psychological footprint is the intentionally designed treatment components. These components are those which providers intentionally use to directly affect patients. In Work Hardening, examples might include job simulation, specific exercises, body mechanics training, or vocational counseling. Individual or group psychotherapy is a part of this factor.

The second factor that contributes to the psychological footprint arises from how caregivers provide the apparent, designed components. To be truly effective, Therapists must consider the psychological messages they convey about patients and treatment. Patients base judgments about their health and treatment progress, in part, on the psychological messages conveyed to them by treatment designs and services. Therapists' inattention to the messages that treatment delivery imparts can sabotage the effectiveness of apparent treatment components.

Programs must appreciate the psychological impact of decisions. The services programs offer and how they are organized help determine the psychological footprint. Programs must select and organize treatment services like manual manipulation, job simulation, functional capacity evaluation, psychotherapy, and stress reduction.

Effective programs establish how they provide intervention for maximum psychological effect. They manipulate treatment frequency, guidelines, duration, length of treatment day, intensity, individual or group treatment choices, single or multiple therapists, type of therapists, tight or loose patient supervision, location and type of physical plant, conference frequency and attendees, degree of flexibility, possibility of follow-up, and whether concurrent return to work is an option. All of these selections have subtle psychological effects which determine the interventions' psychological footprint.

Table 18.3 illustrates how a sample Work Hardening program might configure treatment for a particular patient at one point during the program. The program Therapists make conscious choices, with regard to the psychological effect on the patient at that moment. The program Therapists might make different choices at other times or for other patients.

Alterations in program variables can have a large impact. The change during a program from individual attention to more group instruction can serve as a simple example regarding the importance of patients' perceptions. The change may mean little to Therapists. However, while some patients might agree, others might not. Some patients may think therapy is winding down prematurely and may wonder how soon the program will conclude treatment. These patients may interpret the change as a sign of having plateaued, rather than of having progressed. They may begin to

TABLE 18.3   Work Hardening Service and Organization Illustration

Variable	Choice	Psychological Reasoning
Services		
Manual manipulation	No	Has learned to handle flare-ups
Job simulation	Yes	Creates appropriate mind set
Psychotherapy	Yes	Fear of reinjury facing new job
Stress reduction	Yes	Attends to instruction better
Functional Capacity Evaluation	Yes	Reassures patient for new job
Organization		
Length of day	6 hours	Also studying for GED exam
Intensity	Moderate	Showing fair/good motivation
Individual/Group	Group	Benefits from camaraderie
Supervision	Moderate	Needs redirecting
Conference frequency	Two weeks	Moderate workers' compensation issues
Treatment frequency	Daily	May not do home exercises
Treatment duration	Six weeks	Fearful of reinjury on job
Concurrent work	GED study	Needs for new job with employer

contemplate the need for more invasive treatment. Other patients may exhibit doubts or anxiety. There may be increasing Physician visits or treatment setbacks.

Therapists, so familiar with their program, may fail to appreciate how patients form impressions. Attention to the psychological milieu of therapy gives therapists additional manipulative variables to achieve treatment success. Moreover, Therapists can attenuate unintended psychological effects by careful consideration of the psychological impact of treatment decisions, and through excellent communication with patients. This is important throughout health care, including Physician office visits, Work Hardening programs, surgery planning, and interaction with insurers or employers.

Program Psychological Footprints

Frequently, the crucial differences between programs are their psychological footprints. Health clubs, chronic pain programs, and Work Hardening programs have different psychological footprints. Table 18.4 highlights the elements that contribute to the psychological footprints of these three program types.

Health Club Programs.   At a health club, patients will feel independent and able to set their own program. There is little guidance and less motivational assistance. A health club provides a sense of normalcy and perhaps isolation from the health care system. Patients can return to work concurrent with participation. Since duration is open, there is little fear of failure or pressure to progress at a certain rate. On the other hand, fear of injury may be high.

TABLE 18.4   Elements Contributing to the Psychological Footprint of Programs

	Health Club	Chronic Pain Program	Work Hardening Program
Open duration	+	−	−
Job unknown	+	+	−
Partial return to work	+	−	+
Therapist directed			
Biomechanically based exercise	−	−	+
Psychological intervention	−	+	+
Complex behavioral treatment	−	+	−
Job Simulation	−	−	+

Note. Plus signs represent issues programs address or program attributes, whereas minus signs represent elements not part of the program. Minus signs are not shortcomings; rather, program elements must match patient needs.

Chronic Pain Programs.   These can effectively treat complicated behavioral and motivational problems. Patients receive direct encouragement to dispense with hidden agendas. Most programs have medical and program directors, providing the patients a sense that behavioral and motivational issues are part of their health care. Often, such programs deemphasize biomechanical exercise in favor of behavioral reactivation. Since chronic pain programs usually defer concurrent return to work, they tend to be brief, communicating the need for decision making and action, although creating an artificial barrier between treatment and work. Support during return to work may be absent.

Work Hardening Programs.   For patients without a chronic pain syndrome, but who require more assistance than health clubs, Work Hardening programs offer a Therapist-guided environment to pursue return to work. Patients are likely to feel more secure because exercise is specific for their injuries and jobs. Job simulation encourages return to a vocational focus from a health focus.

Partial return to work opportunities also encourage a vocational focus, providing a sense of immediacy. Time limitation facilitates separation from the health care system. Programs which take patients with diverse injuries help them to put their injuries in perspective.

Nevertheless, patients may present Work Hardening programs with well-known psychological issues inherent in the return-to-work endeavor. These issues include low patient commitment to program goals, failure to see similarities across diverse program participant injuries and situations, and inadequate readiness to separate from the health care system. Well-designed Work Hardening programs can handle these issues, particularly when the program integrates psychological care in a supradisciplinary model.

Patient Screening

Careful patient screening by the full program team, including the psychologist, with input from employers, insurers, lawyers, and case managers prior to admission can determine patients' orientation toward return to work. The team's evaluation might incorporate assessment of patients' desire to return to their previous jobs and employers, past relationships with supervisors, beliefs in availability of financial support for retraining, feelings about thoroughness of acute care and readiness for rehabilitation, orientation toward the Workers' Compensation system, and patients' goals. Evaluation of these factors helps insure that the team is ready to handle issues of patient commitment.

Group Cohesiveness

During treatment, patients may fail to bond with the other participants. Diversity can be a source of material for alert Therapists to use as examples of coping. The utilization of patients as models for each other, with Therapists guiding the process, enhances outcome. Program teams sensitive to the psychology of group roles and configurations can facilitate cohesiveness and support. Furthermore, if patients enter the program in a staggered fashion, experienced patients can aid newer ones as role models, providing peer counseling.

Fear of Discharge

Finally, patients may resist program termination. Programs can attenuate the fear of eventual discharge from the program by patient involvement in decision-making throughout the program. Patients are more likely to achieve a sense of self-sufficiency when they participate in goal setting, agree with the expected rate of progress, and understand program philosophy regarding pain complaints. Participation in team meetings builds trust and programs can use this to empower patients.

Summary

In summary, wise Therapists and programs decide on treatment services and their organization with psychological effects in mind. However Therapists devise programs, they should consider the psychological footprint. The traditional wisdom that "it is not what you say, but how you say it" translates in health care service provision, into a recognition of the crucial nature of psychologically derived patient perceptions.

TREATMENT TECHNIQUES

Regardless of the nature of the program, patients tend to have predictable psychological adjustment issues. Failure to handle these recurring concerns will undermine efforts to improve health or achieve vocational reactivation.

Programs can address psychological issues through a combination of techniques. Help in addressing these issues comes through the provision of:

1. Conceptual frameworks
2. Specific information
3. Skills training

It is important that programs are able to use all three techniques effectively. The decision about which methods to use depends upon the particular issue.

Conceptual Frameworks

Conceptual frameworks provide patients with templates upon which they can organize observations about life. Many people are observant about life events and experiences, but lack a scheme for organizing their raw data observations. When patients lack a format to understand their experiences, they must individually process each event. People with knowledge about how events tend to occur are better prepared and can look ahead with less stress.

By analogy, a quarterback recognizes defensive schemes from past experience. It would be highly inefficient to look at each player, decide the individual implication of each particular player and each player's actions each time, and then decide what play to run based on all those separate bits of information.

Rather, the quarterback compares the crucial elements of the defensive scheme, for the design of the scheduled play, against known defensive patterns. The quarterback knows what defensive "templates" look like; there are preexisting formats.

Similarly, an experienced automobile driver quickly sorts information against previously experienced patterns even at highway speeds. For student drivers, all of the things rapidly happening at once is confusing and overwhelming even at slow speeds.

For patients who have never encountered chronic injury, providing a framework to understand the differences between chronic and acute injury may prove very helpful.[19] Chronic medical problems follow a different course than acute problems, such as a broken leg. The sociological and psychological responses of family, friends, coworkers, employers, insurers, and health care professionals are different. A conceptual framework allows patients to understand the environment in which they now find themselves.

For instance, when friends drop away, patients may feel hurt. Understanding why friends may remain supportive during the brief, acute injury of a broken leg, but may fade away when faced with the chronic life changes of a back injury can facilitate coping by patients.

Programs can provide other conceptual frameworks as well. Patients often have a poor understanding of pain and the nervous system. Explanation of the gate control pain theory[6] or the difference between chronic pain and damage can increase patient understanding of the nonacute care, rehabilitative Work Hardening model.

Specific Information

Beyond acquiring conceptual frameworks, patients may benefit from having specific information in order to address the issues they confront. Patients may require a wide expanse of information. This might include information on medications,[26] sex and injuries,[11,15,33] expressing emotions,[13] Workers' Compensation,[9] disability insurance,[37] communicating with Physicians[12,35,36] or fear of reinjury. Patients often try to handle problems and make decisions with grossly inadequate information.

Specific Skill

Sometimes, just having information is insufficient. Specific skill building is necessary so that patients can apply the information. A program could include instruction and practice in communication skills, techniques to use when interacting with health care providers, and interviewing skills.

In summary, patients face many challenges in managing their injuries. Treatment should provide a combination of conceptual frameworks, specific information, and skills building opportunities to address these challenges.

SPECIAL CONSIDERATIONS

Rehabilitation of injured workers occurs best in a team format, particularly in supradisciplinary teams. Some Therapists, unfortunately, work without the advantages of a complete team. These Therapists must decide on a case by case basis when to consult psychologists. Often these Therapists must confront four issues: when to refer to a psychologist, who to use as a consultant, how to explain the referral to their patients, and cost.

When to Refer

Referral to a psychologist is appropriate in three situations.

1. When psychological issues may be interfering with recovery. The issues may predate the injury or may result from the injury. Regardless, supposedly correct care is failing to achieve the results Therapists anticipate. Logic suggests, in such cases, that Therapists consider factors interfering with the achievement of success, or reconsider the choice of treatment.

For the purposes of referral, the distinction about whether the psychological issues predate injury onset, or not, is a moot point. If the problems hamper treatment, they require attention. The distinction is crucial to insurers with regard to financial liability for treatment, though many insurers now recognize the need to resolve psychological issues, even if they predate injury onset, so that the rest of the care plan can proceed successfully.

There are numerous examples of psychological issues interfering with recovery. The injury may cause marital troubles in an otherwise successful relationship. The marital discord can sabotage treatment due to the lack of spousal support for maintaining a treatment regimen, preoccupation with family finances, and difficulty in the acceptance of new roles at home.

Coping with pain from an injury can tire and depress patients. Depressed, fatigued patients are less likely to do well in treatment. A final example occurs when patients are fearful of reinjury. Patients who are afraid can become withdrawn, distrustful, noncompliant, and resistant to treatment.

In general, health care providers accept the idea that referral to psychologists ought to occur when psychological issues hinder recovery. In Minnesota, this orientation is so well acknowledged that it is codified in the state rules[42] governing the treatment of Workers' Compensation patients. The rules state, "Personality or psychological evaluations may be indicated for evaluating patients who continue to have problems despite appropriate care. . . . These evaluations may be used to assess the patient for a number of psychological conditions which may interfere with recovery from the injury."

2. When the difficulties psychologists address are part of the injury, but do not necessarily interfere with other treatment. Since injuries and pain are multifaceted, it is essential to avoid assigning primary importance to any one treatment strategy, which would be the case if referral to psychologists only occurred when other treatment was failing. Sometimes the aspects of injury most in need of treatment are those psychologists address.

The following two situations illustrate difficulties injuries cause which may not be interfering with other treatment. In one situation, patients may sincerely participate in treatment to regain employment. Their injuries may necessitate career changes that have implications for their identity. Some patients may avoid letting the alteration in self worth interfere with treatment efforts, but the modification, in their sense of self esteem, is clearly due to their injury and deserves treatment.

In the other situation, patients may experience difficulty with sexuality because of an injury. This may have little impact upon return to work. However, for these patients the importance of damage to sexual functioning may be devastating and bears treatment.

3. When problems neither interfere with treatment nor are a part of the injury, therapists may become aware of a patient's eating disorder or difficulty with child rearing. Therapists should recognize problems even when unrelated to the immediate injury and facilitate referral to appropriate caregivers. This is true for referrals to psychologists or anyone else.

Health care providers of all disciplines should facilitate referral for incidental health problems. Coverage for the care of incidental difficulties, psychological or otherwise, may be elsewhere than with the injury insurer.

Therapists can be in a quandary about when to refer specific cases to a psychologist. Three broad categories suggest referral when issues—1) interfere with recovery, 2) stem from the injury, or 3) are incidental to the injury or too general to provide immediate guidance. Box 18.2 provides behavioral cor-

relates. This list is not all inclusive, but the items on it can serve as markers for problems Therapists can watch for in their patients.

Psychological Specialists

For diagnoses or treatment of injured patients who are coping with organic injury or pain, the psychological consultant ought to specialize in a field variously called behavioral medicine, medical psychology, or health psychology. These terms indicate a specialty field dedicated to helping patients with health problems from a psychological perspective. Such psychologists may work with patients having difficulties related to

---

BOX 18.2

Markers for Problems to Refer to Psychologists

Treatment process
_____ Attendance
_____ Compliance
_____ Comprehension
_____ Effort

Chemical use
_____ Medication seeking
_____ Multiple medications
_____ Tolerance
_____ Withdrawal
_____ Illicit drugs
_____ Excess alcohol
_____ Alcohol/illicit drugs for
         pain control
_____ Excess caffeine
_____ Excess nicotine
_____ Driving while intoxicated

Emotional status
_____ Depression
_____ Anger
_____ Bitter/resentful
_____ Fearful

Relationships
_____ Separation/divorce
_____ Conflicts/fighting
_____ Role issues
_____ Not understand patient's
         limits/pain

Somatic issues
_____ Guarding
_____ Pain focus
_____ Fear of reinjury
_____ Misunderstood diagnosis

Acceptance
_____ Treatment shopping
_____ Denial of chronic condition
_____ Multiple surgeries
_____ Multiple treatment failures

Basic functions
_____ Sleep
_____ Appetite
_____ Weight control
_____ Sexuality

Coping style
_____ Suspiciousness/distrust
_____ Sabotaging
_____ Cognitive distortion

Psychosocial history
_____ Illiteracy
_____ Arrests/jail
_____ Head trauma
_____ Low education

Vocational
_____ Rigid goals
_____ Unrealistic retraining goals
_____ Hidden agendas

Financial
_____ Sale of valuables
_____ Bankruptcy

Patient difficulty with team
_____ Case manager
_____ Insurer
_____ Physician
_____ Therapist
_____ Lawyer
_____ Employer

Past psychological difficulties
_____ Outpatient counseling
_____ Inpatient hospitalization
_____ Psychotropic medications

chronic pain, cancer, cardiac problems, kidney dysfunction, etc. Their expertise relates to the interface of psychology and health.

To locate psychologists with such specialties, the referral source could contact various organizations. Some professional organizations encompass specialties with expertise in many different health problems, such as the Society of Behavioral Medicine. Some broader organizations have subsections of psychologists specializing in health psychology (American Psychological Association). State psychological associations may have referral services where psychologists list specialties.

There are also various specialty professional organizations for specific health problems (American Pain Society) and board certifying organizations (American Board of Medical Psychotherapists).

Patient Preparation

If patients misunderstand the reason for the referral, even the best of consultants may be ineffective. Clinical experience suggests that an explanation, preferably including a written handout, can do much to dispel misperceptions. The explanation ought to acknowledge that many people are unprepared for coping with a chronic injury.

Seeing psychologists does not discount the validity of the patients' organic complaints—the pain is "real," but stress, lifestyle changes, and emotional status can affect pain, just as they might effect stomach ulcers or elevated blood pressure.

If psychometric assessment is likely, then advance information could ready patients for the possibility of psychometric evaluation. Finally, referral sources should help allay patients' concerns by relating the specialized nature of the consultants' psychological field of expertise.

Expense

A few Therapists, some patients, and many insurance companies seem to fear the expense of psychological evaluation or treatment. This fear is unfounded when there is an appropriate understanding of team functioning, which should include the insurer, and an understanding of the patients' health problems from a broad perspective. Regardless, psychological treatment saves third party reimbursement sources money by decreasing the utilization of other medical services.[23,31,40] In research literature, this is called the "offset effect."

Many reimbursers take the position that psychological intervention is costly, when actually its absence is likely to increase overall costs. Refusal to reimburse for psychological treatment, therefore, results in increased cost and less effective treatment. The reason for referral for psychological care or treatment is not to save money, but because it is appropriate care for the health of the patient. This standard applies to psychological care as it does to other treatment.

SUMMARY

Improving the health of injured workers and returning them to work is challenging. It is essential that programs incorporate a psychological perspective into their diagnostic and therapeutic armamentarium. Consideration of psychological variables enhances the quality of overall assessment and can be crucial in the achievement of successful treatment. Although many patients are unaware of, or deny, the importance of their psychological history and current status, pain and injury are multidetermined, multidimensional phenomena.

To best help patients, programs should bring to bear the efforts of all players in the rehabilitation sphere. Empowered Therapists access the knowledge and skills of insurers, lawyers, employers and caregivers. To be effective, these players must realize their psychological impact on patients. Teamwork does facilitate rehabilitation, particularly in supradisciplinary teams.

Psychologists can enhance rehabilitation through complete psychological evaluation. Psychometric assessment should be broad-based and should supplement clinical interview. Therapists should expect psychologists to present their findings in an understandable manner, with succinct recommendations.

Comprehensive treatment must address psychological functioning. Therapists and psychologists can provide conceptual frameworks, information, and skills to improve outcome. Such efforts will be most efficacious when there is careful design of the psychological footprints of individual intervention.

Therapists can access psychologists even when they are practicing without the benefit of a regular team. Patient preparation is important when Therapists refer to psychologists. Cost should not be an issue among well informed Therapists and insurers.

Therapists can provide their patients with the maximum opportunity to return to a productive life when they approach rehabilitation from a psychological perspective. Patients will make better gains and Therapists will reap a greater sense of satisfaction, finding their work both more successful and therefore more rewarding.

REFERENCES

1. Bradley LA: Psychological evaluation of the low back pain patient. In Tollison CD, Kriegel ML editors, *Interdisciplinary rehabilitation of low back pain,* Baltimore, 1989 Williams & Wilkins.

2. Bradley LA, Haile JD, Jaworski TM: Assessment of psychological status using interviews and self-report instruments. In Turk DC, Melzack R editors, *Handbook of pain assessment,* New York, 1992. Guilford Press.

3. Cameron AJR, Schepel LF: Psychological assessment. In Kirkaldy-Willis WH editor, *Managing low back pain,* New York, 1988. Churchill Livingstone.

4. Deyo RA: Measuring the functional status of patients with low back pain, *Arch Physical Med and Rehab* 69: 1044–1053, 1988.

5. Deyo RA, Walsh NE, Schoenfeld LS, Ramamurthy, S: Studies of the Modified Somatic Perceptions Questionnaire (MSPQ) in patients with back pain: psychometric and predictive properties *Spine* 14: 507–510 1989.

6. Doerfler LA, Parker JC, Karol RL: Gate control theory and behavioral interventions for chronic pain: beyond the operant approach, JSAS *Catalog of Selected Documents in Psychology* 14: 11, 1984.

7. Doherty C: Beyond Work Hardening 101, *WORK* 1: 62–68, 1990.

8. Fairbank JCT, Couper J, Davies JB, O'Brien JP: The Oswestry low back pain disability questionnaire, *Physiotherapy* 66: 271–273, 1980.

9. Fleeson WP: *Going on comp: How to get through a workers' compensation injury without losing your cool.* Duluth, Minn, 1991 Med-Ed Books & Publishers.

10. Follick MJ, Smith TW, Ahern, DK: The Sickness Impact Profile: a global measure of disability in chronic low back pain, *Pain* 21:67–76, 1985.

11. Gendleman J: Sex and chronic pain: The healing touch, *Lifeline Reprint Series,* National Chronic Pain Outreach Association, 4922 Hampden Lane, Bethesda, MD, 20814, February, 1989.

12. Gendleman J, Hitchcock LS: Communication: Getting the most from your doctor-patient relationship, *Lifeline Reprint Series,* National Chronic Pain Outreach Association, 4922 Hampden Lane, Bethesda, MD 20814 November, 1988.

13. Gottman J, Notarius C, Gonso J, Markman H: *A couple's guide to communication,* Champaign, Il, 1977, Research Press.

14. Hanson RW, Gerber KE *Coping with chronic pain: A guide to patient self-management,* New York 1990 Guilford Press.

15. Hebert L: *Sex and back pain,* Bangor, Me, 1987, IMPACC.

16. Karol RL: *The patient as learner: Improving patient's use of knowledge,* Paper presented at the Conference on Patient Teaching: How Do You Measure Up?, Minneapolis, Minn, May, 1982.

17. Karol RL: *Dealing with mental health issues after brain injury: A user's guide to approaches real and imagined,* Paper presented at Mental Health Issues of Adults with brain injury Conference, Minneapolis, Minn, September, 1991.

18. Karol RL: The occurrence of physical, emotional, and sexual abuse in patients and professional caregivers. *American Pain Society Bulletin* 3: 5–7, 1993.

19. Karol RL, Doerfler LA, Parker JC, Armentrout DP,: A Therapist manual for the cognitive-behavioral treatment of chronic pain, JSAS *Catalog of Selected Documents in Psychology* 11: 15, 1981.

20. Karol RL, Micka RG, Kuskowski M: Physical, emotional, and sexual abuse among pain patients and health care providers: Implications for psychologists in multidisciplinary pain treatment centers, *Professional Psychology: Research and Practice* 23: 480–485, 1992.

21. Keith RA: The comprehensive treatment team in rehabilitation, *Arch Physical Med and Rehab* 72: 269–274, 1991.

22. Keller LS, Butcher, JN: *Assessment of chronic pain patients with the MMPI-2,* Minneapolis 1991. University of Minnesota Press.

23. Kessler LG, Steinwachs DM, Hankin, JR: Episodes of psychiatric care and medical utilization, *Medical Care* 20: 1209–1217, 1982.

24. Lawlis GF, Cuencas R, Selby, D, McCoy CE: The development of the Dallas Pain Questionnaire: An assessment of the impact of spinal pain on behavior, *Spine* 14: 511–516, 1989.

25. Lefebvre, MF: Cognitive distortion and cognitive errors in depressed psychiatric and low back pain patients, *Consulting and Clinical Psych* 49: 517–525, 1981.

26. Lerner, P: A consumer's guide to drugs for people with chronic pain: A series, *Lifeline Reprint Series,* National Chronic Pain Outreach Association, 4922 Hampden Lane, Bethesda, Md 20814. 1988.

27. Mayer TG, Gatchel RJ: *Functional restoration for spinal disorders: The sports medicine approach,* Philadelphia 1988. Lea & Febiger.

28. Melzack R: The McGill pain questionnaire: Major properties and scoring methods, *Pain* 21: 277–299, 1975.

29. Melzack R, Torgerson WS: On the language of pain, *Anesthesiology* 34: 50–59, 1971.

30. Millard RW: The functional assessment screening questionnaire: Application for evaluating pain-related disability, *Arch Physical Med and Rehab* 70: 303–307, 1989.

31. Mumford E, Schlesigner HJ, Glass GV, Patrick C, Cuerdon T: A new look at evidence about reduced cost of medical utilization following mental health treatment, *Ameri J Psych* 141: 1145–1158, 1984.

32. Riley JF, Ahern DK, Follick MJ: Chronic pain and functional improvement: Assessing beliefs about their relationship, *Arch Physical Med and Rehab* 69: 579–582, 1988.

33. Rothrock R, D'Amore G: *The illustrated guide to better sex for people with chronic pain,* Morrisville, Penn 1991.

34. Schwartz DP, DeGood DE, Shutty MS: Direct assessment of beliefs and attitudes of chronic pain patients, *Arch of Physical Med and Rehab* 66: 806–809, 1985.

35. Sometimes, talk is the best medicine, *The Wall Street Journal,* p B1, October 5, 1989.

36. Sternbach, RA: Psychological aspects of chronic pain, *Clinical Orthopaedics and Related Research* 129: 150–155, 1977.

37. Stevens M: Shop carefully for disability insurance, *The Minneapolis Star Tribune,* p. 8M. October 19, 1987.

38. Thomas, CL editor: *Taber's cyclopedic medical dictionary,* Philadelphia: 1985. F A Davis.

39. Turk DC, Melzack R editors: *Handbook of pain assessment,* New York 1992. Guilford Press.

40. White SL: The impact of mental health services on medical care utilization: Economic and organizational implications, *Hospital & Community Psychiatry* 32: 311–319. 1981.

41. Williams AF, Lund AK: Injury control: What psychologists can contribute, *American Psychologist* 47: 1036–109. 1992.

42. Workers' Compensation Emergency Rules for Treatment Standards, St Paul, Minn: Minnesota Department of Labor and Industry, 1993.

19

Vocational Rehabilitation

Richard W. Nelson
Mark L. Anderle

Industrial Therapy Worker Care Spectrum

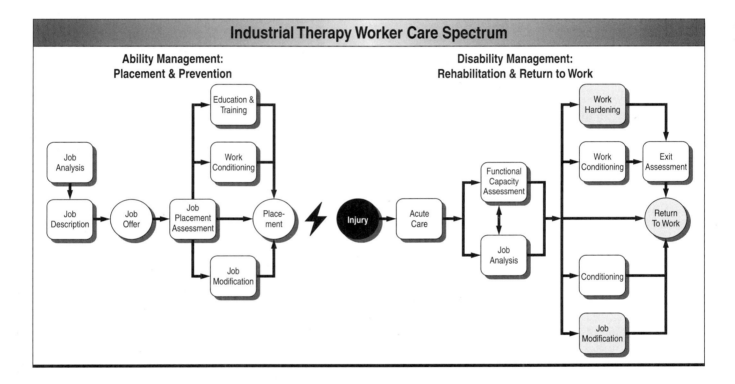

Ability Management: Placement & Prevention

Disability Management: Rehabilitation & Return to Work

Vocational Rehabilitation (VR) is the function of coordinating the people and resources involved in returning injured workers to productive work.

In the context of Workers' Compensation, the Vocational Rehabilitation Consultant (VRC) makes sure the interests of all parties are considered in a potentially adversarial process between claimant and payor, plaintiff and defendant. The VRC is an information resource, a helper, a coordinator, a facilitator, a planner, and a manager. The VRC often provides the forum for diverse parties to come together, resolve differences, and work to achieve the best solution for all, especially the injured worker.

The major benefits of vocational rehabilitation are summarized in Box 19.1.

In this chapter we will give a brief historical account of vocational rehabilitation, its beginnings as a public sector function, the development of private sector vocational rehabilitation in the 1970s and 1980s, the services it provides in the disability management field today, and a glimpse into its future. Relationships with the field of Industrial Therapy will be discussed, with recommendations for both professions.

HISTORY

Early Beginnings

Vocational rehabilitation has been a part of society perhaps since the beginning of mankind. Throughout history family members have assisted one another with various personal needs including emergency medical attention, follow-up care, financial help, return-to-

B O X 1 9 . 1

Major Benefits of Vocational Rehabilitation

Earlier return to work
Reduced disability payments
Controlled and reduced medical costs
Earlier and more fully-restored productivity
Better information flow for decision making
Reduced adversarial relationships in rehabilita-
    tion process
Reduced burdens on families and communities

work support, job searching, self employment, and other types of aid to overcome disabling injuries.

In our early agrarian society, families were more self sufficient. Then the Industrial Revolution led to changes in our society and families, no longer allowing the same degree of flexibility when disabling injuries occurred. Due to increased injuries within an industrial society, and the reduction of death with advancing medical science, a need for more formalized and organized vocational rehabilitation was created.

The Public Sector

In the early 20th century, the State/Federal rehabilitation programs were established, delivering services to the growing disabled population. The original State/Federal rehabilitation program, Public Law 236 in 1920, was established to serve two principle populations, disabled veterans and the industrially disabled.

In the view of one author, it was found to be more dangerous to work in industry than to be a combat soldier in World War I.[5] Over the next 50 years, government programs expanded to serve the needs of the disabled population in America.

Substantial reform began in 1970 when the President appointed a national commission to study the Workers' Compensation laws. That commission issued a report to the President in 1972, a "Compendium on Workman's Compensation," which concluded:[2]

> In general, Workmen's Compensation is not doing an effective job of assuring that workers with work-related disabilities be helped to recover lost abilities and to return to their previous jobs, or where this is impossible, to learn substitute skills. . . . Workmen's Compensation should take a more active role in assuring vocational rehabilitation.

Public sector, government-funded vocational rehabilitation programs attempted to integrate industrially-injured clients into their counselors' caseloads. With increasing caseloads and limited tax funding, the public sector had to give severely disabled populations priority, and could not fully serve industrially injured clients who did not meet the definition of "severely disabled." As a result, many industrially injured were treated without any formal oversight or coordination. A need arose, and private sector initiatives emerged to answer it.

Enter The Private Sector

The genesis and growth of private sector vocational rehabilitation can be illustrated with regard to National Rehabilitation Consultants (NRC), a St. Paul, Minnesota based company founded in February 1970. NRC is recognized within the rehabilitation industry as one of the first, if not the first, private vocational rehabilitation companies in America.

NRC's founder, Richard W. Nelson, had been employed by 3M Company, St. Paul, where he had managed a national program serving severely handicapped people who became employed in their own small graphic services businesses. He presented the idea of private sector vocational rehabilitation to 3M as a unique business opportunity—to oversee injured workers not covered by public sector rehabilitation. When 3M did not pass this idea, NRC was started as an independent firm.

The St. Paul Insurance Companies, headquartered in St. Paul, Minnesota became interested in NRC's proposal to oversee their Workers' Compensation claimants. The superintendent of Workers' Compensation for The St. Paul Companies, referred six test cases to NRC to test whether private vocational rehabilitation would be truly cost-effective. Applying relatively basic rehabilitation techniques, with only the rudiments of a systematic model, NRC sought to return the claimants to work faster, restore productivity earlier, reduce or eliminate wage loss benefits earlier, and justify their hourly fees in the savings.

The approach was simple: interview the client, review their work history, employment skills, medical records, secure a work release from the treating physician, and then design a specific return-to-work plan, including help with job placement.

Within 60 days, four of the six test cases were placed in competitive employment. This encouraging result fueled additional referrals from The St. Paul Companies and other carriers. With this story repeating itself through other start-up ventures in other settings across the U S, private sector rehabilitation, then called "insurance rehabilitation" was gaining momentum.

As interest in vocational rehabilitation by insurance carriers grew, this new industry had become well established by the late 1970s, blending human services with private enterprise to meet the needs of injured workers, employers, and insurers.

Associations

As private sector rehabilitation industry grew in numbers and sophistication, it needed capable leadership as well. In the early 1980s the National Association of Rehabilitation Professionals in the Private Sector (NARPPS) was formed. One of the early leaders of this organization was the late Kevin Karr, founder and president of Karr Rehabilitation Services, Minneapolis. He and other early private sector pioneers helped establish the vision, standards of practice, and credibility for this vital new industry. NARPPS, headquartered in Brookline, Mass., is the leading association to which private VR practitioners belong. Other national associations represent private VRCs, and many states have developed associations or groups.

VOCATIONAL REHABILITATION CONSULTANTS

Profile

Vocational Rehabilitation Consultants usually work in private-for-profit settings. In 1983 there were an estimated 6,000 private rehabilitation professionals in the U S,[5] with approximately 4,000 different firms by 1986.[3]

According to a study prepared for the U S Department of Education in 1987, analyzing proprietary rehabilitation, about 27% of those surveyed worked in individual practice, and 34% were with single-office firms with multiple staff (Box 19.2). About 39% were with larger companies with multiple offices.[2] Some VRCs are employed by insurance companies, larger employers, or medical facilities. Depending upon the size of the VRC firm, about 6% have one or more Physical Therapists on staff, and about 9% have one or more Occupational Therapists.[2]

Credentialing

Credentialing for VRCs varies around the country. Licensure is not typically required for VRCs. Rather, they may need to have educational backgrounds or hold professional certifications related to vocational rehabilitation, counseling, nursing, and allied areas, including physical or occupational therapy. Where a degree is required, the master's degree is increasingly the standard.

BOX 19.2

Proprietary Rehabilitation Profile

Firm type	Percent of firms
Single office firms—	
One person	27%
Single office firms—	
Multiple staff	34%
Multiple office firms	39%

Staff positions employed	Percent of firms
Counselor	89%
Job developer	50%
Nurse	46%
Occupational Therapists	9%
Physical Therapists	6%

Some state governments have established credentialing requirements for VRCs who wish to serve Workers' Compensation clients. These may vary from a very simple registry list, to required certification, educational, and experience criteria. The leading certifications for VRCs are the Certified Rehabilitation Counselor (CRC), the Certified Insurance Rehabilitation Specialist (CIRS), and the Certified Case Manager (CCM), all administered by the Foundation for Rehabilitation Certification, Education and Research, Rolling Meadows, Illinois.

Referral Sources

Most referrals to VRCs are initiated by insurance carriers and self-insured employers.[2] Other referral sources that may grow in importance over time are physicians, other health care providers, Industrial Therapists, attorneys, and employers. Some states require VR intervention for Workers' Compensation claimants who need help getting back to work, but this is becoming less of a factor.

In those states where it is not mandated, VR services are discretionary, and referrals are typically initiated by the insurance carrier or payor, not by other parties. Besides Workers' Compensation, other disability insurers refer to VRCs as well, including Auto No-Fault Liability, Long-Term Disability, and Health and Accident.

Fees

In most cases, fees are paid by the insurance company. Most VRCs charge per professional hour, sometimes on a per unit of service basis as well. Fee regulation is emerging especially in states where Workers' Compensation rehabilitation is regulated by statute.

Services

VRCs will usually serve a caseload of 20 to 30 clients at a time. Services provided by private sector practitioners vary by their firm, expertise, and usually by the local demand from referral sources. According to a survey of 329 private rehabilitation providers in 1987, VRCs provide the following services in their role as case managers:[2]

- Medical care coordination
- Vocational planning
- Job modification consultation
- Job analysis
- Placement
- Job development
- Job seeking skills training
- Labor market surveying

Medical care coordination assures that the most appropriate care is provided, in the most cost-effective manner, for maximum recovery in the shortest possible time.

Vocational planning formulates an agreed-upon pathway for return to work (RTW), consistent with the injured worker's medical treatment and overall vocational capabilities.

Job modification consultation apprises the employer and others about ways to fit the worker's job to the worker, to maximize both employee well-being as well as work place efficiency.

Job analysis assesses the particular job duties, physical demands, and other factors necessary to perform a specific job. Usually written, it is a prerequisite to job modification.

Placement helps the injured worker secure employment, typically with a new employer in cases where the former employer cannot bring the injured worker back in the same or modified capacity.

Job development helps the client use available job search resources and other means to identify specific employers to contact, and assists where possible in contacting employers and creating opportunities.

Job seeking skills training helps the client take charge of the job search through training in proper search techniques, interviewing skills, "selling" oneself, and persistence.

Labor market surveying identifies the employment outlook for a particular occupation, including job entry requirements, compensation, physical demands, hiring frequency, and advancement opportunities.

Standards

Standards of practice are not necessarily uniform across the US, except where VRCs adhere to the standards of their respective certifying body or professional association. By the same token, these existing standards of practice by VRCs have become relatively well established over the years.

VOCATIONAL REHABILITATION CASE PROCESS

Goals

In most cases the VRC's goal is to help their client return to suitable employment, consistent with whatever limitations are imposed by the disability, in the most efficient and cost-effective manner. Early intervention is a key to successful vocational resolution, as illustrated by Table 19.1 and Figure 19.3 discussed later in this chapter.

Participants

The basic participants in the process are the injured worker, employer, insurance company, and medical provider, but the family and an attorney can also be involved in some cases. The insurance company as payor, is typically the last word, but the VRC has the opportunity to influence the process greatly through suggestion and persuasion.

VRC Involvement

With regard to the Industrial Therapy Worker Care Spectrum on page 377, ideally the VRC is involved from the time of injury, until 30 days after the worker has been returned to employment. In reality, involvement begins after several medical visits when it is determined, generally, that "things are not going well" and additional intervention is deemed economically justifiable.

Sometimes the VRC's involvement is for limited services only, but where the VRC is called upon to function as the overall case manager, service delivery usually flows through a series of steps.

Referral

Most cases are referred by the insurance carrier. When circumstances permit, referral by any other party, including the Industrial Therapist, who recognizes need for vocational intervention, is desirable.

Intake and Case Development

Case development is the term applied to the function of gathering information and records, and reviewing it to formulate a good rehabilitation opinion. The VRC will typically interview the client, gather and review medical records, sometimes obtain vocational or functional capacity testing, and otherwise gain necessary background information to fully understand the case.

VRCs should observe data privacy and confidentiality standards at all times. Physical testing, if deemed necessary, is typically referred to a physician or Industrial Therapist. Paper and pencil testing is usually minimal, and is on the wane.

The usual interview takes approximately one hour. Its purposes are to get acquainted, establish mutual goals and expectations, obtain releases for confidential medical records, and discuss areas not typically covered elsewhere, such as work history, the family, social situation, and financial considerations.

Evaluation

Client information is analyzed and compiled in a written report, which leads to a conclusion about the client's employability and a recommended rehabilitation plan. This report is usually prepared for the referring agency, but can be useful for other parties as well. Example report contents are summarized in Box 19.3.

Rehabilitation Plan

Based upon the evaluation findings, good VR case practice then calls for a written plan to direct the desired outcome. The rehabilitation plan should state the vocational goal, specific measurable activities for accomplishing the goal, time frame, and progress check points.

Gaining concurrence on this plan beforehand from the key parties, especially the client, employer, insurer, and health care providers, can make all the difference in a successful outcome. Ideally, each party should sign off on the written plan prior to its initiation. Once endorsed, the plan provides for good communication, accountability, and mutual commitment by the parties who depend upon each other's cooperation. The components of a rehabilitation plan are outlined in Figure 19.1.

Plan Implementation

The VRC case manager's role is crucial for carrying the plan through to successful outcome. In the vast majority of cases, the insurance company as payor has the

---

BOX 19.3

Intake Evaluation Report

Typical subject matter
Personal background
Education and training
Medical information—current and history
Work history and skills
Financial status
Potential to return to former employer
Future employability and vocational options
Recommended rehabilitation plan (given vocational options)

FIGURE 19.1 Components of the Vocational Rehabilitation Plan

❏ **Goal**
Return to work via one of these options
Former employer
• Same job
• Modified job
• New job
New employer
• Job placement
• On-the-job training
• Formal retraining
• Self employment

❏ **Recovery needs**
Treatment to achieve maximum medical improvement, including physical therapy, work conditioning, or work hardening

❏ **Plan activities**
Specific activities for each plan participant, to achieve agreed-upon goal
• Client
• VRC
• Therapist
• Insurer

❏ **Signatures**
Verifying agreement and accountability by each plan participant

final say, but the experienced VRC can exercise a great deal of influence. Typically, the VRC's most effective strategy is not to attempt controlling directly, but acting as a facilitator, contributing information, suggesting ideas, attempting to persuade, watching for problems, and using other low profile methods to keep the process on course. Whether performed by the VRC, or in cooperation with other parties, the rehabilitation plan will typically address medical recovery and return to work.

Medical Recovery.   The client's condition must be medically stable for any reasonable vocational outcome to occur. In a facilitating manner the VRC may suggest medical care or therapy to whatever party or parties they feel can influence the others, and ultimately the insurer-payor to approve the suggestion. The VRC may then coordinate and monitor medical care, ultimately to maximize the injured worker's reemployment. During this phase the VRC may utilize a Functional Capacity Assessment, Job Analysis, Work Hardening, and other care coordination activities to prepare the client for suitable return to work. Before the actual return to work can occur, the VRC needs:

- Stabilized or maximum medical progress
- Written release by the treating physician
- Written clearly defined capabilities

Return to Work.   When medical recovery is achieved, the case fulcrum tips into a vocational mode. Most cases are then resolved by returning to the former employer, where the client last worked. Job modification, Work Retraining, ergonomic restructuring, and employer consulting may be necessary. Essential ingredients for a successful return to work then include:

- A suitable job, consistent with the client's capabilities
- Commitment by the employer and employee to make the best mutual effort for a lasting solution
- Written return to work document or "job offer" from the former employer to the employee formally inviting them back to work
- Follow up by the VRC and allied parties to assure long-term success

Occasionally, returning to the former employer may not be feasible. The employer may not be big enough to offer job modification without undue hardship, or the employer may have gone out of business. Yet if the client has skills that transfer to work elsewhere, then the next logical strategy is job placement with a new employer. However, this alternative presents a more challenging rehabilitation effort, and again calls for a well-prepared, realistic, written plan.

Some clients require new skills to make them more employable, perhaps through on-the-job training with a willing employer, or through a formal school training program. Self-employment is an option for some clients. The VRC is challenged to be flexible and tenacious, always weighing various vocational options against the time, cost, and other resources needed, as well as the likelihood of success.

Monitoring and Follow Up

Once the client is back at work, at maximum activity level, the VRC should follow along for at least 30 days to assure stability and lasting success. Case progress is usually documented in narrative reports, at least monthly, to keep all parties informed. These narratives may report on the employee's attendance record, job performance, physical compatibility with the job, risk factors, and safety measures.

Case Closure

A VRC's greatest satisfaction is preparing a closure report, "Successful Return to Work, Case Closed." The satisfaction of seeing the plan successfully fulfilled, and ultimately the client's vocational life restored, is indeed rewarding.

Some cases close for other reasons, such as simply not being appropriate for further VR services. Some will close because the client is clearly not employable. It is important to be realistic, for the sake of all parties involved.

When a case closure is finalized, for whatever outcome, a good VRC will offer post-closure recommendations for other parties. These might include areas of concern to monitor, or socioeconomic factors that may undermine success in the future. The VRC should notify the parties when VR activity is ceasing, and how they may be reached if any unforeseen problems arise.

TENSION IN THE SYSTEM

Sources of Problems

Sometimes things do not go exactly as planned in the vocational rehabilitation process. In fact, any VRC providing services for Workers' Compensation claimants will eventually see cases literally fall apart, even with the best of efforts and intentions. At such times a VRC must be reminded that Workers' Compensation, as well as other disability compensation systems, is adversarial in nature.

The injured worker and the insurer often view things much differently. One party makes claims to certain things, the other party considers whether to concur, usually with dollars in the balance. At its best, Workers' Compensation is a very imperfect system, often an arena for disagreement, frustration, anger, and win/lose conflict.

Relationship Challenges

Figure 19.2 illustrates the injured worker-focused case management model and the participants involved in the process. As part of the injured worker's rehabilitation team, the VRC facilitates communication and cooperation among all involved parties.

The VRC's challenge is to avoid getting caught in a power struggle, or in someone else's win/lose conflict. The VRC must not think in terms of "winning," nor in helping someone else win, such that someone in turn "loses." As an agent of change, the VRC must remain as unbiased and as creative as possible, in order to remain effective.

A good VRC will carefully balance advocacy issues, sometimes like a skilled tightrope walker, so that what is achieved is a good rehabilitation outcome, not just a good job of advocacy for one party or another. Accordingly, VRCs can work best when other parties, including the Industrial Therapist, serve the case in like-minded fashion.

Role Clarification

Another challenge for the VRC is in the case management role itself. At least three-fourths of VRC companies provide case management.[2] Case management services may vary from one VRC to another. At one extreme, case management by the VRC involves full responsibility for all case planning, coordinating and monitoring services provided by the VRC or others, communicating with various parties, controlling quality, steering the case in appropriate directions, and deciding when to suspend services, including VR services.

At the other extreme, the VRC provides very limited service under someone else's direction with no responsibility for case outcome. Good, realistic VR case management is somewhere in between.

Whether the case is being managed through its medical phase or vocational phase, the VRC may struggle with the question of who takes charge, is it the insurance claim adjuster, the treating physician, the claimant's attorney, or the VRC? Unless so notified at time of referral, rarely will a good VRC assume full case management responsibility automatically.

Legal, contractual, and fiscal responsibilities place the insurance claim adjuster in a designated *claim* management role, which is like *case* management but with a distinct bias toward the cost containment interests of the insurer or payor.

The claim adjuster may delegate cost control to the VRC, based upon the adjuster's own experience, per-

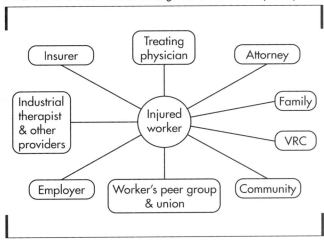

FIGURE 19.2 Case management model and participants.

sonality style, and confidence in the VRC. Such delegation allows the VRC to better balance cost containment with other goals and parties' interests in the case management process.

It is crucial that the VRC clarifies the referring party's expectations at the onset. If the referring source is someone other than the insurer or payor, then even greater care must be taken to avoid presuming too much. It must be noted that the scope of case management practice is determined by the referral source. Thus, parameters which determine the duration and extent of case management involvement can vary.[8]

A competent VRC must understand the claim adjuster's personality style as well as inherent claim responsibility. There is no place for a power struggle between the VRC and claim adjuster in this context. By the same token, this is no place for the VRC to relinquish professional responsibility either. Good communication at the start and throughout the case process will usually enhance a good working relationship for the sake of all parties involved.

COORDINATION WITH INDUSTRIAL THERAPISTS

Benefits of Coordination

Though their roles are distinct, and they may otherwise function unaware of each other, the Industrial Therapist (IT) and the Vocational Rehabilitation Consultant (VRC) can collaborate in vital ways. The IT is typically called in to contribute expertise in areas such as Job Analysis, Functional Capacity Assessment, Work Conditioning and Work Hardening. An injured worker's vocational recovery can be greatly enhanced as the IT and VRC work together in the following areas.

Job Analysis

The Job Analysis (JA) may be performed by the VRC or the IT, often depending on who is called in first. The VRC or IT performs the JA at the work site, assessing the job's physical demands, and identifying how it might be modified for worker compatibility. The JA should be tailored to the complexity of the case, the planning and decision making needs, and the payor's budget.

Functional Capacity Assessment

In the case of the Functional Capacity Assessment (FCA), few VRCs or firms administer them directly, so they rely on ITs to provide this specialized testing[2]. The FCA is an objective, statistically valid measure of the worker's capabilities, removing guesswork and providing a common frame of reference for determining return to work parameters. The Job Analysis and Functional Capacity Assessment together are the foundation for much of the planning and decision making that take place afterwards.

Work Conditioning and Work Hardening

Once the VRC determines the worker is ready to return to his or her former job, or a suitable modified job, the actual return to work can be physically traumatic to a deconditioned worker, especially after a long lay off. Because of its specialized nature, Work Conditioning and Work Hardening are usually referred to outside firms rather than performed by the VRC.[2]

An on-site Job Analysis provides a first-hand description of the anticipated job, so the IT can design the best possible Work Retraining program to prepare the worker for that job. Work Retraining should simulate the client's actual job as much as possible. Then the gradual reconditioning process can have optimal success.

Consultation

The VRC often has a number of issues for which the IT can provide answers. What FCA information beyond physical abilities is useful? When is a standard conditioning program more appropriate than Work Conditioning or Work Hardening? How long should Work Hardening of a particular client take? What maximum functioning level can be anticipated at the end of Work Hardening? What therapeutic or ergonomic advancements can be drawn upon? What creative alternatives might be considered? The IT's experience and expertise can contribute greatly to successful rehabilitation.

Influencing Early Intervention

Aside from the treating physician, the IT may be the best party to recognize need for VR intervention, such as when conflict develops, when the process becomes disorganized, or when loose ends are not being covered. Researchers have concluded that the earlier a person is referred for vocational rehabilitation after being injured, the greater likelihood of return to work.[6]

The most skilled Functional Capacity Assessment or Work Conditioning therapy can be useless to the worker if no VR effort is initiated. The IT is usually in a good position to alert other parties to the need for VR involvement. Thus, the IT and VRC are key players in strategic early intervention.

THE IMPORTANCE OF EARLY INTERVENTION

A simple variable to control is early referral to rehabilitation which has a powerful effect on the desired outcome. National Rehabilitation Consultants (NRC) studied the relationship between referral delay and rehabilitation outcome in its Minnesota VR cases closed from October 1987 through April 1990.[1] A total of 871 cases were categorized according to their time, in months, from injury to NRC referral. Then a count was made of how many cases, within each time group, were reemployed or not reemployed at time of closure.

The reemployed cases included returning to the former employer, placement with a new employer, or self employment. The not re-employed cases were closed due to claim settlement, medical decline, non-cooperation, retirement, death, or referring agency request. The results are summarized in Table 19.1 and graphed in Figure 19.3.

The results support the principle that earlier referrals yield greater success rates. Those cases referred within one month after injury were returned to work at a remarkable 86% success rate. On the other hand, among cases referred beyond two years post-injury only 37% were returned to work.

The costs of referral delays have also been documented. According to a 1985 study by the California Workers' Compensation Institute, delays in initiating or completing vocational rehabilitation services cost an average of $76 to $716 for each month of delay.[4] From the disability insurer's viewpoint, the golden rule of claims management: "The older a claim, the more expensive it is."[9]

TABLE 19.1 Relationship of Rehabilitation Outcome to Referral Delay

Delay from injury to referral in months	Number of cases	Closed reemployed	Closed not reemployed	Total
0–1	190	86%	14%	100%
2–3	278	75%	25%	100%
4–6	118	68%	32%	100%
7–12	86	65%	35%	100%
13–18	54	54%	46%	100%
19–24	38	47%	53%	100%
25+	107	37%	63%	100%
TOTAL GROUP	871	68%	32%	100%

A LOOK TOWARD THE FUTURE

Even in its third decade, private rehabilitation faces some formidable challenges ahead. There are many issues that VRCs and ITs alike must consider as they hope to remain viable in the professional disability market place.

Managed Care

America's health care system is being squeezed, stretched, and shaken up in unprecedented ways. Feeling the pinch of rising costs, insurers and employers have adopted a managed care mind set, much different than years past. Monitoring and controlling health care utilization, including services by VRCs and ITs, is central to managed care. Accordingly, VRCs and ITs must anticipate how managed care will effect the way they practice in the future.

Total Quality

Total Quality Management (TQM) is a theme that characterizes successful organizations in the 1990s, and is positioning them for viability in 2000 and beyond. Corporate executives launch companywide efforts to encourage all employees to improve job performance for the express purpose of better meeting their customers' needs.

In private sector rehabilitation and Industrial Therapy, we as service deliverers must remain keenly aware of higher expectations by the ones we serve—clients, patients, and referral sources. We are being evaluated and compared, and the question is asked, "What are the cost benefits in purchasing services from this provider?" As service providers that compete in a changing market place, it is not enough to simply attract referrals. Those referrals must result in satisfied customers. But as one manager explains, a committed customer is even better:[7]

Satisfied customers feel good as long as their needs are fulfilled; committed customers look beyond short-term pleasures and develop an allegiance to the firm. Satisfied customers are pleased, humored, and fulfilled; committed customers are dedicated and faithful. Satisfied customers remain independent from the firm; committed customers become dependent with the firm through shared resources and values. The totally satisfied customer says, "My

FIGURE 19.3 Reemployment likelihood vs. referral delay.

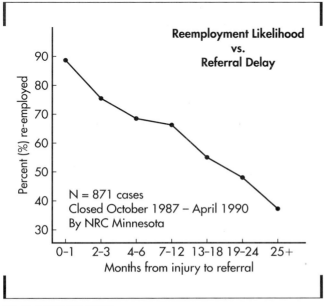

(Courtesy NRC Minnesota.)

needs have been assessed and met, so I feel good about dealing with the firm;" the totally committed customer says, "We have developed interdependencies, shared values, and strategies to the extent that our separate needs can best be met through long-term devotion and loyalty to each other."

VRCs and ITs will do well to look carefully at their customer and referring agency relationships, and determine the true long-term affiliations.

Paradigm Shifts

ITs and VRCs at one time were viewed as resources to help save disability costs, through early return-to-work initiatives. But more and more their services are viewed as costs, burdens on the expense side of the insurers' ledger, rather than a cost-savings mechanism. As the insurance industry shifts its focus, so too must service providers make their own paradigm shifts.

VRCs may no longer enjoy the exclusive role of return-to-work advisors. Many employers are learning how to do for themselves what they previously paid a VRC to perform. Insurance carriers are initiating fewer referrals to VRCs than in the past.[2] Instead, VRCs must look to other sources and other strategies for keeping their practices alive and growing.

Vocational rehabilitation and Industrial Therapy, are simply parts of a larger "disability management" system. If VRCs try to function unaware, or independent of that system, they will struggle to survive. They must recognize their role within the overall system, and determine to preserve value and credibility.

Continuum of Care

When a patient leaves the hospital, clinic, or therapy center after treatment, the health care provider cannot be sure whether treatment continues to progress at the patient's home. Where health care and therapy leave off, the VRC can pick up and maintain continuity. The VRC thus provides a vital link between the treatment setting and the work place.

VRCs characteristically do their best work in the field, at employer work sites, in clinics, and in the community, literally in the client's world. The future will undoubtedly involve increasing collaboration between the health care industry and vocational rehabilitation providers. Together these two disciplines can do more than either one alone.

Health care and Industrial Therapy are moving out of their institutionalized setting, closer to the consumer. They must look for ways to break out of institutionalized practice, and penetrate their patients' world through extended services, such as vocational rehabilitation.

SUMMARY

We have looked back at the beginnings of vocational rehabilitation, its emergence in the private sector, and how it has grown into a major US industry. We have considered how VRCs operate, and the challenging future VRCs and ITs must face. VRCs and ITs should look for ways to collaborate, reinforce each other's roles, and mutually commit to maintaining the highest standards of practice that patients, clients, as well as customers deserve.

REFERENCES

1. Anderle M: A Good Case for Early Intervention, *NRC News & Views,* St. Paul, National Rehabilitation Consultants, 1–2, 1990.
2. Berkeley Planning Associates and Harold Russell Associates: Private Sector Rehabilitation: Lessons and Options for Public Policy, Berkeley, Prepared for US Department of Education, Office of Planning, Budget, and Evaluation, Washington, DC, 1987.
3. Berkeley Planning Associates: Analysis of Rehabilitation Programs in the Proprietary Sector Request for OMB Review, Berkeley, Submitted by US Department of Education, Submitted to Office of Management and Budget 1986.
4. Cain C: Vocational Rehab Costs Soaring, *Business Insurance* Chicago, 1986. Crain Communications, January 13, 1986.
5. Corthell DW, deGroot J: Proprietary Rehabilitation: A Better Understanding, Tenth Institute on Rehabilitation Issues, Menomonie, Stout Vocational Rehabilitation Institute, 1983, University of Wisconsin-Stout.
6. Hester EJ, Decelles PG, Keepper KL: A Comprehensive Analysis of Private Sector Rehabilitation Services and Outcomes for Workers' Compensation Claimants, Topeka, 1989, The Menninger Foundation, 100.
7. Howe RJ, Gaeddert D, Howe MA: *Quality On Trial,* 55, St. Paul, 1992, West Publishing Co.
8. Lowery SL: Qualifications for the Successful Case Manager, *The Case Manager* 3(4):66–74, 1992.
9. North CA: The Golden Rule, *Risk & Insurance* 3(3):52, 1992.

CHAPTER

20
On-Site Therapy

David R. Worth

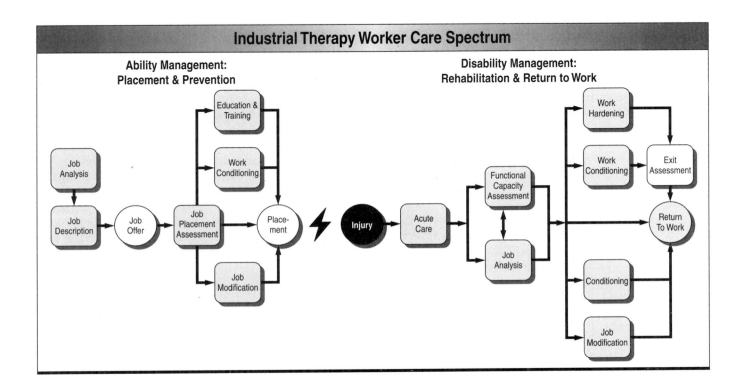

Industrial Therapy Worker Care Spectrum

On-site therapy, where the Therapist contracts services to the employer and provides those services at the worksite, has been practiced for more than thirty years in Australia. This review of on-site therapy from the Australian experience is intended to provide a different perspective for American Therapists, that may enhance insights and provide a glimpse of what the future could hold for certain aspects of this field in the United States.

The chapter will describe the requirements of an on-site Industrial Therapy service, the steps required to set up on-site services, and the differences between on-site and off-site services across the full spectrum of worker care: job placement, job analysis, education and prevention, primary treatment, Functional Capacity Assessment, return to work programs, Work Conditioning, and Work Hardening.

Benefits of On-Site Therapy

On-site therapy benefits the employer's bottom line. Australian subsidiaries of Kodak, the Ford Motor Company, and the Goodyear Tire Company, to name a few, have experienced significant savings in both financial and human terms due to early intervention by the on-site Therapist in the management of work related injuries.[22]

The relationships developed through on-site therapy are more conducive to effective prevention and expeditious rehabilitation. By interacting with management, supervisors, and workers on a regular basis, the on-site Therapist has a more intimate understanding of each job, the risk factors, each worker's capabilities, and the psychosocial issues within the work environment. This close working interaction also helps

385

avoid the adversarial relationships that sometimes develop during the therapeutic and return-to-work process.

Early post-injury intervention, proven to speed recovery in sports medicine,[11] is rendered possible in the industrial setting through on-site therapy. When an injury occurs, the practitioner is able to see the injured worker only hours after the injury, in many cases applying first aid such as that which would occur at a sports venue.

Throughout the worker's therapy, the on-site Therapist can regularly coordinate with shop floor supervisors, giving valuable biomechanical and ergonomic advice, which enables the injured worker to remain at work in a protective environment, throughout the rehabilitation process. Graduated return to work accomplished on-site minimizes the employee's problems of deconditioning and psychosocial barriers, and the employer's problems of disability payments and lost productivity. By actively participating in the return to work program, the on-site Therapist brings about the most cost-effective, efficient and safe placement back to full normal duties.[23]

Disadvantages of On-site Therapy

On-site therapy may not be the best solution in every injury case. In some situations, the amount of force required to pull a lever or lift fixed-size weights cannot be altered to accommodate the injured worker's reduced capabilities. In other situations the worker may require daily supervision of posture, technique, and rates of progression, whereas the Therapist is only on-site two or three days a week. In addition to presenting risk, these circumstances can also prolong the rehabilitation process.

INDUSTRY REQUIREMENTS

The industrial requirements for a systematic approach to occupational injury management have traditionally been dictated by the size of industrial operations, the beliefs and philosophy of the ownership or management, and the nature of the industrial activities. In some situations these requirements are set by the medical profession. In Australia, legislation has also been an important influence in shaping injury management and on-site therapy. As in the United States, legislation typically varies from state to state and applies differently depending on the number of employees in a company.

The nature of a company's industrial activities (heavy labor versus light; unskilled versus skilled) is

important and has an influence not only on the size but also the type of injury management facilities.

In industrial societies, the mutual interests and responsibilities of the workers and the enterprise are typically reflected in the terms of employment. This includes an equal commitment by both parties to occupational health, safety, welfare, prevention of work related illness and injury, rehabilitation, return to work of injured workers, and the provision of a safe, healthy work environment.

Organization of Services

In Australia, workers are generally represented by safety committees and safety representatives. Many of these representatives are trained in first aid and are front line attendees at a work place accident. In small operations, they may be the only person able to assist at the time.

Enterprises of sufficient size will have an occupational health facility on-site, with a nurse in attendance at least during the day shift. Larger facilities and higher risk companies may increase this to more nurses over more shifts. Arrangements are usually made with a local medical clinic or facility, such as an occupational injury clinic or hospital, for urgent medical treatment.

Some companies employ or contract with a medical practitioner to attend the workplace facility on a regular basis. The doctor may be a fellow of the Australian College of Occupational Medicine or equivalent in other countries.

A development over the last three decades in Australia is the contracting of on-site Therapists by employers. These Therapists may be members of the Ergonomics and Occupational Health Special Group of the Australian Physiotherapy Association. They usually have a special interest in the management of work-related injury and illness.

Many of these Therapists are also members of the Ergonomics Society of Australia and New Zealand, and are active contributors to the increasing body of knowledge in ergonomics and how it applies to the prevention of work related injury and disease.

Recent Australian National and State legislative reforms in Occupational Safety, Health and Welfare have included the introduction of Codes of Practice in a wide variety of occupational practices such as manual handling, exposure to toxic substances, and repetitive work. Some of these are published as Approved Codes within the regulations of the Occupational Safety, Health and Welfare Acts, and contain both mandatory and recommended minimum standards of practice. Employers face heavy penalties for failure to comply with these regulations.

Services Provided

Industry requirements of cost effective on-site occupational injury management programs include the following:[18,23]

- Emergency first aid and treatment of injuries
- Preemployment examination of job applicants
- Prevention of injury
- Medical treatment of ongoing disabilities and impairments
- Prevention of time loss due to work-related injuries
- Placement of injured workers in jobs within their capabilities
- Graduated return to normal duties of injured workers
- Reduction of the Workers' Compensation Insurance liabilities
- Presentation of medico-legal evidence at reviews or appeals or within the judicial system
- Counseling injured workers on issues related to their ongoing employment
- Assisting in product design, tool design, and production techniques to help prevent injury and produce a better product.

With regard to legal considerations, because the on-site therapy involves working more closely with management, supervisors, unions, and workers in all aspects of injury prevention and rehabilitation, the Therapist must have a more comprehensive knowledge of Workers' Compensation, Occupational Safety and Health legislation and regulations, and in the US, the Americans with Disabilities Act.

The Therapist may be called upon to give testimony on behalf of either the employee or the employer. In any event, the on-site Therapist must have the same professional liability insurance coverage as the off-site Therapist.

Table 20.1 presents a typical mix of activities in an on-site Therapy affiliation.

The on-site Therapist can play an important role in all of these areas and should decide their level of participation in each. It is insufficient, expensive and

TABLE 20.1 Typical Mix of On-site Therapist Activities

Job review	50%
Acute care	20%
Return-to-work programs	15%
Education	10%
Administration	5%
Total	100%

counter-productive to be involved mostly in clinical treatment. The employer requires expert participation in most of the above activities and expects an enterprise ethos in the Therapist, with an interest in company profitability as well as a strong ethical interest in the patient's welfare.

The occupational health nurse and the doctor may perform preemployment medical assessments of job applicants. These assessments vary widely depending on the medical and fitness requirements of the work. They usually include a general physical examination, review of previous medical history, audiometry, vision testing, and a brief musculoskeletal examination.

SETTING UP ON-SITE THERAPY SERVICES

Contractual Guidelines

There are many ways a Therapist may arrange to provide on-site therapy services. It is important to negotiate a contract which does not have a vested interest in a long list of clinical treatment bookings. The on-site contract should be biased toward prevention of injury, reduction of human and economic cost of injury, efficient and effective resolution of injury and its effects, and the resulting increase in company profitability (Figure 20.1).

The remuneration method should be designed to provide incentives toward:[22,23]

- Injury prevention
- Reduction in time loss
- Early return to normal duties
- Reduction of the Workers' Compensation insurance liabilities

This can be achieved by contracting with the employer to provide consultancy services in return for payment on an hourly fee basis. The company should provide suitable space, consisting of the use of one consulting room; the most basic therapeutic equipment, such as an examination couch, ultrasound machine, and perhaps some basic traction apparatus; and access to basic first aid equipment, including cold packs and a range of strapping and bandages. When the company provides the facilities and materials, the Therapist has minimal overhead costs and may calculate a fair and reasonable hourly rate.

A rule of thumb for on-site hourly rate is 50% of what is charged for stand-alone clinic services. After subtracting the overhead costs of a stand-alone clinic, it may be as profitable to operate the on-site clinic as it would have been to remain in a private clinic.

It is customary in Australia to contract initially for

FIGURE 20.1   The on-site Industrial Therapist should focus on injury prevention, efficient rehabilitation, and reduced injury costs, which in turn increases company profitability.

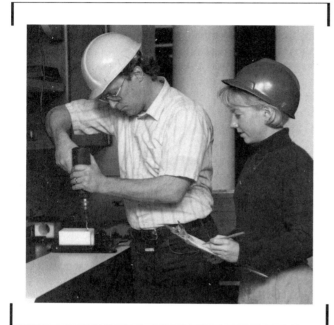

TABLE 20.2   Number of Half-day Therapy Sessions Required per Employee Population.

Number of employees	Half-day Therapy Sessions per week
300	2
1,000	3
3,000	5
6,000	10

Partnering

Where the on-site Therapist is accessible only on a part-time basis and is not present every day of the week, or for all shifts worked, there will be times when that Therapist is unable to provide sufficient intensity of treatment for certain patients. It is therefore wise for the on-site Therapist to build up a relationship with private practicing Therapists nearby, so that referral out for intensive treatment is readily arranged.

It is important that the on-site Therapist has confidence in a network of off-site providers, so that quality assurance is maintained and results of treatment are satisfactory in terms of outcome, cost, and duration.

Perception Management

The on-site Therapist must be seen as an expert in the field of occupational injury management by both the workers and the company as well as unions or employee representatives and employer organizations. This will enable the Therapist to build a high level of integrity and trust between both parties. The Therapist must never be recognized as a "company employee" or as a "plaintiff's advocate."

Injured workers, who find themselves in the midst of the Workers' Compensation system, frequently seek such an advocate, and companies who bear the financial liabilities often seek expert medical opinion which indicates the worker is fit for normal duties. A reputation for independence and for being firm but fair to either side must be jealously and vigorously maintained at all times by the on-site Therapist.

a three month trial of on-site services. If the trial proves mutually agreeable, an annual contract is then consummated. Again, in addition to the space, the company typically supplies most or all of the equipment and materials required.

Staffing Guidelines

Usually no other staffing is required for a single Therapist to conduct an on-site Therapy service. If a number of companies are being supplied on-site Therapy services by a group Therapy practice, it may be necessary to employ staff Therapists, who, following a suitable period of training, may provide Therapy services for the group practice to other companies, on a key customer basis.

Companies employing approximately 300 people benefit from access to an on-site Therapist for two half-day sessions per week. (This assumes all Job Placement Assessments and Functional Capacity Assessments are performed off-site. If not, then more staffing is required on-site than represented below). As this rises to approximately 1,000 employees, accessibility might increase to three half-days per week; 3,000 employees justifies approximately five half-days per week; and 6,000 employees justifies a full time Therapist (Table 20.2).

ON-SITE INJURY PREVENTION

The two most important skills contributing to on-site injury prevention are—1) knowledge of ergonomics and 2) the ability to perform job analysis.

Ergonomics

Ergonomics refers to fitting the job to the person, and deals with making modifications to the way in which the job is performed and the methods by which the worker performs the job. This is referred to as job and method modifications.

Job modifications can involve changes to the whole work environment including tooling, hardware, software, equipment used, and any other components of the external environment and the equipment used by the worker to perform the job (Figure 20.2, *A*).[3,10,12,14,19,24,25]

Method modifications refers to teaching the worker a safer way to perform the job. This entails improving the use of the worker's body, or what is referred to as internal environment involved in the performance of the job (Figure 20.2, *B*).[2,4-6,13-18,21] Method modifications include:

- Symptom avoidance
- Safe materials handling
- Correct use of body mechanics

Symptom avoidance refers to performing job functions in modified ways to avoid exacerbating the injury during healing and rehabilitation. For instance, during treatment, the worker may perform limited lifting strictly through leg flexion with a perfectly erect back. Once the pain or other symptoms have been alleviated as a result of the Therapist's program, the worker can resume performing the full job in more conventional ways, which in this example would permit a return to incorporating some bending at the waist.

Safe materials handling refers to a less risky workstyle which is initiated at the beginning of treatment and progressed to job level performance over the course of treatment.

Symptom avoidance and safe materials handling are often applied at different times in the process of a graduated return to normal duties. Symptom avoidance may be applied while a worker is performing alternative duties and avoiding the painful part of a range of movement. Safe manual handling should of course also be practiced at this time. However, when the worker graduates from alternative duties to normal duties, safe manual handling may remain a vital part of the successful occupational rehabilitation, while symptom avoidance may gradually become unnecessary and inappropriate.

Job Analysis

Job analysis involves the measurement of all the factors which place demands on the attributes possessed by the worker.[2-6,8,10-20,21,24,25] In a return-to-work program, job analysis refers to the techniques for obtaining and presenting job information, which is accurate and

FIGURE 20.2   Job Analysis **(A)** involves an analysis of the equipment (Job Modification) and **(B)** how the worker performs the job (Job Method Modification). This information can then be used in injury prevention and return-to-work programs.

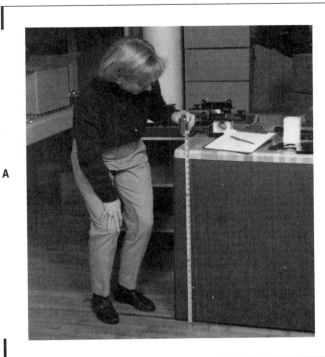

A

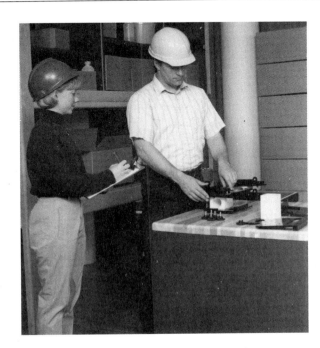

B

inclusive of everything pertinent to the program in a form suitable for use. In terms of injury management, the most important attributes are the physical activities and the equipment used.

The on-site Therapist enjoys a more intimate knowledge of the jobs as a result of ongoing contact and interaction with the workplace, the supervisors, and the workers. The off-site Therapist must work a little harder in job analysis, but fortunately the techniques to do so have been well developed and perfected.

Measurements are required on the frequency, duration, and intensity of the following factors, as listed in the 1983 working draft of the Australian Standard Classification of Occupations[1] and the US Dictionary of Occupational Titles:[7]

Physical Activities

Writing, precision and unskilled hand, coordination, handling, sitting, walking, standing, running, balancing, climbing, pushing, pulling, carrying, lifting to above shoulder height, lifting desk to chair levels, lifting chair to floor levels, reaching at trunk height, reaching above shoulder height, sustained gripping, repetitive gripping, bending, stooping, crouching, kneeling, crawling, squatting.

Equipment Used

Precision tools, semi-precision tools, nonprecision tools, machines, keyboard devices, powered vehicles, worker-powered vehicles.

These factors should be observed, measured, recorded, compiled in a data base, and analyzed for potential improvements in matching worker capabilities and job demands. In addition, cataloging the jobs over time facilitates future job modifications as workers or production processes change.

In addition to activities and equipment, job analysis may deal with a wide range of other job demands. A comprehensive checklist of such demands is presented in Box 20.1, although only a portion of the full set of attributes is relevant to any given job.

The on-site Therapist must have an understanding of the measurement of values on these factors, in order to take into consideration all factors when deciding the suitability of a particular job for a worker.

The Therapist is ideally trained and placed to conduct the job analysis and measurements of the injured worker's functional capacity. The Therapist is therefore the appropriate health professional to facilitate a safe placement in a return-to-work program, by ensuring a precise match of the worker to the job, thus reducing the likelihood of aggravating symptoms or producing a new injury.

A durable placement depends upon the person's capacity to work being greater than or equal to the job demands. Prevention of injury therefore applies to preventing the aggravation of preexisting symptoms or the exacerbation of an impairment with a resulting increase in disability. This form of prevention may be regarded as secondary prevention.

In this way, an injured worker may return to normal duties with minimal risk of reaggravation. This process facilitates the recognition of ergonomic factors likely to be responsible for the production of injuries in other workers, or even new injuries in the rehabilitated worker.

Knowledge of Job Characteristics

In contrast to the off-site Therapist who deals with patients coming from a wide variety of industries, the on-site Therapist deals with patients who come from the same industry and often the same job classification. Therefore, the Therapist rapidly becomes familiar with the characteristics of the tasks within each job at that company, as well as the Job Analysis factors or job demands.

This means that the on-site Therapist has intimate knowledge of the job when the worker first reports an injury. By comparison, the off-site clinician usually has a poor description of the job, offered by the worker at the time of attendance at the clinic.

Knowledge of the job characteristics is one of the paramount benefits of an on-site Therapy service.[22,23] Jobs differ vastly across industry, from high precision repetitive hand work in a cold environment (Figure 20.3, *A*) to very heavy manual handling in excessive heat (Figure 20.3, *B*).

Thorough knowledge of job characteristics assists injury prevention, particularly after approximately one year of on-site therapy service, by which time the Therapist has built up a body of knowledge about the causes of injury from jobs in that industry.

The Therapist should then spend time with management and the design and production engineers, in order to make sound ergonomic suggestions that might lead to a reduction in the number of injuries. Similarly, when management is in the process of investing in retooling for new models or product changes, they may be more receptive to adding investments in ergonomic changes. In addition, they may also be more attracted to the reduced injury savings as a way to enhance the total investment payout of product development (Figure 20.4).

In order to provide sound ergonomic advice, the Therapist must go beyond developing particular skills and knowledge in the field of ergonomics. They must also have a good working knowledge of the local Occupational Health, Safety and Welfare legislation, as

BOX 20.1

Full Listing of Additional Job Demands

Formal preparation
General
Post-school preparation
Higher degree
Postgraduate qualifications
First degree
Diploma
Associate diploma
Paraprofessional qualifications
Trade/post-trade qualifications
Basic vocational

Special requirements
Driver's license
Other licensing
Personal dedication
Individual quality
Updating knowledge
Dress
Visual performance
Auditory perception

Subject matter
Data
Ideas
People
Things

Mental and related activities
Integrating
Analyzing
Planning
Decision making
Reasoning
Mathematical competence
English language

Time constraints
Annual work
Seasonal work
Irregular or shift
Repetitive/mundane
Time deadlines

Informal preparation
On the job training
Experience

Holland interest categories
Realistic
Investigative
Artistic
Social
Enterprising
Conventional

Social activities
Alone
Small groups
Large groups
Informal public
Professional
Top level management
Middle management
Base level supervision
Responsibility size

Environmental location and condition
Travel
Mobility
Location
Conditions

Rewards
Starting salary
Salary ceiling

Labor market size

Industry code

well as particular knowledge about the type of machinery and processes used at that company. What appears to be the ideal ergonomic solution may not be in compliance with regulations, or may not be feasible given the company's existing machinery.

PRIMARY TREATMENT

In the day-to-day practice of an on-site Therapy service, the first contact will be with workers who have suffered an injury or aggravated a preexisting injury.

FIGURE 20.3 A,B   The vast differences in the nature of work and environmental conditions necessitates accurate job analysis for effective injury prevention or treatment.

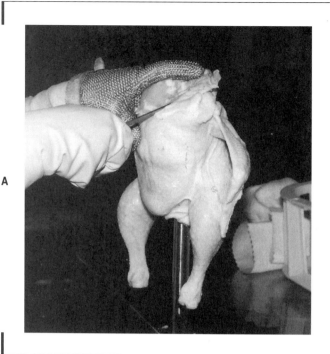

A

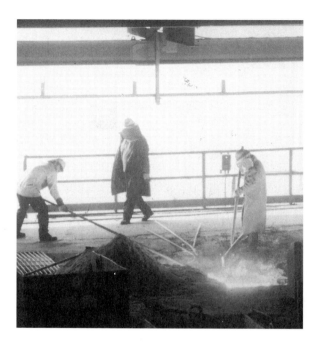

B

FIGURE 20.4   The Industrial Therapist can be a valuable asset to production engineers and management by providing ergonomic suggestions that may lead to injury reduction.

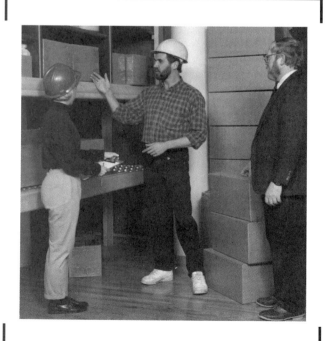

They may also be attending for a follow-up treatment. The on-site Therapist must be prepared to act as a primary contact health care advisor for a worker who has suffered an acute musculoskeletal injury. The Therapist should apply urgent treatment, comparable to the immediate and urgent treatment provided to an injured athlete by a team Therapist.[9]

Urgent treatment may involve application of rest, ice, compression bandaging, and elevation.[11] Similarly, this treatment may involve careful application of early mobilization or, in rare instances, manipulation of joints. The primary aim of urgent primary contact treatment is to minimize physiological damage such as internal bleeding and scarring, and to maximize early healing and restoration of normal function.[9]

Urgent primary contact with injured workers enables the on-site Therapist to make critical early decisions which can result in a reduction in the amount of treatment required. Time loss and loss of function are also reduced when compared to delays caused by the worker leaving the premises to seek primary medical attention. With off-site treatment, there is frequently an additional delay prior to referral to the treating Therapist, or even to a medical specialist for consultative advice or further medical investigation.[22]

While an injured worker has freedom of choice concerning the selection of the most appropriate practitioner from whom to seek primary treatment and ongoing medical care, on-site services should be offered in the first instant, while informing the injured worker of the right to freedom of choice.

In every case, following examination of an injured worker, either for the first time or for ongoing treatment, the on-site Therapist must apply the value-added service of following the worker to the current job. The objective is to ensure that, wherever possible, the injured worker may perform a useful and productive job in the presence of the injury, without aggravating the symptoms or the condition. This can have the effect of decreasing the time taken for full resolution of an injury, comparable to the time taken in returning the injured athlete to active competitive sport.

In this way, further disruption of loss of time from work and the associated Workers' Compensation claim and its medico-legal consequences may be prevented without harm to the worker. Naturally, this has the added benefit of reducing the financial liability to the company, thereby increasing the cost-effectiveness of the on-site Therapy service.[9,22,23]

The secondary benefit of following each injured worker back to the job is identification of ergonomic factors involved in the production of injury, or aggravation of symptoms. This ensures that the on-site Therapist takes part in prevention of injury or re-aggravation of symptoms. Each intervention on the shop floor should be documented as a worksite visit for either ergonomic analysis or job analysis.

This documentation should be filed both in the injured worker's case notes and in a separate ergonomic or job analysis file. In this way, previously made recommendations can be followed up for completion, and a permanent record of the job analysis data is available for use in future cases, involving the same job, or where job demands must be known in allocation of duties.[2–6,8,10,12–21,24,25]

STRATEGIC PLANNING FOR RETURN TO WORK

While it is highly likely that the on-site Therapist has assisted an injured worker to continue working in alternative duties, it is important that during the recovery phase the injured worker is encouraged to participate in a graduated return to normal duties program.

Normal Duties

Normal duties may be defined as the job for which the worker was originally employed, which is often the job in which the worker was injured. This may therefore be described as the "at injury" job. However, normal duties following an injury may not necessarily be the at injury job. Sometimes recovery will never be sufficient

to allow the worker to return to the at injury job, as determined by comparing the injured worker's stable post-injury capabilities to the job demands. Where this occurs, normal duties may arise out of specified or alternative duties, thus expanding the definition.

Alternative Duties

Alternative duties are offered to an injured worker after an initial period of acute, urgent, primary contact treatment and prior to full recovery. These duties are by definition either different from the at injury duties, or are modified at injury duties. They lead to normal duties after further recovery and progression in the worker's ability to perform tasks in terms of frequency, intensity, and duration (Figure 20.5).

Transitional Duties

Transitional duties are tasks which the injured worker is able to perform at the very early stage, when the symptoms are acute and the worker's capabilities are reduced physically, functionally, or by pain. These duties are performed for a short time, usually not in excess of two or three weeks before the worker is able to perform alternative duties.

FIGURE 20.5 An on-site return-to-work program should progress the injured worker through transitional and alternative duties before advancing them to normal duty.

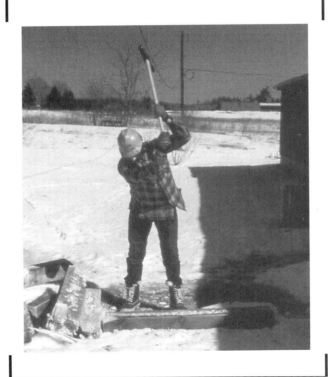

Transitional duties by definition never become either alternative or normal duties. In planning a graduated return to normal duties, the worker should progress through transitional and alternative to normal duties. This transition should be based not only on changes in the signs and symptoms of the condition, but also in functional capabilities as determined clinically, or measured by a reliable Functional Capacity Assessment.

Occupational Goals Analysis

The comparison of an injured worker's functional capabilities to the demands of the at injury job is known as an occupational goal analysis. It is also possible to make a comparison between the injured worker's functional capabilities and the demands of an alternative job, a transitional job, or to the person's functional capabilities prior to the injury.

TABLE 20.3   Occupational Goal Analysis

	Functional Capacity		Job Demands	
Factors	**Preinjury profile**	**FCA profile**	**Ladies hairdresser**	**Alternate duties**
Physical Activities				
Writing	Frequently	Occasionally	Minimal	
Precision hand	Frequently	Occasionally	Frequently	
Unskilled hand	Frequently	Occasionally	Frequently	
Repeated gripping	Frequently	Occasionally	Frequently	
Sustained gripping	Frequently	Occasionally	Occasionally	
Coordination	Frequently	Occasionally	Frequently	
Handling	Frequently	Occasionally	Frequently	
Sitting	Frequently	Occasionally	Not required	
Walk, stand, run	Frequently	Occasionally	Frequently	
Balance, climb	Frequently	Frequently	Not required	
Bending	Frequently	Occasionally	Occasionally	
Stooping	Frequently	Occasionally	Minimally	
Kneeling	Frequently	Occasionally	Minimally	
Crawling	Frequently	Occasionally	Occasionally	
Squatting	Frequently	Frequently	Occasionally	
Repetitive foot	Frequently	Frequently	Not required	
Push	Occasionally 20kg	Occasionally 10kg	Occasionally 5kg	
Pull	Occasionally 20kg	Occasionally 10kg	Occasionally 5kg	
Carry	Occasionally 15kg	Occasionally 5kg	Occasionally 10kg	
Lift chair/floor	Occasionally 12kg	Occasionally 5kg	Occasionally 10kg	
Lift desk/chair	Occasionally 15kg	Occasionally 8kg	Occasionally 10kg	
Lift above shoulder	Occasionally 12kg	Occasionally 6kg	Occasionally 3kg	
Neck movements	Frequently	Occasionally	Frequently	
Neck static				
Equipment Used				
Precision tools	Frequently			
Semi precision tools	Frequently	Frequently	Frequently	
Non precision tools	Frequently	Frequently	Frequently	
Machines	Frequently	Frequently	Occasionally	
Keyboard devices	Frequently	Frequently		
Powered vehicles	Frequently			
Worker powered vehicles	Occasionally	Occasionally		

Definition in terms of an 8 hour workday: Minimally = 0% to 5%; Occasionally = 6% to 33%; Frequently = 34% to 66%; Continuously = 67% to 100%; Not Required (NR) = 0%

The injured worker's best level of functional capabilities prior to injury is referred to as the preinjury profile. The preinjury profile is a list of the highest functional capabilities the worker demonstrated in all of the previous jobs held, for a minimum of three months throughout the employment history.

Table 20.3 is an example of an occupational goal analysis. The two columns on the left indicate the worker's functional capabilities as determined by Functional Capacity Assessments pre and post-injury, and the two columns on the right indicate the job demands as determined by a job analysis.

This form of occupational goal analysis deals only with the physical factors. However, it is possible for a similar comparison to be made for all other factors involved in the work world.

Having determined the occupational goal analysis data, it is possible to plan the recommended treatment goals and return-to-work program. This should be in the form of a strategic plan, as seen in Table 20.4.

Occupational goal analysis is an important tool in the construction of a graduated return to work program. It allows the on-site Therapist to easily recognize those factors which values are less than the requirements of either the alternative jobs or the at injury job, or which differ from the preinjury profile. It is then possible to focus on treatment goals directed towards improving those particular physical capabilities, which have been affected by the injury.

The occupational goal analysis enables the on-site Therapist to make early predictions as to the possibility of the worker returning to the at injury job, or to an appropriate alternative job, within the worker's predicted reduced profile of capabilities. This remaining profile refers to the person's functional capabilities at the time when the injury is stable and these functional capabilities are unlikely to further improve.

It is sometimes possible to estimate the injured worker's functional capabilities, in terms of the physical factors listed in the occupational goal analysis,

TABLE 20.4   Recommended Treatment Goals and Program

CLIENT: Miss C. Client
CLAIM NO: 799c3

	By Whom	By When	Achieved
Goal: Reduction in symptoms and increase in function			
Steps to attain goal:			
1. Strengthen upper cervical flexor muscle groups	Treating Therapist	8/17	
2. Teach upper cervical stabilizing exercises using rhythmical stabilization or cocontraction techniques	Treating Therapist	through 9/17	
3. Strengthen shoulder elevator muscles including deltoid, levator scapulae, upper trapezius	Treating Therapist		
4. Strengthen shoulder stabilizer muscles including rhomboids, mid trapezius, serratus anterior	Treating Therapist		
5. Strengthen thoracic erector spinae muscle groups	Treating Therapist		
6. Relax and lengthen hamstrings, pectorals, and mid cervical extensors	Treating Therapist		
Goal: Graduated return to normal duties			
Steps to attain goal:			
1. Job analysis to identify methods and practices likely to cause exacerbation of symptoms and recommend symptom avoidance strategies	Industrial Therapist	8/20	
2. Teach on-site injury prevention, safe manual handling, symptom avoidance, and postural control	Industrial Therapist	9/15	
3. Document graduated return including:			
a. Commencement 4 hrs/day for 2 weeks	Rehabilitation Counselor	a. 9/17 through 9/31	
b. 6 hrs/day for 3 weeks	Rehabilitation Counselor	b. 10/10 through 10/21	
c. Then normal hours, COMPULSORY 1 hour lunch + 10 minute morning and afternoon break + dinner break 30 minute minimum; Thursday evenings	Rehabilitation Counselor	c. 10/21	
d. Symptom avoidance strategies	Rehabilitation Counselor	d. 9/15	
e. Fail safe immediate response mechanism	Rehabilitation Counselor	e. 9/15	
f. Review by physician at 2 weeks, 5 weeks, and 6 weeks into program	Rehabilitation Counselor	f. 10/1, 10/21, 10/28	
g. Certification by physician as fit for normal duties with no review required after 4 weeks on full normal duties	Rehabilitation Counselor	g. 11/20	

using a detailed clinical examination. The on-site Therapist makes a clinical judgment on the person's capability to perform each of the physical activities. These values should be quantified in frequency, intensity, and duration using job analysis definitions, as they particularly apply to functional capacity definitions.

Sound clinical judgment concerning these values depends on a high level of clinical skill and previous experience in the management of worker's injuries. Such judgments must be recognized as being an experienced Therapist's best clinical estimation of the remaining employment profile.

Where reliable, objective, or defensible data are required, such as in medico-legal instances, or where the on-site Therapist doubts the accuracy of the estimate of capabilities, a Functional Capacity Assessment should be used.[24]

The Functional Capacity Assessment must produce quantified, objective, reliable, and valid data. It should be instrumented and standardized, and contain information concerning repeatability of measurement and predictive validity. A Functional Capacity Assessment should include values on the level of the worker's participation during the assessment, duration of the work day, and scores on all the physical factors in the occupational goal analysis. For purposes of predictive validity, it is important that the Functional Capacity Assessment indicates how the worker is likely to perform on the shop floor, using internal references rather than external encouragement.

Functional Capacity Assessment is useful in obtaining data when:
- An injured worker's capacity to meet job demands is in doubt
- The *definite* functional capacity of an injured worker cannot be estimated by a medical expert
- The residual capacity of a worker must be known to facilitate valid job matching
- An injured worker repeatedly reaggravates the injury
- Work Conditioning or Work Hardening goals require the identification of specific functional weakness
- Evidentiary information is required.

ON-SITE WORK CONDITIONING AND WORK HARDENING

On-site Work Conditioning or Work Hardening is accomplished in the progression through transitional and alternative to normal duties. Using the occupational goal analysis, it is possible to set specific goals for Work Retraining. During the transitional and alternative duties, the injured worker increases endurance and capabilities in those physical factors which were reduced as a result of the injury. Improvement in these factors, as measured by the values, intensity, frequency, and duration, will indicate progress during the Work Retraining process.

On-site Work Retraining differs from off-site in a number of ways. There is little or no need for simulation equipment since the actual equipment is available on-site. Performance at the actual work station is not an approximation of the real world. Many of the psychosocial problems associated with separation from the work routine and peer group are minimized. Finally, from a financial standpoint, on-site Work Retraining involves less disability pay and less lost productivity.

On-site Work Retraining's overriding purpose is, wherever possible, to provide the injured worker a useful and productive job without exacerbating symptoms or the condition. This can decrease the period of rehabilitation, similar to what is done for the injured athlete to speed resumption of competitive activity.

A typical graduated return to work program is documented in Box 20.2.

The Start Up Experience

It is important to recognize and inform the company that upon initiation of an on-site Therapy service, there is likely to be an apparent sudden increase in the registration of people attending the Occupational Health Center for attention to injuries.

It may appear to the employer that the implementation of an on-site therapy service resulted in a minor epidemic of injuries. However, it is important that this occurs in order to identify problems which otherwise remain hidden in workers, who consider they have musculoskeletal disabilities or minor levels of pain as a result of the work they perform.

Furthermore, almost none of these workers will lose time from work and reporting will enable the on-site therapist to rapidly commence a program of prevention.[22] Changes within the work environment will result in the primary prevention of injury and the reduction of workers' complaints. Those workers with some disability will be recognized and treated accordingly, thus reducing their discomfort and increasing their capabilities and productivity.

SUMMARY

The implementation of an on-site therapy service makes the work environment at that particular enterprise a more efficient, effective, and pleasant place for workers, therapists, and management. Productivity levels in the presence of an on-site therapy service usually increase,[22] and this measurable effect should be taken into account by the Therapist when the on-site contract is renewed and cost effectiveness analyzed.

BOX 20.2

Graduated Return to Work Program

Name   :   C. Client
Address   :   36 Church Road, Swansea, S. Aust. 5107
Claim number :   79923/01
Injury   :   Neck injury, motor vehicle accident
Date of injury : May 21
Employer   :   Besthair Inc.
Address   :   93 City Road, Adelaide, S. Aust. 5000
Supervisor   :   S. Supervisor
Area manager :   M. Manager
Starting date :   Monday August 17

Goal: **To implement a safe graduated return to normal duties at the job of hairdresser.**

Weeks 1 and 2 (20 hours currently approved by Physician)
  Monday to Friday:

- Perform back-up service to other hairdressers
  No clients booked.
- 9:50 AM–12 noon
- 12 noon–1:00 PM (Lunch)
- 1:00 PM–3:10 PM
- Total contact time at worksite
  5 hours 20 minutes (including 1 hour lunch break)

Restrictions of Weeks 1 and 2: Set breaks for 10 minutes every hour.

Week 3 Increase in productivity and intensity (30 hours—
  subject to Physician's approval)
  Monday to Friday

- 8:50 AM–12 noon 2 clients booked
- 12 noon–1:00 PM (Lunch)
- 1:00 PM–4:10 PM 1 client booked

Restrictions of Week 3: Two 10 minute breaks to be taken in morning and two 10 minute breaks to be taken in afternoon. Client to be able to ask for assistance when needed.

Weeks 4 and 5 (30 hours)—Client to commence working
  on Saturday and to have a day off in lieu
  (suggested day Friday)
  Monday to Saturday

- 8:50 AM–12 noon 3 clients booked
- 12 noon–1:00 PM (Lunch)
- 1:00 PM–4:10 PM 2 clients booked

Restrictions: Same as Week 3

Week 6 (38 hours) Normal duties, approximately 40
  clients
  One rostered day off Monday, Tuesday, Wednesday or
  Friday at employer's discretion in lieu of working late
  Thursday evening and all day Saturday.
  Monday, Wednesday, Friday, Saturday

- 9:00 AM–5:00 PM up to 8 clients booked

Thursday

- 9:00 AM–8:00 PM (approx. 11 hours—up to 10
  clients booked including 1 hour lunch, 30 minute
  break)

Restrictions: 10 minute breaks every 2 to 3 hours.

Treatment program
Client to continue treatment with Therapist while undertaking graduated return to normal duties program.

Reviews: 1. Physician
  a) At completion of 2 weeks, (August 28) to determine if Client can increase hours to 6 hours per day (30 hours)
  b) At completion of 5 weeks, (September 21) to determine if Client can increase hours to 35 per week (normal hours)
  c) At completion of 4 weeks on normal hours, (October 21)

Continued

BOX 20.2—*cont'd*

2. Fail-safe response mechanism be implemented to address any issues/problems/interruptions immediately so return to work process is not impeded
   a) Contact Rehabilitation Consultant
   b) Medical expert to attend worksite on same day to resolve issue

Signatures:

Client _____

Employer _____

Therapist _____

Physician _____

Rehabilitation Consultant _____

It can be seen from this brief overview of on-site therapy that the skills learned by Therapists in undergraduate training and developed in more traditional clinical experiences, are rearranged to provide a focus on the work world. The key to success in on-site therapy is value-added, cost-effective, occupational injury management directed towards restoration of function.

REFERENCES

1. Australian Standard Classification of Occupations, Department of Employment, Education and Training and Bureau of Statistics, Working Draft, Canberra, Australia, 1983.
2. Berns TAR, Milner NP: TRAM-A Technique for the Recording and Analysis of Moving Work Posture. In Milner NP, editor: Methods to Study Work Posture, *Ergolabs Report* 80:22–26,1980.
3. Chaffin, DB: Manual Materials Handling and the Biomechanical Basis for Prevention of Low-Back Pain in Industry-an overview. Am Ind Hyg Assoc J 12:989–996,1987.
4. Corlett EN, Madeley SJ, Manenica L: Postural Targeting; a technique for recording working postures. Ergonomics. 22(3):357–366, 1979.
5. Corlett EN, Manenica L: The Effects and Measurement of Working Postures, Appl. Ergonom. 11(1):7–16, 1980.
6. Corlett EN, Bishop RP: A Technique for Assessing Postural Discomfort. Ergonomics. 19(2):175–182,1976.
7. Dictionary of Occupational Titles. U.S. Department of Labor, Employment and Training Administration, Washington, DC, 1977.
8. Drury CG, Law CH, Pawenski CS: A Survey of Industrial Box Handling. Hum. Factors 24(5):553–565,1982.
9. Esser TJ: Gathering Information for Evaluation Planning. National Institute of Handicapped Research, Department of Education. March 1980.
10. Garg A, Saxena U: Container Characteristics and Maximum Acceptable Weight of Lift. Ju. Factors 22(4):487–495,1980.
11. Gould J, Davies G: Orthopedic and Sports Physical Therapy: The CV Mosby Company, 1985.
12. Grieve DW: The Postural Stability Diagram PSD: personal constraints on the Static Exertion of Force. Ergonomics. 22(10):1155–1164,1979.
13. Holzman, P: ARBAN-A New Method for Analysis of Ergonomic Effort. Appl. Ergonom. 13(2):82–86,1982.25. Herring, SA: Sports Medicine Early Care. Contemporary Conservative Care for Painful Spinal Disorders, pp 235–244, 1991. Lea & Febiger.
14. Johnson J: Therapist in an On-Site Occupational Rehabilitation Program—A Case Study. Work 3(3):73–76. 1993.
15. Karhu O, Kansi P, Kuorinka, L: Correcting Working Postures in Industry: a practical method for analysis. Appl Ergonom. 18:199,1977.
16. Karhu O, Harkonen R, Sorvali P, Vepsalainen P: Observing Working Postures in Industry. Appl. Ergonom. Vol. 12(1):13–17, 1981.
17. Keyserling WM, Punnett L, Fine LJ: Trunk Posture and Back Pain; Identification and Control of Occupational Risk Factors. Appl. Ind. Hyg. 3:87–92, 1988.
18. Keyserling WM: Postural Analysis of the Trunk and Shoulders in Simulated Real Time. Ergonomics. 4:569, 1986.
19. Legg SJ: Cardiovascular and Spinal Strain of a Complex Materials Handling Task in a Confined Space: Influences of Protective Clothing and Physical Training. Trends Ergonom. Hum. Factors 819–825, 1986.
20. Lytel RB, Botterbusch KF: Physical Demands Job Analysis: A New Approach. National Institute of Handi-

capped Research, US Department of Education. March 1981.

21. Priel VZ: A Numerical Definition of Posture. Hum. Factors. 16(6):576–584, 1974.

22. Rankin Occupational Safety and Health, North Adelaide, Queensland, Australia.

23. Schwartz G, Galvin D, Watson S, Dickinson S: An Employer's Guide to Obtaining Physical Therapy Services, A Study by the Washington Business Group on Health. Healthcare Management and Physical Therapy. APTA - Private Practice Section. pp. 1–51. 1988–89.

24. Smith JL, Jiang BC: A Manual Materials Handling Study of Bag Lifting, Am Ind Hyg Assoc J 45(8):505–508,1984.

25. Winkel J: On the Manual Handling of Wide-Body Carts Used by Cabin Attendants in Civil Aircraft, Appl Ergonom. 14(3):162–168,1983.

21
Assessing Physical Impairment

Tom G. Mayer

Industrial Therapy Worker Care Spectrum

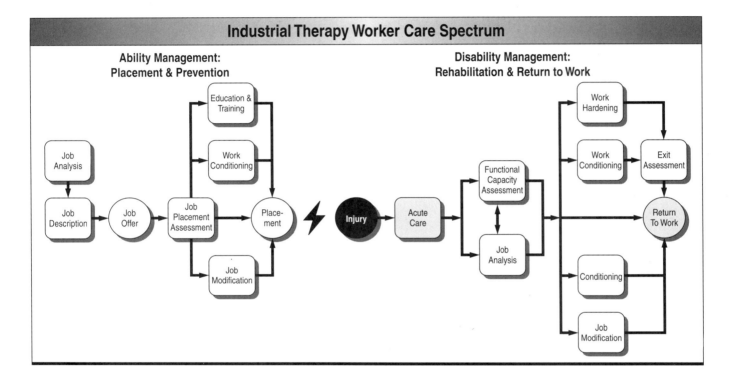

Health providers are often asked to grant the legal system a rating of impairment for a patient who has been injured in a personal or industrial accident. An ethical problem arises because the rating of impairment is, at best, a very inexact "science," and yet is intended to lead to a monetary award for the patient whose amount is contingent, at least in part, upon the rating. This creates a situation with the potential for abuse and exploitation in which litigation may be encouraged, and the physician placed in an unaccustomed role as arbiter between adversarial parties.

Problems generally remain mild as long as the medical provider is only expected to submit documentation on observations of patient activities. They become more complex when judgments regarding an actual numerical rating, specifically tied to a monetary award, are expected of the health provider, along with self-evaluation of the rating's objectivity. The goal of

this chapter is designed to increase the reader's awareness of the problems and partial solutions that have evolved in this area.

History

The tradition of financial reward for accidental loss of life and limb goes back hundreds of years. There is some evidence that Greek warriors' families were compensated in the event of a wartime heroic death more than 2,000 years ago. Likewise, there is solid evidence that the first *scheduled awards* were provided to injured pirates. Fixed payments were provided for specific injuries, prioritized according to the perceived resulting loss of function, for instance, the loss of a right arm compensated higher than loss of a left.

Interestingly, pirate injury compensation occurred

only in the event of a successful attack with recovered booty, and after the captain had received his share (but prior to distribution of other shares). Medieval knights may also have been compensated for going to war by their lords in the event of injury or death, but these rights did not extend to conscripted serfs.

As the Western world's feudal agricultural economy gave way to a rapidly advancing Industrial Revolution, new complexities began to emerge. The traditional obedience, loyalty, and mutual obligation between a landlord and his sharecropping subjects began to move toward a money-based economy of voluntary labor and purchased services. Raw capitalism produced many examples of unsafe working conditions, with tensions between profit-oriented employers and exploited employees rising throughout the eighteenth and nineteenth centuries.

Seeing the success of a progressive injury compensation system for his military, and the crucial link between "blood and iron" of a military-industrial complex that foreshadows the twentieth century, Germany's Bismarck established the first system of workers' compensation in the 1880s. For the first time, civilian workers and their families did not have to face ruin after a disabling industrial accident. Instead, the system provided for three crucial principles:

1. *Medical intervention* specifically designed to ameliorate the effects of the injury and rapidly return the patient to productivity.
2. *Wage replacement* at a percentage of the workers' original salary to maintain a basic standard of living while healing occurred.
3. A final compensation for death or dismemberment.

In the United States, more than two decades later, similar programs evolved in certain states, creating the first US Workers' Compensation laws just prior to the Great War. The development of these laws was patchy and eclectic, with the last state finally coming on board in 1949, about 40 years after the first state laws. Several federal laws, generally tied to interstate commerce issues (railroad, maritime, post office and other federal agencies, and civilian military) also emerged, and evolved in very different ways, but more or less providing injured workers similar rights and benefits.

A crucial factor often not generally recognized in the public discussion of Workers' Compensation, is that the benefits provided to injured workers are conditional. They are contingent upon a very great benefit being provided to the employer (a benefit always provided *de facto* to the military); that is, *limitation of liability.*

In the unconstrained nineteenth century situation, most individuals sustaining an injury would become "charity cases." A few might successfully sue for negligence and win. Such victories were rarely a bonanza in a world with a tradition of legal support for the privileged. The breakdown of the traditional employer/employee feudal obligation, and an increasing ground swell of a rebellious multitude for private, as well as public rights (associated with multiple nationalist revolutions in the Age of Enlightenment) led many employers to be more aware of the legal implications.

The limitation of liability for negligence, so rarely discussed, is generally considered to be a far greater benefit to employers today than a century ago. All discussions of worker benefits must keep this fundamental compromise between employer and employee in mind, because herein lies the basis for the irreconcilable adversarial relationship.

CONCEPTS OF IMPAIRMENT EVALUATION

At least a rudimentary understanding of the terms *impairment, disability, handicap,* and *employability* is needed.

Disability is an *administrative* term and refers to an individual's inability to perform certain activities of daily life, such as gainful employment, customarily accessible to the general population.

Impairment is a *medical* term and represents an alteration of the patient's usual health status that is *evaluated by medical means.*

Handicap occurs as a consequence of an *impairment,* presenting a barrier to performance of an activity of daily living (such as the demands of work), which may be overcome by *reasonable accommodation.*

Employability represents another administrative process affected both by *disability* and *handicap.* Any decrease in employability as a consequence of an injury may result in *economic loss* to the patient, potentially leading to a monetary award. One factor in this award is the perceived damage to the patient's health status (or *impairment*), the determination of which the physician is generally deemed responsible.

Several additional concepts in the assessment of permanent impairment must be understood as follows:

1. Causation and compensability
2. Healing period
3. Functional capacity and work limitation
4. Permanent impairment rating

Causation and Compensability

The concept of *causation* is the crucial one upon which all elements of the system hinge. Depending upon the legal precedents established within a given *compensation injury venue* (not necessarily Workers' Compensation), an evaluation of the cause of the accident and whether it is *compensable* must take place. Even in today's most conservative venues, compensability is usually subjected only partly, or not at all, to the test of employer negligence.

In the most labor-oriented venues, virtually any medical claim ascribed to working hours or working conditions may be accepted as compensable ("stress claims," claims for cardiovascular disease, psychiatric conditions). Until an evaluation of causation establishes compensability, benefits of any kind are generally not awarded. Conversely, once compensability has been accepted, even conditionally, this decision is rarely reversed.

Healing Period

The concept of a healing period is crucial to the evaluation of permanent impairment, and virtually always involves a decision of, or documentation by, the health provider. The concept currently in use in most venues has evolved from a confluence of extremes. Employers would generally pay temporary total disability or temporary partial disability (TTD or TPD) benefits only until the patient was "healed" and any permanent impairment identified.

The healing period was generally considered the length of time it took for a fracture of soft tissue injury to heal, which meant that (except in cases of extreme central neurologic injuries) employers were discontinuing TTD indemnity benefits within 2 to 4 months of injury. In contrast, injured employees generally contended that the healing period was only complete when symptoms were completely resolved (becoming "pain-free"). This difference of opinion over a reasonable healing period made mediation by administrative agencies, even with adequate physician documentation, very difficult.

Pressures by insurance carriers (as representatives of the employer) and plaintiff attorneys (as representatives of injured workers) tended to have a polarizing effect upon the patient's physicians, with medical documentation often as extremely unscientific as the contending views.

Over time, the concept of maximum medical improvement (MMI), maximum medical recovery (MMR) or permanent and stationary (P&S) developed. MMI is defined in a number of ways, but comes down to an essentially medical determination of the point at which all reasonable medical treatments designed to "improve or cure" the condition, and in which the condition is not expected to change over a foreseeable period of time (6 to 24 months) is established. At this point, the patient should be at the "highest functional level," and therefore have overcome all correctable *temporary impairment*, leaving only the residual *permanent impairment*. The patient should be at the highest functional level of capability, with defined handicap and plan for

reasonable accommodations vocationally. Unfortunately, in practice, this is frequently not the case.

Functional Capacity and Work Restrictions

The third crucial factor in impairment/disability evaluation involves the concept of *functional capacity* and *work restrictions*. Limitation of an individual's ability to participate in gainful employment (disability) is affected by the loss of physical function (impairment), as well as the other employability factors (age, gender, education, transferable skills, job demands). Since most monetary awards are legally tied to *permanent disability*, multiple factors extraneous to purely medical impairment determinations are involved in the decision on indemnity benefit.

The most objective determination of the patient's ability to participate in activities of daily living, namely specific functional activities (bending, lifting, running, carrying, reaching), become crucial references to the degree to which one individual is considered more disabled than another, in the presence of similar levels of permanent impairment. Unfortunately, though improving, objective methods of determining functional capacity, and matching to specific job demands, remain in a stage of early development.

Permanent Impairment

The final issue is the method of determining *permanent impairment* as distinguished from *permanent disability*. In addition to the factors previously discussed, many state and federal venues have used two other tests to establish monetary awards for permanent disability. *Wage loss* has often been projected, based on employability, prior wages, and occasional unique formulas. The drawback of these methods is the essentially subjective basis for predicting lifetime loss of income based on limited facts.

Inability to work has also been used as a *sine qua non* of certain laws, but again suffers from the subjectivity of this determination. Of all the methods, it has the additional disadvantage of creating the most adversarial environment, in which the injured worker is placed in a position of demonstrating all the things that they cannot do, rather than being motivated to demonstrate the highest functional level and desire to return to work.

It is for this reason that pressures have been accelerating to utilize medical input into permanent impairment, tied to generally-accepted guidelines, as the critical factor of greatest weight in the determination of permanent disability leading to specific financial payments. In the case of traditional *scheduled awards* (loss of an eye or a hand) the medical evidence is usually clear and incontrovertible. However, in the case of more obscure conditions, generally involving chronic pain, leading to nonscheduled or general injuries, the greatest controversy arises.

DEVELOPING IMPAIRMENT ASSESSMENT SYSTEMS

Placing a numerical value on impairment, like any schedule, represents an administrative rather than a scientific determination. The following are several factors that are generally considered in providing a rating guideline for impairment.

Objectivity

Rating of *permanent impairment* occurs after the declaration of *maximum medical recovery* (or determining the condition to be P&S or MMI). What constitutes factors in impairment evaluation is the topic of considerable controversy, although it is agreeable that these factors should be covered as fully as possible in the medical report provided by the examining physician. Typical *impairment* factors of varying objectivity utilized in musculoskeletal impairment assessment include symptom report, structural alteration (often identified by imaging tests), range of motion, neurological loss, other physical examination findings (such as loss of strength, cosmesis) and, more recently, other functional capacity measures.[1,2,10,11,13,18]

While most rating guides incorporate all but the last factor in some way (with either "analog" or "digital" methodology), the goal of the objective rating of impairment is usually to relate the effects of a specific injury to body functioning as a whole.[3-5] This makes functional capacity inclusion desirable, but begins to invade the province of disability evaluation.

Currently, functional capacity measurements do not appear to be sufficiently standardized to be appropriate for inclusion in rating systems, which are attempting to condense the relevant impairment factors into a simple number. There is no argument that relevant physical examination factors are necessary to substantiate the patient's symptomatic complaint. This validation must be included in the examiner's documentation.

Consistency and Cost

The administrative "Disability System" would most desire the rating physicians to produce perfect consistency. That is, that two physicians employing the same standardized process would always deliver exactly equivalent ratings. Administrative and friction costs are reduced if the number of evaluations in a given case can be reduced. This cost-consciousness fuels the pressure to produce a numerical scale, even though all physicians realize that expressions of alteration of human functioning and health status cannot scientifically be neatly condensed. Thus, some variability between physician's ratings, regardless of the system utilized, is to be expected, but must be minimized. A creative tension between desire for objectivity and consistency will always exist within any rating system.

Fairness

This abstract concept refers to the relationship between the measured impairment rating, and the actual alteration of health status and physical function experienced by the patient. This issue is usually of far greater interest to the employee/patient and the examining physician, than it is to the administrative Disability System, which health providers seek to serve.

Fairness is closely related to the ability of a numerical rating to quantify the actual degree of functional loss. In the musculoskeletal system, this is clearly more likely to be accomplished when there is simple visual access to discrete anatomical units, along with a "normal" contralateral comparison (knee, foot, or hand). By contrast, absence of visual access and contralaterality (such as in the spine) creates barriers to observing functional loss. It should therefore not be surprising that greater progress has been made in achieving wide acceptance of rating methodology for the upper extremity than for the spine.

Relevance and Accuracy

Any factor included in a rating guide should be relevant to comparison of results of an injury to functional loss. Amputation of an index finger is a clear example of a highly relevant factor, while discovery of degenerative changes in a spinal disc or glenohumeral joint may represent only age-related change. Such imaging findings may often document premorbid alterations, and may have little relevance to the site causing symptoms which lead to functional loss.

The concept of relevance is closely linked to that of accuracy, which refers to the closeness of any measured quantity to the true quantity. A simple two-armed goniometer may be highly accurate in defining elbow flexion/extension, but the same device applied to compound regional (lumbar) and hip mobility involved in flexion at the waist, may be grossly inaccurate.

The recognition of compound motions involved in spinal movement has led to substantial advance in accuracy of its determination. Inclinometric motion measurements have therefore superseded simple goniometric measurements in assessing spinal range of motion in the *American Medical Association Guides to the Evaluation of Permanent Impairment*.[1,2]

Other physical examination factors (such as strength and cosmesis) remain the province of upper extremity impairment evaluation, because their accuracy cannot be assessed against a "gold standard" in the spine, even though their relevance to functional loss would be high. The future of impairment evaluation will likely emerge from improved methodology for measuring functional loss through more relevant and accurate systems of quantifying the physical examination.[4,6,7,9,10,12–18]

Convenience and Timeliness

Convenience to the practicing physician is an area of controversy. Busy practitioners may resent utilizing an impairment rating system requiring expenditure of time in providing medico-legal information to the *Disability System* in Workers' Compensation and personal injury cases. Such nonmedical administrative demands often discourage younger physicians from involvement with these cases. By contrast, there is a perception that the physician regularly involved in Independent Medical Examination (IME) may unnecessarily complicate the evaluations.

In California (which is unique in demanding that physicians evaluate disability, rather than impairment), reimbursement for a single IME may exceed the total reimbursement provided to the treating physician managing the patient's medical recovery. Such monetary disincentives reinforce concerns about qualifications to perform impairment ratings, leading to formation of multi-specialty certifying organizations.[4–5]

As this chapter goes to press, the perceived extraordinary nonproductive cost of such examinations in creating noncompetitiveness for the California economy, has resulted in bipartisan legally-mandated controls on frequency and reimbursement for such evaluations that are drastically altering the California system.

Rapid and radical changes in compensation injury law in several large venues (Texas, California) recently, demonstrate the strong relationship between financial awards (particularly permanent disability) and other major political forces encompassing the disability system.

The treating physician, in attempting to provide a timely impairment evaluation, may also be frustrated by the perceived need to employ services of allied health personnel (because of limited physician training) in order to prepare a numerical rating, which they feel bears little relationship to treatment of patients. Lack of education on medico-legal and administrative concomitants of medical practice in compensation injuries is a serious barrier to a physician being comfortable with this aspect of medical care.

THE THERAPIST'S ROLE

Although the major role in assessing physical impairment is still primarily the Physician's, Therapists can make an important contribution to the overall process. Measuring range of motion and administering Functional Capacity Assessments are the two key areas where Therapists can offer significant value.

Range of Motion

In most approaches to assessing impairment, range of motion (in combination with other physical examination and other diagnostic findings) is an important measurement in determining impairment ratings. Physicians then apply experienced interpretation to all of these factors and determine an official percentage for the purpose of determining the settlement.

Therapists can offer a service to physicians by providing accurate, objective measurements of range of motion using goniometers, inclinometers, and other measurement devices and approaches. This allows the physician time to attend to other medical needs, and places the Therapist in position for referrals regarding the rehabilitation program to follow.

Functional Capacity Assessment

Currently, determining impairment involves a considerable amount of professional interpretation and opinion. As a result, the parties may often incur extensive time and legal expense resolving perceived differences. As Functional Capacity Assessments become increasingly standardized and reliable, however, their objectivity may begin to expedite settlements and yield significant reductions in time and expense for all parties concerned.

Accordingly, there is a significant opportunity for Therapists to offer increasingly standardized FCAs that can bring objectivity to impairment and disability ratings.

METHODS FOR ASSESSING PERMANENT IMPAIRMENT

It is beyond the scope of this chapter to comprehensively review different methods for assessing impairment. We have alluded to certain common methods and primary references. The reader is referred to these primary sources for further information. In summary, the impairment evaluating physician is expected to obtain a rating by evaluating one or more of the following categories, according to the specific rules of the compensation injury venue, as follows:

1. Persistent symptoms
2. Physical examination-based characteristics (including physical capacity performance measurements of the injured area)
3. Functional capacity whole-person task performance measurements
4. Diagnosis of the patient's condition

Persistent Symptoms

Though patient symptoms are usually excluded as ratable factors for obvious reasons, in practice there are almost always subtle implicit or explicit considerations of symptoms in nonscheduled impairments. In the case of scheduled awards, where obvious loss of a body part (dismemberment), creates the impairment, symptoms are usually less important. This is not simply due to the observability of the injury, but to the fact that there is usually little controversy about such awards.

In contrast, situations in which pain is the predominant remaining symptom, accompanied by little objectively-observable relevant pathology, pain complaints always subtly influence the evaluator. The severity of complaints may actually be built into the guideline, as when a specific diagnosis is provided greater impairment in a "digital" graded determination based on whether patient symptoms attributable to that diagnosis are mild, moderate, or severe.

The lack of absolute objectivity in nonscheduled injuries, as well as a tendency over the past 50 years to broaden compensability rights as a social decision, makes it inevitable that symptom complaints will remain a critical, but often unspoken, factor in impairment assessment.

Physical Examination

Physical examination methods vary in perceived objectivity and relevance as discussed previously. Physical examination findings in impairment assessment may involve such easily observable factors as scarring of the skin (cosmesis), or the presence or absence of pulses or passive joint motion (preferably an easily-manipulable extremity joint like a finger or elbow).

In most cases of dispute, less "objective" methods must be used. These methods generally can be summed up as requiring some human performance component. Voluntary action, or self-report of a specific performance end-point, become crucial to the examination. Examples of the former are "neurologic" tests

such as myotomal strength of an anterior tibial or quadriceps musculotendinous unit, grip strength, any *active* range of motion measurement (spine or extremities), or "machine measurement" (pulmonary function or trunk strength tests).

The second category generally involves limitation of some activity by patient report of pain or incapacity, such as that which occurs in a straight leg raise or bowstring test for evaluating stretch of an irritated sciatic nerve.

Both types of tests become controversial because of the perception that monetary disincentives will create reduced effort for the patient's performance in these situations as a consequence of human nature.[9,14,15] Consistency tests and "fake factors" are built into some of these measurements to reduce the probability of such behaviors, or assist the examiner in recognizing them.[1,2] Such methods are often inconclusive, necessitating complex judgments by the examining health provider to insure some degree of validity. Conversely, in the most controversial areas of impairment assessment, physical performance measures usually have the greatest face validity.

Functional Capacities

In only a few situations are *functional capacities* specifically tied to assessment of permanent impairment. In most cases, the inclusion of these methods reflects a fundamental intermingling of the concepts of impairment and disability, since functional human performance measurement (bending, running, lifting, reaching, pushing, climbing) is related to specific work activities of daily living.

These assessments generally require extremely complex measurement methods, and are therefore tests most subject to patient effort. Unlike physical examination tests, effort in functional assessment is usually harder to recognize. The unique California system is probably the best example of use of such methodology.[4,5]

Diagnosis

At this point in time, probably the most popular way for reluctant treating physicians to discharge their unwanted obligation to determine impairment, is a diagnosis-based model. Making a diagnosis is fundamental to instituting any form of treatment, and is universally understood and performed by physicians as a prelude to treatment, documentation, and reimbursement. It is the simplest way to provide a rating, although issues of accuracy, fairness, test discrimination ability, and objectivity often challenge this method. Because inter-rater reliability is high and cost is usually low, such measures may be favored in certain cases.[2,8]

At this time, the American Medical Association *Guides to the Evaluation of Permanent Impairment* (editions 3 or 4) is the most popular manual used for impairment assessment. All 13 organ systems are represented, making it the most comprehensive impairment system available, and utilized to one extent or another in the majority of both state and federal venues.

The methodology is highly eclectic, varying from purely physical exam and function-based systems to nearly pure diagnosis-based systems, or a variety of combinations in between. It is not surprising that this diversity may even play out within a single chapter, as in the musculoskeletal chapter (which is used approximately 80% of the time that the *AMA Guide* is employed).

Systems for measurement in upper extremity, lower extremity and spine are very different, employing a variety of mixtures of diagnosis-based and physical examination (human performance)-based systems. It is considered a "living document," in which perceived success of one edition leads to alterations in a subsequent one.

Measurement Example

For those unfamiliar with the *AMA Guide*, the following example pertaining to Lateral Flexion (lateral bending)

of the dorsolumbar region is offered for illustration in Figure 21.1 and Box 21.1.[2]

Certain states, such as California and Minnesota, have evolved their own systems in a desire for greater flexibility in indemnity management. Additionally, the Social Security Administration has its own impairment evaluation system, performed administratively by full-time examiners, based on physician records, which review combinations of symptom, diagnosis, and physical examination-based measures.

If impairment is felt sufficient to potentially permit eligibility for benefits, a secondary test is provided that compares perceived patient functional capacity against job demands for which the individual may, by virtue of age, experience and education, be eligible. If no match is found, benefits are provided for Social Security Disability Income (SSDI) or Supplemental Security Income (SSI), with associated Medicare or Medicaid benefits respectively. Such benefits may continue for a lifetime. Essentially, both the California and Social Security systems evaluate disability rather than impairment.

For these reasons, controversy will continue to exist over the variety of impairment rating systems available in diverse administrative venues, and the progressive changes made in advancing the science.

FIGURE 21.1 Two-inclinometer measurement technique for lumbosacral lateral bend. **(A)** Set the inclinometers at T12 and over the sacrum in the frontal (coronal) plane with the inclinometers set at 0° in the erect position. **(B)** With the subject bending maximally to the right, subtract the sacral inclinometer reading from the T12 reading to obtain the right lumbar lateral bending angle. Carry out the procedure on the left side.

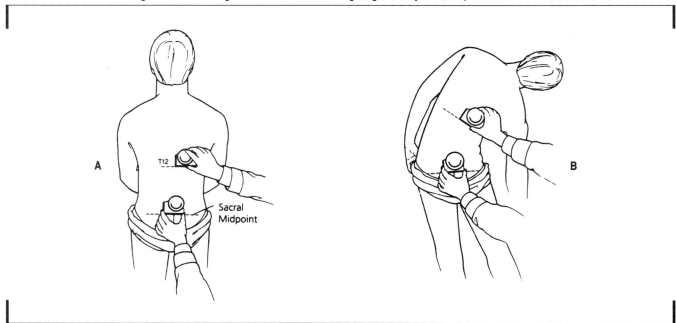

(With permission from *Guides to the Evaluation of Permanent Impairment*, ed 4, Chicago, 1993, American Medical Assoc.)

BOX 21.1

One-inclinometer Technique
Use an automated device that can determine compound joint motions and indicate the involved angles.

1. With the subject standing erect with the knees straight, locate and place skin marks over the T12 spinous process and the sacrum. Place the inclinometer aligned in the coronal plane over the T12 skin mark and set the first 0° reading. Move the inclinometer to the sacrum and set the second 0° reading.
2. Ask the subject to bend the trunk maximally to the right, and record the sacral (hip) flexion angle. Move the inclinometer to the T12 skin mark and record the angle. Then ask the subject to resume the neutral position, and calculate the lumbar right lateral flexion angle.
3. Set the 0° readings first at T12, then over the sacrum. Ask the subject to flex fully to the left, and determine the angles at the sacrum and T12. Calculate the lumbar left lateral flexion angle.
4. Repeat the procedure three to six times. To be a valid set, three of six measurements should lie within ± 5° or 10% of the mean, whichever is greater. The final impairment estimate is based on the best (least impairing) angle of a valid set.
5. Consult the Abnormal Motion part of Table 82 (p. 130) to determine the whole-person impairment.

Example: In a 55-year-old man who complains of persisting back pain, T12 angles for right flexion are 20°, 20°, 30°, and 25°. Matching sacral (hip) lateral flexion measurements to the right are 15°, 5°, 10°, and 10°. Subtracting, the lumbosacral right lateral flexion angles are 5°, 15°, 20°, and 15°, respectively. The first measurement is discarded, and the next three measurements fulfill validation criteria. The best right lateral flexion angle is 20°, and the impairment is 1% (Table 21.1).

Ankylosis
Ankylosis in lumbosacral spine lateral flexion generally represents a scoliosis and usually produces only limited impairment. Mark the T12 and sacral spinous processes and ask the subject to stand in the most erect position

TABLE 21.1 Impairment Due to Abnormal Motion and Ankylosis of the Lumbosacral Region: Lateral Flexion

Abnormal Motion
Average range of lateral flexion is 50%;
the proportion of total lumbosacral motion is 40%.

a. Right lateral flexion from neutral position (0°) to:	Degrees of lumbosacral motion Lost	Degrees of lumbosacral motion Retained	% Impairment of the whole person
0°	25	0	5
10°	15	10	3
15°	10	15	2
20°	5	20	1
25°	0	25	0
b. Left lateral flexion from neutral position (0°) to:			
0°	25	0	5
10°	15	10	3
15°	10	15	2
20°	5	20	1
25°	0	25	0
c. Ankylosis Region ankylosed at:			
0° (neutral position)			10
30°			20
45°			30
60°			40
75° (full flexion)			50

possible that corrects the deformity. Using the simple measurements made in the coronal plane, subtract the sacral (hip) inclination from the T12 inclination and record the ankylosis angle or the angle of restriction.

THE FUTURE

The future of impairment rating will include ever-closer approximations of the measured value to the degree of functional loss sustained by the claimant with altered health status. No system can be effective, if not accompanied by appropriate interest and education on the part of the practicing specialist utilizing the guidelines.

There is clearly no single "best way" to condense

the multiple factors involved in human functional loss into a single number, but it is hoped that this chapter will provide the reader with an understanding of some of the complex issues involved in formulating a rating system.

Some anatomical areas obviously lend themselves to more objective, quantifiable measurement than others, but the effort to improve relevance and accuracy in documenting functional loss continues. With no "ideal system" on the horizon, the physician who provides medical documentation to the Disability System should be aware that the medical reports, particularly those at the time of conclusion of treatment, remain the single most important factor used by administrators to assess permanency and *degree* of functional loss.

In turn, these decisions may often lead to financial awards (Workers' Compensation or personal injury lump sum settlements) or permanent disability payments (Social Security Disability Income or ongoing Long-Term Disability). The impact of these payments on patient's future behavior and productivity is incalculable, and produces a staggering, if not always desired, responsibility for the physician providing the impairment rating. In financial terms, the impact to taxpayers or an insurance carrier of a single patient evaluation, may exceed $1 million over a lifetime.

Impairment rating is a critical activity for which many health care providers can anticipate greater involvement. Changing Workers' Compensation methods, and a search for cost containment, as well as increased fairness, leads legislators to depend, to an ever-greater extent, on the medical evaluator for determining financial and other permanent disability benefits. Education on the history, principles, and methods of impairment evaluation are essential for health providers to adequately discharge responsibilities. No system is infallible, which means that medical opinion and judgment will inevitably be required, and controversy and disputes will always occur. The future will certainly bring change in this rapidly evolving field.[1,11]

REFERENCES

1. *American Medical Association Guides to the Evaluation of Permanent Impairment*, ed 3, Chicago, 1990, American Medical Association.

2. *American Medical Association Guides to the Evaluation of Permanent Impairment*, ed 4, Chicago, 1993, American Medical Association.

3. Brand R, Lehmann T: Low Back Impairment Rating Practices of Orthopaedic Surgeons, *Spine* 8:75–78, 1983.

4. Clark W, Haldeman S, Johnson P, Morris J, Schulenberger C, Traumer D, White A: Back Impairment and Disability Determination: Another attempt at objective reliable rating, *Spine* 13:332–341, 1988.

5. Clark W, Haldeman S: The Development of Guideline Factors for the Evaluation of Disability in Neck and Back Injuries, *Spine* 13:1736–1745, 1993.

6. Dvorak J, Antinnes J, Panjabi M, Loustalot D, Bonomo M: Age and Gender Related Normal Motion of the Cervical Spine, *Spine* 17:S393–S398, 1992.

7. Kohles S, Barnes D, Gatchel R, Mayer T: Improved Physical Performance Outcomes Following Functional Restoration Treatment in Patient with Chronic Low Back Pain: early versus recent training results, *Spine* 15:1321–1324, 1990.

8. Lohman W, editor: *Permanent Partial Disability Schedule*, St Paul, Minn, 1992. Minnesota Department of Labor & Industry.

9. Lowery W, Horn T, Boden S, Wiesel S: Impairment Evaluation Based on Spinal Range of Motion in Normal Subjects, *J Spinal Dis* 5:398–402, 1992.

10. Mayer T, Dowdle J: Impairment-Disability Evaluation, *American Aca Orthopedic Surgeons Bulletin* 40(2):12–13, 1992.

11. Mayer T, Mooney V, Gatchel R: Contemporary Care for Spinal Disorders: concepts, diagnosis and treatment, Philadelphia, 1991, Lea and Febiger.

12. Mayer T, Tencer A, Kristoferson S, Mooney V: Use of Noninvasive Techniques for Quantification of Spinal Range of Motion in Normal Subjects and Chronic Low-Back Dysfunction Patients, *Spine* 9:588–595, 1984.

13. McBride E: Disability Determination, *J Bone Joint Surg* 44A:1441–1446, 1962.

14. Newton M, Waddell G: Trunk Strength Testing with Iso-Machines, Part 1: review of a decade of scientific evidence, *Spine* 7:801–811, 1993.

15. Newton M, Thow N, Somerville D, Henderson I, Waddell G: Trunk Strength Testing With Iso-Machines, Part 2: experimental evaluation of the Cybex II back testing system in normal subjects and patients with chronic low back pain, *Spine* 7:812–824, 1993.

16. Shorbe H: Disability Evaluation, *J Bone Joint Surg* 44A:1447–1456, 1962.

17. Troup J, Hood C, Chapman A: Measurements of Sagittal Mobility of the Lumbar Spine and Hips, *Ann Phys Med* 9:308–313, 1968.

18. Waddell G, Somerville D, Henderson I, Newton M: Objective Clinical Evaluation of Physical Impairment in Chronic Low Back Pain, *Spine* 17:617–628, 1992.

The Management of Industrial Therapy

22

Regulations and Regulatory Agencies

Susan M. Brookins
Robert B. King

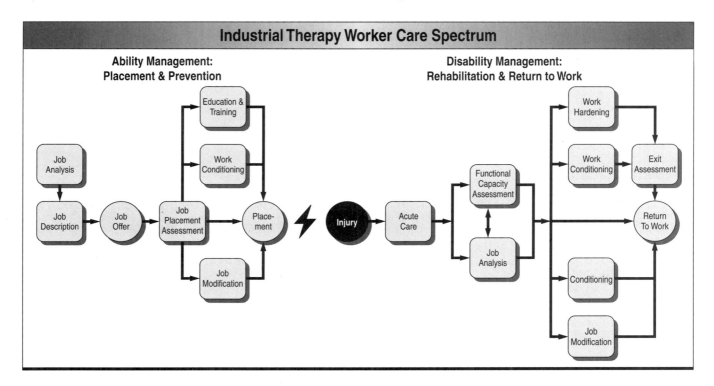

Industrial Therapy Worker Care Spectrum

The first segment of this chapter will deal with the Commission on Accreditation of Rehabilitation Facilities (CARF). It will begin with an overview of CARF, then discuss the presurvey process and the actual site survey. This will be followed by a description of how the typical Industrial Therapy team would be involved in preparing for CARF certification of their facility.

CARF is currently the only accrediting authority for the specialty of Work Hardening programs. (It is not, however, currently involved in accrediting Work Conditioning programs. After July 1, 1995 the standards will encompass a greater variety of Occupational Rehabilitation programs including: Acute Occupational Rehabilitation, and Category I and II Work Specific Occupational Rehabilitation.) CARF is a nationally

recognized private, not-for-profit organization. The Commission's focus is to promote within the field of rehabilitation quality services for persons with injuries or disabilities.

The remainder of this chapter deals with other regulatory agencies and legislation specifically with regard to Workers' Compensation, the Occupational Safety and Health Administration (OSHA), the National Institute of Occupational Safety and Health (NIOSH) and the Americans with Disabilities Act (ADA).

The chapter will discuss how these impact the provision of Industrial Therapy (IT). Each of these areas will be dealt with briefly in the order mentioned above. A basic understanding for each of these areas will be provided, recognizing that a much greater in-depth understanding beyond the scope of this chapter is necessary to provide IT in a competent manner. The information provided on Workers' Compensation, OSHA, NIOSH, and the ADA was extracted from government publications from the respective agencies referenced at the end of the chapter.

CARF

History of CARF

Historically, the Commission's formation evolved from the efforts of two organizations—1) the Association of Rehabilitation Centers and 2) the National Association of Sheltered Workshops and Home-bound Programs. In 1966 these two organizations merged their efforts and incorporated as the Commission on Accreditation of Rehabilitation. At this time the newly formed Commission entered into an agreement to obtain administrative support from the Joint Commission on Accreditation of Healthcare Organizations. This affiliation was terminated in 1971 when CARF became an independent entity.

Organizational Structure

CARF is currently comprised of both sponsoring and associate memberships representing 40 national organizations involved in services for persons with disabilities. The Board of Trustees of the Commission is composed of one representative of each of the sponsoring members as well as an equal number of members-at-large appointed by the Board of Trustees.

This Board of Trustees is the Commission's authoritative body whose responsibilities include the adoption or modification of standards, as well as the determination of the accreditation status of surveyed organizations. The Board of Trustees is also responsible for the approval of basic policies and fiscal issues which govern the operation of the Commission.

Purposes

The bylaws of the Commission identify its purposes. Threaded through all the established goals and objectives of the Commission is the focus on improving the quality of services provided to individuals with disabilities. To accomplish this the Commission provides the rehabilitation community with a forum through which rehabilitation specialists can participate in setting standards and improving programs.

In addition to organizations seeking accreditation, CARF offers an independent, impartial, and objective system of reviewing the organization's performance based on relevant standards with consultative feedback. Through this process, organizations are assisted in assessing their strengths and weaknesses. The accrediting process then directs the organization toward growth and development, by providing guidelines for upgrading services in conformance with standards developed by the rehabilitation community.

Accreditation By Peers

The accreditation process is one of peer review. For the most part surveyors are professionals working in organizations which are accredited in the field. Peer review is used to promote both accountability and consultative support to organizations as part of the survey process.

Individuals eligible for selection and training as a CARF surveyor must have experience in the field of rehabilitation and be current or recent practitioners. These individuals are selected on the basis of their professional and programmatic leadership and experience. Once selected, the potential surveyor participates in an intensive training model which includes a simulation of an actual site survey. Following completion of this training, the surveyor participates in two surveys as an intern, prior to being appointed as a CARF surveyor.

Genesis of Work Hardening Accreditation

The establishment of CARF standards for Work Hardening programs came from interest in the field from providers and funding sources requesting that standards be established. In 1988 a National Advisory Committee was established by CARF to develop standards for Work Hardening programs. Fifteen professionals representing predominately the fields of Occupational Therapy, Physical Therapy, Vocational Services, and Psychology served as members of the Committee. A draft of the guidelines for Work Hardening programs was then sent out to the field for feedback in the spring of 1988 for feedback. The final standards were approved in December 1988, published in January 1989 and became effective in July 1989. The first program was surveyed in July 1989 and by June 30, 1994, 312 Work Hardening programs had been accredited by CARF.[2]

The Commission recognizes and accepts the responsibility of keeping the standards relevant. In order to address the rapid growth and innovations that have characterized Work Hardening programs, the Work Hardening section of the standards was reviewed, revised and updated in the winter of 1991 and again in 1994. These new guidelines were again sent out to the field for feedback and then finalized. The most current revised standards will be effective July 1, 1995.

Growing Importance of Accreditation

The Commission promotes the use of standards and accreditation to enhance the quality of service delivery. Certain state agencies have mandated that organizations be accredited, in order to receive referrals for Work Hardening services and to be eligible for reimbursement.

THE ACCREDITATION PROCESS

Initiating The Process

The initial steps in the accreditation process are for an organization to:

- Make a commitment to become CARF accredited
- Review the Standards Manual and interpretive guidelines
- Do a self assessment of comparing their standards of practice to those outlined in the manual

When the organization is satisfied that it substantially meets these standards, it is ready to submit an application for the accreditation survey. This application documents information regarding the organization and the program for which accreditation is sought. The application is then reviewed by the Commission for its appropriateness. Once the application is validated, surveyors with expertise in the appropriate field are chosen and a survey date is set.

The Site Survey

There are five phases of the site survey process:

- The orientation conference
- A tour of the facility
- A review of the documents
- Interviews
- The exit conference

The survey team conducts a site survey visit during which they provide an in-depth assessment of the organization's conformance with CARF standards. Using a consultative approach, the survey team assists the organization in improving the quality of their services.

The Orientation Conference

An orientation conference is held to provide an overview of the survey process, as well as establish a tentative schedule for the survey visit. At this time the organization is given the opportunity to meet the survey team members and provide them with some information about its own history, programs, and future plans.

Tour of the Facility

After the orientation conference, the organization is asked to conduct a brief tour of the physical facilities. At this time the surveyors are already visually inspecting the facility according to the criteria set in Section 1 of the Standards Manual regarding accessibility, health, and safety.

Document Review

During the balance of the site survey process, the surveyors observe the program and review documents in order to determine conformance with the standards. The organization is reviewed against three sections of the Standards Manual:

Section 1.   Organizational Standards which addresses issues relevant to:

1. Consumer focus
   - Purpose
   - Consumer based planning
   - Accessibility, health, and safety
2. Leadership
   - Goverance, organizational structure, and ownership
   - Organizational management
3. Information, analysis, and decisionmaking process
   - Information management
   - Program evaluation
   - Assessment of program quality
   - Fiscal management
4. Human resources
   - Personnel
   - Personnel development

Section 2.   Program Standards Part I which addresses issues relevant to:

Promoting service quality
- Rights of persons served
- Intake
- Orientation
- Individual planning
- Referral, exit/discharge, follow-up

Section 3.   The third section reviewed includes standards to be applied to the specific program being surveyed. The standards specific to the Work Hardening program are in Section 2 of Program Standards Part II. According to the program description, Work Hardening is:

"A highly structured, goal oriented, individualized treatment program, designed to maximize the persons' ability to return to work. Work Hardening programs are interdisciplinary in nature with a capability of addressing the

functional, physical, behavioral, and vocational needs of the person served. Work Hardening provides a transition between the initial injury management and return to work while addressing the issues of productivity, safety, physical tolerances and work behaviors. Work Hardening programs use real or simulated work activities in a relevant work environment in conjunction with physical conditioning tasks. These activities are used to progressively improve the bio-mechanical, neuromuscular, cardiovascular/metabolic, behavioral, attitudinal, and vocational function of the person served." [1]

The standards for Work Hardening identify the need to have the program available five days a week. Entrance and admission criteria need to be established and the Work Hardening process defined. According to the standards, the evaluation process should include psychosocial and physiological factors and should reflect the demands of competitive employment. The interdisciplinary team is defined as being:

"Characterized by a variety of disciplines that participate in the assessment, planning, and/or implementation of a person's program. There must be close interaction and integration among the disciplines so that all members of the team interact to achieve team goals." [1]

In the case of Work Hardening programs, the core team is to include an Occupational Therapist, Physical Therapist, Psychologist, and Vocational Specialist. The standards identify the need to include the employer, insurance company, and family in the process.

The Work Hardening program must include a number of components:

- Real or simulated work
- Strength and endurance development for work tolerance
- Safety education

In addition, the standards call for specific practices and disciplines to be incorporated in the program:

The program should include work site job analysis as needed, keeping the employer apprised of the worker's status in regard to return to work.

Worker behaviors and attitudes must also be taken into consideration.

There should be some mechanism to identify the person's transferable skills if return to work at the same job is not feasible.

There should be specified exit or discharge criteria and an established discharge policy.

The program should have a designated competent manager vested with the responsibility and authority to maintain the integrity of the program's standards.

There should be dedicated space and equipment that simulates a work environment in order

to achieve the goal of reintegrating the worker into the work community.

Finally, two outcomes should be measured: the level of employment and discharge status.

Interviews

Besides reviewing documents to determine conformance with the Standards, surveyors also conduct interviews with program clients, since the Standards clearly focus on the importance of input from those served. In addition, input is also solicited from administrative representatives, governing board members, staff members, community representatives, referral sources, funding sources, and consultants.

These interviews are scheduled so they do not interfere with the daily operations of the organization. Some interviews may be conducted over the telephone if it is not convenient for the person to come to the facility.

The Exit Conference

When all team members have completed their survey review, they meet to discuss their collective findings and prepare for the final step in the survey process—the exit conference. During this conference, the survey team members share their findings with the organization. The organization determines who will be present at this conference. This presentation may be taped if the organization so chooses.

In essence, the organization receives an oral report of what the survey team submits in writing to the CARF office. The organization will be told in what areas they have demonstrated strengths and in which areas recommendations are made in order for the organization to come into conformance with the standards. The survey team may also make suggestions as to areas in which the organization may improve the quality of service. Following this presentation, time is allotted for reaction and questions from the organization.

THE CERTIFICATION DETERMINATION

The survey team does not advise the organization regarding the certification outcome during the exit conference. This decision will be made by the Accreditation Committee of the CARF Board of Trustees after their review of the survey report. The survey team provides the Commission with a detailed written report of their observations during the survey. This report is reviewed, edited, and typed by the CARF staff then submitted to the CARF Board of Trustees for an accreditation decision.

The full report and outcome is generally received by the organization in four to six weeks. It is the organization's responsibility to respond to the CARF office by submitting a corrective action report which identifies their plan to address the recommendations made. This report is due in ninety days.

Possible Accreditation Outcomes

At the conclusion of the CARF Board review, they may issue any one of several outcomes:

- Three year accreditation
- One year accreditation
- Nonaccreditation
- Twelve month abeyance
- Six month deferral

A three year accreditation is the most coveted result, which acknowledges that the organization meets the accreditation criteria and substantially fulfills the standards.

A one year accreditation substantiates that the organization meets the accreditation criteria, with evidence of deficiencies in relation to some of the standards, but also with the evidence of capability and commitment of the organization to become compliant.

Nonaccreditation is a judgment that the organization has major deficiencies relative to the standards. It should be noted that when the Accreditation Committee of the Board of Trustees determines not to award accreditation, there is an appeal process available to the organization.

Two options are available to the organization when found to have critical problems precluding its accreditation: a twelve month abeyance or a six month deferral.

A twelve month abeyance is for organizations seeking accreditation for the first time. If the organization is judged to have the capability and commitment to become compliant, it is given an opportunity to conform within the time frame of twelve months. No accreditation decision is rendered until the conclusion of the abeyance process.

A six month deferral is an option offered to those organizations who have been previously surveyed and who demonstrate the capability and commitment to address CARF recommendations. The only difference is the more limited timeframe.

Return visits are scheduled for follow-up reviews of the organizations which have completed the twelve month abeyance or six month deferral periods. Usually one member of the original survey team revisits the organization for one day as a continuation of the survey process. The organization must present evidence of its conformance with the critical recommendations of the abeyance or deferral reports.

Reaccreditation

Approximately six months prior to the expiration date of an accreditation, the Commission will send the organization a new application, and the process starts all over again.

PRESURVEY PREPARATION

The Decision To Seek Accreditation

In some States CARF accreditation is mandated in its Workers' Compensation legislation. Without accreditation no reimbursement for services will be provided. Where it is not mandated, the first decision an organization must make is whether or not to seek CARF accreditation. Figure 22.1 indicates factors that might go into that decision. This decision is not always a simple one. There are associated expenses, as well as programmatic, legal, and reimbursement issues to be considered.

In addition to expenses associated with staffing, space, and equipment to meet the standards, the costs of the survey application and process must also be considered. Once accredited, there are on-going costs in time and money to maintain the standards of program evaluation, safety, program management, program components, documentation, and quality assurance.

Programmatic issues enter into the decision, such as the requirement that four "core" team members be present, including Occupational Therapist, Physical Therapist, Psychologist, and Vocational Specialist.

The organization has to weigh carefully their goals in seeking CARF accreditation. One benefit however, should not be overlooked. The process itself compels an organization to critically look at its standards of service to the clients they serve. The Standards provide guidelines for measuring this quality of service.

Compliance Status

Once an organization decides to seek accreditation, it should be able to demonstrate standards of practice essentially in compliance with the accreditation criteria and Standards of the Commission. An important requirement is that the organization provide services that are up to standard for six months in order to demonstrate their compliance. The appropriate policies need to be in place, appropriate documents and reports generated, as well as all the required case documentation.

Preparation

The author suggests that the organization establishes a task force empowered to prepare the organization for

FIGURE 22.1   Factors that go into the decision to seek CARF accreditation.

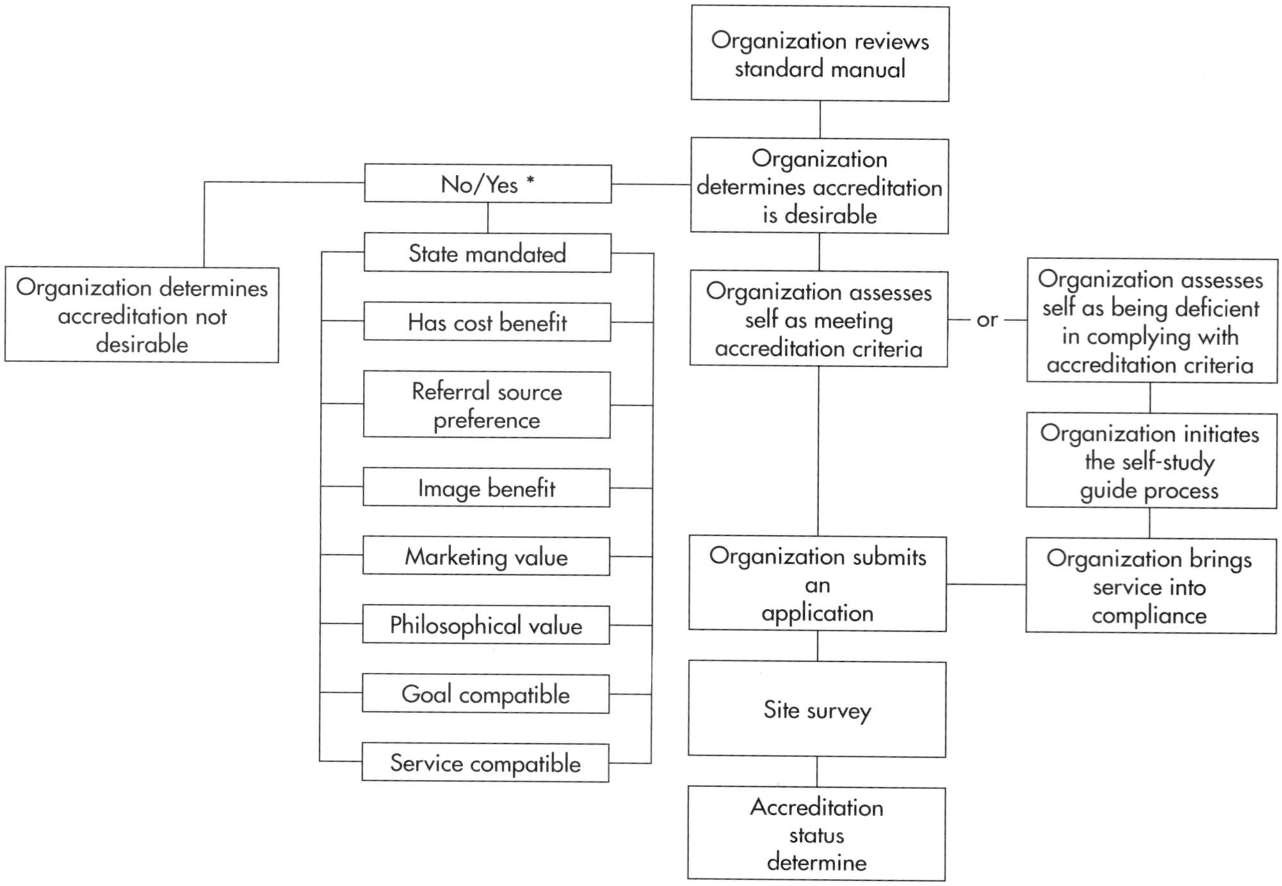

the accreditation process. One helpful document for this process is the *Self Study Questionnaire*. This questionnaire and an application can be obtained from the Commission by writing:

Commission on Accreditation of
Rehabilitation Facilities
101 North Wilmot Road, Suite 500
Tuscon, Arizona 85711

Documentation

One way to address readiness for the survey is to delegate members of the task force specific sections of the Standards to prepare for the survey.

What Management Should Document

Representatives of management should probably prepare the organization for Section 1. The documents most commonly needed to demonstrate compliance with each of the following standards are as follows:

A. **Purposes**
Bylaws, articles of incorporation, other related legal documents
Brochure(s)
Handbook for persons served
Service program descriptions disseminated externally and internally
Records of public information activities
Mission statement

B. **Governance, Organizational Structure, and Ownership**
Bylaws, articles of incorporation, other related legal documents
Governing body minutes and attachments to minutes from meetings
Committee minutes and attachments to minutes from meetings
Roster of governing body members with affiliations and dates of beginning and expiration of terms
Conflict of interest policy and facilitating procedures if governing body is a board

List of names and addresses of owners, partners, officers and directors, as appropriate

C. **Organizational Management**
Legally required licenses, certificates, and reports from such licensure or certification reviews or surveys
Governing body minutes and attachments to minutes from meetings
Committee minutes and attachments to minutes from meetings
Description of chief executive's role
Evaluation of chief executive's performance
Table of organization with dates of establishment and review
Minutes of administrative, managerial, supervisory, and other staff meetings
Administrative policies and procedures manual(s)

D. **Information Management**
Governing body minutes
Management reports, including program evaluation management reports, financial statements, fiscal reports and the results of program quality assessment
Department head meeting minutes
Minutes of administrative, managerial, supervisory, and other staff meetings
Administrative record keeping policies
Reports of results provided to staff and administration
Record retention policy

E. **Program Evaluation**
Governing body policy statement on program evaluation
Governing body minutes
Minutes of administrative, managerial, supervisory, and other staff meetings
Description of program evaluation system
Program evaluation management reports
Organizational brochures, advertisements, etc.
Reports of program evaluation results provided to the governing body, staff and organization's various publics including consumers, purchasers, contributors, and supporters.

F. **Consumer-based Planning**
Documentation containing short- and long-range goals and objectives
Documentation of assessment of consumer needs
Planning documents which include marketing activities

G. **Personnel Administration and Staff Development**
Job descriptions for staff

Policies and procedures to act upon the results of reference checks
Roster of consultants with consultant qualifications
Affiliation agreements
Documentation of frequency of use of consultants and affiliation mechanisms
Personnel policies
Personnel records
Inservice training agenda and minutes
Affiliation agreements with universities and colleges for internship programs
Documentation of participation in and dissemination of information from local, state, and national programs related to the mission of the organization

H. **Fiscal Management**
Governing body minutes and attachments to minutes from meetings
Committee minutes and attachments to minutes from meetings
Policies and procedures for recording, reporting, and control of earnings, expenses, assets and liabilities
Annual budget
Annual audit report with accompanying recommendations and management letter
Policies for administration of funds
Fiscal records and reports including payroll, purchasing, and financial statements
Policies regarding cash management including investment of funds, mechanisms to meet working capital and contingency needs, and cash control
Reports of determination of costs of services or activities
Long-term contracts and agreements to provide services
Schedule of fees for service
Annual fiscal description
Description of risk protection program that includes the file or summary of insurance coverages indicating types, dates, and amounts with limits of coverage
Policies and procedures regarding acknowledgment and receipt of donations, contributions, and bequests
Copies of a sampling of acknowledgement letters
Policies and procedures regarding identification and accountability of expenditure of funds belonging to persons served

I. **Physical Facilities, Health, and Safety**
Copies of fire, health and safety inspection reports
Reports documenting corrective action resulting from fire, health, and safety inspections

Plan for fire and other emergencies

Minutes of safety committee meetings

Records of tests of emergency procedures

Plan for hospital or physician referral

List of person(s) trained in first aid, other emergency care procedures, and fire suppression

Copies of incident reports which include accidents, allegations of abuse, etc.

Policy regarding sale and/or use of smoking products in all locations

Policy and program for prevention and control of infection and adherence to local immunization requirements

Records of equipment maintenance and calibration

Vehicle inspection and maintenance reports, where applicable

Documentation of vehicle operator training and current licenses

Plan for vehicle accidents and road emergencies

What Other Staff Members Should Document

Other members of the task force should prepare the documentation for Section 2. Clinicians can certainly address these standards. The documents most commonly needed to demonstrate compliance with each of the following standards are as follows:

A. **Intake and Orientation**

Entrance and admission criteria for each program

Intake policies and procedures

Individual case records

Records of persons declared ineligible for services

Orientation procedures

B. **Assessment**

Evaluation procedures

Individual case records

C. **Individual Plan Development, Implementation, and Management**

Policies and procedures for case coordination

Individual case records

Minutes of team meetings

Human rights policies

Policies governing the use of restrictive procedures

Policies governing medications

Affiliation and consultation agreements

D. **Referral, Exit or Discharge, and Follow up**

Individual case records

Release of information forms

Exit or discharge criteria for each program

Exit or discharge procedures

Follow up procedures

E. **Records of Persons Served**

Individual case records

Case record review committee minutes

Case record policies

F. **Assessment of Program Quality for Persons Served**

System for review of the persons' programs

Minutes or reports of review findings

Individual case records

Program Compliance

Lastly the task force needs to prepare the organization for the specific programs for which they are seeking accreditation. Representatives of management should probably prepare the organization for these standards. The documents most commonly needed to demonstrate compliance with the standards of this section include:

- Entrance and admission criteria for the program
- Individual case records
- Affiliation or consultation agreements
- Evaluation reports including Functional Capacity Assessments and evaluations of attitudinal and behavioral factors
- Evidence of personnel credentials (degrees, licenses)
- Exit or discharge criteria for the program

Resource Expenditures

As one can well imagine, the services of support staff are critical in this preparation period. A great deal of time is required in generating and assembling all the required documents. The preparation time frame is six months at a minimum, but the author suggests the organization consider a twelve month period to alleviate pressure and enable more completeness.

Each organization must evaluate the time it will require to prepare for the survey process. One must recognize that the organization has to delegate preparation tasks to the most appropriate staff members. Then, they must be given the necessary support and time to complete their assignments. The number of persons involved depends greatly upon the size of the organization.

For clarification of questions or concerns which may arise, do not hesitate to call the CARF office in Tucson. Some organizations seek outside consultants to assist them in the assessment of their readiness for the survey. Organizations must realize that these consultants do not represent CARF, and they cannot guarantee an accreditation outcome. The Commission reserves the right to be the only authorized resource.

Figure 22.2 illustrates suggested time frame to be allotted for the accreditation preparation process.

For those seeking accreditation for programs, the author wishes all success and encourages that the approach to the process be a learning experience and an opportunity to increase the quality of programs for the service of all clientele.

OVERVIEW OF OTHER REGULATORY AGENCIES AND LEGISLATION

Summary Regulations and Legislation

Workers' Compensation's purpose is to transfer the financial burden of a work related injury from the employee to the employer. OSHAs intent is to assure safe and healthful working conditions by requiring employers and employees to reduce work place hazards and implement new or improved safety and health programs.

NIOSH was set up to develop and establish occu-pational safety and health standards, and to engage in research and experimental programs through contracts, grants, or other arrangements. ADA was enacted to eliminate discriminatory hiring and employment practices with regard to disabled individuals.

Workers' Compensation, OSHA, and NIOSH all encourage the employer to control the risks associated with employment. ADA on the other hand pressures employers to give equal opportunity to higher risk populations. All of these regulatory laws and entities require specific employer behaviors. In many cases, however, jurisdictions overlap, provisions are in conflict, and there is little coordination between regulatory bodies.

Potential Impact of ADA

Many employers seeking to hire healthier, lower risk employees have used medical exams or musculoskeletal screens to eliminate job applicants with musculoskeletal deficits, poor body mechanics, insufficient strength, heart disease, or AIDS. Some have also

FIGURE 22.2   Suggested time frames to be allotted for the accreditation preparation process.

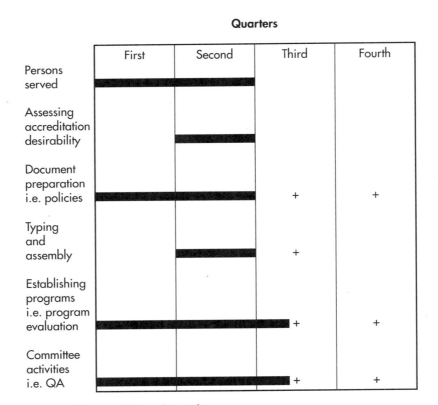

Note + indicates additional time if necessary

consulted Workers' Compensation records to determine any histories of job related injuries or illness.

The implementation of ADA renders all of these strategies illegal. Employees must now be evaluated based on their ability to perform job related functions, not on an assumed risk of injury or a prognosis regarding a current medical problem.

The potential to increase employers' healthcare costs relative to compliance with the ADA is obvious. Individuals who have had previous back problems, or musculoskeletal problems are more likely to reinjure those areas performing job related functions, than those individuals who have not had a previous injury. Yet ADA takes such histories out of consideration.

Many employers are taking a "wait and see" approach to monitor how firmly EEOC enforces the preemployment assessment restrictions stipulated in Title I of the ADA. But employers should recognize that it is only a matter of time before their best strategy will be to comply with both the letter and the spirit of the law.

Therapist Opportunities

For Therapists, these new provisions will increase opportunities to provide industrial therapy services such as physical agility tests, job analyses, and job placement assessments.

It is reasonable to expect that employers will gradually take greater control over the management of their employees' injuries, by developing a process of treatment with rules which providers must follow, if they desire to be players. In this regard, the opportunities that exist for providers of occupational health services are considerable. Analyses and assessments that are statistically reliable and valid can help employers determine essential job functions, write job descriptions, and properly test applicants' and employees' capacities. Therapists can also counsel employers regarding issues of accessibility and reasonable accommodation.

The ADA also opens new avenues for training seminars such as sensitivity training to foremen, supervisors, and employees with regard to people with disabilities and the ADA. Seminars with regard to risk management, attitudes, and motivation are all very viable and valuable services.

Impact on Therapy Services and Reimbursement

At the same time, Industrial Therapists should anticipate that healthcare cost containment will mean tighter reimbursement policies. This will require increasing quality of care while decreasing costs.

The challenge is to develop methods of treatment that meet stricter criteria while remaining economically viable. This means using personnel other than PTs and OTs to cover certain aspects of the practice, so that more highly paid Therapists can concentrate on services only they can provide. New services should be developed that can be provided with minimum additions to capital or staff. The result may be discounted fee schedules to remain price competitive.

In any scenario, reimbursement will eventually be based upon outcome. If providers of occupational health care cannot provide payors with authoritative statistics, demonstrating overall cost savings for specific treatment protocols and outcome criteria, they will encounter great difficulties. Quality and outcome to the payor will depend on the lowest cost to resolve the case.

To the extent that employers will provide feasible emergency and rehabilitation services on their site, multidisciplined work hardening will be reserved for only the most severely involved individuals experiencing delayed recovery. Work simulation will be via reasonable accommodation and early return to work. Both physical agility tests and post offer screening represent great opportunity for the IT to be of service to the employer and the applicant, or employee.

The Liability Issue

Another important issue concerns liability for violations of the ADA. Clearly, it is the employer's responsibility to comply with the ADA. However, Industrial Therapists should accept an ethical and moral obligation to ensure that the employer has been informed of ADA obligations with regard to the services provided.

The impact of these new regulations and legislation are far reaching and comprehensive. Employers face a new set of challenges. Therapists have a broad range of opportunities to assist employers and other entities, in complying and adjusting to the changed environment.

WORKERS' COMPENSATION INSURANCE

Opportunities and Challenges

Industrial Therapy will continue to evolve as a result of changes in the Workers' Compensation system. The continued rise in Workers' Compensation rates and the need for employers to cut costs presents challenges for the industrial professional.

The Industrial Therapist is in an ideal position to help employers through prevention programs, job analysis, on-site therapy services, Functional Capacity Assessments, and return-to-work programs. By collecting data and establishing injury trends, the Industrial

Therapist can help identify problem jobs. Outcomes based reimbursement will reward Therapists who can provide effective treatments.

In order to take advantage of these opportunities, the Industrial Therapist will need to keep abreast of advances in treatment programs, and in the policies and procedures of the Workers' Compensation system.

History

Prior to the industrial revolution, the US was an agriculturally based economy. Nonfarming related jobs were generally located in small shops with many tasks performed by hand. Workers were considered independent free agents, responsible to find and keep employment. It was assumed workers understood the risks associated with their employment and were responsible for their own safety, and in some situations, the safety of coworkers.

The latter half of the nineteenth century brought some significant changes associated with the Industrial Revolution. Rapid industrial expansion created numerous new jobs, so employment was relatively easy to obtain. Many of those new jobs required the use of complicated, powerful, and potentially harmful machines. Probably many workers did not understand the risks involved with these new jobs, therefore, the "assumption of risk" was no longer appropriate.

Under these conditions, when a worker sustained a work related injury, the employer could be sued for damages. The employee had to prove the employer was liable, and since the employer's responsibility related only to work place safety and not the employee's actions, this was nearly impossible. It has been estimated that in the early 1900s only 6% of workers injured on the job received financial relief. Clearly, a need for change existed.

A system was devised whereby the injured employee would waive the right to sue the employer for damages and, in turn, the employer would assume responsibility for the injury, regardless of the circumstances. New York was the first state to enact a Workers' Compensation Law in 1910. Other states rapidly followed.

General Overview

Workers' Compensation laws vary from state to state. Therefore, it is very important to understand the Workers' Compensation laws of the state in which services are being provided. There are some common features among all the states.

The purpose of Workers' Compensation is to transfer the financial burden of a work related injury from the employee to the employer. The costs for Workers' Compensation is paid by the employer to a state Workers' Compensation fund or an insurer. These costs of course are passed along to the consumer. Some states permit the employees or employers to choose between the Workers' Compensation system and civil courts to settle claims arising from work related injuries. This choice must be established before an accident occurs.

Each state determines the kind of employment and types of injuries covered. Worker's benefits are usually determined by the State and listed on a schedule. This schedule includes compensation benefits to replace lost salary, a fixed dollar amount for the loss of various body parts, monetary compensation for bodily disfigurement, and death benefits. In certain situations an employee may appeal a decision made by the Workers' Compensation Commission Board to that Board or through a civil court.

Information regarding state Workers' Compensation laws can be obtained by contacting the Workers' Compensation Commission listed in the phone book. It is usually listed under the "State Government" section under "Workers' Compensation" or as a sub listing under "Department of Labor and Employment." Other useful information regarding Workers' Compensation can be obtained from the State Insurance Commissioner or the library.

Clinical Significance

The Workers' Compensation system of the 1970s was a very Therapist-friendly system. There were numerous patients available to be treated who were covered by Workers' Compensation, and this number seemed to grow almost daily. Workers' Compensation historically paid for "physical problems" caused by "physical causative agents."

If a worker stuck a hand in a press (physical agent) and sustained a crushing injury to the hand (the physical problem), Workers' Compensation paid for Physical Therapy and Occupational Therapy to restore function to the hand. In 1970 Workers' Compensation benefits paid claims amounting to about $3 billion nationally.

Over the next several years benefits were extended to include mental problems caused by physical causative agents. If the individual with the hand injury is unable to return to the job for fear of reinjury (a mental or emotional problem), retraining (vocational rehabilitation) may be necessary, and is covered by Workers' Compensation.

Impact On Providers

Rehabilitation clinicians' interest in treating work related injuries increased in the early 1980s. Workers' Compensation benefits were expanded to include mental factors (job related stress) causing physical problems (ulcers) and mental factors (job related stress), causing mental problems (inability to work) due to the stress.

Work Hardening, practically unknown to Workers' Compensation payors in 1980, became very familiar to clinicians and painfully familiar to all Workers' Compensation payors by the late 1980s. Personnel, equipment, and other costs to provide services rapidly escalated, resulting in commensurate increases in fees for services provided, and contributing to a general rise in healthcare costs. A growing number of underinsured and uninsured people received care that had to be subsidized by the fully insured. Attorneys' fees added to the cost of settlements.

In response, Health Maintenance Organizations (HMO), and Preferred Provider Organizations (PPO) were beginning to proliferate, requiring a discounted fee schedule by their providers. All of these factors have applied pressure on providers and payors.

Many providers and payors reacted by shifting costs to Workers' Compensation cases. By 1980 Workers' Compensation benefits totaled $13.6 billion—a 453% increase over 1970. Workers' Compensation coverage was extended to almost any procedure, modality, or service. Documentation requirements were minimal and reimbursement was generally based upon a fee for service. By 1989 Workers' Compensation paid benefits amounted to $34.3 billion, equal to one-third of US business profits being spent on health care.

It is no wonder Workers' Compensation reform has become a major issue. Workers' Compensation payors' efforts to manage this situation began with requiring more detailed documentation to use for case management, including utilization review. This was followed by a series of fee schedule revisions designed to limit disbursements for rehabilitation services. These systems include reimbursement based upon relative value units, establishing maximum reimbursement rates per treatment or per case for services rendered. It won't be long before services will be reimbursed based upon outcome. It is possible that reimbursement may be paid as agreed if the outcome is achieved and less, or no, reimbursement if the desired outcome is not reached.

The trend for the future will continue to be an expansion of illnesses and injuries covered by Workers' Compensation. As more specialized jobs are developed and workers are confined to fewer job tasks, we may discover types of over-use injuries heretofore not recognized. Eye and neck strain caused by constant viewing of a video display terminal is one possibility.

Efforts to control disbursements will be through case management, stringent reimbursement rates and procedures, and by encouraging employers to improve worksite safety. Workers' Compensation will undergo many reforms but will probably remain state con-

trolled. It is probable that Workers' Compensation and OSHA will work more closely to coordinate their activities.

OSHA AND NIOSH

Opportunities and Challenges

OSHAs standards and regulations for work place safety will continue to broaden over time, and will continue to increase focus on ergonomics. As a result, employers will be looking for assistance to prevent OSHA citations and fines. This provides a multitude of opportunities for the Industrial Therapist in the areas of job design, modification, ergonomics, employee selection, placement, training, risk assessment and management, and health care administration.

General Overview

On December 29, 1970 Congress created the Occupational Safety and Health Administration within the Department of Labor. The act, officially known as Public Law 91–596, was amended November 5, 1990 by Public Law 101–552. OSHAs purpose is to assure safe and healthful working conditions for working men and women. It does this by requiring employers and employees to reduce work place hazards and to implement new or improve existing safety and health programs.

Through grants and other means OSHA encourages research into occupational safety and health. It established a reporting and record keeping system to monitor job related illnesses and injuries. OSHA has also been empowered to provide standards for the work place environment and the means to enforce them.

The act covers all employers and their employees in fifty states, (state and local governments are not covered under OSHA), but does not include self-employed persons, farms where employees are only the immediate members of the farm employer's family, and working conditions that are regulated by other federal agencies and statutes.

The Development of OSHA Standards

The Secretary of Labor is empowered to promulgate occupational safety and health standards. This may be done on OSHAs own initiative or in response to petitions from other agencies such as Health and Human Services (HHS), the National Institute of Occupational Safety and Health (NIOSH), state and local governments, any national or recognized standards producing organization, employer or labor representative, or any other interested person.

Such standards may be altered on the basis of information obtained by the Secretary. As part of this process, OSHA is required to conduct research experiments and demonstrations relating to occupational safety and health including all of the various factors involved with employment.

NIOSH, the National Institute of Occupational Safety and Health was set up in 1970 by the same act that established OSHA. The institute was originally directed by the Secretary of Health, Education, and Welfare, which has been renamed Health and Human Services. The institute is authorized to develop and establish occupational safety and health standards, and to engage in research and experimental programs through contracts, grants, or other arrangements.

One of the most valuable publications produced by NIOSH is the "Work Practices Guide for Manual Lifting" which can be obtained by contacting:

NIOSH
Publications Dissemination, DSDTT
Division of Standards
4676 Columbia Parkway
Cincinnati, Ohio 45226

For information on other occupational safety and health problems,

call 1-800-35-NIOSH (1-800-356-4674)

This 183 page guide provides many important things to know about manual lifting. It discusses several methods of addressing manual lifting at the work place including: epidemialogical, biomechanical, physiological, and psychophysical approaches. The reference also addresses administrative, engineering controls and recommendations, and must be read by any provider of Occupational Health Services.

Once OSHA has established a standard, it publishes it in the Federal Register as an "advanced notice of proposed rule making," or as a "notice of proposed rule making." This will give the public and other interested parties at least 30 days to respond. Such interested parties may request a public hearing on the proposal. OSHA then publishes the full text of any standard, amended or adopted, and other pertinent information in the Federal Register.

OSHA may bypass this process and establish a temporary standard if they feel workers are in grave danger due to exposure to toxic or hazardous substances. OSHA will then go through the normal process, and the temporary standard will be replaced by one that is permanent. Within 60 days of the rules promulgation, anyone adversely affected by an OSHA standard may file a petition with the US Court of Appeals for a review of the standard.

An employer may ask OSHA for a variance from a standard if they cannot fully comply by the effective date. The request for variance is based upon the inability to comply due to shortages of technical personnel, materials, or equipment, or the belief that the employer's own standard meets or exceeds the standard being promulgated by OSHA.

A temporary variance may be granted for a period of one year and renewed twice, each time for six months. If an employer is able to prove the conditions, practices, and means of operation provide a safe and healthful work place, as effectively, or more so than would be the case in complying with the OSHA standard, a permanent variance may be issued.

Compliance

Employers have the responsibility to be familiar and in compliance with mandatory OSHA standards. These standards include minimizing or reducing work place hazards to make the work place a safer environment; informing all employees about OSHA and their rights and responsibilities; and providing all of the documentation and other activities required by OSHA.

Employers of eleven or more employees must maintain records of occupational injuries and illness as they occur. The obligation to comply with these requirements would pertain to a Therapist if they employ 11 or more employees. The purpose of these records is to enable the Bureau of Labor Statistics to define high hazard industries, and to inform employees of the status of their employer's record.

For the purposes of recording injuries and illness, OSHA requires employers to maintain OSHA form #200, "Log and Summary of Occupational Injuries and Illness." Each and every recordable occupational injury or illness must be reported on this form within six working days from the time the employer is informed of it.

Fatal accidents must be reported within 48 hours. If this log is maintained at a central location by a computer, the employer is permitted up to 45 calendar days to have a hard copy present at the satellite location. This form would assist an IT in better understanding the needs of the business and how to design services to meet those needs, by reviewing the injury record.

Enforcement

OSHA is authorized to conduct work place inspections by OSHA Compliance Safety and Health Officers. Inspections may be conducted without advanced notice, and are normally prioritized in order of importance. The highest priority are situations where imminent danger is present. This is defined as any condition where there is a reasonable certainty that a danger exists, which can be expected to cause death or serious physical harm, before that danger could be eliminated through normal enforcement procedures.

The second priority is given to the investigation of accidents in which there are fatalities, or catastrophes resulting in hospitalization of five or more employees.

The third priority is given to employee complaints of alleged violation of OSHA standards or unsafe or unhealthy working conditions. In researching the complaint, the compliance officer explains to the employer why the place of business was selected for inspection. An authorized employer and employee representative is given the opportunity to attend this opening conference and to accompany the officer during the inspection.

After the opening conference, the inspection takes place. After inspection, a closing conference is held by the compliance officer with the employer or employer representative. The results of the inspection are discussed with the employer. These findings are then relayed to the area OSHA Director to determine what citations, if any, will be issued, and what penalties will be proposed.

OSHAs fines can be quite substantial and occasionally exceed the million dollar figure. OSHA, therefore, commands considerable attention from the employer community. Employees are becoming more inclined to complain to OSHA regarding work place safety.

In an effort to better define what constitutes a safe working environment, OSHA is establishing ergonomic guidelines which will send companies scurrying to perform analyses to make sure they are in compliance. This provides opportunities for ITs to perform job site analyses, physical agility tests, pre and post offer functional and musculoskeletal screens, training seminars and other services depending upon technical and selling expertise.

Ergonomics is the next frontier for OSHA, which in combination with OSHAs growing authority will cause an increase in the amount and frequency of fines. Consequently, there will be increased motivation for employers to look for assistance in job design, employee selection, training, risk, and health care management, all of which represent areas of opportunity for Industrial Therapy services.

Information regarding OSHA is available by writing:

> OSHA Publications Office
> 200 Constitution Avenue, NW
> Room N-3101
> Washington, DC 20210

There are 25 OSHA approved state plans. These are also available from OSHA at the above address.

AMERICANS WITH DISABILITIES ACT

Opportunities and Challenges

The enactment of the ADA has required employers to evaluate their human resource practices. This law provides equal employment opportunities for the disabled by making it illegal to discriminate against a qualified individual if they can perform the essential functions of the job with or without reasonable accommodation.

The opportunity for the Industrial Therapist lies in helping employers to objectively and accurately determine the "essential functions" of each job, the functional capabilities of each worker, and the accommodations required to bring the two into alignment. Accordingly, efforts to comply with the ADA will significantly expand the demand for preoffer Physical Agility Tests, postoffer Job Placement Assessments, Job Analyses, ergonomic audits, job design, and job modification.

General Overview

In the preface to the Americans with Disabilities Act it is stated that:

> *The U.S. Congress has estimated that there are 43,000,000 Americans that have one or more physical or mental disabilities. Discrimination against these individuals exists in areas including employment, housing, and access to goods and services, to name a few. Congress has also determined that as a group, people with disabilities occupy an inferior status in our society. This costs the government billions of dollars in unnecessary expenses resulting from dependency on government programs and nonproductivity.*

Therefore, Public Law 101–336, better known as the "Americans with Disabilities Act of 1990," (ADA) was signed into law by President George Bush on July 26, 1990. The purpose of this law is to give disabled Americans equal opportunities in employment, and accessibility to goods, services, and programs provided by either public or private entities.

The ADAs definitions and terminology conform to the definitions and terminology in the Rehabilitation Act of 1973, and use the same enforcement provisions of Title VII of the Civil Rights Acts of 1964. As revised, the ADA is essentially a civil rights act for the disabled.

This law affects everyone living in the US in one way or another. The rules and regulations implementing this law are not specific, leaving them open for more than one interpretation. This causes difficulty in complying with the letter and the spirit of the law. In some legal circles the ADA has been facetiously called the "lawyer relief act."

The fear and trepidation regarding this law are most pronounced among those who are least knowledgeable about its provisions. This is also true with health care clinicians who must comply with the provisions of this law as employers, providers of care, and advisors to industry.

As providers of IT it is necessary to thoroughly understand the provisions of this law as it affects the structure and administration of the services provided. In attempting to sell IT services, knowledge of ADA will be tested by the people to whom services are being proposed. Failing the test, can lose the business.

The ADA has far reaching effects. It has been said that the best way to predict the future is to create it. An in depth understanding of ADA provides an opportunity to do just that. Most employees are familiar with the first definition of disability (a physical or mental impairment that substantially limits a major life activity). It is well known that the preceding law has not covered an individual with a sprained ankle. The ADA expands the definition of disability.

If an employer refused to hire an individual with a sprained ankle out of a concern that the ankle would limit the ability to perform the job, that employer would be treating this individual as disabled, and the applicant would be covered under the ADA.

Another instance pertains to reasonable accommodation. Many employers still insist on an injured employee being fully recovered and able to perform all job functions before returning to work. The ADA requires that an employer allow an injured employee to resume work if that employee is able to perform the essential functions of the job, with or without reasonable accommodation. This opens opportunity to provide services on the employer's site to assist the injured employee to return to gainful employment much earlier than would otherwise be the case.

This will be the next revolution in "Work Hardening." The employer benefits from reduced costs associated with a faster return to work. These opportunities require an in depth knowledge of ADA and flexibility to design services that will meet the needs of the employer.

The law may not be as complicated as it might initially seem. So it is hoped that by reading this chapter, Therapists will have a basic knowledge of the ADA and be motivated to become very knowledgeable with regard to the provisions.

There are five parts or "Titles" that comprise the ADA:

Title I
Equal employment opportunity for individuals with Disabilities.
Effective: July 26, 1992 for employers with 25 or more employees
July 26, 1994 for employers with 15 or more employees

Title II
Nondiscrimination on the basis of disability in state and local government services.
Effective: January 26, 1992

Title III
Nondiscrimination on the basis of disability by public accommodations and in commercial facilities.
Effective: January 26, 1992

Title IV
Telecommunications: Service for hearing-impaired and speech-impaired individuals.
Effective: July 26, 1993

Title V
Miscellaneous Provisions

These Titles will be reviewed in enough detail to give you a solid foundation in understanding the ADA and how the ADA effects the provision of clinical services and hiring practices. Titles I and III will be presented in more detail than Titles II, IV, and V, as they have greater impact on IT.

These titles create the need for the employer to determine what they must do to comply with the Law. The employer or business operator must meet accessibility requirements and comply with hiring and employment regulations. If an employer chooses to comply with the Law, the choices are to study the law independently, use an internal expert, or hire a Therapist.

Please be aware that what follows is a summary. Therapists should obtain additional information regarding the ADA by contacting the source indicated at the end of the description of each Title.

Title I Provisions

Summary Parameters

Purpose: To provide equal employment opportunity for the disabled by making it illegal to discriminate against a qualified individual with a disability for employment if such individual can perform the essential job functions with or without reasonable accommodation.

Who is Covered: Employers, employment agencies, labor organizations or joint labor-management committees with 25 or more employees as of July 26, 1992. Those with 15 or more employees are covered as of July 26, 1994. The US Government, Indian tribes, and tax exempt private membership clubs are exempt.

Opportunities and Challenges

Efforts to comply with Title I of the ADA will significantly expand the demand for Job Analyses to establish the essential job functions, and to determine job modifications that may be made to reasonably accommodate a disabled individual. In addition, since the ADA allows Physical Agility Testing preoffer, the Industrial Therapist can help the employer develop a compliant testing scheme.

Qualified Individual

A qualified individual is someone who meets the requisite education, experience, skills, and other job related requirements of the position held or desired to be held, and who can, with or without reasonable accommodation, perform the essential job functions.

Disability

There are three categories of "disability" against which the applicant or worker is protected from discriminatory employment practices. Industrial Therapists will be called upon to help determine if a person is limited in a major life activity through orthopedic exams and Functional Capacity Assessments.

In addition, the increasing emphasis on Job Analysis and essential job functions will make hiring and placement decisions more objective, accurate, legally defensible, and fair.

The first category of protected disability is physical or mental impairment that substantially limits one or more of the major life activities (walking, seeing, learning) of an individual. Physical or mental impairment includes any physiological disorder, cosmetic disfigurement, or anatomical loss involving nerves, muscles, bones, or vital organs.

Disability does not include physical characteristics such as left-handedness, hair color, obesity (in most cases), or height or personality traits such as a quick temper, or poor judgment. Also excluded are conditions that are not physiological disorders, such as pregnancy, cultural or economic disadvantages, or illiteracy.

Fractures, sprains, and colds are usually temporary

in nature and are not therefore considered to be disabilities. However, complications arising as a result of these conditions might cause a longer than usual rehabilitation time and result in significant limitations in one or more major life activities, and therefore be considered a disability.

Mitigating circumstances are not to be considered in the determination of impairment. A lower extremity amputee who is able to walk with the use of a prosthesis is still considered to be disabled because without the prosthesis he would be substantially limited in the major life activity of walking.

It is clear that protection under ADA is made on a case by case basis considering the impact an impairment has on that individual's major life activities.

The second category of protected disability is when a person has a record of a substantially limiting impairment. PT and OT are two disciplines mentioned in the regulations as a source of records attesting to a disability, which could be through a Functional Capacity Assessment. The purpose of this category is to protect those who may have had a history of a disease or disorder which is presently cured, controlled, or in a state of remission.

This will protect from discrimination, those with a history of cancer, heart disease, or other disabling ailments. It will also protect those who may have been misdiagnosed in the past for a learning disability or psychological disorder. "Official records" attesting to such histories include school records, Workers' Compensation files, and medical records.

The third protected category of disability is discrimination due to fears, myths, and stereotypes about a particular condition. Such prejudice may come from the employer who denies a promotion due to the employee's high blood pressure on the notion that the increased stress might cause a heart attack.

Or the prejudice may stem from the attitude of others, as in the case of a burn victim whose facial disfigurement is thought to preclude jobs involving public contact. The prejudice may also be toward a condition that is not disabling but thought to be so, such as HIV. Employment decisions prejudiced by any of the above invalid notions would be in violation of the ADA.

Essential Job Function

This term means those functions which are necessary to perform a particular job. The Industrial Therapist can be part of a team that determines which job functions are "essential" to each job on a case by case basis. By bringing objective, reliable measurement protocols to this process, Therapists can play a key role in developing job descriptions that are compliant with the ADA, and if necessary, legally defensible.

"Essential job functions" do not include "marginal" job activities which are desirable but not essential to the job. There are several reasons why a job function may be considered "essential:"

1. The position exists to perform that function. An individual hired as a transcriptionist must be able to type. It's the reason the job exists.
2. There are a limited number of others to whom the function can be distributed. Answering the telephone would also be an essential function for the transcriptionist mentioned above, if there were no one else available to perform that function.
3. The function is highly specialized. If a large part of a business's clientele are Spanish speaking only, being bilingual may be an essential function.

The ADA and its regulations provide several examples of evidence to be considered in determining whether or not a job function is essential. The list below is not all inclusive and not prioritized in terms of importance. Items not included on the list may be equal in importance to those on the list. Evidence to be considered in determining essential job functions include:

1. The employer's judgment. EEOC (Equal Employment Opportunity Commission, the enforcement agency for ADA Title I) will rely on the employer's judgment regarding identification of essential job functions. While the EEOC does not intend to second guess the employer's production standards, the validity of those standards may be checked.
2. Written job descriptions. Job descriptions are not *required* by the ADA but will probably be *necessary* in defending the employer's determination of essential job functions. Caution is given to make sure job descriptions are accurate. The EEOC may also perform a "reality check" to validate the tasks described.
3. The amount of time spent performing the function. If an employee spends the majority of their time performing a particular function, it is strong evidence that the function is essential.
4. The consequence if the particular function is not performed. Even though a firefighter may only have to carry a person out of a burning building occasionally, it would be an essential function due to the consequence of not performing the function.
5. The terms of a collective bargaining agreement. This may affect what are considered to be the essential functions of a job.
6. The work experience of past and current employees performing similar jobs.
7. Other relevant factors which include the nature of the work procedures and the organizational structure. An employer may require employees to work in teams, each employee performing only one task, but on a rotating basis, so that each employee is required to perform all of the tasks over a period of time. In this case, all such functions would be considered essential as long as this is consistent with business necessity.

It is important to determine the essential job functions on a case by case basis. Considering the usual job functions for Therapists—taking a history; performing an evaluation; interpreting the data; establishing and implementing a treatment plan—which would be considered essential? The answer depends on the specific situation.

In a one person department, it may be that a Therapist's responsibility is to provide passive range of motion, set up the exercise equipment, assist the patient in exercise routines, prepare the hot packs, and assist the patient into the whirlpool. In a large department these functions could be distributed to a number of Therapist Assistants, aides, or other personnel, so that a disabled person could be assigned performable tasks. In the one person department, a disabled person may not be able to perform the essential functions.

It is also very important to define the essential functions in terms of the expected outcome, not in the method to achieve that outcome. In the case of a Therapist, documenting the results of an initial evaluation is an important function. It would be inappropriate to say that the Therapist must write the evaluation in the patient notes, since it would be possible for a manually impaired person to dictate the notes to a stenographer or to a word processor that understands the spoken word. The important thing is to note that recording the results of the evaluation is the essential function and not the means of achieving that outcome.

The point of this section is that even though job descriptions are not required by the ADA, employers would be better positioned to comply with the Law if they had written job descriptions. It must be kept in mind that a job description is not required to identify essential job functions. This is an opportunity for the Industrial Therapist to assist the employer by performing a job analysis. The Therapist should be able to assist in that exercise equipped with an understanding of the rules governing the determination of essential functions, and knowing that "essential functions" are a moving target.

Reasonable Accommodation

This term refers to modifications or adjustments to the job or work environment to enable an impaired individual to enjoy an equal employment opportunity. The Industrial Therapist can assist in assessing the nature and cost of accommodations by comparing Functional Capacity Assessment results with a Job Analysis, possibly incorporating ergonomic analysis, and making recommendations accordingly.

Reasonable accommodation also includes an equal opportunity for disabled individuals to apply for the job. All information regarding the job should be in accessible formats. This may include accessible entry for the mobility impaired, braille application forms or a reader for a blind person, a sign interpreter for a deaf person, and oral applications and tests for dyslexic individuals.

If an advertisement for a job lists a phone number as the only method to obtain information, a telephone relay service or TDD (telecommunication device for the deaf) must be provided. The principle to remember here is to be sure the application and testing procedures emphasize abilities and measure job related functions.

The employer is required to make accommodations only for known disabilities. If unaware of a need, the employer cannot be held responsible. It is generally the responsibility of the person who needs an accommodation to inform the employer. The employer is responsible to inform all applicants and employees of their obligation to request reasonable accommodation.

When a reasonable accommodation is requested the employer may request documentation of the functional limitations justifying the request. Such documentation can be obtained from a variety of sources including Functional Assessments performed by Physical and Occupational Therapists.

Job application forms should not ask any questions related to disability. The following questions cannot be asked:

Have you been hospitalized in the last five years?
Have you ever been treated for a mental illness?
Were you absent from work in the last year?
Check off the following diseases or illnesses that you have had (followed by a checklist).

In job interviews, applicants may be asked questions about abilities, but not about disabilities. Before an offer of employment, an employer may not inquire from any source regarding the applicants illness, disabilities, or Workers' Compensation history. It may be in the best interest of both the employer and the job applicant to administer a physical agility test which will be described later.

If skill tests are administered, they must be related to essential job functions, and they must be administered to all applicants. Job requirements including attendance requirements may be described to the applicant and the applicants may be asked if they can meet those requirements.

The exception is that where an obvious disability might likely affect the applicant's ability to perform an essential job function, the individual may be asked to tell or show how they would perform that essential function.

A man with an obvious hip disarticulation (and no prosthesis) may apply for a job as a brick layer which requires walking across narrow scaffolding. He may not be asked about the nature, severity, or prognosis of the disability, but he may be asked to tell or show how he would negotiate the scaffolding. This is permitted even if the employer does not require every applicant to demonstrate this ability, because this particular applicant's obvious disability would appear to prevent the performance of an essential job function.

If this same applicant applies for a job as a typist, the employer may not ask him to describe or demonstrate how he could perform typing functions, unless all applicants for this job were asked to do so. That is because the obvious disability is not related to typing performance. The key is to ask questions in terms of ability.

The employer is also responsible to provide reasonable accommodation to permit a qualified employee with a disability, to perform the essential functions of the job they hold, or desire to hold. Such accommodations may include making facilities accessible to disabled individuals, redistributing marginal job functions, modifying job schedules, reassignment to a vacant position (reassignment is an accommodation available to employees but not to job applicants), or providing unpaid leave for necessary treatment.

For a Therapist who is unable to perform transfers, it may be a reasonable accommodation to require an aide or some other personnel to assist them in that procedure. These and any other accommodations must be determined on a case by case basis.

Equal Access To Benefits and Privileges

The employer is also responsible to provide equal opportunity to enable an employee with a disability, to enjoy the benefits and privileges of employment equal to nondisabled employees in similar roles. In addition to equal opportunity regarding pay and promotion, this means access to lunch rooms, employee lounges, exercise rooms, meeting rooms, company sponsored social and educational events, participation in insurance programs, vacation, and other benefits.

In companies with employee fitness programs or facilities, the Industrial Therapist can be an advisor regarding modifications that will enable disabled employees to have equal access and benefits.

There are several funding sources available to assist employers in making reasonable accommodations to comply with ADA.

1. Eligible small businesses (defined as a business with gross sales of $1 million or less or with 30 or fewer employees) may take a tax credit for 50% of the cost of "eligible access expenditures" that are more than $250, but less than $10,250. This amounts to a maximum tax credit of $5,125 per year. This tax credit applies to accommodations to comply with Title III as well.

2. Any business may take a full tax deduction, up to $15,000 per year, for expenses of removing architectural and transportation barriers. Both the tax credit and the tax deduction are available to eligible small businesses but double dipping is not allowed. For an expenditure of $24,000, a tax credit would be taken for the first $10,250 of expenditures amounting to $5,125.00. The remaining amount could be deducted ($13,750) from taxable income.

3. Other funding sources can be found by contacting appropriate state or local organizations.

A point to ponder is whether an on-site graduated return to work program constitutes a period of "reasonable accommodation" that qualifies for deductions and tax credits.

Undue Hardship

Undue hardship is a defense that an employer can use for not making an accommodation. An undue hardship is an action that requires "significant difficulty or expense" in relation to the employer's size, resources available, and the nature of the operation. This includes any action that is unduly costly, extensive, substantial, disruptive, or that would fundamentally alter the nature or the operation of the business.

As with many other provisions of the ADA, undue hardship must be determined on a case by case basis. In general, a larger employer would be required to make accommodations requiring greater effort or expense than a smaller employer.

Using Job Placement Assessment in combination with Job Analysis and possible FCA and ergonomic analysis, the Industrial Therapist can work with engineers and financial people to objectively develop and cost out reasonable accommodation alternatives.

The cost of the accommodation used in determining undue hardship is the actual or net cost to the employer. The funding sources available to assist employers in making reasonable accommodations, including tax credits and tax deductions described earlier, funding from other sources, and even the assistance from the individual requesting an accommodation are subtracted from the total cost in determining whether or not the accommodation presents undue hardship.

Thus, only the net cost to the employer is considered in determining undue hardship.

In addition to cost, the effect that the accommodation would have on the over all operation of the business is also considered in determining undue hardship. Suppose an individual with a visual impairment applies for a job as a waiter in a dinner theater. As an accommodation, he might request the lights be turned up so he can write down dinner orders. Even though this accommodation would require little if any extra money, the effect of turning the lights up in a dinner theater would fundamentally alter the nature of the business and therefore would be considered an undue hardship.

Another example would be an individual who requests that the temperature in the work environment be elevated to accommodate a disability. If this temperature would create an uncomfortable environment for other employees, this would be considered an undue hardship. However, in complying with the letter and the spirit of the law, the employer may be required to provide a separate space with a suitable temperature for that individual.

An employer may not claim an undue hardship because the morale of nondisabled employees would suffer, as a result of creating a reasonable accommodation for a disabled employee. An employer may not claim an undue hardship, because the cost of the accommodation is high in relationship to the disabled employees' salary.

Direct Threat

"Direct Threat" means that an individual poses a significant risk of substantial harm to themselves, or others, that cannot be eliminated or reduced by a reasonable accommodation. However, even if a Direct Threat is thought to exist, reasonable accommodation to reduce this risk must be considered.

The Industrial Therapist can provide defensible medical evidence that can be interfaced with other objective documentation, to support a Direct Threat determination. The Therapist may then participate in objectively analyzing whether reasonable accommodation is possible, to eliminate the Direct Threat circumstances.

Direct Threat as a defense for not providing a reasonable accommodation, or in denying employment must meet certain criteria:

1. There must be a significant risk of substantial harm, and not merely a slightly increased risk. An individual who has suffered from narcolepsy for the past 20 years might seriously endanger his or her own life, as well as the lives of others, if they were employed as a crane operator. However, that same person

would not pose a severe threat if employed in a clerical job.

2. The risk must be current and imminent, not speculative or remote. The fact that an individual might suffer from degenerative disk disease five or ten years in the future is not significant enough risk (not imminent) to be considered a Direct Threat. The determination of Direct Threat must be based upon the most recent medical evidence including documentation from medical doctors, psychologists, rehabilitation counselors, physical or occupational Therapists, and others who have expertise in the disability involved and or a knowledge of the individual with a disability.

There are four criteria that must be considered in determining Direct Threat with each being a threshold test for the next. In other words an individual must meet all four criteria to be considered a Direct Threat. These criteria are as follows:

1. Duration of the threat
2. The nature and severity of the threat
3. The likelihood that harm will occur
4. The imminence of the harm that might occur

The duration of the threat must qualify as long term. A sprained ankle probably would not qualify, whereas AIDS would. As with many of its provisions, the ADA is not specific with regard to what constitutes adequate duration to meet this test.

The nature of the risk relates to the pathology and the extent to which it affects job function. A back injury will affect job function if the job involves heavy lifting. It will not in the case of a sedentary job.

As to the likelihood that harm will occur, there must be a high probability, but again the ADA is not definitive.

As with many aspects of the ADA, Direct Threat must be established on a case by case basis, with full knowledge of the criteria for its determination.

Medical Examinations and Inquiries

The ADA governs permissibility of medical testing preemployment and post employment.

Physical Agility Tests

These tests are not considered to be medical exams and therefore can be done at any point in the hiring process. The EEOC does not specifically define a physical agility test. By law, agility tests need not be job related or consistent with business necessity unless they tend to screen out individuals or groups with disabilities. It would be hard to defend, however, that a physical agility test does not discriminate against some disability group. It might be wise, therefore, to voluntarily design agility tests that are job related and consistent with business necessity.

The Industrial Therapist can help develop physical agility tests that objectively relate to essential job functions as determined by Job Analyses. Properly designed, the Physical Agility Test may also provide baseline data of preinjury status, and may be an input in determining direct threat and reasonable accommodation parameters.

If an employer is going to use an agility test prior to an offer of employment, the employer must ask all individuals in that particular job category to submit to the same test. An exception to this rule is when an individual with an obvious disability may be asked to show how they would perform a particular job, without the employer being obligated to request this demonstration of all candidates.

Physical agility testing prior to an offer of employment will entail more testing than a post offer test. Accordingly, preoffer agility tests are cost-justified only where the job involves difficult or critical job demands and the tests are affordable. A physical agility test would be appropriate for an employer who has a job category that requires employees to manually lift 75 pounds from waist height and place it over their shoulders (and no reasonable accommodation can be made). An agility test probably would not be justified in a job category that does not have such strenuous demands.

Preoffer

Prior to an offer of employment an employer may not require a job applicant to take a medical exam, respond to medical inquiries, or provide information about Workers' Compensation claims. An employer may not ask an individual about a disability even if it is very obvious (such as an individual who has an upper extremity amputation). However, an employer may describe to such an individual the essential job functions and ask the individual to tell, or show, how they would perform these tasks.

Post Offer

After an offer of employment has been made, the employer may require the employee to undergo a medical exam and make employment conditional upon passing the exam. At this point the IT could provide a valuable service for both the employer and the employee by administering a musculoskeletal and functional screen. The purposes would be to:

1. Collect base line information which should be used should the employee become injured. The obvious purpose is to determine the injured employee's preinjury status and the

employer's responsibility regarding medical treatment and rehabilitation

2. To determine if a Direct Threat exists
3. To determine if an accommodation is necessary, and what it would be
4. To determine if the employee is capable of performing certain job functions, especially if a physical agility test was not performed prior to an employment offer being made

Drug Testing

At the preoffer stage, the employer is permitted to request drug testing, as this is not considered to be a medical exam. Individuals who are engaging in the illegal use of drugs under the Controlled Substance Act are not protected by the ADA. This also includes the illegal use of controlled prescription drugs such as amphetamines which are legally prescribed but also "controlled" because of the potential for abuse.

Alcoholism

Under the ADA an alcoholic is a person with a disability. Nevertheless, the ADA does not prevent efforts to combat the use of drugs and alcohol in the workplace. The employer may prohibit the use of drugs and alcohol in the workplace. The employer may require that employees not be under the influence of alcohol or drugs in the workplace and require that employees who illegally use drugs meet the same production standards that apply to other employees.

An employer may deny employment or discharge an alcoholic if the use of alcohol adversely affects job performance. Such an individual would be considered "nonqualified." It is important to note that the employer may not discipline an alcoholic employee more severely than it would a nonalcoholic employee.

Enforcement

The enforcement agency for Title I is the Equal Employment Opportunity Commission (EEOC). Any individual or group of individuals may file a complaint with the EEOC if they feel that discrimination on the basis of disability has taken place. If there is no EEOC office, the EEOC can be called toll free at 1-800-669-4000 (voice) or 1-800-800-3302 (TDD). A complaint must be filed within 180 days of the alleged discriminatory act. In certain cases this may be extended up to 300 days.

The Industrial Therapist's involvement can work in the company's favor in defending against complaints. First, enlisting the services of Industrial Therapists represents a good faith effort to comply with ADA regulations. Second, the Industrial Therapist's objective measurement, analysis, and recommended accommodations represent a sound line of defense against frivolous or fraudulent claims, or attempts to manipulate the law.

The information that will be requested by the EEOC is the charging party's and the employer's name, address, and telephone number, the charging party's disability, the details and date of the discrimination, the names of any witnesses, and the issues involved.

Discrimination charges may be filed on more than one basis. A person may be the victim of sex, race, and disability discrimination simultaneously. In such a case, the employer would be responsible to pay for damages due in each of the areas.

The EEOC has up to 180 days to reach a decision. They may determine that certain remedies are necessary to rectify the discrimination. These remedies may include hiring reinstatement, repromotion, front pay, back pay, reasonable accommodation and the payment of fees for attorneys, expert witnesses, and court costs. In addition, a complainant may request a right to sue letter, and punitive damages may be awarded where intentional discrimination is found. These damages are based upon the size of the employer according to the following schedule in Table 22.1.

It should be noted that punitive damages may not be awarded to the charging party, if an employer can demonstrate that they made a good faith effort to comply with providing reasonable accommodation. Motivation of employers to comply with Title I of the ADA will increase in direct proportion with the vigor with which the EEOC enforces this section.

The first lawsuit under ADA was settled for $572,000 which seems like a rather stout fine. Other lawsuits are pending and it does seem that the EEOC intends to aggressively pursue enforcement. It is important to remember that Therapists must also comply with this law.

TABLE 22.1   EEOC Discrimination Settlements Punitive Damage Maximums

Number of employees	Damages not to exceed
15–100	$50,000
101–200	$100,000
201–500	$200,000
500 or more	$300,000

Title II Provisions: Public Services Summary Parameters

Purpose.   To ensure nondiscrimination on the basis of disability in the provision of services by State and local government.

Who Is Covered.   "Public Entities" means State or local government including state legislatures and courts, police and fire departments, the department of motor vehicles, employment and any other instrumentalities of state or local government.

Therapist Opportunities

The Industrial Therapist can be a valuable member of a team that develops and costs out accessibility accommodations, to either implement the best ones, or provide defensible documentation where undue hardship is present. The Therapist can also help public service entities modify policies, procedures, and practices to equalize access by disabled people.

General Overview

State and local governments may not deny an individual participation in a service, program, or activity solely because the person has a disability. This may require modifications in policies, procedures, and practices that allow individuals with disabilities equal access, unless doing so would result in a fundamental alteration in the service. All facilities should be accessible and may utilize the furnishing of aids, auxiliary services, and special benefits beyond those determined by the regulations unless an undue burden exists.

Some areas of accommodation could include relocating a service to a more accessible area, providing an aid or assistant for an individual with a disability, or providing services at an alternative site including an individual's home. This also includes telephone emergency services (911 services) to be accessible by individuals with speech or hearing disabilities.

Public transportation services must also be accessible including over the road and most rail operations. All public transportation vehicles acquired after February 26, 1992 must be accessible and usable by individuals with disabilities. Public transportation using a prescribed route according to a fixed schedule, must provide paratransit and other special services to individuals with disabilities. These services must be comparable to the nondisabled service in its level of service and response time.

Those eligible for the paratransit service include people who need the assistance of another to board, ride or disembark from any vehicle on the system, those who need a wheel chair lift, and any individual with an impairment which prevents travel to a boarding or disembarking location.

There are considerable extensions granted for key light rail stations that require substantial structural changes. In these situations two thirds of key stations must be accessible within 20 years, and a 30 year total extension may be granted for certain extraordinary and expansive structural changes.

Services must be provided in an integrated setting unless separate or different measures are necessary to insure equal opportunity. No special charges may be levied on individuals with disabilities for costs associated with measures to assure equal opportunity. Necessary safety requirements may be imposed, provided they are based on actual risks.

Title II Specifics

The regulations implementing Title II were produced by the Department of Justice and are organized into seven subparts, A through G.

Subpart A—General.   There are two main categories of programs or activities covered by this regulation. One involves situations in which there is public contact, including telephone contacts and use of public facilities. The other involves activities administered by the entity including programs that provide state or local government services or benefits.

Subpart B—General Requirements.   The services, programs, or activities provided to individuals with disabilities must be equal to those provided to those without disabilities.

Subpart C—Employment.   This requires that a public entity not discriminate on the basis of disability for employment, regardless of the size of the public entity.

Subpart D—Program Accessibility.   This requires that public entities make programs accessible in all cases, except where to do so, would result in a fundamental alteration in the nature of the program, or an undue financial and administrative burden.

Subpart E—Communications.   This section requires public entities to take such steps as may be necessary to insure that communications with applicants, participants, and members of the public with disabilities are as effective as communications with others. This section specifically requires the availability of telecommunication devices for the deaf (TDDs). These are devices that enable an individual with a hearing or speech disability to communicate with the nondisabled. This subpart also requires that telephone emergency services, including 911 services, be available to those individuals who use TDDs and computer modems.

Subpart F—Compliance Procedures.   Any individual who believes that discrimination on the basis of disability by a public entity has taken place, may file a complaint. The complaint must be filed within 180 days from the date of the alleged discrimination unless an extension is granted.

The appropriate agency shall investigate each complaint and attempt an informal resolution. Barring that, it may issue a letter of findings including the facts and conclusions of law, a described remedy for each violation, and a notice of complainant's rights to file a private lawsuit.

If the public entity declines to cooperate, the designated agency shall refer the matter to the Attorney General.

Subpart G—Designated Agencies.   The Assistant Attorney General will coordinate Federal agency compliance with respect to state and local government, providing the policy and guidance to implement requirements of this part. The following are the designated agencies responsible for implementing the compliance procedures of Title II.

1. Department of Agriculture, for agricultural activities.
2. Department of Education, for educational activities and libraries, excluding schools of medicine, dentistry, nursing, and other health-related schools.
3. Department of Health and Human Services, for health and social service activities, including schools of medicine, dentistry, nursing, other health-related schools, "grass-roots" community services, and preschool and day care programs.
4. Department of Housing and Urban Development, for state and local public housing activities, assistance and referral.
5. Department of Interior, for natural resource management activities including parks and recreation, environmental protection, energy, historic and cultural preservation, and museums.
6. Department of Justice, for legal and regulatory activities including law enforcement and correction, industry and finance, consumer protection, small business and all other government functions not assigned to other designated agencies.
7. Department of Labor, for labor and work force activities.
8. Department of Transportation, for all transportation activities including automobile licensing and inspection.

Functions not specifically assigned to designated agencies may be assigned by the Department of Justice.

Information pertaining to Title II can be obtained by contacting:

Office on the Americans with Disabilities Act
Civil Right Division
U.S. Department of Justice
P.O. Box 66118
Washington, DC 20035–6118

(202) 514-0301 (Voice)
(202) 514-0383 (TDD)
(202) 514-6193 (Electronic Bulletin Board).

Title III Provisions: Public Accommodations and Services Operated By Private Entities

Summary Parameters

Purpose.   To insure that no individual is discriminated against on the basis of disability by any person who owns, leases or operates a place of public accommodation.

Who Is Covered.   Any private (nonpublic) entity operating a commercial facility, excluding noncommercial residential facilities, facilities exempt under the Fair Housing Act of 1968, railroad vehicles, religious organizations and private membership clubs. (Public entities are covered by Title II).

Definitions

Commerce means any trade, transportation, travel, or communication relating to the exchange of goods or services.

Commercial facilities are nonresidential facilities involved in commerce.

Public Accommodations include the following:
- Place of lodging
- Establishment serving food or drink
- Place of entertainment
- Place of public gathering
- Sales or rental establishment
- Service establishment
- Station or depot for public transportation
- Place of public display or collection
- Place of recreation
- Place of education
- Social service center establishment
- Place of exercise or recreation

Therapist Opportunities

As with public services access, the Industrial Therapist can help private entities develop and cost out accessibility accommodations to either implement feasible ones, or provide defensible documentation in instances of undue hardship. The Therapist can also initiate new relationships with private sector establishments by offering seminars on ADA compliance strategies.

General Overview

Private places of public accommodation number over 5 million establishments, including dining, lodging, entertainment, recreational, and retail facilities, clinics and hospitals, private schools, and day care centers. They all must provide to the disabled, goods and services that are equal in quality and accessibility to those available to the nondisabled. This may require reasonable modifications to facilities or policies and procedures.

Movie theaters must provide seats without arms for individuals in wheel chairs, and establishments that do not allow pets must allow seeing eye dogs. Book stores may be required to provide auxiliary aides and services such as telecommunication devices for the deaf, video text displays, reader's tape text, braille materials, or large print materials.

Perhaps the greatest impact of Title III is with regard to removing architectural and structural barriers. Existing facilities must remove physical barriers, such as curbs and narrow passages if achievable without undue burden. If not, steps must be taken to arrange accessibility through alternative means, such as providing goods and services at the door or sidewalk, home delivery, or relocating activities and services to more accessible areas.

Extra charges for these services may not be imposed upon individuals with disabilities. The use of undue burden as a defense will be interpreted very strictly, because alternative accommodations are viewed as readily achievable. The government provides tax relief for public accommodation costs associated with removal of barriers. (As previously described in Title I).

Noteworthy under Title III, a healthcare professional may not refuse treatment to a disabled individual if they are competent in the area for which the individual is seeking care. A back specialist could not refuse to treat an HIV positive back injury patient, but they could refuse to treat an HIV positive burn patient because they are not competent in treating burns.

Any alteration that takes place must comply with the 86 page ADA Accessibility Guidelines (ADAAG) that accompany the regulations for implementation of Title III. This includes very specific guidelines with regard to dimensions, accessibility, obstructions, ramps and stairs, windows and doors, elevators, and lavatory facilities. In addition to compliance regarding alterations, the path of travel to the altered space must also comply with the ADAAG, unless the costs to do so exceeds 20% of the cost of the original alteration.

Compliance with the ADAAG is required for any new construction, where the building permit is dated after January 26, 1992, and the building is occupied after January 26, 1993.

Enforcement of Title III

The enforcement agency of Title III is the Department of Justice and the office of the Attorney General. Individuals may file a complaint with the Attorney General who is authorized to bring lawsuits in cases of public importance where there is a pattern of discrimination.

Private parties may also bring lawsuits to obtain court orders to stop the discrimination. While no monetary damages are available to the complainant in such suits, a reasonable attorney's fee may be awarded. In suits brought by the Attorney General, monetary damages may be awarded not to exceed $50,000 for a first violation or $100,000 for any subsequent violation.

Title IV Provisions: Telecommunications

The purpose is to insure the nondiscrimination on the basis of speech or hearing disabilities in the provision of telecommunication services. Each common carrier providing telephone voice transmission services shall provide telecommunication relay services.

Definitions

Common carrier is any service engaged in interstate communication by wire or radio. Telecommunications Relay Services are services that enable an individual with a hearing or speech impairment to communicate by wire or radio.

The Communications Assistant is essentially a relay operator, that is an intermediary between the individual with a speech or hearing disability, and the individual to whom they are communicating.

Voice Carryover is a reduced form of telecommunication relay services where the person with a hearing disability is able to speak directly to the person at the other end. The Communications Assistant types the response back to the person with a hearing disability. The Communications Assistant does not voice the conversation.

Hearing Carryover is a reduced form of Telecommunications Relay Services where the person with the speech disability is able to listen to the person at the other end, and in reply, the Communications Assistant speaks the text as typed by the person with a speech disability. The Communications Assistant does not type in any conversation.

FIGURE 22.3   Americans With Disabilities Act hiring process flow chart.

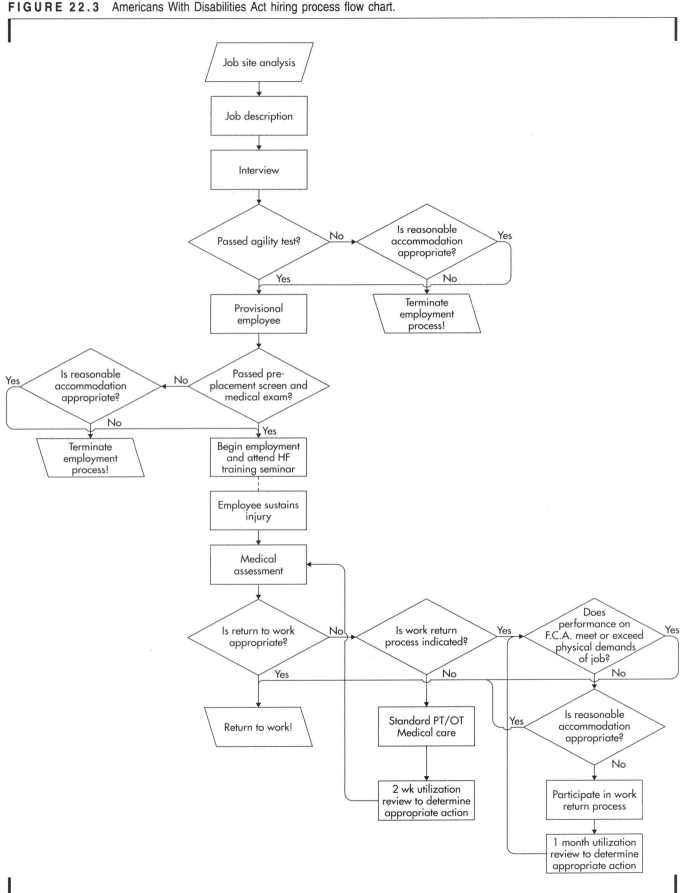

(Copyright: Robert B. King)

General Overview

This title insures the availability of telecommunication services to individuals with speech or hearing disabilities. Standards for this include a twenty four hour availability of the service, cost of the service being equivalent to standard voice communication, the speed of transmission being equivalent to normal conversation and the availability of emergency services such as 911.

Enforcement

The FCC is the enforcement agency. All complaints must be filed with the FCC, and the FCC shall resolve any complaint within 180 days after the complaint is filed. Such complaint should list the name and the address of the complainant, the name and address of the defendant against whom the complaint is made, a complete statement of the facts including supporting data where available, and the relief sought.

Information pertaining to Title IV can be obtained by contacting:

Federal Communications Commission (FCC)
Secretary's Office, Room 222
1919 M Street NW
Washington, DC 20554

Telephone (202) 632-7000

Title V Provisions: Miscellaneous

The purpose of Title V is to describe the ADA's relationship to other laws, and to discuss the prohibition against retaliation and coercion by those involved in any action related to this law. It also includes definitions of conditions not covered by the ADA such as sexual behavior disorders (homosexuals, transvestites), compulsive disorders (compulsive gamblers, kleptomaniacs), and illegal drug users. Title V also outlines alternate means of dispute resolution such as settlement negotiations, facilitation, mediation, fact finding, and arbitration.

Title V information can be obtained by contacting EEOC. If there is no EEOC office, the EEOC can be called toll free at 1-800-669-4000 (voice) or 1-800-800-3302 (TDD).

SUMMARY

The present and future hold considerable challenges, and every challenge brings opportunity. As demonstrated in Figure 22.3, the opportunities offered for Industrial Therapists in the hiring process is increasingly influenced by regulatory agencies. To take advantage of the opportunities that exist, one must be aware of the factors described in this chapter, which requires in-depth understanding. This chapter gave a brief overview of some of those factors.

REFERENCES

1. 1993 Standards Manual for Organizations Serving People with Disabilities, Tucson, Arizona; 1992. Commission on Accreditation of Rehabilitation Facilities.
2. 1994 Operations Analysis of 1993 Survey Activities, Tucson, Arizona; 1994. Commission on Accreditation of Rehabilitation Facilities.

BIBLIOGRAPHY

1. 1990 Reference Manual for Commission Surveyors, Tucson, Arizona; 1990. Commission on Accreditation of Rehabilitation Facilities.
2. American Law Encyclopedia Vol 12: 413–419
3. Ellexson MT: The Impact of CARF Standards on the Practice of Work Hardening, Work 1: 69–72, 1990.
4. Policies, Procedures, and Process for Site Surveys, Tucson, Arizona; 1991 Commission on Accreditation of Rehabilitation Facilities.
5. Social Security Bulletin, Annual Statistical Supplement, 1991.
6. US Social Security Administration Annual Statistical Supplement to Social Security Bulletin.
7. US Social Security Administration; Social Security Bulletin, May 1991.
8. US Health Care Financing Administration; Health Care Financing Review, Fall 1991.
9. US Social Security Administration; Social Security Bulletin, Spring 1992.

APPENDIX II

Documents available through the CARF Office:
Interpretive Guidelines for the Standards Manual.
Standards Manual for Organizations Serving People with Disabilities.
Self-Study Questionnaire for Organizations Serving People with Disabilities.
Directory of Accredited Organizations Serving People with Disabilities.
Program Accessibility in Organizations Serving People with Disabilities.
Market-Based Planning: A Tool for Organizations Serving People with Disabilities.
Program Evaluation: A First Step.
Program Evaluation: A Guide to Utilization.
Program Evaluation: Utilization & Assessment Principles.

23

Ensuring and Monitoring Client Safety

Linda M. Demers

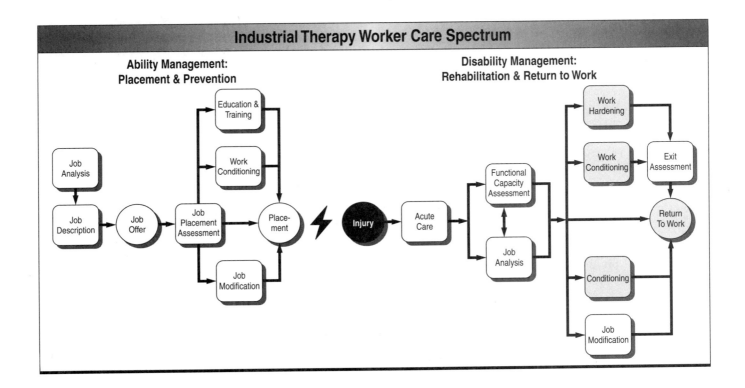

Industrial Therapy Worker Care Spectrum

Ability Management:
Placement & Prevention

Disability Management:
Rehabilitation & Return to Work

Very often, when an injured client enters the Work Retraining center, a review of the client's history will reveal that the injury occurred because of unsafe work practices. Therefore, the challenge of rehabilitation also becomes the challenge of changing habits which may have become deeply ingrained through the years.

The rehabilitation specialist may also encounter production standards, piecework, incentive work, and peer pressure. Nevertheless, the specialist must find a way to balance the needs of industry with the needs of the worker to remain safe and still make a good living within the framework of the workforce.

Idealistically, the goal of Work Retraining is for

100% of discharged work-injured clients to reenter the workforce with perfect safety practices. Realistically, this is not going to happen. The pragmatic goal of the Work Conditioning or Work Hardening center is to change what can be changed through practice and education, with an emphasis on translating these learned skills into all aspects of the client's life, including the work environment.

This chapter will discuss the conditions, policies, and procedures necessary for operating a safe facility, providing safe Therapy programs, and facilitating the development of safer work environments and workstyles.

ENSURING A SAFE OPERATION

A safe facility is made up of a safe environment, a well-trained staff, and safety-oriented policies and procedures.

Physical Environment

In the ongoing effort to provide an effective, safe, pleasant working environment for Work Retraining clients, ventilation, illumination, and noise levels must also be considered. Ventilation is probably one of the most difficult environmental controls to build into a rehabilitation facility. There are many jobs which produce noxious fumes. Unless specialized ventilation is designed into a rehabilitation facility, these jobs cannot be fully simulated. This is not necessarily a weakness in the Work Retraining center concept.

The basis for Work Simulation is to provide a safe, supervised environment in which the injured worker can effectively and functionally rebuild damaged tissue to the level necessary to safely return to the work environment. Work Simulation provides as much true to life simulation as is reasonable, then carries on with muscle group simulation which will adequately retrain the client for return to work.

Staff Training

One of the best ways to insure safety is to provide safety training to all staff members who will have contact with injured workers.[11] Staff members working in the Work Simulation center will require special knowledge of the Occupational Safety and Health Administration (OSHA) standards specific to many jobs. This does not mean that they will have to memorize these standards, but that they will need to look up any unfamiliar standards when a client in an unfamiliar industry is admitted for rehabilitation.

Standard Policies and Procedures

Once job simulation commences, all safety practices for that industry must be observed. Clients are often resistant to wearing protective equipment or following the established guidelines, but the rehabilitation center would be held negligent if these safety practices were not enforced and a client was injured.

If a client is sanding with an electric sander, ear and eye protection are required, along with a dust mask if ventilation is in question, or if there are particles floating in the air to be breathed into the lungs. The setup must also assure that the particulate matter and noise is confined, to protect the other clients in the Work Retraining center (Figure 23.1).

FIGURE 23.1 Clients must use protective equipment during their work hardening rehabilitation to comply with OSHA standards.

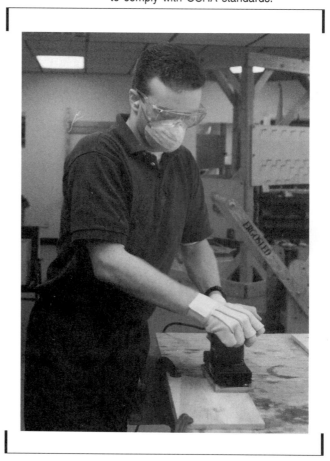

Physical Emergency Procedures

Staff should be familiar with all means of egress, and all exits should be pointed out to clients during the orientation process. Illustrated evacuation charts should be posted by each exit. Emergency exits should be clearly marked throughout the center.

In case of fire, all personnel should be knowledgeable about the use and locations of fire extinguishers, hoses, and alarms. Check with your local fire department to see what kind of training is offered in your community.

If an evacuation is required due to fire, bomb threat, earthquake, flood, tornado, or hurricane, procedures should address the following:
- Who will take charge?
- Where will everyone meet?
- How long should it take?
- Who will make the necessary call(s)?

Centers located in areas of the country where inclement or inhospitable weather creates a hazard for evacuees, should have a designated sheltered area where they can report until it is safe to return to the building. These arrangements should be made ahead of time to keep chaos to a minimum if and when these emergency plans need to be put to use.

Medical Emergency Procedures

Medical emergency procedures will vary considerably among rehabilitation facilities due to the setting (within a hospital, independent single discipline with or without physician access, or within a medical building).[1] In a hospital setting, physicians are usually on-site and can be reached with an emergency code page. In a private setting, off site, an ambulance may need to be called. No matter where the center is located, however, personnel must receive basic first aid and cardiac life support training.[2]

When procedures are written to prepare for medical emergencies, be sure to include the following:
- Who will take charge?
- Who will initiate CPR?
- Who will make the emergency call(s)?
- Where is the emergency equipment kept?
- Who will check the equipment and how often?

The best way to assure that all personnel are qualified in basic life support is to make arrangements with the Red Cross to come to the facility and train everyone at the same time. The initial training session requires six to seven hours, but subsequent refreshers take much less time (Figure 23.2).

Long periods of time often occur between use of any of these emergency procedures, so written guidelines must be set up for personnel to review to assure familiarity with the procedure. This periodic review also ensures that the procedure is still accurate. If the original medical procedure was to call the hospital emergency room and a physician has now joined the group for 20 hours per week, then the new procedure should reflect a change of plans for the time when immediate physician involvement is available.

Drugs and Medications Policies

Along with the emergency medical and evacuation procedures, there should be policies and procedures addressing use of medication or products which have the potential to impair the Work Retraining client's judgment, during participation in the Work Retraining process. A generic statement regarding the acceptability of the use of medication or products that do not impair the client's judgment, balance, coordination, or sensation may suffice. The policy may read as follows:

> Because the safety of our clients is of the utmost importance to us, the use of medications or products which have the potential to

FIGURE 23.2 All Work Retraining personnel should be trained in basic first aid and CPR. (From Armstrong Medical Industry, Inc., Lincolnshire, Ill, 1994.)

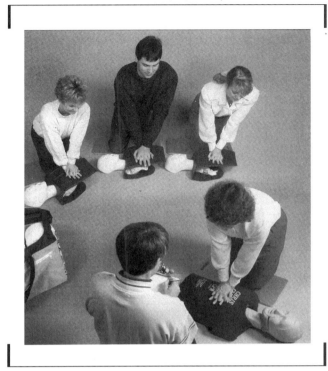

impair the judgment, balance, coordination, or sensory input of the client is prohibited.

The Physician's Desk Reference (PDR) will be the reference of choice when investigating these concerns.

Enforcement of this policy will largely depend on the observation skills of the trained professional working with the client.

If there is any question that the Work Retraining client is not safe, immediate action, following the procedures established for this situation, must take place. Procedures for this situation should include:
1. Confronting the client with the concern
2. Use of a private space to protect the client from embarrassment
3. The method to be used to question the client
4. Presentation of the facts to assist the client's decision making regarding Work Retraining participation

Because of the personal and legal sensitivity required when dealing with this situation, which may involve drug or alcohol abuse issues, personnel may require specialized training. For those less comfortable with this role, it is a good idea to have the option of deferring to someone skilled in handling this subject.

It is important to be careful not to accuse anyone of

anything. Clients with diabetes may have a breath odor which leads to mistaken conclusions. A false accusation of wrong doing is not only insulting to the client, but may also have legal ramifications.

What options does the Therapist have if drug and alcohol issues are hindering the progress of a client? This is one of the most difficult issues to deal with, because it feels controllable but is really an issue that is totally up to the injured worker.

The first step in dealing with this issue is to recognize that fact. Approach the client with concern rather than accusations: "Do you have a medical problem which would give your breath an odor?" If the client is a diabetic, assist that client in seeking intervention if the diabetes is not under control. If the client says there is no medical problem, investigate further. Explain the detrimental effects of caffeine, nicotine, and alcohol to the client.

Insuring the client's safety through the use of building and medical emergency policies and procedures is probably familiar to anyone who has worked in the rehabilitation field. Dealing with the work injured population brings with it, the additional responsibility of improving the client's safety practices and transposing these behaviors into the real work situation.

ASSESSING CLIENT SAFETY ISSUES

Assessment Overview

Improving client safety begins by performing a Functional Capacity Assessment (FCA) on every client who enters the Work Hardening program.[6] This assessment discloses many pertinent details about the client's safety practices and the ability to learn new behaviors. Are the body mechanics safe? What kind of attitude is displayed regarding safety practices? What is the employer's role?

Does the worker know how they became injured and why? Do they blame someone else for the injury, or are they taking personal responsibility? Do they know their limits? Do they over or under achieve? It is important during this evaluation process to observe if the client is angry, complacent, feeling self pity, or is assertive and proactive with care.

If they own splints, pain control devices, or assistive devices, do they use them appropriately and consistently? How easily does the client follow instructions? Do verbal instructions appear to be easier to follow than demonstrated instructions, or is it best when these are given in combination? Is the client easily intimidated when presented with something new?

Besides the obvious provision of safe work capaci-

ty parameters, the Functional Capacity Assessment provides the rehabilitation specialist with abundant information about who this injured worker truly is and how to most effectively approach them when initiating rehabilitation in the Work Retraining center.

Body Mechanics

Are the worker's body mechanics safe? The FCA provides the opportunity to observe the client in a multitude of body positions while performing everyday tasks. Observe if the client holds the object too far from the body, struggles with it, and if the proper natural responses to find a better way occur.

As the FCA progresses, note if fatigue influences changes in body mechanics. As the conversation flows, note if the client verbalizes exactly what is being exhibited. When asked the method used to lift, many clients say that they have had body mechanics training at work and know all the right answers; but when put into an uninstructed activity, natural lifting techniques reveal that the knowledge of proper body mechanics is in theory only.

Once the injured workers' safe parameters have been determined, a decision is made regarding the most effective means of providing rehabilitation. Can the employer provide for all of the client's needs through a modified duty program, or are the client's body mechanics so poor that they will result in future injury without retraining in body mechanics?

If the client demonstrated fair body mechanics throughout the assessment but needs to learn some modifications to make them safer, this can frequently be accomplished through short sessions of body mechanics education. If the employer has modified duty available and the employee's capabilities fit these modifications, the worker may return to the workforce full time while continuing body mechanics training after hours. If this option is not available, the employer may provide part time safe modified duty and allow the client to attend daily body mechanics training sessions with a qualified professional outside the work setting.

Environmental Factors

Was the injury caused, not by a cumulative trauma mechanism due to poor mechanics, but rather by an unsafe environment resulting in a one time serious trauma? These type of injuries, usually called accidents, are often the result of carelessness on someone's part. Good examples of these types of injuries are those caused by slipping on spilled oil which was not wiped up, climbing on a chair with wheels on the legs to reach a high shelf, or falling on a wet floor someone neglected to mark as wet. If this appears to be the case, then a job analysis should be carried out to evaluate the work conditions.

After obtaining the necessary information regarding the inherent safety of the work environment, a functional capacities match can be performed against the results of the analysis. Wherever there are discrepancies, alternate work methods should be considered. Can the worker alternately sit and stand rather than be required to stand all day? Can the worker use a different tool? Can the worker alternate between tasks throughout the day, as long as they still complete the work by the end of the day?

Attitudinal Factors

What kind of attitude is displayed regarding safety practices? Is it laissez faire, or does the client flaunt the number of Occupational Safety and Health Administration (OSHA) regulations that have been broken during his or her work career? Most workers are somewhere in the middle, obeying some practices and ignoring others. Determining the worker's attitude is a critical piece of the puzzle when searching for contributing factors to the injury. Also, because the safeguards built into the FCA are often self determined, the assessor must keep a watchful eye and constantly reinstruct if the client is not heeding common sense rules of safety.

Education and Prevention Issues

Does the worker know how he or she was injured and why? During the Functional Capacity Assessment, there is ample opportunity to delve into the client's recollection of the events leading to injury. Even though it may have been several months since the original injury occurred, clients frequently remain mystified as to why it happened. The client is doomed to repeat the events leading to injury if a different approach is not learned.

Does the client know self limits? Clients who disregard the body's warnings, or never learned to pay attention to these signals, are dangerous to themselves and those around them. To determine the client's participation level during the assessment, the KEY Method, for example, evaluates the "validity components" to determine if the client over or under achieved. This participation level is a reflection of the client's ability to accurately judge end range capabilities when compared to body responses. The KEY Method FCA uses statistically based protocols, supported by reinjury rate studies, to make this determination.[3,9]

The client's ability to follow instructions and the best method of giving those instructions for that individual are also important factors gleaned from the

assessment. This tells the Assessment Specialist if a lack of understanding of safe practices at work may have been a contributing factor in the client's work injury.

Within a work environment, written memos are sometimes the method used to disseminate new information. Sometimes workers can read but their comprehension is poor. This can be embarrassing to admit, so the worker never tells anyone of the inability to understand the new instructions. This, combined with the right set of circumstances, can lead to an injury.

If the client owns assistive devices, it is important to determine that they know the proper usage. Often, injured workers speak with other injured workers, who identify something they have used that worked for them. The client then runs to the medical supply store and buys the item. However, incorrect use of this device could lead to an unsafe situation.

The client may purchase a cane. When a Therapist is not involved, the finer points of fit and proper use to facilitate a gait pattern that is as close to normal as possible are not addressed. So the client chooses a cane that is ill-fitting lengthwise and proceeds to use it on the wrong side of the body. Because of the length, it does not provide the support that it should. Because it is used on the wrong side of the body, it promotes an abnormal gait pattern and low back pain. This becomes a self-perpetuating cycle of misuse of soft tissues that leads to further problems.

Although education does not necessarily occur during the assessment process itself, this insight will influence the recommendations resulting from the assessment. If the client does not realize that back strain was caused from repeatedly bending forward from the waist with locked knees, they will continue to perform their daily activities at home and at work using this method.

Employer's Role

What is the employer's role? Is the worker being held to standards that are impossible to meet? What is the supervisor's attitude towards the workers? During the FCA process, the assessor should be acquiring a sense of the work environment. This is through the eyes of the worker, but regardless of whether this is skewed or not, it is how the worker sees his or her plight.

Many Workers' Compensation laws now make the employer responsible for returning the injured worker to work in some capacity if at all possible. Also at issue is the Americans with Disabilities Act (ADA), which is already being wrestled with in the courts. Ultimately, the dynamics between the worker and the employer can make or break an attempt at successful return to work.

Psychosocial Factors

Is the worker angry, and blaming someone else for their injury? Is the worker proactive and assertive in the activities and care? If the worker is angry and blaming, there may be a tendency to sit back and wait to be cared for. This kind of injured worker can easily get lost in the system for months at a time and may continue to deteriorate.

The assessor's recommendations following the FCA may call for a more proactive, structured approach to moving this client along. Without this, the client could be suddenly rediscovered in the system and may be tossed back into the work environment haphazardly.

One of the primary roadblocks to safe return to work is poor work feasibility.[10] Work feasibility is those combined qualities which make a worker a desirable employee, including timeliness, productivity, appropriate dress, and social skills. The injured worker once demonstrated all of these qualities in order to remain employed. However, once a worker is out of work and out of a routine, days are filled with other activities, other interests develop, and skills are lost very quickly.

The longer the client is unemployed, the more these issues arise. When the worker cannot arrive on time for appointments, this is a timeliness issue. The worker must maintain a respect for safe, appropriate dress for the environment. When an injured worker is isolated, after a time, the ability to appropriately communicate is lost. If the injured worker demonstrates multiple work feasibility deficits, a full time Work Hardening program is critical to a successful, safe return to work.

Summary of Assessing Client Safety Issues

If feasibility is not an issue and body mechanics are fine, and the employer can accommodate the employee, the work environment must be addressed through a job analysis and adjustment prior to the worker's return to work. Usually, a worker's injury is caused by a combination of factors which can be rectified through education, practice, and heightened awareness. But the first step to this process is an objective Functional Capacity Assessment to provide a strong base from which to build.

SAFETY PRINCIPLES IN REHABILITATION

Work Conditioning and Work Hardening

If the injured worker requires a full course of Work Hardening prior to returning to the workforce, the rehabilitation team should proceed on the assumption that it takes twenty-one consecutive days to change a behavior, as noted in the book *Psychocybernetics*.[5]

Begin by insuring the client's safety through the use of the safe work parameters established during the Functional Capacity Assessment. A safe "rule-of-thumb" starts the client working at 50% of occasional parameters.[2] Although technically the client should be able to work at 100% of occasional parameters without reinjury, during entry into the Work Retraining program the worker can feel barraged with a massive amount of new information and significantly increased activity at the same time.

To prevent the feeling of being overwhelmed and discouraged, the client is familiarized with the program at a lower level. When the program is tolerated without objective signs of "flare-up," it should be quickly increased to the maximum demonstrated safe capabilities. This method is safe, effective, and immediately allows the client to experience success.

Client to Therapist Ratios

To this point, the client has had an FCA, been admitted into Work Conditioning or Work Hardening, and begun body mechanics training, stretching for body awareness, and pacing techniques. Throughout this procedure, the client is constantly supervised by a qualified professional who is there to problem solve, support, and instruct. The professional to injured worker ratio in this program should reflect the amount of supervision needed.

At Milliken Physical Therapy Center (MPTC), a division of Sportsmed's facilities, a ratio of one professional to five clients is the acceptable level.[7] There are times when this is not adequate. When a group of clients have difficulty, fewer clients are scheduled per Therapist. The ratio must assure that each client can be adequately supervised and that clients have immediate access to a professional for any questions. This promotes safety for each client, while providing an environment to experience success.

There are many clients who enter Work Retraining programs who are functioning at a very low formal educational level, sometimes fourth or fifth grade, and will require more one-to-one attention for a longer period of time. Each time these clients are introduced to something new, the plan should be to spend more individual time assuring that they understand the concept and can safely perform it independently.

This process does not have to be disruptive to the daily schedule; these new concepts should be scheduled for introduction during quiet times during the Work Hardening day. During the planning phase of this type of client's care, review the FCA results to see what was learned about the client's comprehension skills and the best method of instruction: verbal, demonstration, or both.

Body Mechanics Training

Although proper body mechanics is a regularly debated topic among professionals, there are common grounds considered safe, by most people.[8] Holding the object close to the body, pushing rather than pulling, and testing the weight prior to lifting are some of these. Body mechanics and posture are introduced to the clients very early in the Work Retraining program.

The client must have twenty-one consecutive days of practicing newly learned behaviors in order for them to develop into habits prior to discharge. Learning these skills is hard work, but when the injured worker persists, this persistence is well rewarded. Usually, the client remarks on feeling improved once these methods become more habitual. As the worker learns these new, safer work methods, he or she also becomes a crusader, promoting these methods to others.

The newly-admitted Work Retraining client is learning stretching techniques that provide feedback about the body. This is often a new concept, and is not readily accepted or understood. However, it is a critical step to the client's beginning safer work practices.

Often, work-injured clients describe forcing through the work day, concealing physical pain so as not to jeopardize the job. If this has been the practice through years of work, the habit of turning off the body's warning signals can be a difficult one to break. The client who works through the warning signs believes that the company will really appreciate such a good work ethic.

It is important to think back to the FCA and review the client's participation level, or as KEY Method calls it, validity of participation.[3] In KEY Method's participation level determinants, this client would probably test at the "conditionally invalid" level, indicating being unsafe at that level due to not knowing their safe limits.

Those clients who are at a "valid" participation level do know their safe limits. Therefore, when they enter the rehabilitation program, this concept will not have to be taught.

On the other hand, the underachiever or "conditionally valid" client will need assistance to work through their fear and discomfort. This client will be slower to try new body mechanics and feel less sure that this is really the proper, safer work method. This is a client who requires more "TLC," but is one of the most successful groups in Work Hardening.

While the approach may be different when teaching body mechanics to each of these individuals, in all cases, the objective information provided by the FCA can point to the most effective direction.

Gaining Credibility With Clients

As the work injured client acclimates to the new environment and adjusts to what is expected, a cama-raderie develops with the rest of the group. It is important to allow pleasantries to develop, while maintaining a firm hand on all safety issues. Because there is strength in numbers, any particular client may use the newly found camaraderie to impress upon the rehabilitation specialists, that health professionals are foreign to the real work environment and just do not understand.

If this occurs, schedule a job analysis at the client's workplace immediately. If the health professionals directing the clients are not viewed as credible in their roles, clients will not learn from them, and safety is greatly compromised. To be successful in providing Work Simulation services, a job analysis is needed anyway.[9] It is almost impossible to provide accurate job simulation through someone else's description of what the client does at the worksite. Too often, small but important details are left out.

By admitting that there is not a full understanding of the client's job, but being willing to learn, the Industrial Therapist can gain a tremendous amount of credibility with the clients. Through maintaining a firm hand on what is expected and providing consistency and mutual respect, the Therapist can encourage the reemergence of the internal locus of control in each client.

The clients begin to assume responsibility for themselves in all aspects of their lives. Knowing the pain and disruption injury has caused, they begin to take steps to prevent it from happening again. Although the clients may initially rebel at the new body mechanics and protest that they just cannot do it that way on the job, the integration of stretching and improved body awareness eventually leads to a natural assumption of body postures that feel good.

Clients also note that once the new methods feel more natural and they do not have to think about them so much, the methods seem to provide more strength, so they feel less likely to "bull" through the tasks.

Therapist Role Models

Once the clients have been taught proper body mechanics, are practicing them daily, have established a new body awareness through stretching, and are convinced that the staff has some idea of what their jobs entail, the health care professional's daily activities should set an example of the behaviors clients are being asked to adopt. For their own safety, and to remain credible, Work Retraining professionals must practice what they preach.

Assistive Devices

Although the Work Retraining center is set up to simulate a work environment and to avoid the use of equipment and techniques conventionally thought of as part of the medical model of care, use of assistive devices is encouraged when necessary to facilitate the rehabilitation process. Each Work Retraining center must set its own policies regarding acceptable devices. The following information should be considered when setting up the policies at the facility:

1. Can the device be used at home, or does it require a professional to administer?
2. Can the device be used on the job without interfering with the job duties?

3. Is the device easily portable and small enough so as not to draw attention to its use?
4. Is the device specifically designed to meet the needs of the client in a day-to-day setting?

Acceptable assistive devices may include TENS units, back belts, anti-vibration gloves, working and resting splints and braces, ambulation devices, portable hot and cold packs and ice massage popsicles, cervical and back pillows, shock absorbing shoe inserts, and anti-fatigue mats (Figures 23.3, *A, B, C*).

When assistive devices are used, the client assumes

FIGURE 23.3 A, B, C   Assistive devices are encouraged in the Work Conditioning or Work Hardening center when they are necessary to facilitate the rehabilitation process.

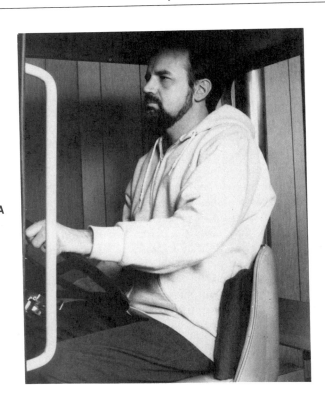

A

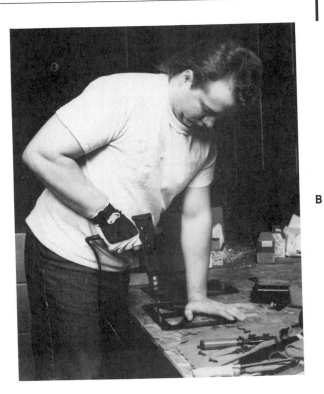

B

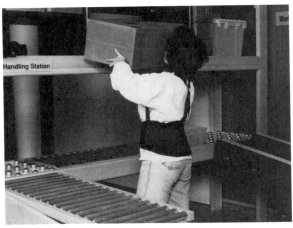

C

the responsibility for bringing the device to and from home, and for applying it in a timely manner. The client must self-identify when the device is needed and initiate its use. This is all part of the process of the client internalizing the locus of control while resuming self care responsibilities, and is part of the education mechanism of self awareness, feeling the body's warning signals.

Safety Training

The training of the worker in safe work practices is an integral part of the Work Retraining program.[6] One can never assume that workers have had the necessary training or that they have fully integrated the information provided within a work setting.

In some settings, education regarding safety on the job is handled through written memos which are never read or understood. There is little or no time provided for questions to be answered, or the atmosphere is not conducive to information gathering. When someone is injured or OSHA becomes involved because of an excessively high rate of injuries at the worksite, the education process changes to a method that addresses all workers' learning styles regardless of education level.

The good news is that today many employers are going beyond the "letter of the law" and providing safety training which addresses everyone's needs soon after hiring. This prevents bad habits from forming.

The Work Retraining center must set an outstanding example for training in safety and proper work techniques for clients. A full job analysis and identification of the specific needs of that client are necessary to face the challenge of teaching and enforcing safety with each individual client. The safety techniques taught should include:[2]

1. Pacing to insure quality productivity in a timely manner
2. Push rather than pull
3. Do not manually lift when there is an assistive device available
4. Use the two-man lift whenever the weight of an object warrants it
5. Test the weight of an object prior to lifting
6. Use mini-break stretches during highly repetitious or static positioning jobs
7. Use proper body mechanics whenever possible
8. Keep work as close to the body as possible
9. Counterbalance or suspend heavy or vibrating equipment
10. Wear clothing appropriate to the setting
11. Keep work areas clear of debris
12. Maintain equipment including blades, electrical cords, and guards
13. Use safety equipment such as safety glasses, ear plugs, hard hats, and steel-toed boots, in the proper settings

The above list is far from all-inclusive, but sheds light on the many unique procedures that Work Conditioning and Work Hardening professionals must have knowledge of in anticipation of meeting the client's needs.

Job Simulation

How does muscle group simulation work? Following receipt of a job description obtained through job analysis, each job task is reviewed for muscle group use. Productivity tasks are then assigned which simulate these tasks. The idea is to simulate the job tasks to the extent that the client is safe to perform them, based upon the results of the FCA.

If a client pushes pallets as part of the job, the push/pull sled will be loaded and the client will push and pull the sled in a safe manner as part of the program. If the client reaches forward to perform the job tasks, work may be done on developing safe performance capabilities using the upper body ergostation. If the client lifts and carries from one area to another, the same is done during Work Hardening. If the client works with fine motor, static posturing, some wood burning may be done (Figures 23.4, *A, B, C*).

Work Simulation professionals are not required to have a working knowledge of all tools and jobs that could possibly enter a Work Simulation program. The responsibility placed on the provider, is to know where to find the necessary information and then make a judgment as to whether this specific piece of equipment and work process can be safely used within the Work Retraining center environment. Often, job movements can be more readily simulated through equipment more familiar to the Work Simulation specialist. The primary consideration is always the guaranteed safety of the client with the most realistic portrayal of the job.

There are times when it is appropriate for a client to bring tools to the Work Retraining center even though the Work Simulation professionals have never used them. While there, the client is the only person allowed to use the tools, and must use all protective equipment required under OSHA regulations including guards, goggles, ear plugs, protective clothing, or face mask.

Proper ventilation may also become a prime consideration. If the client works with tools and products which produce excessive dust particles or noxious fumes, the ventilation system in the Work Simulation room must be able to keep the air clear of these byproducts.

Sometimes it is best to simulate the muscle group use with another functional activity acceptable to the client (Figures 23.5, *A, B*). It can feel somewhat uncom-

FIGURE 23.4 A, B, C The job analysis identifies the job tasks which can be reviewed for muscle group use. Work Simulation center activities are then assigned to simulate these tasks.

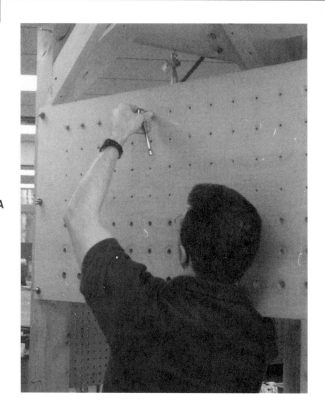

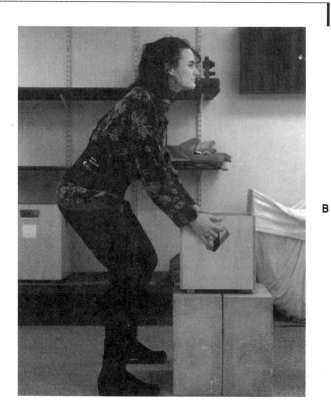

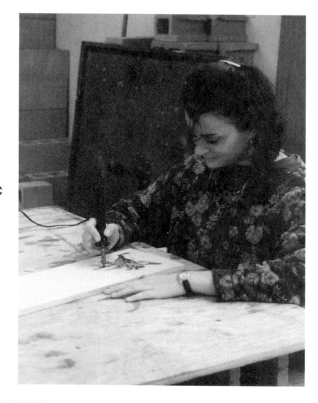

FIGURE 23.5 A, B   When work place equipment is unavailable or deemed unsafe for the Work Retraining center, job movements can be simulated through equipment more familiar to the Work Simulation specialist.

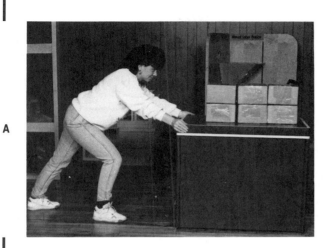
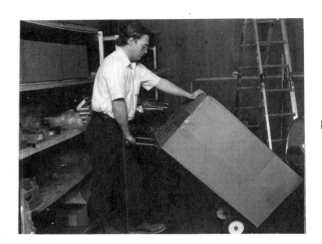

fortable having clients work with unfamiliar tools, but as long as all safety practices are followed, there is no reason for anyone to become injured at the Work Retraining center. The provider of Work Simulation services must first be convinced that this client is a professional in the field of work and has a strong working knowledge of tools.

Carelessness is never acceptable. If the injured worker is skilled at the trade, the tools are an extension of those skills. As long as the tools are treated with respect and inspected regularly, it may be an appropriate choice for optimum rehabilitation.

Should the Work Simulation professional determine that safety would be compromised by allowing a client to use a particular tool, then the decision can be made to not allow it. If safe use of tools is a feasibility issue that is being addressed during the Work Hardening program, the client may not be permitted to perform certain tasks requiring the use of those tools until this feasibility issue improves.

When setting up the policies for equipment use, look at the types of jobs from which the facility is likely to treat workers. One may decide to provide a set of tools and equipment to fit these categories so that their maintenance and inspections are assured.

For woodworking trades, a facility may supply various hand and power saws, drills, hammers, and ladders—whatever the staff feels comfortable supervising. The client's responsibility is to identify the tools with which he or she is accustomed and to use those tools as intended. As with any professional procedure, use customary protocol and follow a set of safety procedures, and breach of safety should not be an issue when tools are used.

Illumination needs vary considerably from jobsite to jobsite. To meet these needs, the Work Hardening center can provide spot lighting and groups of overhead lighting placed on dimmer switches.

Noise levels may become an issue when dealing with power equipment, especially in a smaller Work Simulation center. Care must be taken to protect the hearing not only of the clients using the equipment, but also of those clients exposed in the surrounding area. Ideally, noisy areas should be adequately separated from quieter areas, but there must be sufficient Work Simulation personnel to maintain the safety ratios discussed earlier.

There may be times when clients other than those using the tools may be requested to wear hearing protection. If the Work Retraining facility is part of a larger complex, the center must be designed with added noise buffers. The Work Simulation center is never a quiet area, even when power equipment is not being used.

Summary Safety Principles in Rehabilitation

The general environment in the Work Retraining center should radiate confidence, caring, individualism, and success. Safety may not be the most exciting aspect of providing Work Conditioning or Work Hardening services, but it is at the root of everything that is done. When working with clients, talk to them about providing a "safe, productive return to the workforce."

Safety is the subtle theme of every Work Retraining program. To keep clients safe, teach them to work with safety in mind, provide a safe physical environment in which to rehabilitate, provide safe equipment with which to work, teach Work Simulation personnel safe practices, perform an FCA to obtain safe beginning parameters, perform a final FCA to obtain safe return to work parameters, write or confirm the client's Work Retraining programs for the next day only after observing what worked for them today, and treat each client as an individual with individual needs.

Return to Work

How does the Work Retraining professional assist the client with the transition into the real world? Clients will ask this question very early in the Work Hardening process, especially if they perceive that their safety efforts will be thwarted at the workplace.

Alleviating Fears

One of the best methods for addressing the client's fears is to provide a thorough Work Conditioning or Work Hardening orientation. During this process, the client is educated regarding the philosophy behind Work Retraining, and is then provided with the opportunity to share fears and beliefs. These fears may include the inability to make a living. This threatens the client's core survival instinct.

Under Maslow's Hierarchy of Needs, food, shelter, and safety are base level needs. When clients believe the job may be jeopardized, they will often do anything they perceive they need to in order to remain employed. These clients will be most difficult to safety train.

Correcting Perceptions

If the clients' perception is that the safety techniques that are being taught will decrease production, and only those workers who can maintain the pace will remain employed, that client will be reluctant to address the safety issue. The specialist needs to be sensitive to this and work with the employer and the client to improve this situation. Early formation of a cohesive team approach, including the rehabilitation team and the employer, alleviates the Work Retraining client's apprehension of being left to fend alone when the physical rehabilitation process is complete.

The client must believe in the ability to practice the new skills without ridicule or difficulty from the employer. Otherwise, the client will perceive safety efforts as a utopia that is out of reach, and will not integrate these new behaviors. Ongoing work with the team is the answer to success when assisting this client to integrate these concepts of safety.

With the employer's involvement, the client's Work Simulation program can specifically address the work rate issues through time tests and pacing, while maintaining safety during the process. If weighted activities are the issue, gradual increases using safe body mechanics will be integrated. A good, clear exit interview will demonstrate to the client the success achieved in meeting the goals of the program for both safety and work parameters.

Enlisting Team Involvement

Initial employer contact is frequently sought through performance of a job analysis. This job description information is critical to the transition process when the client is ready for discharge. As mentioned earlier, it is also used when the job simulation phase of Work Retraining is initiated. When the Work Simulation professional performs a job analysis, first hand knowledge is gained about the attitude regarding safety at the worksite. With this knowledge, the Work Simulation professional can reassure the client that all safety issues will be addressed.

Communication with the injured worker's team is the key to success for the client. If the client cannot return to full duty, a relationship has already been established to transition the client into the workforce. All special needs should be addressed.

A rehabilitation or vocational specialist may also be involved with the injured client. These counselors usually become involved when it is doubtful that the client can return to the original job following physical rehabilitation. If the counselor is involved with the client prior to, or at the time that the facility is providing Work Hardening services, this valuable team member becomes part of the safety network, assuring the client of a safe transition back into the workforce.

SUMMARY

Ensuring the safety of Work Conditioning or Work Hardening clients requires a conscious effort to build safety into every aspect of the process. It begins with the planning of the facility, the training of personnel and the attitude of the team. It is carried out throughout every fiber of the Work Retraining program. Finally, the commitment is renewed each time a client is successfully and confidently returned to the workforce with new skills to safely perform the required duties.

REFERENCES

1. CARF: *CARF Standards Manual,* Tucson, 1992, CARF.
2. Demers LM: *Work Hardening: A Practical Guide,* Stoneham, MA, 1992, Andover Medical Publishers.
3. Key GL: The 99% Success Rate Study, Minneapolis, 1989, KEY Method.
4. Matheson LN: *Work Capacity Evaluation: Systematic Approach to Industrial Rehabilitation,* Anaheim, 1987, ERIC.

5. Maxwell L: *Psychocybernetics,* New York, 1989, Pocketbooks.

6. May VR, Stuart R, Soderburg G: Rehabilitating the Injured Worker: A Physical Capacity Evaluation and Work Hardening Model, abstract, *Phys Ther* 65(5), 1985.

7. Milliken Physical Therapy Center, Actual Staffing Records, Scarborough, Me, 1993.

8. NIOSH: *Lifting Guide to Manual Materials Handling,* Cincinnati, 1993, NIOSH.

9. Personnel Decisions Inc: A Study of Statistical Relationships Among Physical Ability Measures on Injured Workers Undergoing KEY Functional Assessments, Minneapolis, 1986, Personnel Decisions Inc.

10. Peters P: Successful Return To Work Following a Musculoskeletal Injury, *AAHON Jour* 38(6).

11. Tramposh AK: Work-Related Therapy for the Injured Reduces Return-To-Work Barriers, *Occup Health Safety* 57(4) 1988.

12. Work Hardening Guidelines . . . in an Occupational Therapy Setting, *Am Jour Occup Ther* 40(12), 1986.

24

Economic Considerations of Industrial Therapy

Cherilyn G. Murer

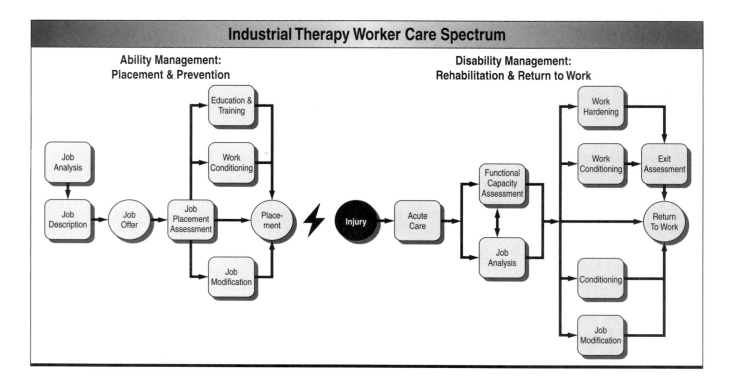

Industrial Therapy Worker Care Spectrum

Worker's disability is a staggering liability to American industry. Faced with soaring healthcare costs, lost productivity, and disability claims, employers are aggressively seeking to return workers to their jobs. This is the objective of Industrial Therapy. Indeed, rehabilitation is now generally accepted as the most effective remedy for injured workers and the most judicious use of disability dollars.

Notwithstanding employer and insurance companies' growing support for Industrial Therapy, not all programs are successful. A multitude of factors can contribute to a program's lackluster performance. Many times a staff's inability to document appropriate clinical outcomes (returned to work) is a major factor contributing to a program's failure. Not all providers have sufficient resources and expertise to withstand the

competitive challenges and rigors of a results-driven industry.

Operating a successful Industrial Therapy program entails much more than combining patients with staff. Successful Industrial Therapy programs follow sound economic practices. These include:

- Establishing project feasibility
- Developing a product line orientation
- Conducting financial planning
- Marketing outcome-oriented programs

FEASIBILITY

The development of an Industrial Therapy program requires an extensive commitment from administration and staff, significant resource expenditures, and some risk. Prior to such an undertaking, therefore, it is critical to determine the realistic viability or feasibility of the venture. A feasibility study conducted over the course of ten to twelve weeks can prove to be very beneficial as it identifies opportunities, strategic options, and a context for developing specific programs and services. The information gained through the study can serve as a foundation for establishing financial projections.[1,5,6,8]

When conducting a feasibility study, it is wise to use a broad range of methodologies to obtain the necessary information. These methodologies include, but are not limited to:

- One-on-one interviews with key referral sources—physicians, case managers, insurance carriers, employers, and Workers' Compensation attorneys

- Focus group sessions with insurance carriers, union representatives, or employers
- Competitive analysis of rehabilitation services in local and regional markets
- Review of national and local reimbursement and industry trends affecting rehabilitation
- Situational analysis of existing programs and services (if applicable)
- Analysis of market demand and community perception of rehabilitation programs and services

While there is no one mix of indicators which must be present to predict success of an Industrial Therapy program, the Key Feasibility Indicators of Industrial Rehabilitation (Box 24.1) provide a general guide for consideration. The more "yes" answers, the more feasible it is to pursue further development. More than 18 "yes" answers indicates a strong grounds for devel-

---

BOX 24.1

Key Feasibility Indicators of Industrial Rehabilitation

- Does the state mandate (Certification of Need) CON for outpatient rehabilitation services?
- Do private practice therapists offer industrial rehabilitation within your community?
- Do private practice therapists, with their industrial programs, control less than 50% of the market share?
- Are there clear guidelines differentiating Work Conditioning from Work Hardening?
- Are payor sources apt to use a fully integrated Work Hardening approach over the limited Work Conditioning programs?
- Is there a lack of market entry by national for profit chain providers?
- Does the physician community recognize the benefits of work hardening?
- Does the physician community recognize the benefits of chronic pain management?
- Are there identifiable physicians practicing pain management?
- Have physiatrists been accepted by the medical and payor communities?
- Will you be able to allocate requisite financial resources?
- Do you have requisite political support to proceed in a timely fashion with consensus driven expectations?

- Are you willing to practice outcome oriented management?
- Is this program part of a comprehensive outpatient rehabilitation center?
- Is this program part of a larger health system?
- Is the program located in a city of over 200,000 people?
- Can the work force be categorized as primarily blue collar?
- Is there a dominant industry employing at least 50% of the available work force?
- Do unions play a significant role in area industry?
- Do workers' compensation laws recognize rehabilitation?
- Does the state mandate the provision of rehabilitation services?
- Are insurance case managers used within the system?
- Are case managers influential in the decision making process?
- Is there a lack of state operated and owned rehabilitation services?
- Does the state mandate (Commission on Accreditation of Rehabilitation Facilities) CARF accreditation?

opment of an Industrial Therapy program. Ten to 18 "yes" answers suggests that an Industrial Therapy program may be very appropriate for development. An Industrial Therapy program may not be appropriate for consideration at this time if there are less than ten "yes" answers.

Location and Design

In addition to reviewing the key indicators of Industrial Therapy, the location and design of the program should be assessed.[5,6,8] During the feasibility study, many factors must be taken into account, such as space allocation, location, accessibility, availability of parking, and overall design of the programs. Generally, the physical design and location accessibility of the program are considered to be the primary determinants in generating referrals.

It is most beneficial to locate the Industrial Therapy program in a nonhospital outpatient environment, and to allocate 2,500 to 7,500 square feet to accommodate Functional Capacity Assessment and Work Simulation stations. However, product line parameters and services offered will ultimately determine space requirements (Figure 24.1).

The nonhospital outpatient environment has a number of advantages. First, Industrial Therapy clients are not commingled with chronically ill or injured patients, whose presence might divert emotional focus or compete for staff attention and equipment use. Second, being outside the hospital setting fosters more independent thinking and encourages self motivation. A distinct environment provides a tailored product for this specific patient population.

FIGURE 24.1 Providing Industrial Therapy clients with an environment specialized to their needs is more conducive to success.

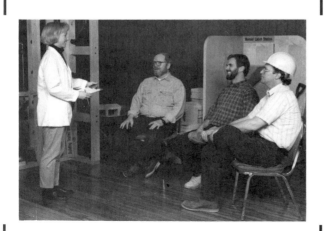

While it is not pragmatic to describe every appropriate data gathering methodology of a feasibility study, some of the more salient components include interviews, focus group sessions, and competitive analysis.

Interviews and Focus Groups

One-on-one interviews and focus groups are excellent means to obtain the information necessary to determine the demand for an Industrial Therapy program. This information assists in identifying actual needs and in determining the specific product lines to be offered by the program.

One-on-one interviews provide knowledge and insight from a broad cross section of people involved in Industrial Therapy. Typically, these interviews have virtually no costs attached. As a result, they can be used extensively to elicit information from anyone who might contribute information to your feasibility study —physicians, case managers, insurers, or employers.

A workable approach is to start with a known resource and then "network" to other sources suggested by the initial interviewees. These "information" interviews also initiate contacts that can lead to referrals when the program is eventually launched.

The purpose of focus groups is to elicit objective opinions from the participants with regard to program demand, design, specific client characteristics or injuries, competition, overall perception of rehabilitation, and future support.

The advantage of focus groups over one-on-one interviews is that the interaction between participants stimulates more ideas and insights than the individual interview. The focus group is also a mechanism to market the future program and to convey to the audience, the seriousness of the provider in developing and enhancing services.

The focus group facilitator is the key to the focus group's success. The facilitator must direct the topic of discussion, involve all participants if possible, and present an atmosphere which allows a free exchange of ideas, opinions, and comments.

A focus group should consist of ten to twelve homogeneously grouped participants (insurance people, union people, or employers). It should be noted that careful consideration should be given to inviting individuals to the focus group session. The participants should have similar backgrounds and compatible viewpoints as to the expectations of a rehabilitation program.

The following is an example of some general questions which can be asked in focus groups or one-on-one interviews:

1. Identify the services and features which are most attractive to you about an Industrial

Therapy program.

2. What are you doing now to meet the needs that those services and features address?
3. Are you generally satisfied with existing programs? Why or why not?
4. In your opinion how frequently might such an outpatient rehabilitation program be utilized? Which areas of specialization would have the most utilization? Which would have the least utilization?
5. Are there any aspects you don't like about the proposed program?
6. Are there other services which should be considered for development as well?
7. What would be the ideal location for such a program?

Questions regarding desired payment structure, client injuries, and specific rehabilitation services should also be included, but designed according to the particular characteristics and needs of the individuals participating in the session.

Competitive Analysis

Competitive analysis is imperative to the feasibility study as it provides a comprehensive view of present and potential competition, and allows for a more realistic determination regarding the establishment of the Industrial Therapy program, the future product line development, and the marketing strategy.[5,6,8]

Competitive analysis should focus on local and regional facilities and programs offering similar rehabilitation services with particular regard for the following:

- Market penetration
- Image perception
- Significant growth or expansion
- Facility design, aesthetics, and location
- Referral community satisfaction with services
- Staff expertise
- Patient profiles and statistics
- Affiliations with other hospitals, programs, and universities

This information can typically be obtained through telephone and personal interviews, focus groups, on-site tours of competing facilities, and a review of brochures and informational materials.

It is often advantageous to develop a matrix to display visually the various competitors' strengths and weaknesses relative to programs offered, accreditation standing, medical directorship, and location. Comparison of Area Providers (Table 24.1) has been completed using fictitious information to demonstrate how such an exercise clearly depicts the competitive picture.

PRODUCT LINE DEVELOPMENT

Prior to developing an Industrial Therapy program, it is important to analyze and define the product lines to be offered. A product line is a group of coordinated, compatible, and specialized programs which are struc-

TABLE 24.1 Comparison of Area Providers Matrix

Name of Facility	CARF Accred.	WH	CP	HC	VOC	FCA	BACK	Other Specialty Programs	Med Dir Specialty
Hospital XYZ	X	X	X		X		X	On-site work sim	Ortho
Rehab Center		X	X		X	X	X		None
Medical Rehab Center	X	X	X	X		X		Ergonomics	OCC Med
ABC Hospital	X	X			X		X		Physiatry
Institute for Rehabilitation		X	X	X	X	X	X		Ortho & Anesthesiology
General Rehab Services		X			X				Physiatry
Memorial Hospital	X	X				X	X		Physiatry

Key
WH = Work Hardening, CP = Chronic Pain, HC = Hand Clinic, VOC = Vocational Evaluation, FCA = Functional Capacity Assessment, BACK = Back Rehabilitation.

tured to provide optimal services to a specific population and a referral base.[5,6,8]

One product line might be Work Hardening, within which would be programs for Work Conditioning, Job Simulation, and Psychological Counseling.

Each product line should address the complete range of needs in each area of Industrial Therapy, to ensure the full knowledge and experience necessary for clinical specialization and quality of care. Without complete product lines in each specialization, the program may underserve the market's breadth of needs, and lose the competitive edge crucial to sustaining viability in today's healthcare market. Indeed, effective product line strategies are an important economic consideration.

The delineation of product lines can be based upon information obtained from interviews and focus groups conducted during the feasibility study. Employers, insurance carriers, and Workers' Compensation attorneys will likely indicate which services they desire, and the competitive analysis will provide key information as to the demand and availability of such specific programs and services.

Within Industrial Therapy programs there are a number of possible product lines which can offer comprehensive rehabilitation programs and services for injured or disabled workers. In fact, many product lines can be integrated by cross utilizing staff and resources, and by coordinating services to reach a common outcome or goal.

As indicated in Figure 24.2, the primary product lines in a typical Industrial Therapy program are: Functional Capacity Assessment, Job Analysis and Job Placement Assessment, Education and Prevention,

FIGURE 24.2   Sample product line options.

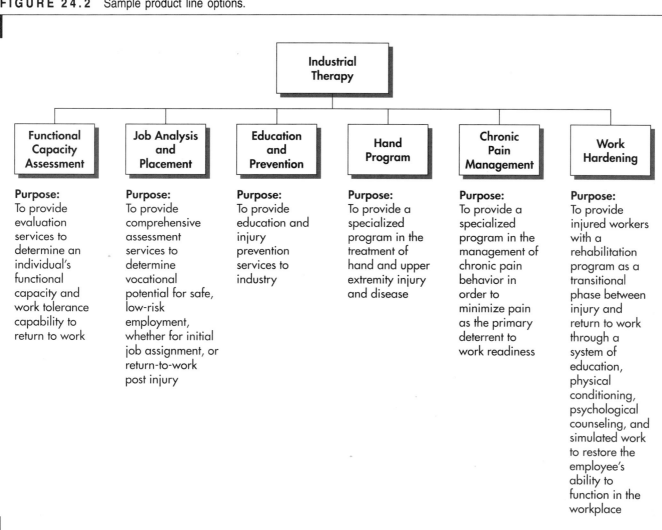

Hand Clinic, Chronic Pain Management, and Work Hardening.

FINANCIAL PLANNING

The number one economic consideration of Industrial Therapy programs is:

Are the resources expended appropriate given the resources generated?

To answer this question, one must step back and determine the financial viability or cost/benefit of operating the program. This can be achieved by analyzing the staff requirement, resource expenditure, and revenue generating ability of each product line. A cost/benefit analysis such as this provides a foundation for developing realistic financial *pro formas* and judging product line accountability.[2,3,4,5]

A portable mobile assessment unit in an automobile is another way to broaden market penetration without requiring additional permanent facilities (Figures 24.3, *A*, B). Work Hardening can be initially conducted on-site at the employer's facility. These are just a few examples of how to phase services into fully-owned, fully-staffed, fully-equipped Industrial Therapy services.

When evaluating the financial viability of product lines, it is necessary to determine the staffing, space, and equipment required to operate the program efficiently and competitively. Again, these in-vestments can be owned, leased or subcontracted as financial considerations permit. There are no fixed formulas for these decisions—they will vary depending upon:

- Product lines offered
- Forecasted number of clients
- Management expectations
- Acceptable risk
- Preferences of the clinical decision maker
- Market demographics
- Competitive environment

There are various guidelines for determining the requisite mix of staff, space, and equipment. For instance, CARF standards for work hardening require a mix of staff that includes:[9]

- Physical Therapist
- Occupational Therapist
- Vocational Specialist
- Psychologist

Phase-In Approach

In evaluating expenditures for staff, space, and equipment, it is important to know that these financial commitments do not have to be made all at once. They can be phased in gradually, commensurate with revenue growth and cash flow. Staff can be subcontracted part time until the case load justifies full time employment.

Space for product lines like Hand Clinic and Back School can be arranged at local public schools, or at the company's facility. Functional Capacity Assessments can be subcontracted until utilization justifies the

FIGURE 24.3 A, B A mobile functional capacity assessment is just one option to help broaden market penetration without requiring additional costs and space.

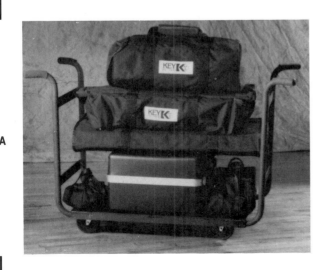
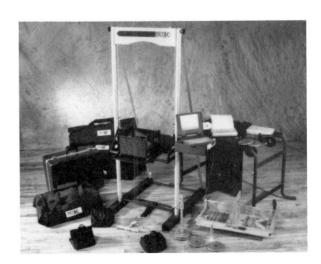

A

B

BOX 24.2

Sample Full Time Equivalent Clinical Staff Allocation Per Product Line (Minimum Standards)

Product line	Full time equivalents
Functional Assessment:	
FCA and Job Placement Assessment	1 PT or OT
Job Analysis and Placement:	
Job Analysis	1 Voc specialist or PT or OT
Counseling and Placement	1 Voc specialist or placement specialist
Hand Clinic:	
	1 Hand therapist (OT or PT)
	.5 COTA
	.5 Aide
Work Hardening:	
	1 PT or OT
	.5 Psychologist
	1 Sales/case manager
	.5 Exercise physiologist
	.5 Aide
Chronic Pain:	
	.5 Exercise physiologist
	.5 PT
	1 RN/case manager
	.5 Psychologist
	.5 Voc specialist or counselor (on contract as needed)
	.5 Physician
Education and Prevention:	
Back School and Cumulative Trauma Prevention	1 PT
	1 PTA
	.5 OT
	1 Aide

---

equipment purchase. Clinical Staff Allocation (Box 24.2) indicates the generally-accepted number of clinical staff for various product lines. These figures can be used as one benchmark in evaluating your staffing needs.

Once decisions have been reached regarding the minimum number of staff needed per product line, a cost benefit analysis of each product line can be conducted. Since 55 to 66% of total expenses are typically for staff, viability can be determined on the basis of staffing alone. The format in Boxes 24.3 and 24.4 may be used to accomplish this goal.[2,3,4,5,7]

A general guideline is that the ratio of revenue to salary expense should be in the range of 2:1 in order to cover operating expenses, overhead, cost of capital, and return on investment.

The following are key issues to resolve after conducting the cost/benefit analysis illustrated in the aforementioned boxes:

1. Is the proposed program space sufficient to accommodate the projected average daily census?
2. Is there sufficient diversity in the anticipated client mix relative to chronic condition and acuity?
3. Is the ratio of gross revenue to salary expenses satisfactory and in keeping with goals and expectations?

BOX 24.3

Projected Cost/Benefit Analysis Program—Work Hardening

Number and Type of Staff	Approximate Compensation Salary and Benefits
1 Sales/Case Manager	$ 40,000
1.5 Physical Therapist	$ 81,000
1.5 Occupational Therapist	$ 81,000
1.5 Clinical Psychologist	$ 93,000
2 Exercise Physiologists	$ 74,000
2 Aides	$ 44,000
1 Vocational Specialist	$ 43,000
2 Technicians	$ 62,000
2 Support Staff	$ 52,000
.5 Physicians	$ 70,000
15 Total Full Time Equivalents (FTEs)	$640,000

Number of clients per year	240
Average Daily Census (ADC)	20
Average Length of Stay (ALOS)	6 weeks
Number of rotations per year	8.6
Charge per day	$ 245
Average charge/client	$ 7,350
Projected revenue Work Hardening	$1,764,000
Average revenue per staff	$ 117,600
Average salary	$ 42,666

Ratio of gross revenue:
program salary expense 2.75:1

BOX 24.4

Projected Cost/Benefit Analysis Program—Chronic Pain Management

Number and Type of Staff	Approximate Compensation Salary and Benefits
.5 Physician	$ 70,000
1 Physical Therapist	$ 54,000
1 Occupational Therapist	$ 54,000
2 Clinical Psychologists	$125,000
1 Exercise Physiologist	$ 37,000
.5 Vocational Specialist	$ 24,000
1 Sales/Case Manager	$ 40,000
.5 RN	$ 24,000
1 Support Staff	$ 26,000
8.5 Total Full Time Equivalents (FTE's)	$454,000

Number of clients per year	120
Average Daily Census (ADC)	20
Average Length of Stay (ALOS)	8 weeks
Number of rotations per year	6.5
Average charge per patient	$ 7,500
Projected revenue	$900,000
Average revenue per staff	$105,882
Average salary	$ 53,411

Ratio of gross revenue:
program salary expense 2:1

---

4. Is the ratio of client to dedicated staff acceptable?
5. Are all assumptions realistic and able to be achieved? If not, what modifications can be made:
   a. Increase or decrease average daily census?
   b. Identify core staff and modify FTEs while maintaining integrity of care?
   c. Decrease or reduce compensation?
   d. Increase fees per patient?
   e. Add new services that can be implemented with the same staffing?
6. What variables, if any, should be considered for modification?
7. Should this program be implemented given the financial and staffing variables?

This system of analysis allows management to view both the *macro* and *micro* picture and upon this basis determine success potential of product lines and the overall program.[2,3,4,7] After determining each product line's viability through cost benefit analysis, it is necessary to develop a financial *pro forma* for the entire Industrial Therapy program.

The *pro forma* should include all anticipated expenses and revenues for operating all product lines under the program. The expenses should be detailed by month. It is also important to calculate the adjusted bad debt and any contractual arrangements or discounts, if applicable.

To assist in developing the financial plan, Box 24.5 provides an example equipment list. Figures 24.4 and 24.5 provide a financial summary and detailed format for a one year *pro forma* covering monthly revenue and expenses for the total outpatient Industrial Therapy program. Figure 24.6 provides a format for monthly revenue projections by product line.[2,3,4,7]

Financial projections for the start up phase should

BOX 24.5

Example Industrial Therapy Equipment List

Equipment Need	Approximate Cost
Functional Assessment:	
FCA system	$25,000–35,000
Job Placement Assessment (usually included in FCA)	—
Upper extremity add on to FCA	1,000–1,500
Job Analysis and Placement:	
Job Analysis equipment	3,000–4,000
Education & Prevention:	
Audio visual and 3 models	2,500–3,000
Hand Program:	
Acute care equipment and materials	3,500–5,000
Chronic Pain Management:	
Education and prevention equipment (AV + models included in above)	—
Biofeedback system	3,000–4,000
Work Hardening:	
4 Basic stations	30,000–40,000
Conditioning equipment	15,000–20,000
Other specialized equipment	5,000–10,000
Total	$88,000–122,500

assume negative profit for the initial months until revenues catch up with expenses. Projections should also include cash flow, as cash outlays for equipment and working capital need to be recouped by the monthly bottom line profit indicated in Figure 24.5. Box 24.6 provides a format for the program's monthly cash flow projections.[2,3,4,7]

A line of credit might have to be established to cover this lag in cash flow, especially during the first six months of operations. Interest expense would increase accordingly.[2,3,4,7]

MARKETING

The best research and financial planning are irrelevant unless the program has a strong marketing component. As more providers enter the rehabilitation field, mar-keting plays an increasing and significant role in assuring the economic success and stability of any Industrial Therapy program.[5,6,8]

Marketing strategies and tactics are covered in greater detail in Chapter 27, but it is important to discuss some of the key economic considerations.

In order for an Industrial Therapy program to capture a large share and presence in the competitive market, it is imperative to implement a strong marketing plan. The marketing plan should be time-delineated, focus on developing market share in key Industrial Therapy product lines, and establish one year and three year plans outlining:

- Status of the present and future market
- Overall program image and direction
- Marketing tactics to be used
- Budgeting allocation
- Persons responsible for implementation
- Means of monitoring and revising to the plan on a quarterly basis

Each organization's marketing plan should be prepared with an awareness of the present and future dynamics in the industry, competitor strengths and weaknesses, the organization's current market share and potential market share, and the organization's strengths and weaknesses relative to the competition. Market share is a critical variable to examine.

When considering market share, plans should look not only to a reallocation of the current utilization "pie," but also to increasing the size of that pie by addressing demand for services not currently being met by existing providers.

While a program may have distinct and well-identified opportunities to capture a significant share of the existing market, future growth and viability depends upon identifying and pursuing new market sectors currently unserved or under-served.

This concept of market creation is especially promising in Industrial Therapy. Focus groups with third-party carriers and employer representatives indicate much room for improvement in existing programs, particularly Work Hardening, and a belief that most programs do not truly offer a comprehensive breadth of services.[7]

Key characteristics of a comprehensive system of Industrial Therapy that would meet the expected needs of carriers and employers, are outcome orientation, and responsive to the issues of the injured worker.[7]

Industrial Therapy is a dynamic and changing business. Success in delivering programs to injured workers will require that providers adopt an entrepreneurial approach to developing and managing their operations. By focusing on creating new markets, addressing the needs of the unserved or underserved,

FIGURE 24.4 Industrial Rehabilitation program financial summary.

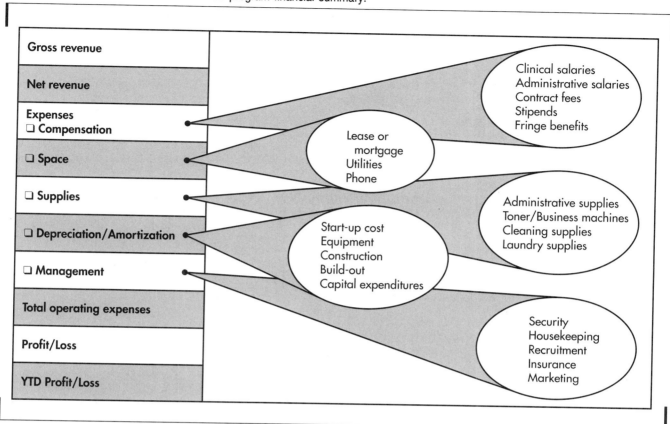

(Courtesy Murer Consultants.)

BOX 24.6

Start-Up Cash Flow Projection Format

Month:	Prelaunch	1	2	3	4	5
Revenue:						
Gross revenue:						
Less ABD						
Net revenue						
Total expense						
Profit <loss>						
Cash flow +/−						
Cash flow YTD						

Prelaunch cash outflow:
Facilities/leasehold $ _____
Equipment _____
Prepaid expenses _____
Working capital _____
Other _____

Total prelaunch _____

FIGURE 24.5   Detailed one year pro forma covering monthly revenue and expenses for an outpatient Industrial Therapy program.

Sample Pro Forma
Year_____

Prepared by: Murer Consultants

Month:	1	2	3	4	5	6	7	8	9	10	11	12	Total	
Revenue: Gross Rev. Less ABD														**Revenue:** Gross Rev. Less ABD
Net Rev.														Net Rev.
Expenses														**Expenses**
Salaries Clinical Adm. per.														Salaries Clinical Adm. per.
Fringe ben.														Fringe ben.
Med. dir. fee														Med. dir. fee
Rent/space exp.														Rent/space exp.
Computer depreciation														Computer depreciation
Med. eqpt. depreciation														Med. eqpt. depreciation
Offc. eqpt. depreciation														Offc. eqpt. depreciation
Leasehold/ buildout depre.														Leasehold/ buildout depre.
Pre-open exp. amort.														Pre-open exp. amort.
Eqpt. maint./ service														Eqpt. maint./ service
Medical supply														Medical supply
Marketing														Marketing
Educa./travel														Educa./travel
Adminst. supply														Adminst. supply
Housekeeping														Housekeeping
Recruitment expense														Recruitment expense
Phone/leasing/ mon./chrg.														Phone/leasing/ mon./chrg.
Misc. software														Misc. software
Laundry														Laundry
Video/ptnt. edn.														Video/ptnt. edn.
Insurance														Insurance
INTEREST														INTEREST

TOTAL EXPENSE
Profit (Loss)
Profit (Loss) YTD

TOTAL EXPENSE
Profit (Loss)
Profit (Loss) YTD
HCFA Contr. Adj.

Year_____   Net Margin

© Murer Consultants 1992

(Courtesy Murer Consultants.)

and educating the market to new solutions, the market creator can set the standard of expectation for the industry.

The implementation of aggressive marketing re-quires significant resources. In addition to strong sup-port and commitment from administration and staff, a realistic and well reasoned budget and plan must be developed. To do so, it is important to consider the

FIGURE 24.6 Sample format for monthly revenue projections by product line.

Prepared by: Murer Consultants

Month:

Product line	1	2	3	4	5	6	7	8	9	10	11	12	Total
Total pts													
Total revenue													

© Murer Consultants 1992

(Courtesy Murer Consultants.)

marketing needs and opportunities for each product line and apportion the dollars accordingly.

Each product line plan should take into consideration the client, insurance company, employer and other significant referral sources in determining the appropriate amount of, and best allocation of, marketing funds.

Refer to Chapter 27 for more detail on developing and executing marketing plans.

SUMMARY

To ensure the long term success and profitability of Industrial Therapy programs, it is imperative to consider the numerous factors which will impact the program's financial and market status. A decision to develop or maintain a program which can excel in today's marketplace requires: careful research; strategic, financial, and marketing planning; product line development; and significant commitment and vision from administration and staff.

Notwithstanding the importance of the economic considerations of Industrial Therapy, the bottom line is still dependent on returning the worker to work in a timely and cost efficient manner.

REFERENCES

1. Breen GE, Blankenship AB: *Do-It-Yourself Marketing Research*, McGraw-Hill.
2. Brigham EF, Gapenski LC: *Intermediate Financial Management*, 1990, Dryden Press.
3. Flamholtz EG, Diamond MA, Flamholtz DT: *Financial Accounting*, 1986, MacMillan Publishing.
4. Garrison RH: *Managerial Accounting, Concepts for Planning, Control, and Decision Making*, 1988, Business Publications.

5. Gumpert D: How to Really Create a Successful Business Plan, *Inc. Magazine,* p 1–174, 1990.

6. Kotler P: *Marketing Management, Analysis, Planning, Implementation, and Control,* 1988, Prentice Hall.

7. Murer Consultants, Joliet, Ill. Findings from focus group research among third party carriers and employers.

8. Porter ME: *Competitive Strategy, Techniques for Analyzing Industries and Competitors,* 1980, The Free Press.

9. 1993 *Standards Manual for Organizations Serving People with Disabilities,* Tucson, Arizona, 1992, Commission on Accreditation of Rehabilitation Facilities.

CHAPTER

25

Transition to Industrial Therapy

D'Arcy Bain

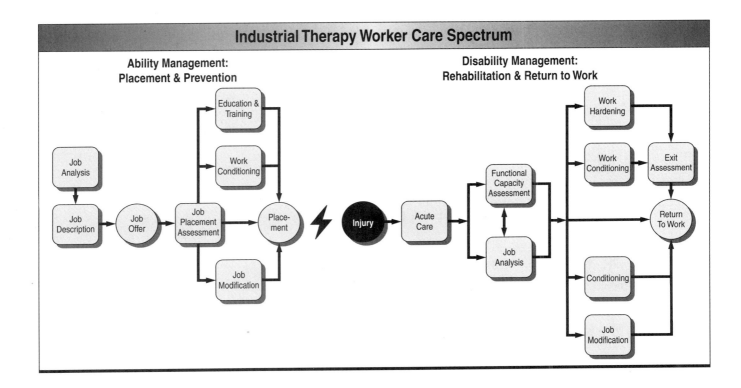

Industrial Therapy Worker Care Spectrum

To start out in Industrial Therapy requires an entrepreneurial spirit. The Therapist will encounter many differences relative to traditional therapy. There is a whole new group of customers, tougher measurement and performance standards, and an abundance of new technology to meet them. The programs must be aggressive, active, well planned, and effectively marketed. The approach must be goal-orientated in all aspects of management, business practice, and patient care.

Industrial Therapy is not a decorative add on. It is work and must reflect that. It requires a self-starter who has more than a 9 to 5 work ethic. But the satisfaction and rewards are well worth the effort.

Expanding an existing business into new areas requires considerable knowledge about the differences that will be encountered. The steps required to make the transition involve careful planning and management of capital resources, staffing, marketing funds, and cash flow.

Accordingly, this chapter will provide a base of knowledge regarding the differences between traditional therapy, sports therapy and Industrial Therapy. It will then outline the steps involved in developing an Industrial Therapy practice as an outgrowth of an existing PT practice, including an equipment checklist, expansion guidelines, and marketing suggestions. The chapter can also guide those conceptually contemplating starting an Industrial Therapy practice.

TRADITIONAL, SPORTS, AND INDUSTRIAL THERAPY

Industrial Therapy involves differences in who the customer is, the treatment processes, the return-to-function context, the treatment site, legal and regulatory rules, measurement standards, programs, performance standards, equipment, and marketing requirements. Table 25.1 summarizes these differences relative to traditional and sports therapy. (Differences in treatment process and equipment are too numerous to include in Table 25.1, so they will be covered separately later in the chapter).

TABLE 25.1 Traditional, Sports, and Industrial Therapy Major Differences

	Therapies		
Issues	*Traditional*	*Sports*	*Industrial*
Person treated	Patient	Athlete	Employee Client Claimant
Referred by/reports to	Physician Family	Physician Family Health team Coach/team	Physician Family Health team Employer Insurance company Vocational Rehab. Case Manager Attorney Workers' Comp. board
Payor	Health insurer	Health insurer Athlete	Workers' Comp. insurer Employer
Goal-return to . . .	Normal life	Sports play	Work
Legal and regulatory exposure	Moderate	Light	Heavy
Measurement standards	Some measurement and profess. opinion	More science	Statistically intense
Outcome orientation	Informally defined— "do your best"	Moderately defined— return to play ASAP	Clearly defined—Return to maximum function quickly, with minimum risk of reinjury, cost-effectively
Programs offered	Pain relief Range of motion Strengthening Education-general	Traditional Emergency care Aggressive treatment Transition treatment Preseason cond. Postseason cond. Education-sports specific	Functional Capacity Assessment Job Task Analysis Job Placement Assessment Job Site Analysis Education and prevention Work Conditioning Work Hardening
Site of treatment	Hospital Private clinic Rehab facility	Hospital Private clinic Team facility: university, pro, or amateur	Hospital Private clinic Rehab facility Work Hardening Center Work site Company offices
Age group	0 to 80 years	8 to 55 years	18 to 65 years
Marketing	Very little	Some	Intense

FIGURE 25.1 A, B, The transition from the patient as passive recipient in a clinical setting to an active participant in real-world settings.

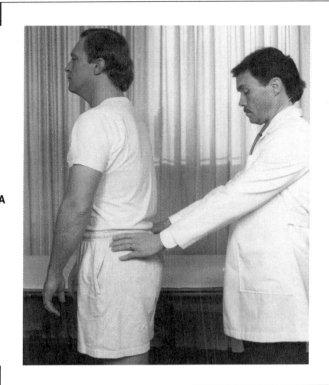

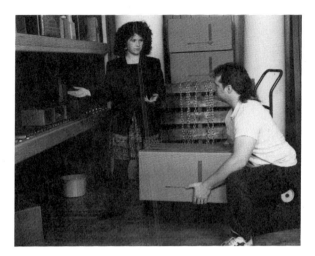

A

B

THE PATIENT AND PROCESS PARTICIPANTS

Traditional Therapy

Traditionally, Therapists in institutions or private clinics begin patient contact upon the physician's referral or the hospital's standing orders (post-operative programs).[4,16] The patient can be anyone who has had surgery or an injury, and the Therapist typically reports to the doctor or referring party.

Sports Therapy

The Therapist typically has a more on-going relationship with the sports organization or team. The association does not always begin through a doctor's referral as is the case in traditional therapy. Referrals may also initiate through a school athletic director or coach, or through a professional team's front office. The patients are almost exclusively athletes. Status and progress reports are typically reviewed with the athlete and the coach as well as other medical and team management personnel.

Industrial Therapy

In Industrial Therapy the patient is typically referred to as the "client," and is an injured worker. In this con-text, there is an expanding complexity of referral sources and reporting relationships. The referral might come from any one of a number of sources including the doctor, insurance company, employer, or vocational rehabilitation consultant, to name a few.[11] Although the insurance company most typically exercises the final decision, because they pay the bills, the decision-making process is often shared by a number of participating parties interacting as a team.[11]

TREATMENT PROCESS

Table 25.2 outlines the major differences in treatment process between Traditional, Sports, and Industrial Therapy.

Traditional Therapy

In Traditional Therapy, treatment is provided in three main stages—1) acute (injury healing), 2) rehabilitation, and 3) reintegration.[16] The acute stage is that time period from 0 to 21 days of wound treatment, pain management, and infection control.[10]

The rehabilitation stage includes out-patient clinic treatment designed to return the patient to independence. This treatment incorporates range of motion,

TABLE 25.2 Traditional, Sports, and Industrial Therapy Treament Processes Differences

	Therapies		
Issues	*Traditional*	*Sports*	*Industrial*
Initial steps	Therapist takes history and asks questions	Therapist reviews with team doctor, coach, and athlete.	Therapist conducts FCA, JA, or JPA, then specifies RTW Goals and treatment process
Treatment process	Acute care: In or outpatient Outpatient rehab Education	Acute care: In or outpatient On-field rehabilitation Prevention and education	Acute care: In or outpatient On-site, or rehabilitation center Prevention, training, and education Work Conditioning Work Hardening
	Outpatient reintegration	In practice reintegration	On-site reintegration
Real-world simulation	Light	Heavy	Heavy
Psychosocial inclusion	Little	Moderate: motivation to return to play	Heavy: Self esteem Attitude adjustment Peer relationships Family and social issues
Treatment "team" orientation	Little	Moderate: Doctor, Athlete Therapist, Coach	Heavy: Doctor, Worker, Therapist, Employer, Peers, Family, etc.

strengthening, and preparation for return to activities —work, sport, or independent daily living.

The reintegration stage is when therapy is gradually phased out and the patient's return to independence is phased in.

In traditional therapy, upon referral from the physician or from hospital personnel, the therapist typically takes the patient's history and questions the patient to understand his or her personal situation, work situation, and hobbies. Treatment goals are established to restore the patient's independence. Great attention to simulating the exact postures, movements, and resistances involved are frequently not done as long as the patient is independent.

Treatment consists of pain relief, general range of motion, strengthening, and education. Social or psychological factors impacting progress and return to function are not typically considered or managed in the process, unless it is of great concern.

Sports Therapy

Sports therapy is more aggressive and active than traditional therapy, even in the acute stage of recovery from athletic injuries. The athlete is advised to continue aerobic conditioning during acute treatment if possible, and attend practices to ensure a better transition

to return to play. This "active" acute stage makes the rehabilitation stage progress with ease.[9]

In the sports rehabilitation stage, psychology and motivation play an important role, so that when the athlete is ready to return, they are prepared mentally as well as physically. For amateur athletes, therapists have to "pull back on the reins" to ensure that they do not try to progress too quickly.

To ensure safer return to play with minimum risk of reinjury, the therapist observes and evaluates the athlete's performance on the field in a controlled situation (the practice) before permitting return to the game situation. Being on the field to guide the athlete through to full activity is an essential part of the process. In addition, being on the field gains the athlete's respect and confidence that the therapist understands the sport and knows what is to be.[9]

It is very important to have the resources and consensus on adhering to these principles of rehabilitation:

1. Earliest possible intervention and early start of acute care rehabilitation
2. Aggressive, active, participating rehabilitation
3. On-field presence and observation during the reintegration phase until full capabilities are restored
4. On-site preventative programs to reduce injuries

Industrial Therapy

Industrial Therapy can be seen as more complex than sports therapy in a number of areas.

Goal orientation is not only toward enhancing the worker's capabilities to fit the job, but also toward modifying the job to safely fit the worker.[11] Greater control over outcomes is attempted through more scientific and reliable methods of testing, evaluation, and simulation.

On-site analysis, treatment, and prevention are used to ensure results translate to successful outcome. Procedurally, there is an increasing emphasis on a team approach, in which the doctor, therapist, case manager, insurer, and even family and peers work together for maximum coordination and success.

Medically and legally, Industrial Therapy is a more adversarial process—worker's physician and company physician, claimant and payor, plaintiff and defendant, —and the therapist has a greater involvement in resolving disputes and facilitating teamwork.

Psychologically, greater attention is paid to such factors as the worker's self esteem, positive or negative attitude, peer group relationships, and family, social, and financial situations.[9] There are methods for detecting malingerers so that they can be dealt with appropriately through treatment or case management.[11,12] It is also important that negative attitudes do not undermine the morale and progress of others.

Patient conversations, apparent negative advice and comments to each other should be monitored. Those not wanting to return to work may consider this structured program and supervision an infringement of the right to be idle, and may be looking for opportunities to profit through litigation.

In summary, the Industrial Therapy treatment process is more comprehensive, job site driven, outcome based, science intensive, team oriented, and holistic than traditional and sports therapy.

RETURN-TO-FUNCTION CONTEXT

Traditional Therapy

Although there is some effort to understand the patient's job, social and leisure life, and hobbies, the emphasis is on returning to capabilities and activities in general, rather than to specific movements, resistances, frequencies, and endurance in a specific environment. This generalized emphasis also results in a focus on individual body parts rather than on the whole body.

The therapist relies on the doctor's instructions, the patient's input, personal observations and measurements to determine treatment goals and the plan.

Treatment is typically in a hospital or clinic outpatient area. There is little or no in-home, on-field, or on-the-job analysis or treatment. Prevention programs are often in a classroom at the hospital or other medical facility, usually for health care employees, and tend to be generic in nature.

Sports Therapy

Sports therapy uses on-field assessment, then progresses from the controlled practices, to specialty teams, to active competitive play. Return to activity is monitored and adjusted on the field during the transition until the athlete is ready to participate at full levels. Players may be tested on Cybex, Dynatrac, or Kincom systems, but on-field performance is the final determinant on whether they can return to competition.

This increases confidence in the recovery stage, reduces the risk of reinjury, and better prepares the athlete to resume safe play.

Industrial Therapy

The focal point in Industrial Therapy is the job site and the work station. The analysis of the total environment (physical and psychosocial) and of all the job tasks is more thorough and scientific. All the components of the Worker Care Spectrum—Functional Capacity Assessment (FCA), Job Analysis, Job Placement Assessment, Work Conditioning, and Work Hardening—attempt to represent real world conditions in order to better control outcomes. There is growing recognition that analysis, treatment, and the return-to-work transition are enhanced by proper simulation and interaction (Figures 25.2, *A, B, C*).

LEGAL AND REGULATORY

Traditional Therapy

With the doctor or hospital referring and managing the case, traditional therapists have not tended to become entangled in liability suits or Workers' Compensation litigation. The therapist may recommend return to activity, but the final say, and hence the liability, lies primarily with the referring physician or hospital.

Sports Therapy

Sports therapy involves the least amount of legal and regulatory intrusion. The therapist typically shoulders more decision making responsibility, but there is less propensity for the kinds of law suits, litigated insurance claims, and discrimination suits found in traditional or industrial therapy.

FIGURE 25.2 A, B, C   The transition from a hands-on focus on the injured body part to more scientific procedures that more closely simulate real-world function.

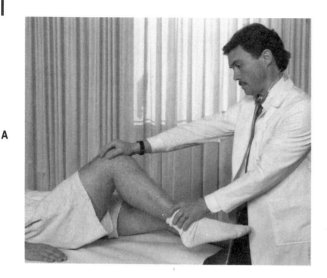

A

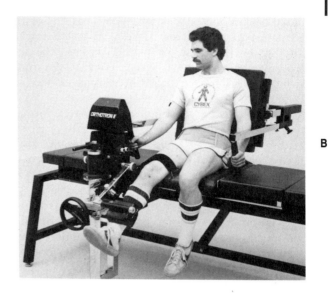

B

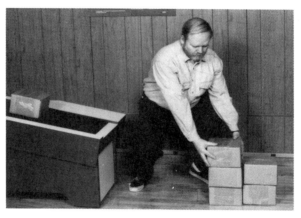

C

(25–2B From Gould: Orthopedic and Sports Physical Therapy, ed 2, St Louis Mosby.)

Industrial Therapy

Industrial Therapy is surrounded by a growing amount of legal and regulatory complexity.[2,5,8,14,18,19,21] The majority of cases to date have involved Workers' Compensation and liability claims. New OSHA Regulations and the Americans with Disabilities Act are sure to increase the involvement.

These aspects are covered in greater detail in other chapters, but it is important to note here the overall implications. In Industrial Therapy, there is a growing necessity to justify or defend treatment and recommendations with statistically reliable data.

If a worker becomes injured, the employer might have to show, in court, that the FCA and the Job Placement Assessment were thorough and proper. Or, if the worker is deemed unable to reassume the job, the employer might have to show that the Job Analysis is relevant and that no accommodation can be made without undue financial hardship.[3,6,13,17,20]

Some Therapists may view such issues as reasons to avoid Industrial Therapy. Others will see them as a new source of demand for their services, and will derive a great deal of satisfaction helping employers and their employees reap the long term benefits intended by these legal and regulatory measures.

MEASUREMENT STANDARDS AND OUTCOME ORIENTATION

Traditional Therapy

Traditional therapy has been driven by medically-based standards of evaluation and measurement. In traditional medicine, physicians have focused on returning the individual to "normal." All physician orders derive from evaluations comparing to normal, such as "blood count is normal, electrocardiogram is normal," or "no significant abnormalities." Medicine learns what "normal" is, and directs treatment to either increase or decrease the readings until they are once again "normal." Unfortunately, there are times when the numbers are normal but the patient is not ready to return to full function (Figure 25.3 *A, B*).

In determining the patient's ability to return to normal home, recreational, or work activities, traditional therapy uses the guidelines of pain free range of movement, strength, and the patient's input. Doctors and therapists rely on observation, experience, and intuition. Lack of objective measurement or outcome definition can result in discontinuing treatment too early, or prolonging treatment beyond what is necessary.

In traditional therapy, fixing the injury has often taken precedence over developing precise measurements of job demands and functional capabilities. In the last ten years, however, employers, claims payors, regulatory bodies, the courts, researchers, and others have demanded more objective independent reproducible assessment systems.

Technology has emerged to meet these demands as academic credentials have increased to masters and doctorate degrees, which in turn has spurred university research and given rise to greater specialization in areas such as orthopedics, sports medicine, and now Industrial Therapy.

Adoption of these new technologies by traditional therapists has been only gradual, as the demand increased and their budgets allowed.

FIGURE 25.3 The transition from a range-of-motion goal **(A)** to a job performance capability goal **(B)**.

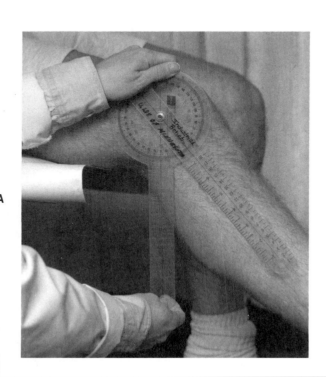

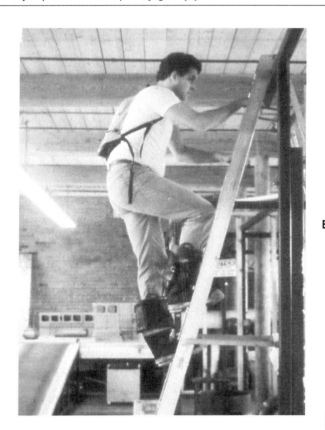

Sports Therapy

In sports therapy, athletes are at the extremes of the measurement ranges and often outside the learned normal variances of strength, range of motion, and endurance. These extremes gave rise to new measuring devices like Cybex, Kincom, Dynatrac, and various movement analysis systems. Sports medicine has also used many scientific assessment units to evaluate performance, but many like the EKG, EMG, or EEG are unidimensional and of limited use in determining whether the athlete could return to dynamic play.[10]

To more fully meet their needs, sports Therapists have developed on-field dynamic tests that are functionally related to specific sports. The Therapist has the athlete do segments of the sport, with each skill broken down into its demands for strength and range of motion. Treatment can then be focused on the areas preventing the athlete's return to play. These on-field tests, although still subjective, improve the coach's and medical team's ability to assess the athlete's readiness to resume full competition.

Sports therapy has been the testing ground for many new developments in objective measuring devices and subjective testing, to assess the individual's ability to return to an activity. Industrial Therapy has drawn from many of these approaches.

Industrial Therapy

Industrial Therapy's growing requirements for more objective measurements and predictable outcomes has brought about steady improvement in technology and in statistical applications.

Return to work assessment systems with static lift stations reliably assist return to employment decisions. Since these assessments do not relate to the job's actual components, it is like testing a swimmer on a bicycle.

Industrial Therapy requires more reliable, reproducible, objective, measurement systems. When the employer, doctor, insurance carrier, or lawyer asks if the employee/patient/claimant/client can return to work, the Therapist needs a measuring system that can provide a reliable answer, one that might have to hold up in court. This need has been answered by the Functional Capacity Assessment.

The market offers several FCA systems that are dynamic and demonstrate a track record of safely returning workers to work (Figure 25.4). Most systems test the common 22 to 26 work related activities, some are computerized, others are reproducible and reliable, and all have varying degrees of medical-legal acceptance.

The company's reputation, compliance with other agencies such as CARF, length of time in business, and satisfied users are all considerations. Additionally, the system should produce an income similar to patient contact, so that it is not a drain on overall fees.

Some FCA systems require two days of testing which can be a costly diversion of time from clinic patient contact. There are, however, systems that deliver state-of-the-art reliability in a four-hour full-body evaluation (KEY Method). These systems enable therapists to do the analysis and reporting yet still maintain patient contact on the same day. With the addition of Job Task and Work Site analysis (Taskmaster TM), the complete picture can be assembled in one day.

The FCA is a marketable tool that satisfies industry's need for more reliable measurement and predictability. It is the baseline measurement of capabilities that provides the foundation for the other analyses and prescriptions in the Worker Care Spectrum described in Chapter 1 and elsewhere. It is the heart of an Industrial Therapy program. It provides the credibility required to interface with therapists, physicians, vocational rehabilitation consultants, and industry.

FIGURE 25.4   A functional capacity assessment relates the worker's capabilities to norms that enable the therapist to set goals, develop a rehabilitation plan, and predict outcomes.

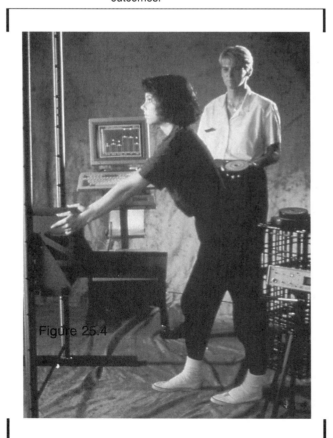

PROGRAMS

Traditional Therapy

Traditional therapy offers programs in pain relief, range of motion, strengthening, and education. In addition, there are programs that focus on specific body parts such as hip replacement rehabilitation, medial collateral ligament repair, and William's flexion exercises for the back. Prevention programs are not typically involved.

Sports Therapy

Conditioning programs—preseason, post-season, and on-going—have proven instrumental in reducing the frequency of injury and enhancing the injury healing stage. Regular conditioning, if maintained during rehabilitation, accelerates the athletes' healing process and return to play.[1]

On-site (on-field, in the gym) services in sports therapy are the most valuable. The therapist gains complete knowledge of the sport, the physical needs of each position, and the fitness profile needed for the sport—strength, flexibility, power, and endurance. There are preseason evaluations to ensure that individuals are physically ready to participate.[7]

Some clinics open training facilities to the general public during off hours and off season. Positioned as a fitness center offering professional conditioning programs for the weekend athlete, these programs ensure more economic use of the equipment and space.

Industrial Therapy

Industrial Therapy is significantly more program-oriented than traditional or sports therapy. The many components of the Worker Care Spectrum give an indication of the multifaceted and interactive nature of IT. Some of these programs can be adapted from traditional and sports therapy programs. Others have to be created from scratch.

Starting at the preemployment point and moving through the Worker Care Spectrum, a brief summary of the programs offered in a typical Industrial Therapy practice are as follows.

In the hiring process, the Americans with Disabilities Act bars any capabilities testing before making a job offer, except for an "agility test," which is a potential loophole in the regulations because it can include literally hundreds of tests. Besides this exception, capabilities testing is prohibited until the applicant has been offered a job and accepts the offer. At this point it is permissible to do a Job Placement Assessment (JPA).

The JPA is enhanced if a Job Analysis has been performed so that an applicant's capabilities can be optimally matched to the actual job requirements. New equipment and training in proper methods are required to offer these programs. See the equipment list later in this chapter for more information.

The next program in the spectrum might be education to instill safe work habits, or work conditioning to reduce the risk of injury. Education programs stressing prevention, posture, relaxation, stretching and strengthening exercises may be adapted from traditional or sports materials, by adding slides showing employees at work stations. The presentation can be enhanced by focusing on employees and work stations with high injury rates.

Industry also needs a Repetitive Injury Prevention Program for afflictions such as carpal tunnel syndrome. Ergonomic programs, such as seating for drivers or office workers, can be valuable additions to the total offering.

If a worker becomes injured, once initial healing is complete, a Functional Capacity Assessment is performed to provide a measurement of post-injury status to determine if the person can return to work, or whether they require rehabilitation. If rehabilitation is indicated, the FCA in combination with job analysis can help determine reasonable return-to-work goals. The combination of these analyses ensures that injured workers can be returned to jobs that match their capabilities safely.

Work Conditioning programs can be implemented using existing exercise, weight, and aerobic equipment, although equipment that simulates the actual job functions should be added. See the equipment lists later in the chapter for more detail.

Work Hardening programs at a facility are essentially Work Conditioning with the addition of social and psychological considerations during the therapy. Work Hardening attempts to replicate the work environment with special task simulation equipment, and with sessions of several hours to further simulate the work day experience.

A Work Hardening session of two to four hours requires a facilitating environment, variety in day to day activities, and appropriate education sessions such as lifting postures, relaxation techniques, life style modification, and stress control to keep the client motivated and prepare for reentry into the workforce. Negative attitudes and malingerers (detected by invalid participation levels in FCAs) must be identified and dealt with very early.

On-site Work Retraining can function as a graduated return-to-work-program. It gives the employer, employee, and union the confidence that the client is going to be able to do the job and that the client is being given every opportunity to return safely. It also gives the supervising Therapist an informal dialogue with management, supervisors, foremen, and workers. On-site Work Retraining can also be a viable approach prior to investing in a Work Retraining facility.

One disadvantage of an on-site Work Retraining program is that the Therapist must travel to each company to instruct and supervise the activities, and cannot work with as many clients simultaneously.

Industrial Therapy has several other areas that supplement and enhance an existing traditional or sports therapy practice. For instance, most traumatic hand injuries occur in industrial settings, so this is a specialty area that can be added to both attract new industrial clients, while strengthening the overall patient base. Another program that accomplishes the same result is therapy for upper limb cumulative trauma disorders. Some FCA systems have special upper extremity and hand protocols to assist efforts in these areas.[12] In implementing these programs, it is important to have qualified Therapists to provide sufficient credibility.

PERFORMANCE STANDARDS

Traditional Therapy

In traditional therapy, the direction that comes with the referral might be general such as "assess and treat," or a more specific prescription for pain relief, range of motion, or strengthening. The Therapist's goal is to raise the patient to "the highest possible level of independence."

Often, the patient's program is concluded with little or no objective evaluation as to the ability to perform the previous job. The patient might be released from therapy upon reaching strength and range of motion goals based on the capabilities of the uninjured limb.

Sports Therapy

In sports therapy, the ideal is to restore the athlete's skills to the preinjury level. In professional sports, where recovery time impacts income, there is pressure to accomplish recovery as quickly as possible, sometimes at the risk of reinjury. In amateur sports with no impact on income, there is seldom a compromise medical-legally on the decision of when to return to play.

The progression for athletes is that they go into practice first. If there are no problems reported or demonstrated they can return to play. Typically the Therapist observes and evaluates the ability to run,

catch, jump, stop, start, or shoot, duplicating the sport to which the athlete wants to return.

Industrial Therapy

Industry does not just want an employee healed, which was acceptable under traditional therapy programs. They want the employee returned to maximum job performance quickly, cost effectively, and with minimum risk of reinjury. If the worker is unable to assume the former job functions, the employer will require assistance in finding a suitable alternative, which may include job modification. Employers want their employees to realize that the company has their physical well being and safety in mind. Enlightened companies understand the benefits of having productive healthy employees with low incidences of injury.

EQUIPMENT

Box 25.1 outlines the equipment additions involved in the transition from traditional therapy, to sports therapy, to Industrial Therapy.

There is some cross-over of equipment, but Industrial Therapy is a specialization that requires special equipment for FCA, JPA, Job Analysis, Conditioning, Job Simulation, and Work Hardening. In some cases more weight stations and aerobic stations are required to maintain two to four hour programs.

The cross-over from traditional therapy is a much greater step than from sports therapy, but it is not a risk if there are already sound administrative structures and effective therapy programs in place (Figures 25.5, *A, B, C*).

Equipment and materials for in-house education programs on anatomy, lifting techniques, posture, lifestyle changes, weight-control, nutrition, and pain control are readily accessible from commercial sources in most areas of the country. These programs, conducted in a class format, enhance the client's positive outlook and progress toward returning to work.

MARKETING

Traditional Therapy

In traditional therapy, most patients come from doctor or hospital referrals. This reduces the need to market one's practice broadly, however, the therapist has less control over maintaining a steady flow of patients when dependent upon a small universe of referral sources.

BOX 25.1

Equipment Requirements
Transition From Traditional to Sports to Industrial PT

Traditional therapy equipment package

Transcutaneous electrical nerve stimulator
Electrical muscle stimulator
Interferential current therapy
Short wave diathermy
High voltage galvanic
Laser
Ultra sound
Traction
Ice/heat
Strengthening—Pulley, free weights, latex tube
Stretching   —Mats, poster, handouts
Aerobic   —UBE, bike, treadmill, stepper, rower
Education   —Neck and back programs (slides
                 and O/H projector)

Sports therapy equipment package

Same as traditional therapy equipment package, with these additions:
Exercise—Multi-station or separate station stack
             weight units
          —Some eccentric equip., proprioceptive
             training
          —Heavier free weights
Aerobic —3 to 4 Stations for variety and multi user
             concept

Industrial therapy equipment package

Same as sports therapy equipment package with these additions:
Functional Capacity Assessment system
Job task/job site analysis equipment—video camera,
    scale, tape measure, dynamometer, pedometer,
    clamps, data collection unit, etc.
Work Hardening (job simulation equipment):
    —Light assembly conveyer
    —Shovel pit
    —Material handling station
    —Construction station (plumbing, electrical)
    —Push/pull station
    —Driver's station
Work Conditioning—(Use traditional and sports PT
    equipment)
Education
    —Neck and back (customized for specific indus-
      tries)
    —Repetitive stress injury prevention program
    —VCR and TV (for education and interactive
      videos)
Time clock

Sports Therapy

In sports therapy there is more latitude and control over professional relationships and referrals. Although patients may be initially referred by a team doctor, frequent and on-going contact with players, coaches, trainers, and managers puts sports therapists in a position to be the preferred choice for future needs. These team relationships may also lead to treating family members' injuries as well.

Industrial Therapy

Marketing is covered in great detail in Chapter 27. As one of the most important elements in the transition to Industrial Therapy, however, some comments are appropriate in this chapter's discussion.

Not everyone is able to approach industry to offer products. Being out of the clinic and meeting industry face to face is very difficult for some individuals. Some practitioners have the opinion that marketing is unprofessional, however, clients do not come running to the therapist's door.

Marketing can make or break success in Industrial Therapy. This becomes apparent early in the transition. Industrial Therapy is not an activity that a therapist can just dabble in.

Industry and the client have critical needs that are taken very seriously. Communicating the availability of solutions to these needs requires time, treading in areas which may not be comfortable, and incurring extra expenses for marketing material. The therapist must study the policies, terminology, and politics of this practice, then learn how to be persuasive through the media that most effectively reach this audience. Those who have to compete should meet the game face on and prepare for the challenge.

Industrial Therapy requires thoroughly researching the industrial area referral base. This involves

FIGURE 25.5 Some equipment for Industrial Therapy programs transfer from traditional **(A)** and sports therapy **(B)**, while other equipment is developed uniquely for Industrial Therapy **(C)**.

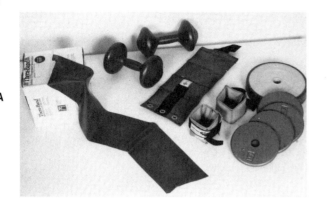

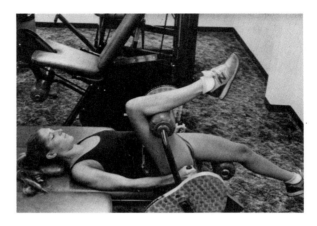

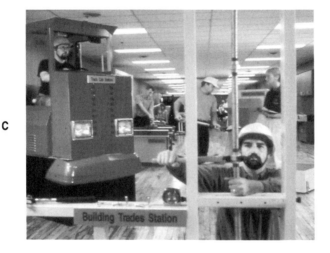

(25.5, **B** From Gould: Orthopedic and Sports Physical Therapy, ed 2, St. Louis, 1990 Mosby.)

determining target companies' sizes, number of employees, frequency of injuries, types of claims, costs of claims, length of time employees are off work, and all other details that will help tailor products to meet companies' needs.

Industry purchases everything through marketing and sells everything through marketing. Competition takes place on industry's playing field or not at all. And to be effective, marketing must be directed to all the players—company physicians, insurance companies, employers, unions, Workers' Compensation Boards, occupational health nurses, safety officers, employees, and the public.

As the rehabilitation process becomes progressively more cost and outcome-driven, the key message to these parties is "economics."

Good communication skills, in written as well as

the presentation medium, are necessary. Graphic designers and writers can help produce professional brochures. Some equipment manufacturers provide brochures that can be customized with practice information to enhance exposure and image.

Writing is critical to appeal to both skilled medical professionals and the industrial community which understands little medical terminology. Health care providers will want a technical or feature focus, while industry management will want to know the costs and the benefits the company will gain.

Industry has to be called on several times (three to five) before they will buy into the product even on a trial basis.[14] This means marketing activities may not bear financial fruits until months after the initial contact.

The Therapist has to become comfortable outside

the clinic, in industry settings speaking to managers, employees, and unions, and in technical settings when meeting with doctors, nurses, or health care management.

Communication with the market must be frequent, and service continuous in order to remain competitive. To strengthen on-going relationships, customers should be told about additional services: exercise programs, safety training, education, FCA's, Job Analysis, Job Placement Assessments, Work Conditioning, and Work Hardening. There are few loyalties in industry. Those who let up on service lose market share and become a statistic.[14]

Location is an important marketing decision. Location options should be approached realistically. In most instances the best locations are areas near, or in industrial parks[14]—not in a downtown area, and not in the suburbs.

An important consideration is that it is possible to build on an already credible track record but not on a weak practice. It is also important to study the components of Industrial Therapy we have discussed in this chapter, and to become familiar with prospects' needs. It is best to master the knowledge before attempting to communicate with prospects.

A checklist follows in the next section and helps to ensure that all the bases are covered. Thorough planning is recommended in order to perfect the strategy and enhance the chances of success.

An added benefit in Industrial Therapy practice is the opportunity to start handling all of a company's employees and their families for motor vehicle injuries, sports, and domestic accidents. This again, only gets new patients in the door. After that, treatment must be excellent, aggressive, and goal-orientated. When clients are served well they will recommend the service to others.

MAKING THE TRANSITION

It is hoped that the foregoing has helped provide a better understanding of the differences encountered in making the transition to Industrial Therapy. Attention now turns to the steps involved in that transition.

Planning

The most important first step in any venture is a thorough job of homework. The key information required to prepare a proper plan is summarized as follows:

Financial Projections and Feasibility
- Revenue projections from base of referral sources
- Space requirements for administration
- Space requirements for classrooms

- Space requirements for equipment
- Work Conditioning
- Work Hardening
- Equipment costs
- Functional Capacity Assessment System cost
- Man-hour commitments required to develop this practice
- Advertising and marketing expenses
- Operating costs (salaries, expenses, telephone)

Revenue Potential By Product
- Functional Capacity Assessment
- Special Purpose Assessment
- Job Placement Assessment
- Job Site/Work Task Analysis
- Work Conditioning
- Work Hardening
- Education sessions
- Medical-legal reports
- Expanded traditional therapy clientele

This information should be organized in the form of a *pro forma* that, ideally, yields a break-even in 24 to 30 months. For a detailed discussion and example, see Chapter 24.

Transition Steps

If planning indicates an acceptable level of feasibility, risk, and payout potential, the transition can proceed. There are many tasks involved in the transition, but the following are the major ones in summary form.

1. Evaluate existing equipment with reference to the equipment checklist in Box 25.1. Some existing equipment is transferable, but additional purchases might also be required.
2. Evaluate existing education programs to see if there is a fit. If a Repetitive Stress Injury Prevention program is not in place, it will have to be added.
3. Improve the practice's knowledge base as to:
   - Exercise prescription, strengthening, and aerobics
   - FCA
   - Job task and work site analysis
   - Work Hardening
   - Ergonomics standards, garments, and appliances
   - The politics within the Workers' Compensation system
   - The politics of insurers, employers, and unions
   - Americans with Disabilities Act
   - CARF standards
   - OSHA regulations and NIOSH standards
   - Other industry regulations

4. Design programs specific to workers' needs and the job site:
   A. Conditioning
      - Back strengthening
      - Neck strengthening
      - Upper limb strengthening
      - Lower limb strengthening
   B. Work Conditioning
      - Back strengthening
      - Neck strengthening
      - Upper limb strengthening
      - Lower limb strengthening
      - Education—neck, back, and repetitive stress injury
      - Task simulation equipment.
   C. Work Hardening
      - Back strengthening
      - Neck strengthening
      - Upper limb strengthening
      - Lower limb strengthening
      - Education—neck, back, and repetitive stress injury
      - Task simulation equipment
      - Incorporate psychosocial aspects
   D. Education
      - Neck
      - Back
      - Repetitive stress injury

5. Purchase a comprehensive FCA/FCE system. Initially these services may be contracted to a provider of FCAs.

6. Review the existing patient list and inquire if their physicians or employers want FCAs, job task, or work site analysis. The best prospects initially are existing cases.

7. For every patient who is being seen for traditional therapy:
   A. Make sure they are familiar with the full range of services offered. Word of mouth recommendations are often the most valuable.
   B. Obtain the name and address of their employer when they initially register at the clinic.
   C. Send out a card to the employer stating that their employee is being treated. This is a good time to request a job description that itemizes the physical demands of the job as framework for returning the worker to the job safely.
   D. Alternatively, telephone the occupational health nurse or safety officer to ask for a job description.
   E. Follow up with a visit to the company to

offer specific services and products, such as:
   - Job task and work site analysis for high injury areas
   - Education programs for prevention and reduction of injuries
   - Job Placement Assessments
   - FCAs for employees on Short Term Disability before they go on Long Term Disability
   - FCAs for employees on Long Term Disability, or two hour Special Purposes Assessments if they have previously had a four hour FCA. This will ensure things are not regressing.

8. Offer services to physicians who have industrial clients:
   - Mention FCAs, Job Placement Assessment, Job Analysis, Work Conditioning, Work Hardening, prevention, and all the other programs on the Worker Care Spectrum.
   - Make Industrial Therapy programs easily accessible so that referrals are as effortless as possible.
   - Ensure that services are helpful to their practice so that they have a "good feeling" in referring their patients.
   - Give them a tour of the facilities and provide more information on the spectrum of programs offered.

9. Develop an effective advertising and marketing program. A key change in the transition to Industrial Therapy is an intensified marketing emphasis. This topic is covered in considerable detail in Chapter 27, but a detailed brochure on the approach to the market is outlined below:
   - Practice mission statement—future direction and focus
   - Staff credentials, track record, major strengths, and uniquenesses
   - Services offered in Industrial Therapy
   - What to expect from treatment programs offered
   - Benefits of services to doctor, schools, unions, and companies
   - Benefits to the employee

10. Cold call employers—visit similar industries and talk about services used by competitors especially stressing results. Offer products and services, and follow-up.

11. Follow-up . . . Follow-up . . . Follow-up—Securing a client may require three to five con-

tacts before there will be a trial of services. Then, services must be delivered as promised. Industry expects on-going follow up and attention so as to feel like a valued customer. If industry is not continually courted there will be no loyalties. Industry judges the program by its impact on budget and therapy services are considered an expense. Good communications with the industry are necessary to ensure a long term relationship.

12. Develop outreach preventative education programs. These are good introductory programs because they require little or no additional space, and may be handled with existing staff. These programs begin orienting the company toward prevention and job-site-based thinking. The Therapist can initially implement these programs single-handedly until revenue builds and staffing is affordable:
    - Neck programs
    - Back programs
    - Stress management
    - Repetitive stress injury prevention
    - Job task and work site analysis

13. Offer services to companies to evaluate their employees on Short Term Disability (STD) and Long Term Disability (LTD) with FCAs. Stress the financial benefits of returning the client to work—reduced premiums and regained productivity. The FCAs should also generate demand for Job Analyses and Job Placement Assessments which in turn will feed into Work Conditioning, Work Hardening, and Education.

14. Plan to make additional financial commitments as the practice grows. In addition to an FCA system, requirements include exercise equipment, education programs, space, staff (certified athletic trainer, exercise physiologist, physical education instructor, kinesiologist, an occupational or physical Therapist Assistant) and/or the time to cover these functions until it is affordable to hire them.

15. When daily Work Conditioning or Work Hardening clients start to number eight to ten and it is affordable, hiring additional staff not only enables continued expansion, the staff can also assume supervisory responsibilities, so that clients can receive more individualized attention.

16. Set up on-site Work Retraining programs as an intermediate step prior to investing in a fully equipped and staffed center. This allows the Therapist to introduce and demonstrate Work Retraining benefits to employers, employees,

and insurers prior to making major investments.

17. Introduce Work Hardening at the clinic. Strong planning and rapid growth is important to justify the specialized staff and equipment required.

18. Do not become stereotyped as only interested in rehabilitating injured workers, or as a hard driver. Balance the practice's image by offering preventative education programs in the plants, in order to be viewed as a supplier of positive, safe, helpful, preventative programs.

    Develop a positive image in the Work Conditioning and Work Hardening areas so that a forcing, task master type of feeling does not develop. Take steps to ensure that clients are enthusiastic and goal-orientated toward returning to work safely and efficiently.

SUMMARY

Industrial Therapy involves a number of dramatic differences relative to traditional and sports therapy: a wider diversity of customers, a greater insistence on reliable measurements and predictable outcomes, more legal and regulatory involvement, a broader assortment of programs, more specialized equipment, and more intense marketing.

Some might view these differences as reasons to avoid involvement in Industrial Therapy. Others would see them as opportunities—to expand potential referral sources, control a steady influx of clients and patients, justify treatment with convincing statistical proof, expand the breadth of services, and have a greater impact on the physical wellness of workers and the financial wellness of the companies that employ them.

Building from either traditional or sports therapy, one can progressively integrate an Industrial Physical Therapy model. A Functional Capacity Assessment system provides the initial foundation of reliable measurement and predictable outcomes. This in combination with Job Analysis and Job Placement Assessment begins to feed into Work Conditioning and later, Work Hardening.

The transition is advanced with outreach programs (education, financial planning, and research) that have two advantages. They require little investment, and they establish working relationships and trust with employers and workers.

Investments in manpower, equipment, and facilities are phased in to expand products and services to this growing client base.

Present exercise equipment is adapted to develop a

Work Conditioning program. Work Hardening can be introduced as an on-site program with the employer, developing later into a full facility model.

Marketing is the most important concept that philosophically must be adapted to make Industrial Therapy a success.

In the final analysis, Industrial Therapy is a vital development that addresses the worker's need to pursue safe, injury free employment, and the employer's need to maintain a healthy, productive workforce to successfully thrive in today's global competitive arena.

REFERENCES

1. Arnheim DD, Klafs CE: Modern Principles of Athletic Training, St Louis, 1981, Mosby.
2. Barlow WE, Hane EZ: A Practical Guide to the Americans with Disabilities Act, *Personnel Journal*, June 1992.
3. Campion MA: Personnel Selection For Physically Demanding Jobs: review and recommendations, *Personnel Psychology* 36:527–548, 1983.
4. Deyo RA: Historic Perspective on Conservative Treatment for Acute Back Problems. Contemporary Conservative Care for Painful Spinal Disorders, Philadelphia, 1991, Lea & Febiger.
5. EEOC: Technical Assistance Manual for the Americans with Disabilities Act, IV–5, IV–12.
6. Ergonomics Guides: Ergonomics Guide to Assessment of Metabolic and Cardiac Costs of Physical Work, *Amer Ind Hyg Assoc J* 32(9):560–564, Aug 1971.
7. Gould JA: Orthopaedic Sports and Physical Therapy, St Louis, 1990, Mosby.
8. Greenberg SN, Bello RP: The Americans with Disabilities Act—what you don't know can hurt you, *Occup Ther Forum*, June 12, 1992.
9. Hazard RG, Matheson LN, Lehmann TR, Frymoyer JW: Rehabilitation of the Patient with chronic Low Back Pain. Occupational Low Back Pain: assessment, treatment and prevention, St Louis, 1991, Mosby.
10. Herring SA: Sports Medicine Early Care. Contemporary Conservative Care for Painful Spinal disorders, Philadelphia, 1991, Lea & Febiger.
11. Key GL: Key Functional Assessment Training and Resource Manual, Minneapolis, 1991, KEY Method.
12. Key GL: KEY Method Work Hardening Training Manual and Access Kit, Minneapolis, 1991, KEY Method.
13. Keyserling WM, Herrin GD, Chaffin DB: Isometric Strength Testing as a means of Controlling Medical Incidents on Strenuous Jobs, *J Occup Med* 22(5):332–336, 1980.
14. Kotler P: Marketing Management, Analysis, Planning, Implementation, and Control, New York, 1988, Prentice Hall.
15. Lotito MJ, Allen JC: Legal Report: Answers to commonly asked ADA questions, *Society for Human Resource Management*, Summer 1992.
16. Mayer TG: The Shift from Passive Modalities to Reactivation, Contemporary Conservative Care for Painful Spinal Disorders, Philadelphia, 1991, Lea & Febiger.
17. Park KS, Chaffin DB: Prediction of Load-Lifting Limits for Manual Materials Handling, *Professional Safety* 45–48:1975.
18. Preston G: Legal Issues and concepts of Disability, Contemporary Conservative Care for Painful Spinal disorders, Philadelphia, 1991, Lea & Febiger.
19. Sivestri SM, Zimic DL: An Employer's Compliance Checklist, A look at the practical aspects of compliance with the ADA, *Federal Bar News J* 39(1):1992.
20. Snook SH, Irvine CH: Maximum Acceptable Weight of Lift, *Amer Ind Hyg Assoc J* 332–329:1967.
21. US Department of Justice, Civil Rights Division: The American with Disabilities Act, Questions and Answers.

26

Legal Issues in Industrial Therapy

Philip C. Moe

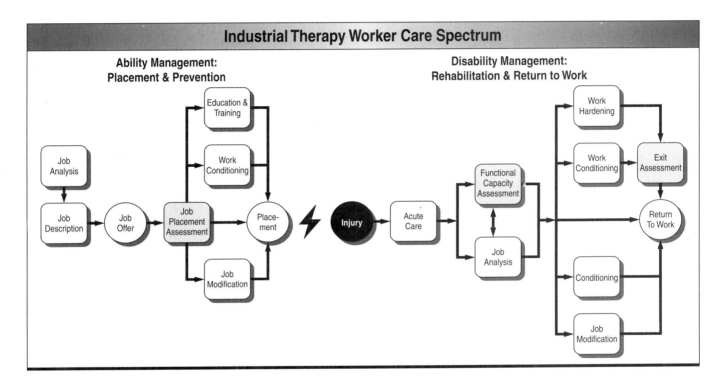

Within the professions of Physical and Occupational Therapy today, it is widely accepted that the field of Industrial Therapy includes a high level of exposure to litigation and to the litigation process. Therapists working in industrial medicine are responsible for providing information and making decisions which have far-reaching implications for the lives of their patients, the insurance and business communities. It is their responsibility to provide information that is as accurate, objective, and reliable as possible for the purposes of making these decisions.

Often the information provided by an Industrial Therapist can make the difference in a decision between returning to work, reeducation, or possibly total disability for life. These decisions have far-reach-

ing consequences for society, and the information provided is likely to be highly scrutinized by the legal community.

This critical information typically comes from a Functional Capacity Assessment, the performance outcome of a Work Hardening program, or a combination of the two, and is used according to a specific hierarchy of importance.

Initially, the most critical factor is the ability to accurately determine the participation level of an individual. If found to be manipulative or grossly underachieving, many lawyers will refuse to represent that individual, physicians will drop him or her as a patient, and most insurance companies will start proceedings to discontinue benefits or terminate settlement negotiations. Issues regarding this determination are discussed in Chapter 13, Functional Capacity Assessments.

If an individual is found to be working up to true safe capability levels, that worker is deemed to be fully participating or a "valid participant." Given this determination, the first preference is to ascertain whether or not it is medically safe for the return to their regular preinjury job with the same employer.

This most amicable outcome involves the least incidence of legal involvement. Here, the litigation or insurance settlement is determined by the amount of medical impairment, except in personal injury cases ("tort" cases), where pain and suffering may also be considered.

The method of determining impairment varies from state to state, but the impairment rating is often incorrectly and inappropriately labeled a "disability rating" (see definitions in working glossary Box 26.1).

The next preference is a return to work with the same employer, but at a different or modified job. In this case, the incidence of legal involvement increases somewhat. There may be some additional disability payment involved, to make up for possible wage loss or the loss of some physical capability. Legal representation is typically required in order to be awarded a significant disability payment.

If the individual is unable to return to work within current capabilities and skills, the next step is to consider some type of retraining or other education to provide the skills necessary to become employable again. Having moved another step up in complexity, legal involvement increases in likelihood.

Finally, if a combination of an individual's age, medical condition, education, skills, and experience lead to a determination of unemployability (often litigated), that individual may be considered totally disabled (Table 26.1).

Given the significance of these decisions, Industrial Therapists have a responsibility to the professional community and a moral obligation to society, to be well prepared in the way that they present information to the business, medical, and legal communities.

LEGAL CONSIDERATIONS IN ASSESSMENT AND TREATMENT

The bulk of the information sought or in question in the majority of litigation cases involving Industrial Therapists is provided from the areas of Functional Capacity Assessment, Job Placement Assessment, and Work Hardening. The information must be reliable, and the processes of assessment and treatment must be safe.

Information Reliability

There is a certain comfort in being able to rely on information, research, and protocols that have been developed, tried, and tested by other professionals. There are several nationally-recognized and accepted methodologies which are currently used in Industrial Therapy, as well as some equipment manufacturers whose equipment is readily recognizable and used in Work Conditioning and Work Hardening programs.

One value of these nationally-recognized programs is that they adhere to very specific and detailed protocols in the use of the equipment and the administration of any assessments based on their equipment. This means that each activity has very specific and detailed instructions on how to carry out the activity, what equipment to use, and exactly how that equipment is to be used. Many practitioners will argue that rigid protocols take away their professional discretion. However, any researcher will assert that variation in data collection produces unusable data.

Another important consideration in the area of reliability is the validity of the client's participation. Validity of participation is a critical factor in the testing procedures, whether in the post-offer preplacement testing, or in a post injury Functional Capacity Assessment.

This measure enables the Therapist to verify honest performance even when it is at a very low level. Reliable measures of a client's true attitude and motivation enable responsible judgments that can stand up in legal proceedings.

Liability Considerations

It is exceptionally important to use specific, acceptable assessment and treatment algorithms, when available, that are diagnosis-specific, in order to reduce the possibility of injury to the client or error on the part of the Therapist. The provider can be liable for injury

TABLE 26.1 Outcomes of Injury Cases

Outcome	Desirability	Incidence of Legal Involvement
Same employer/ same job	Highest	Lowest
Same employer/ different job	Second highest	Second lowest
Retraining and education required	Second lowest	Second highest
Unemployable/ totally disabled	Lowest	Highest

arising from not having protocols, not following them, having faulty equipment, or misusing the equipment.

There is also case law establishing liability on the part of an examining medical provider for injuries caused during an examination, injuries resulting from a negligent examination, and financial injuries resulting from an inaccurate assessment (Rothstein, 1984). Since the client is in the hands of the Therapist, liability resides there as well.

In a Functional Capacity Assessment to determine safe return to work guidelines, it would certainly be inappropriate and a legal risk to encourage a client to work beyond what they have already indicated to be the tolerance limit. These issues of Therapist interference in assessments, or the misuse of equipment, underscores the importance of very specific and detailed practice protocols and parameters.

In a Job Site Analysis, the Therapist should take care to use protocols that are well accepted or documented. Making up one's own methods on the scene, or improvising without supporting precedent exposes the Therapist to liability if they pronounce the job safe and an employee is subsequently injured. For extra protection, it is highly advised to have the supervisors and employees sign an agreement allowing the analysis and recommendations.

In Prevention Programs, like low back or upper extremity injuries, the Therapist should make sure teachings are research based and well documented. Inventing one's own principles exposes the Therapist to liability for subsequent injuries.

In Work Hardening, it would be inappropriate for a participating carpenter to engage in activities that might create increased radicular signs in a low back diagnosis. The individual may be highly motivated to return to the construction field and want to perform the activities that would assist in return to work. This should not be allowed at the risk of any further neurologic insult. Should this occur, there would certainly be some liability on the part of the treatment program.

Job Placement Assessments are probably the most rapidly changing area of Industrial Therapy at this time. With the onset of the Americans with Disabilities Act (ADA) and its overriding regulations, many changes continue to occur within the preemployment arena.

Under the umbrella of the ADA, there is no longer any room for preemployment, preoffer medical examinations. There is some latitude to perform preemployment, preoffer skills testing, provided the tests are for essential job functions, and are administered to all applicants. There can be no medical evaluation until a job offer has been already made.

Under the ADA, an employer may choose to administer exercise or strength testing, rather than a job trial or job simulation. Whether preoffer or post offer, such tests must be relevant to essential job functions, and must be administered to all applicants or hirees.

> *"These types of strength or exercise tests typically use standardized protocols and standardized equipment. The results are also generally reported on a computerized print out and these results need to be comparable to the averages of other individuals of the same age and gender"* (Schultz, 1993).

FEES

An important issue for the Industrial Therapist is the need to have a preestablished fee schedule for such things as consulting, depositions, and expert testimony. Setting these fees is a function primarily based on the worth of service in the marketplace and the alternative income that could be generated in the clinic during that same period of time.

Other factors include the expertise that the Therapist has developed (education, training, published articles, number of assessments) in the particular area at issue, and the fact that, to some degree, testifying under oath puts the Therapist's reputation on the line.

In the author's experience, many Therapists are somewhat reluctant or unwilling to charge the level of fees that are appropriate for the services that they are rendering, and often neglect to charge for travel and other expenses. Physical Therapy has long been a service-oriented profession, which may explain why there is a tendency for many Therapists to want to "give their time away."

How Fees Are Set

Typically, fees are set on a sliding scale, depending on the level of the service being given. At the bottom of the legal services fee scale are the charges for consulting in legal matters, which may vary, whether it is provided in-house or on-site, such as, at a factory.

The next level on the scale is for depositions, with fees varying based on whether the deposition is taken within their own clinic, or at another facility. The fees are higher yet if they are appearing live in an actual hearing process, and are the highest when appearing in a public courtroom.

On the whole, when compared to the fees charged by physicians, Therapists are a real bargain as far as the attorneys are concerned, providing information that is essential, objective, and sometimes more useful than what physicians might provide. It is not unusual for an orthopedic surgeon to charge upwards of $400 to $500 an hour for a deposition. Some therapists set rates based on a percentage (50 to 60%) of what local physicians charge.

Most physicians and some Therapists charge very high rates for live testimony in the hearing process, primarily to discourage regular occurence, and also because they feel that there is some increased amount of pressure and more valuable expertise associated with live testimony.

What Fees Cover

Fees should be set up in such a fashion that they include preparation time as well as the actual consultation or testimony time. This author charges $100 per hour for consultation services or educational seminars to industry. If an attorney has a question regarding a claim or a particular legal situation, the charge is also $100 an hour for those services.

If a case is being disputed and expert testimony is required, the fee will start at $200, which includes preparation and the first half hour of testimony. Following the completion of the first half hour of testimony, the fee is broken down into quarter hour increments, billed at $50 per quarter hour. If the services are required away from the clinic, travel time is charged at the $100 per hour rate, and all travel expenses incurred are also reimbursed. If the services require absence from the clinic for an entire day, the fee becomes $2,000 per day plus expenses.

If medical records are requested, prepayment is required prior to providing the records. Written authorization is also required from the client for distribution of information.

Whatever the actual fee schedule, it is important that it is clearly communicated, understood, and accepted prior to entering into any deposition or hearing process.

MEDICAL RECORDS AND REPORTS

In the realm of Industrial Therapy, it is not unusual to have a number of interested parties requesting medical records on the same individual. A general rule is that whoever is actually paying for the therapy services (FCA, JPA, JA, Work Hardening) is entitled to the results. An individual client also has a right to their own records without charge. The client does need, however, to sign a consent form to obtain his or her own records.

In any Workers' Compensation case, the employer is also entitled to the medical information. In Workers' Compensation cases, the insurance company is considered to be acting as an agent of the employer. The employer is paying for the services and is therefore entitled to the information.

A trend on the rise is a tendency for attorneys to encourage clients to come in and pick up their own records. This enables the attorney to obtain all of the information necessary without incurring a fee.

An important consideration in dealing with medical records is that if a medical record is referenced during testimony, then that record's entire file is now open and available to both attorneys for full inspection. This means that any loose papers, any handwritten notes, any stick-on notes that may have been put into that record at one point or another, now become a part of that patient's record, and are completely available.

The implications in this instance are two-fold. First, Therapists must be very careful about what information they include during testimony. Second, Therapists must be very careful about the nature and wording of information put in clients' files.

TESTIMONY

This section will focus on three basic areas with respect to giving testimony:
1. General preparation
2. Preparation for testimony
3. The testimony itself

General Preparation

In general, it is extremely important to begin by having well-established protocols and guidelines to follow consistently for each client that is treated. It is essential to know these protocols, to understand the rationale and the support behind them, and to be able to explain the results of adherence to these guidelines in a clear and concise manner.

In the specific case of Functional Capacity Assessments, it is important to be well aware of all the activities involved in the Assessment and how they interrelate with each other. The ability to interface the client's or patient's diagnosis with pain reports, pain behaviors, heart rates and body mechanics, as well as the consistency of these items throughout the Assessment, will establish the basis for the validity and reliability of information.

It is essential to be able to relate the sequences of the activities that patients are expected to perform and how those activities relate to their diagnosis. Further, the Therapist must be able to explain, in chronological order, how these activities progress, without having to refer to notes or cheat sheets.

If it is necessary to rely on information from the patient's chart or narratives, this information should be quickly and efficiently accessible. It is also becoming increasingly important to be aware of any possible supporting literature that helps to substantiate recommendations and protocol reliability.

Before testimony, the Therapist should review the

clinical research and data sources that support the testimony to be given. This would include information relating to the specific diagnostic groups at issue in the proceedings, the return to work capabilities of like populations, and outcome studies of the program referenced in the testimony.

Preparation For Testimony

Proper preparation before giving testimony is crucial to the avoidance of pitfalls in the litigation process. In general, the process of preparing for testimony remains the same, regardless of the services or information at issue. The underlying principles of preparation do not vary much, whether you are defending a Functional Capacity Assessment, a preplacement screening process, JPA, or a Work Hardening program.

There was a time when subjective information could be presented in court without much difficulty, due to attorneys' inexperience or unfamiliarity with the field of Industrial Therapy. It was possible to make mistakes in testimony without serious consequences, since the Therapist was regarded as the only expert on the subject. This definitely is no longer the case, as there is now a highly educated legal community with respect to medico-legal issues.

If the attorneys have any questions about the information or the expert involved in a case, they will more than likely hire their own expert to review the case and to provide them with additional information and the proper line of questioning.

Attorneys today are also quick to obtain any literature that may be involved with the case, so that they can use that literature as a potential source for questioning in a deposition or trial. Failure on the part of the testifying Therapist to keep up on current literature and research could lead to some very embarrassing moments in court.

Organizing The Records

Just prior to giving testimony, one of the first things the Therapist needs to do is to organize the client chart or other information. This may include dictation or handwritten notes, statistics collected from various equipment manufacturers, correspondence from insurance companies, attorneys, or other medical personnel involved in the care of the patient, test results pertaining to the patient, and finally, handwritten information and forms that have been completed by the client. All of this information needs to be readily accessible to the Therapist and organized in a very neat fashion.

A cardinal rule for data collection and storage is that *nothing should be put into a chart that is not intended to be submitted as evidence in court.*

Once client records are referenced during the testimony process, they become "fair game"—the opposing attorney can request to review the records (if they have not already done so), read from them in court, and also submit them as evidence. If records and client information are maintained in a sloppy or careless manner, it would not be unusual for the hearing examiner, judge, or jury to surmise that the clinic may also have been slipshod in the way that the information was obtained. It is strongly recommended that records be reviewed thoroughly and committed to memory, as much as possible, prior to entering into a deposition, or appearing in court. It is highly advantageous not to refer to them during the testimony process.

When reviewing information, it is helpful to highlight important facts such as specific and clear test results, pain reports or pain behaviors, and inconsistencies in behavior or performance. If any correspondence has been drafted pertaining to the client, it is important to know what was said and why any conclusions were reached.

If, during a review of the information, any mistakes or discrepancies are discovered, it is essential to immediately notify all interested parties prior to giving any testimony. Lack of advance disclosure of mistakes may seriously undermine the Therapist's integrity, reputation, and objectivity, as well as the integrity of the Industrial Therapy profession itself.

The many Therapists throughout the country who are involved in various aspects of Industrial Therapy could be severely compromised if inaccurate information is presented by fellow professionals claiming to be experts in their field.

The Therapist's Status As A Witness

Therapists may be called upon to establish themselves as a more qualified expert than other witnesses who may have more advanced professional degrees. In medical cases, it is not unusual for the Therapist to present testimony along with specialists in such fields as orthopedics, neurology, or neurosurgery. Under these circumstances, it is important to establish that Industrial Therapy is a unique field of expertise just as the physicians' specialties are unique to them.

The Therapist has a discrete body of knowledge which is not taught in any other medical profession. Absence of physician credentials renders the Therapist's testimony no less important in a court of law. The Therapist simply needs to establish the fact of unique expertise in the area of Industrial Therapy, more so than any of the other witnesses presenting testimony.

When a physician's testimony is in conflict, the Therapist needs only to state that there are differences of opinion and that the Therapist's position stands on the information presented. After all, if the facts were so clear as to present no conflict, then there likely would be no hearing process in the first place.

Understanding The Context Of The Testimony

Finally, it is essential to have a good understanding of the venue in which the testimony is given. There is a big difference between testimony given in a trial in the presence of a hearing examiner or judge, versus testimony given in a deposition.

During the hearing process, the judge is able to control the questioning by ruling on objections entered by each attorney, thereby influencing the questions that may be asked and answered.

In the deposition process, this judge is not present and, therefore, any and all questions must be answered. A clever attorney may ask questions designed to fluster, trip up, and diminish the witness's credibility. Later in the process, a judge will be called upon to rule on any objections that may have been lodged during the deposition, and to determine whether or not the answers given will be allowed to remain on record and be used as evidence in the hearing process.

Hearing processes, as well as depositions, may vary from case to case. In a Workers' Compensation setting, there is no jury involved in the initial litigation process. Testimony will be given before a hearing examiner, who rules on any objections lodged by either attorney, and also determines the amount of weight given to the various testimony presented.

In a private sector setting or in a "tort" proceeding, the initial hearing is generally held in a public court room, with a judge present to rule on the objections lodged, and on the admissibility of particular pieces of evidence. In a tort proceeding, there is also a jury, who then collectively weigh the evidence presented and arrive at a conclusion.

Depositions

There are three basic types of depositions (Figure 26.1):
1. A deposition for discovery
2. A deposition to be presented at a trial
3. A video deposition to be presented at a trial

Discovery depositions are used by both attorneys in order to determine what type of information the opposition is planning to present. It is as important and as official as testimony given directly in front of a jury. Once this information is obtained, the attorneys will reevaluate their case, perhaps readjust strategies, or enter into negotiation and possible settlement. A discovery deposition may or may not be used in trial.

Depositions for trial generally are taken in lieu of having the individual actually appear live in the hear-

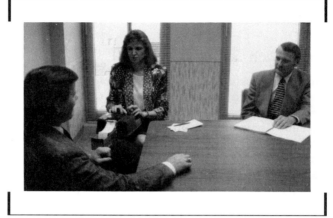

FIGURE 26.1   Depositions are given away from the courtroom and are presented in written or video form in the actual courtroom proceeding.

ing process. In this case, the deposition is taken and the written record is submitted as evidence in the hearing process.

Video depositions are common in jury trials. The deposition is videotaped and replayed in front of the jury, rather than having the witness appear live. In the event of a videotaped deposition, a neat and professional appearance is essential.

In all cases, any testimony given during a deposition will be done under oath, in the presence of both opposing attorneys, and in the presence of a court reporter who will record accurately all of the information presented.

Prior to giving the deposition, it will be necessary to prepare a *curriculum vitae* which outlines educational experience, work history, and subsequent specialty training, to establish status as an expert witness. This document must be prepared in advance, with copies readily available to both attorneys, as well as a copy to be submitted into evidence.

On the business side, the party requesting the deposition must be contacted, as they are the party to be billed for the services. It is important to have the paying party receive and accept a fee schedule prior to giving testimony. Whenever the Therapist is established as an expert and is expected to provide expert information or explanation, it is the obligation of the requesting attorney to pay the expert witness' fees.

Subpoenas

When subpoenaed to testify, there is no obligation on the part of either side to pay a fee, but fees are sometimes paid for services that go beyond what subpoenaed testimony requires. As a subpoenaed witness, the Therapist is obligated only to provide treatment information as to the procedures carried out and the information collected. If the Therapist is not paid a supplemental fee, there is no obligation to present any detailed explanation of these procedures.

If there is not an agreement to provide supplemental fees as an "expert witness," the Therapist may be considered a "fact witness." The court pays a modest stipend (under $50) for such appearances.

Even when a supplemental fee is involved, some therapists prefer to be subpoenaed because it helps them appear objective and neutral in the case.

Giving Testimony

The first thing that will be requested, before giving any testimony is to raise your right hand and take an oath, swearing to tell the truth, the whole truth, and nothing but the truth. It is not unusual to find that the attorneys involved are not necessarily interested in the "whole" truth, but only in that information that favors their particular position in the case. It is important to remember this oath when formulating answers so that the whole truth is indeed conveyed rather than a presentation of half truths.

Name, profession, and place of employment will be first stated upon request. The attorneys then have the option of either agreeing to accept the *curriculum vitae* as presented, or have the therapist actually answer all questions pertaining to education and experience to be submitted as written testimony. At this point, the preliminaries are usually over, and questioning pertaining to the particular case will begin.

Testimony Guidelines

It is essential when giving testimony to follow some basic guidelines:
1. Look and sound professional
2. Be clear, objective, and to the point
3. Pause before answering a question in order to allow the attorneys to lodge any objections
4. Do not be afraid to admit not knowing an answer
5. Do not become angry or frightened
6. Do not attempt to memorize your testimony
7. Answer only the specific questions being asked (the less said, the less the attorneys have to use in formulating further questions)
8. Remain neutral—do not take sides
9. Be consistent at each trial, and between trials
10. View involvement as an opportunity to educate

When presenting testimony, it is very important that the therapist looks and sounds professional. One needs to dress professionally, and in such a fashion that nothing detracts attention from what is being said. When speaking, "aahs" and "ums" could create doubt. Statements such as "that is correct" or "yes," are used rather than "yah" or nodding of the head.

Not knowing an answer to a question is an admission of honesty and vulnerability and may, in fact, increase credibility with the judge or the jury.

The ability to maintain a calm and controlled demeanor will also lend to increased credibility. Remember that the attorneys are, in fact, simply attempting to carry out their jobs as effectively as possible.

One should not attempt to memorize any testimony, but simply respond to each question being presented. It is essential to be prepared prior to taking the stand in order to be viewed as a credible witness and be of value to the litigation process. With respect to the litigation process, remember the "Rule of Five Ps—Prior Preparation Prevents Poor Performance."

In order to remain neutral with respect to the hearing process, one should simply support the information gathered and the process by which the information is gathered. Take care not to be manipulated, avoid going out on a limb and speculating outside your area of expertise for the testimony may become vulnerable and easily discredited by another professional.

If forced to speculate on an answer, such as in the case of a hypothetical situation being presented, one should be sure to qualify the answer by saying that it applies only to the hypothetical situation and not to any other situation that might be described.

With respect to giving testimony in general, it is absolutely crucial that one maintains consistency, not just in the testimony of a particular case, but across the board from case to case. Inconsistent or contradictory answers constitutes conflicting testimony, which can result in impeachment. If the attorney can show that one thing is said in the deposition and another during the hearing process, a request that the therapist be impeached as a witness can be made, thereby losing credibility and having the entire testimony thrown out.

One cannot allow influence by other individuals asking questions or by the particular side that has engaged one's services. The therapist may be required to give testimony on the part of a defense attorney in one case, and on the part of a plaintiff attorney in another case. The therapist's testimony needs to remain consistent with respect to procedures and findings to maintain credibility within the field.

Finally, the opportunity to provide testimony in a proceeding is also the therapist's opportunity to educate as to what he or she does and how that information affects the case involved. If the therapist is unable to effectively communicate that information to the judge or to the jury, failure with respect to professional involvement and responsibility to that case will result. When presented with clarity, both sides in the case will appreciate the testimony and may seek services in the future.

Attorney Tactics

The therapist must be aware of the attorney who asks rapid-fire questions that call for repeated similar answers. It is not unusual to be asked five or six questions in a row that require a positive response, and then suddenly be slipped a question that requires a negative response. If not keenly aware of this process, one may inadvertently provide an incorrect answer that will be regretted at a later time.

Another common practice is the presentation of a double question, in which the attorney poses two questions within one statement. The tendency is to simply focus on and respond to the second half of the question, leaving the impression that the answer is also accurate for the first half.

The attorney might ask, "Isn't it true that Mr. Jones' heart rates were consistent and he had difficulty lifting above his shoulder?" The answer must separately address both issues. If the client's heart rates were *not* consistent but he *did have* difficulty lifting to shoulder level, a yes answer to the question would improperly represent the heart rate information.

In another tactic, the attorney may start out a question by suggesting that a particular piece of information is a fact when the fact may not be accurate at all.

The attorney might ask, "In your recommendation that Mr. Jones could safely perform the job, did you assess and recommend 35 pounds as his safe lifting capability from floor level?" If the recommendation had been misstated, the answer would have two parts. "I *did not* recommend that Mr. Jones could safely perform the job. However, I *did* assess and recommend 35 pounds as his safe lifting capability from floor level."

If the information to be presented has the potential of being exceptionally damaging to the opposing attorney's case, they will more than likely go to great lengths to either discredit the therapist as a witness or to discredit his or her information. This underscores the importance of having accurate, objective protocols for what to do, and a sound rationale for those protocols.

It is not unusual for an attorney to attempt to discredit the therapist by starting a line of questioning in an unfamiliar area. At this point, the therapist simply needs to remind that attorney that it was already established at the outset of the testimony, the background, education, and the area of expertise the therapist can provide.

CASE EXAMPLES

The following examples illustrate what can happen with poor or inappropriately administered assessments.

Case A: Functional Capacity Assessment Injury

One case in which this author was consulted as an expert involved an alleged injury during the administration of a Functional Capacity Assessment. In this case, the claimant was asked to perform activities already deemed medically inappropriate by the treating physician. The claimant was further encouraged to perform beyond the identified physical tolerance, and equipment was used in a manner grossly different than its manufactured intention and outside of its established protocols. The end result was an alleged new injury during the assessment.

The injury was allegedly reported to the Therapist during the assessment, but not documented. It was documented the following day, but only after the patient had already undergone a considerable amount of treatment. A medical malpractice suit was successfully prosecuted against the Therapist.

This case involved a number of issues including poor documentation, the lack of specific treatment protocols, an inadequate adherence to the ones that were established, and inappropriate use of equipment.

Case B: Improper Functional Capacity Assessment

Another case in which this author was involved concerned a Therapist who was not credentialed in any particular method. He had apparently decided to pick and choose various components from various different assessment methods, throwing them all together into what he called his own method. The result was an assessment performed by an individual with inadequate education, no treatment protocols, no database, and no ability to establish any validity to the results.

The results of that assessment were totally undermined by the completion of an established Functional Capacity Assessment, and in the end, the claimants lost the case entirely and did not receive any monetary award.

B O X   2 6 . 1

Working Glossary [1,2]

Defendant   A person who is sued by a plaintiff for causing an injury.

Defense lawyer   A lawyer who represents the defendant.

Deposition   A statement given under oath, which is recorded and preserved by stenographic or other means. A deposition may be a discovery deposition or an evidence deposition, or used for both purposes.

Disability   An alteration, expressed in non-medical terms, of an individual's capability to meet personal, social, or occupational demands, or to meet statutory or regulatory requirements. The gap between what the individual is required to do and what they are able to do.

Discovery deposition   Usually conducted by the attorney NOT representing your patient, and used to "discover" what happened (i.e. diagnosis, treatment, and prognosis).

Evidence deposition   Generally taken to be used as a script to be read to the jury in trial, instead of that witness being at the trial personally. More formal and structured by the attorney in his pattern of questioning. Usually conducted by the patient's attorney, with cross-examination questions by the defendant's attorney.

Expert witness   A witness who has special experience, training, or education and is allowed to give opinions about specialized matters within an area of expertise.

Fact witness   A person who testifies as to their own actions or his perceptions of other occurrences.

Impairment   An alteration, expressed in medical terms, of an individual's health status. That which is wrong with the health of an individual.

Plaintiff   One who brings a lawsuit or claim for damages as the result of alleged negligence of someone else (the defendant). The patient is usually (but not always) a plaintiff.

Reasonable medical opinion   In one's opinion, something that is *more certainly likely than not likely* to be true now or to reasonably occur in the future.

These examples should be of concern to all Therapists. If these types of situations are not corrected or eliminated, the field of Industrial Therapy, along with the Therapists and the facilities they represent, could be considered the next "gold mine" by the litigious community.

SUMMARY

Industrial Therapy involves a great deal of exposure to legal issues and proceedings, with far reaching implications for the patient, insurer, and employer. Therapists have a vital responsibility to provide information that is objective, accurate, and reliable. This is accomplished in part by using proven equipment with specific detailed protocols.

Procedures must also be supported by clinical research, data sources, and the clinic's own outcome studies.

Therapists may be called upon to provide written or video depositions, or appear as live witnesses in hearings or court proceedings. Most of the information required stems from Functional Capacity Assessments, Job Placement Assessments, and Work Hardening Programs.

For these purposes, the Therapist's testimony carries no less weight than that of physicians in the eyes of the court. The Therapist is uniquely qualified to provide expert testimony in the field of Industrial Therapy, just as physicians are uniquely qualified in their respective fields. The Industrial Therapist's services are indispensable, and compensation should reflect that value.

Preparation for a deposition or live testimony requires thorough homework and mastering of the material. Appearance, professional delivery, clarity, conciseness, neutrality, candor, and most importantly, consistency can be as important as content in influencing the proceedings.

As an important and expanding role, services to parties in legal proceedings is a calling that demands the best of what Therapists can offer in the interest of workers, employers, insurers and the legal system.

REFERENCES

1. Engelburg AL, editor: Guides to the evaluation of permanent impairment, ed 3, Chicago, IL, 1988, American Medical Association.
2. Burns RJ, Ford BM: Depositions and court appearances: assisting your patients with the legal aspects of their injuries, Sioux Falls, SD, 1993.
3. Horsley JE, Carlova J: Testifying in court: A guide for physicians, Oradell, NJ, 1983. Medical Economics.
4. Rothstein MA: Legal issues in the medical assessment of physical impairment by third-party physicians, *J Legal Medicine* 5(4): 542–547, 1984.
5. Schultz D: Medical Examinations Under Title I of the ADA: the role of the physician, *NARPPS* 8(3): 101–114, 1993.

CHAPTER

27

Marketing Industrial Therapy Services

Ronald E. Bates

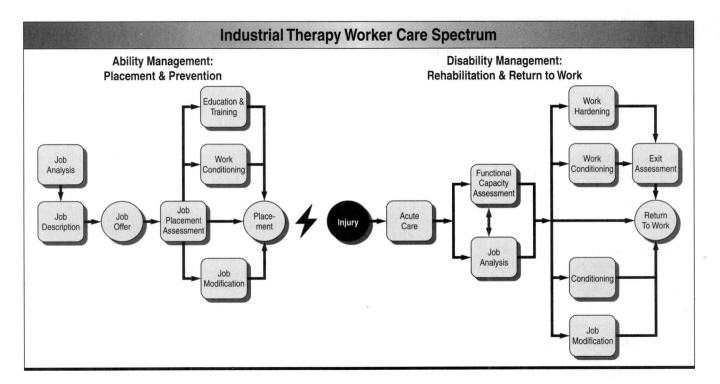

Industrial Therapy Worker Care Spectrum

Marketing one's health care practice or services is a relatively new phenomenon in health care. Some health care practitioners feel that marketing detracts from their professionalism and that health care is not something to be "advertised" or "sold." But marketing can be viewed in another light. It brings more objectivity to the way people choose providers and promotes steady improvement in the quality of care. It is also an opportunity for those who have found a "better way" to tell the world about it and persuade them to adopt their methods. In short, marketing can be a means to facilitate improvement and progress in Industrial Therapy.

Background Literature

To supplement the information provided in this chapter you may want to immerse yourself in the language of business and marketing by reading about it. Some suggestions; Alvin Toffler's *The Trilogy of Future Shock, The Third Wave* and his most recent book *Powershift* will give you a two-decade view of trends and the changing values and culture of the provider/consumer matrix.

The winning team of Patricia Aburdene and John Nesbitt have been collaborating on social insight books since 1982 with the introduction of *Megatrends*. Their most recent book, *Megatrends for Women*, will update you on the new role of women regarding their impact both as consumers and providers of products and services for the remainder of this century.

Two other business and marketing gurus not to be missed are the old master Peter Drucker, and the new master Tom Peters.

Next Steps

We can now turn to describing the marketing process in general and illustrate specific ways to use it in building an Industrial Therapy practice.

Defining Marketing

There are as many definitions of marketing as there are marketing textbooks.[6] For our purposes, it is defined as a process that first determines what people (the market) want, and then directs resources to fulfill that demand. In marketing a product or service the therapist will first assess the demand to ensure that employees, equipment, and money are deployed to deliver exactly what the market needs.

A marketing approach is very different from a manufacturing approach. With a manufacturing approach, the first step is to produce the goods or services and the second is to seek buyers. This approach fails to take market demand into account and as a result, the selling process often leads to large inventories of unwanted goods, services, and employees. If an organization measures the market demand first and then produces goods and services to fill the market's need, output is "presold" to the marketplace, thus eliminating waste.

In many ways, marketing is very similar to therapy treatment. In both, there is a series of pathways designed to give two parties, the provider of the service (the therapist) and the receiver of the service (the client), what they both want. In both cases, a set of standardized steps is followed leading to that end. The marketing pathway culminates in a "solution" for the buyer and compensation for the producer. The treatment pathway culminates in wellness for the patient and satisfaction for the therapist.

Like therapy, marketing is a process, not a rote prescription—each industry is different; each employer is different; each work force is different; each job is different. So, every marketing program, like every physical rehabilitation program, is a unique process addressing a unique set of conditions.

Marketing Components

Marketing can be further defined as all of the activities that contribute to bringing a buyer and producer together for fulfillment through the transfer of goods or services. The most important step in the marketing process is the point at which the sale is consummated. In Industrial Therapy, that event usually occurs in the face-to-face personal selling process. There are many activities which precede consummation of a sale. Accordingly, this chapter will discuss those steps that are

necessary before turning to personal selling. Box 27.1 lists some of the steps that lead the therapist to this point.

The steps are distributed between two phases: developmental and executional. In the developmental phase, the therapist determines what the market wants and designs or tailors products and services to fill that demand. In the executional phase, resources are directed to bring the therapist and prospective customer together through a selling process.

The developmental phase should always precede the executional phase—a therapist should always find out what the market wants before anything else is done. The next sections will examine this important foundation-building phase called "development."

BOX 27.1

Developmental phase
1. Market analysis (to determine demand)
2. Competitive analysis (to identify the competitor's strengths to better position your products)
3. Product development (to leverage strengths where demand exists)
4. Product research (to ensure your "products" meet demand)
5. Product positioning (to identify the product's most persuasive reason for being)
6. Budgeting (to determine the resources that should be devoted to marketing)

Executional phase
1. Marketing and sales personnel staffing
2. Pricing (to maximize long term returns)
3. Mass media advertising (to reach broad-based targets)
4. Direct mail communications (to reach decision influencers)
5. Telephone campaigns (to gain immediate response)
6. Public relations/press releases (for third-party coverage)
7. Product and service brochures (to facilitate selling)
8. Speeches and presentations (for exposure and image building)
9. Newsletters (for awareness and knowledge leader image)
10. Health fairs (for exposure and networking)
11. Logos (for company identity)
12. Personal selling (to close the sale)

THE DEVELOPMENTAL PHASE

Although the steps described and detailed below may seem formidable, a thorough understanding of them is critical to the success of your marketing effort. The most common mistake people make is to fall in love with a product or service idea and rush into the marketplace without firm confirmation of the demand. In fact, a study by the internationally renowned consulting firm of Booz-Allen and Hamilton found that the success or failure of an enterprise can be traced to decisions made in the very early stages of the venture.[1]

Market Analysis

General Information Needs. Industry books and journals can provide a good overview of major trends in the market. It is a good idea to set aside several hours a week to read the books and journals covering Industrial Therapy. This base of information can be supplemented through informal discussions with therapists, physicians, insurance agents, and company benefits personnel. Engaging in frequent informal discussions with those involved in Industrial Therapy is a good way to be aware of new trends and opportunities in the marketplace.

With this base of information, a therapist should be able to identify groups which will be a good target for marketing efforts (e.g. companies, physicians' practices, insurance agents, law firms). Selection of these targets should be based on information regarding the total referral potential, the penetrability of the target, and the expected ease or difficulty of working with the organization. The greatest source of referral potential may have to be bypassed if it is nearly impossible to gain entry or if they are too difficult to work with.

Detailed Information Needs. When this base of general information has been established, the next step is to gather more specific information about the organizations that are to be targeted for the practice's products or services. The therapist will want to obtain information for each target organization, including:

- Who is in charge of buying Industrial Therapy products or services?
- What does their buying decision process look like?
- What do they see as their own or their organization's problems or needs?
- What are they doing now to address these problems or needs?

- What Industrial Therapy products or services do they currently use?
- How satisfied are they with current Industrial Therapy products or services?
- How do they evaluate the performance of current Industrial Therapy products or services?
- Are there any prejudicial attitudes or perceptions that must be overturned before the Industrial Therapy products or services can be accepted?

Information Networking. Networking is an effective and inexpensive way to gather information about a prospective client or organization.[2] If a particular company is the target, the networking process can be started with someone—*anyone*—who might have *some* information about that company. After finding out everything this first contact person knows about the target company, including what or who influences its buying decisions, they may then be asked who else might be contacted to obtain additional information. By networking from individual to individual, it is possible to gain a wealth of information about any given company or organization and become better prepared to launch a successful marketing effort.

Networking can be initiated with an acquaintance who works somewhere in the company or someone who is a sales person calling on that company. In most cases, benefits managers, human resource personnel, and other decision makers in the organization are receptive to an informational interview, particularly if the person requesting the interview has been referred through the networking process. People are generally flattered when someone is interested in their company and are happy to be a source of helpful information and advice.

Networking can be delegated to a support person or subcontracted to a marketing research or consulting firm. Some of the networking and interviewing should be done by the therapist; there is no substitute for getting first-hand information.

Identifying Buying Influencers. The starting point in any marketing process is people. The first step in information gathering is to identify all of the people who will influence the decision to purchase the products and services to be offered.[6] The decision may be influenced by corporate executives or staff, outside physicians, hospital personnel, or insurance agency personnel. It is important to identify all of these people and to understand the decision process as thoroughly as possible.

The Decision Process. In some organizations, particularly small ones, the owner or CEO makes the buying decision. In most organizations, however, CEOs and corporate officers prefer to delegate decision making to their staff. These people do the initial screening of the products and services being offered. If they find the offerings may be of significant benefit to their organization, they will arrange a meeting with someone in their group who has a higher level of decision making authority. This process can continue up the line until the person with the authority to make the decision decides to contract with the therapist.

Middle managers who are consulted or involved in the decision making process must be courted during the selling effort or they can derail any progress that might be made with higher level managers. It is usually a mistake to attempt to sell at the top and hope to be accepted by middle management. Contact at the top can be helpful, but the people with the most influence on the buying decision are not necessarily the highest ranking people in the organization. Middle managers are often the key to the initial purchasing decision and the long term relationship with the organization.

It is important to understand how all levels of management influence the decision to purchase and make their decision. How do they evaluate the performance of current Industrial Therapy services? How did they first decide to use or not to use Industrial Therapy services? What were the key considerations? What would persuade them to consider other approaches to Industrial Therapy? These are the buying process issues that must be understood in order for the therapist to successfully sell Industrial Therapy products and services.

Need. Once those who influence the decision to purchase Industrial Therapy products and services are identified and their decision making process is determined, then the therapist must understand the organization's unmet needs and how to address them. What are their biggest problems? What is the source of the greatest amount of organizational pain? Do they understand the cause of these problems and the solutions that are available?

The most common barriers to making a sale are that the organization:

- Does not perceive it has a problem
- Believes its problems are "givens" that must be tolerated
- Misidentifies the cause
- Misidentifies the solution
- Does not believe that a solution is possible

Some organizations may not realize that certain work stations pose ergonomic risks or that their hiring and job placement practices are in violation of the ADA. Other organizations may not be aware of how unpleasant their situation is, and how preferable a different set of circumstances would be. If an organization's employees are experiencing injuries, the organization may feel it is an unavoidable consequence of their industry or that the injured workers are simply malingerers. An injury-free organization may reject an employee fitness program because they do not realize how dramatically these programs can boost productivity.

Accordingly, when it comes to identifying and discussing needs, the selling process often involves educating potential clients regarding solutions to problems of which they were not aware.

Outcome Study Support. Assuming the prospect can be persuaded to consider alternatives to the status quo, the therapist may be required to produce hard proof that the products or services can yield the solutions and benefits promised. This underscores the need to monitor and document outcomes of the practice's therapy programs. It is important to know how programs have impacted such statistics as injury rates, work loss days, return-to-work time frames and percentages, and overall health care costs. See Chapter 3 for more information on outcome studies.

Current Services. In most cases, making a sale involves persuading the target organization to replace a current product or service with the one being offered. In some cases the product or service being provided is an alternative to a competitor's solution. In other cases, the product or service replaces "doing nothing" about the problem. In either case, there is a certain comfort level with the status quo and a certain uneasiness with the untried or unproven. In some instances the organization may have tried a similar Industrial Therapy service that did not work, and they may be reluctant to experiment any further.

When approaching the organization, it is important to know what Industrial Therapy services they have tried or are currently using, how satisfied they are with the progress they are making, and how they evaluate whether a program "works" or not. This information enables the therapist to avoid proposing solutions that are already in place and working, and to tailor the suggested program toward untapped areas of opportunity.

Competitive Analysis

In gauging the market demand for products and services, it is also important to assess the presence and strength of competitors. Wherever there is great demand, there are usually many competitors trying to fill that demand. As a late entrant in a crowded field, it is difficult to displace those who have been there for some time.[11] Even when there are compelling reasons for a prospect to switch to a new product or service, they will resist change when the status quo solution is, or seems to be, working for them. In most cases, when entrenched competition is present, the best strategy is to pursue another company or industry segment or to present a product or service that represents a ground floor opportunity. The therapist will not want to attack entrenched competitors, but will instead want to find untapped market potential where it is possible to build one's own entrenched position over time.[9]

Sustainability. An additional consideration is whether entry into a segment, even if on the ground floor, is one that can be sustained. The therapist must determine the strengths and weaknesses of his or her practice relative to that of the competition.[9] For example, an Industrial Therapy practice with no prior ergonomic experience may come up with a brilliant new ergonomic program, but a practice more strongly entrenched in ergonomics can easily copy the idea and out-muscle the innovator. An Industrial Therapy practice must enter only those areas where a competitive advantage can be sustained.

Product Development. Armed with knowledge of the demand for various products and services, those who will influence the buying decision, their decision process, and the competitive environment, the next step in market development is to design and tailor specific products or services to fill that demand.

Tangibility. "Services" are often difficult to sell due to their intangibility. When a company buys a machine, the CEO can walk back to the production floor and see what the company got for its money. When a company buys a service, it is more difficult to perceive what has been gained from the investment. For this reason, it is important to present Industrial Therapy services to prospective customers in the most tangible way possible. To accomplish this, all Industrial Therapy services should be "packaged" into discrete "products" that the user can "grasp" conceptually and "buy."

For example, rather than offering to come in and charge hourly rates to teach safe lifting practices, the therapist should package these services into a "Safe Lifting Program" presented in tangible product-like terms such as the program's phases, components, specific steps, evaluation points, measurement tools, reporting systems, outcome analyses, and time frames. The more tangible these services seem, the more comfortable prospective customers will be in evaluating and buying them.

It helps to prepare a professionally printed brochure or fact sheet for each "packaged" service. Simply giving something to a prospective customer that they can hold in their hands, can enhance the perception of tangibility.

Features and Benefits. Selling involves communicating reasons why the prospect should purchase the product or service. In presenting the program it is important to remember that prospective customers are not buying the features of the product or service; they are buying the benefits. Therefore, communication should focus on the benefits involved. If the service is a back prevention program, for example, the communication should emphasize reduced injuries, less work loss, better performance from employees, and lower Workers' Compensation ratings. The specific features of the program should be mentioned as support for the promised benefits.

The Development Process. With a thorough understanding of the market demand, the Industrial Therapy practice is ready to initiate the development of products and services to fill that demand. Box 27.2 shows a typical product or service development process.

A good way to begin this process is to gather staff members, colleagues, trusted advisors, and even friends to participate in an initial idea generating session. Anyone with experience and knowledge of Industrial Therapy or its components can make a valuable contribution to this process. It is also important that the group represents a cross-section of professional and managerial disciplines. Participants should be thoroughly familiar with the results of the market and competitive analyses (Box 27.2, Phase I) so that the ideas are relevant to the market. The group should be urged to come up with as many ideas as possible. Many ideas may build on products and services already offered or may suggest modifications to an existing product or service that will help to address a specific need.

It is important not to reject any ideas during this creative process. Criticism or negativity can stifle creativity. In addition, "bad" ideas on the table are often a good way to stretch thinking and may serve to stimulate thought and produce good ideas.

BOX 27.2

Industrial Therapy New Product and Service Development Process

1. Opportunity identification
   Market trends
   Practice strengths/weaknesses
   Competition strengths/weaknesses
2. Product and service concept development
   Idea generation
   Preliminary feasibility screening
   Product or service concept description
   Initial concept research
3. Comprehensive feasibility analysis
   Medical/therapeutic
   Legal/regulatory
   Marketing
   Competitive
   Projected referrals/clients/fees
   Investment and operating expenses
   Financials
   Go/no go
4. a. Final product development
      Medical/therapeutic
      Program design
      Implementation and delivery plan
   b. Positioning development
      Identify prime prospect
      Identify major benefits
      Identify major competitors(s)
      Communication strategy
5. Initial pilot phase
   Final marketing plan
   Marketing and sales materials production
   Marketing support and selling
   Initial customer implementation
6. Evaluation
7. Expansion

Preliminary Feasibility Screening.   Once the group has generated all the ideas it can, then and only then should the group start weeding out the weaker ones and building up those that are more promising. The feasibility of implementing an idea should be a part of this screening process and should include preliminary evaluations of the medical, therapeutic, and financial benefits, a competitive analysis, and the marketing potential of the idea.

After the initial development and evaluation of a new idea, it is a good to get feedback from those who may be purchasing and/or using the new product or service in the future.

Product Research

Feedback on product and service ideas can be obtained by using the same kind of one-on-one interview with potential clients that is used for market analysis. Also, potential clients can be gathered into focus groups to discuss product and service ideas.[2]

Whether conducting one-on-one interviews or leading focus groups, the therapist should present each new concept (product or service) in an appealing format such as that of a brochure, advertisement, or flier. General questions that can be asked are:

- To whom, if anyone, does this product or service appeal?
- What, if anything, is being done to serve the same purpose?
- Would it replace what is being done now?
- What are the key advantages of this product or service?
- What are its shortcomings?

Of course, each practice will have its own unique issues to be covered with questions like:

- Is this product or service compatible with your current perceptions of (name of practice)?
- What other organizations (hospitals, physicians' practices) would you expect to offer a product or service like this?

Professional marketing research services, if affordable, may be contracted to help with this phase. They can provide advice on the pros and cons of various research approaches as well as how to present the concepts, frame the questions, and interpret the results. They will try to sell their services to conduct the interviews or focus groups. If the price is reasonable and affordable, this professional assistance would be ideal. Be cautious of anyone trying to talk the practice into an expensive "sophisticated" research study. There is no mystery or magic in asking questions and finding out what people are thinking. If professionals are not affordable, this can be done in-house. The important thing is to get some feedback on the product or service ideas so that they can be as fine-tuned and on-target as possible before a great deal of money is spent to further develop, plan, equip, stage, and launch them into the marketplace.[2]

Comprehensive Feasibility Analysis.   If research feedback is promising, the next step is to perform an in-depth analysis of the feasibility of each new product or service candidate. The kinds of questions that should be addressed include:

- Is the product or service within the medical or therapeutic expertise of the practice?
- What are the legal and regulatory requirements? Are they affordable?
- Is there sufficient market demand?
- Are the requisite capital and operating resources affordable?
- What is the current presence or absence of competitors?
- Does the product or service fit with the practice's existing sustainable strengths or advantages?
- Does the product exploit competitors' weaknesses?

The medical and therapeutic parameters should be exhaustively evaluated. Legal and regulatory issues should be addressed, possibly with the advice of attorneys. A forecast of referrals, clients, and fees should be formulated and compared to the capital and operating expenses. An analysis of the competition and the comparative strengths and weaknesses of the product or service should be made. Only after a product or service idea passes these criteria should it be considered for market introduction.

Budgeting

Determining how much of a practice's resources should be devoted to marketing products and services to prospective clients is one of the most difficult decisions to make.[3-5] In theory, marketing expenditures should be increased as long as each dollar being spent brings back more than one dollar to the bottom line. Practically speaking, the large number of variables in the marketplace make it impossible to scientifically determine the optimum spending level with complete accuracy.

Published advertising-to-sales ratios for industries involved in activities similar to Industrial Therapy can be a useful benchmark in the budgeting process. Examples of these ratios can be found in Table 27.1.

There are also a number of considerations that can assist the therapist in determining an appropriate marketing budget. They are as follows:

- *How large is the market?* Budget requirements increase with the number of prospective clients and the degree of geographic dispersion.
- *Is competition present?* Fewer competitors means fewer dollars required to capture prospects' attention.
- *How much is the competition spending?* The more the competitors spend on marketing, the harder it is to obtain an effective "share of voice."
- *What marketing tools are to be used?* If the specific vehicles for your message (i.e. magazines, newspapers, direct mailings) can be determined, they can be costed out to derive the budget.
- *How much can be afforded?* The cost of equipment, operating budget, and other expenses may place a certain and unavoidable cap on the marketing budget.

In the process of budgeting, a practice might decide to pursue a smaller market. The practice might decide to focus on a locally-based or smaller niche, to go where competition is absent or not spending, or to find ways to use less expensive marketing tools to get the job done. The important point to remember is to follow a rational, step-by-step budgeting process and to weigh the considerations listed above.[3-5]

When budgeting funds for marketing, it is important to develop a detailed twelve month plan that includes all the marketing tools and programs anticipated. Even if the practice is not sure of all of these elements, it is preferable to put some assumptions on paper and then monitor and adjust the plan over time. A common mistake many organizations make is to set up a loosely-defined marketing fund and spend it piece-meal as ideas or opportunities come along. This approach tends to spread resources in a disorganized fashion, resulting in a fraction of the impact that would be achieved with a better orchestrated plan.

TABLE 27.1 Advertising Dollars as a Percentage of Gross Sales and Gross Margins

Industry	Ad dollars as a percentage of sales	Ad dollars as a percentage of margin*
Business services	3.1%	12.7%
Educational services	4.7%	10.7%
Hospitals	.6%	2.5%
Management consulting	.2%	.5%
Nursing services and facilities	1.0%	5.0%
Research labs	1.0%	7.1%
*Margin = net sales dollars minus cost of goods		

THE EXECUTIONAL PHASE

Executional activities have to do with "selling" in one way or another. Most often, people tend to think of selling in terms of one person giving a sales pitch to another over the phone or in person. In this chapter, we will refer to that form of selling as "personal selling." It should be emphasized, however, that advertising, direct mail, press releases, and other devices are also forms of selling, and that a mix of such selling tools in connection with personal selling will generate more new clients that either one alone.

The Selling Process

The Rule of Five. A therapist seldom expects to achieve his or her goal after one treatment. In the same way, a marketer's objectives are not usually met after just one intervention. Multiple interventions lead the buyer through the mental steps that are necessary to reach a buying decision. This series of steps is often referred to as the Rule of Five. The Rule of Five consists of the following steps:

1. Curiosity
2. Awareness
3. Understanding
4. Familiarity
5. Decision

During this process, marketing activity should be driven according to which step is being accomplished by the buyer. Marketing efforts may be heavier or lighter for certain steps depending on the product or service and how the market views it. Relatively new ideas will require stronger emphasis on building curiosity and awareness. When ideas already have high awareness, focus should be placed on explaining the product and establishing a sense of familiarity. Each step sets the stage for the next one to be accomplished.

Personal Selling versus Direct Mail and Advertising. McGraw-Hill Research found that it takes an average of eight selling contacts to consummate an industrial sale.[8] There are a wide variety of products and services offered by the Industrial Therapist and some will require more selling steps than others. The important thing to remember is that selling is a multiple step process.

For each step in the selling process, the Industrial Therapist could use personal selling. However, personal selling is labor intensive and, therefore, expensive. To appreciate just how expensive a marketing effort based solely on personal selling would be, add up the cost to employ one sales person for a year, fully equipped with a car, office space, supplies, support staff, and expense account. A conservative figure would be $50,000. Divide this figure by the number of sales calls that person could make in a year consisting of 250 working days. If the salesperson can make two calls per day, total calls per year are 500, and the cost per sales call is $100. This is a very conservative estimate considering that the average industrial sales call is now estimated to cost over $250. Using a 50 cent brochure or a 19 cent postcard to make some of those contacts makes a lot of sense.

In addition to economic considerations, communication materials such as a brochure or postcard will increase the number of prospective clients that can be reached in any given time frame. If it takes eight contacts to make a sale, and through personal selling, only 500 contacts can be made per year (two per day), the average number of sales per year would be:

$$500/8 = 62.5 \text{ sales per year}$$

If communication materials were used for five of the eight required contacts, the number of sales could be almost tripled:

$$500/3 = 166.67 \text{ sales per year}$$

Using printed materials to perform some of the prospecting enables the therapist to reach a much broader market with the same number of sales people.

Apart from the economic savings and efficiency of direct marketing, communication materials can often accomplish the objectives of certain steps in the selling process more effectively than personal selling. For instance, preceding the initial personal contact with a mailing is preferred over making a cold call. A mailing can help to break the ice and peak the prospective client's curiosity before a sales call is made. In some instances, people will not take a sales call seriously until they have seen information about the practice in print.

The therapist's selling plan should include multiple points of contact, using a combination of communication materials and personal selling to move prospective clients through the selling process.

Table 27.2 outlines one example of a selling process. The specific selling process used for each Industrial Therapy practice and each product or service will vary. The structure of the selling process should always be flexible enough to allow for modification over time as the effectiveness of the tools and approaches at each step is monitored.

Prioritizing Steps and Materials

Many times the ideal selling process calls for a lead mailing, a comprehensive brochure, a fact sheet, and a number of other printed pieces. However, few practices or companies can afford to develop and produce all of these materials at the outset. Materials must be prioriti-

TABLE 27.2   Example Selling Process

Step	Selling Tool/Purpose	
1	Mailing:	Generate awareness and curiosity
2	Telephone sales:	Call, qualify, then get an appointment
3	Information mailing	Cover the basics to develop an initial understanding
4	Personal appointment	Further understanding and familiarity
5	Leave-behind brochure	Detailed understanding and familiarity
6	Follow-up mailing(s)	Gain acceptance
7	Follow-up phoning	Get invited back to make a proposal
8	Present proposal	Action: close the sale
On-going post sale		Support the customer

zed so that the most crucial ones can be developed and produced first.

One way to determine which materials might be most important is to analyze where selling efforts are most difficult or meet with the most resistance. If prospective customers have not heard of the practice and are not interested in talking about it, initial funds should be spent on generating awareness and curiosity (Table 27.2, Step 1). On the other hand, if they agree to talk but do not believe the practice can deliver, funds may be focused on follow-up mailings that build credibility by chronicling successful case histories (Table 27.2, Step 6). Working through the selling process, the therapist will begin to learn where resources are most needed and how efforts can be modified to be more effective.

Selling Process Principles

While the specific steps and materials used during the selling process will differ for each practice, product, and service, there are some basic principles that should be followed.

The First Principle.   During each step of the selling process, the therapist should not think in terms of closing the sale. Objectives at each step of the selling process should be set in terms of advancing the sale through curiosity, awareness, understanding, and familiarity.

The Second Principle.   At each step of the selling process, the therapist should work toward building a relationship with the prospective client. It is important that the prospect trusts and likes the person making the presentation.

The Third Principle.   Do not make the promise too big. There is a natural inclination to position a product or service in the most positive way possible—to prom-

ise the most dramatic improvement or to represent extraordinary progress. However, most people are afraid of change, even when the change will be undeniably beneficial. Products and services should be positioned as a logical extension of principles and practices that are already being followed. As long as the product or service represents some significant improvement over the status quo, there is no reason to present it as a great magnitude of difference.

Marketing and Sales Staffing

Having arrived at the best mix of personal selling and supporting materials it is then possible to determine the staffing requirements necessary to launch the marketing effort. The personal selling function may be performed initially by the therapists on staff who can devote a portion of their time to converse with new prospects. Development and production of communication materials such as brochures and advertisements can be contracted to a marketing communications firm or advertising agency. However, the practice will need to designate a staff member to act as contact and supervisor for materials development and production.

Pricing

Everyone recognizes that pricing is an important factor in survival and profitability. Any enterprise must price its offerings in such a way as to maximize bottom line profit. In some cases, this involves a high price and low volume approach. In other cases, a low price paired with a high volume is more successful. Every practice must look at the prospects' interest in their products and services, their ability to pay, and competitive pricing before making this decision.[3-5]

In studying start-up ventures, the Strategic Planning Institute in Cambridge, Mass. found that the highest long terms returns on investment were achieved by those who charged a premium price for their products and services, and promoted quality.[11] In fact, in virtually any product or service category today, the perceived quality leader is also a premium-priced option.

Pricing can also be used as a tool for communication. When approaching a prospective client, it is important to resist the temptation to "fire sale" products or services. This approach calls quality and credibility into question. The Industrial Therapist will always be better off with the message, "the fees are a little higher, but the quality is worth the difference."

Mass Media Advertising

Advertising in local or national magazines, industry journals and trade publications, yellow pages, and newspapers is used primarily to establish and maintain awareness.[6] As mentioned earlier, selling efforts will be more productive if the prospective customer has heard of the practice, product, or service and has seen it in print. Many prospects interpret such exposure to signify that the advertised entity is a bona fide "player."

When evaluating media, the therapist should consider the following:

- Target prospect cost per thousand
- Percent of target prospects reached
- Message impact capability of the media vehicle
- Perceived prestige or credibility of the media vehicle

Cost per thousand is a common measurement used to compare the efficiency of one type of media over another.[7] This figure is calculated by dividing the total cost for space or time by the estimated readership or audience in thousands. All other things being equal, the media with the lowest cost per thousand should be chosen. However, all other things are not equal.

The cost per thousand of printed media depends on the size of the ad. The lowest cost may be achieved by running a 1/64 page ad in the newspaper. Whether anyone will notice the ad is another matter.

The percent of target reached is also important. For example, outdoor billboards have an extremely low cost per thousand. However, only a small fraction of a market drives by any given outdoor billboard. By the time enough boards are purchased to reach a significant percentage of the market, the cost differential relative to newspaper or electronic media is considerably narrowed.[7]

Message impact varies by media. Television, with the use of color, motion, and sound is usually the most effective way to generate awareness and memorability. Magazines or newspapers are usually next in impact. People actively read printed media and spend a good deal of time reading the advertising as well. Radio tends to be a background medium to which people do not actively listen, so it is difficult to command people's attention or register strong selling points over the radio. One emerging exception is radio talk shows. In this case, the audience is actively listening and advertising messages can have more impact. Outdoor billboards have only a few seconds to reach passing motorists, so they are not able to communicate complex messages. They are, however, effective in reinforcing messages that have been established through other media.

The prestige or credibility of the media is a consideration often overlooked in the rush to minimize cost per thousand. Sometimes the authority of the leading daily newspaper or regional business magazine is worth a significant premium in cost per thousand over less expensive options.

It is important to mention that in some instances, mass media advertising is not warranted or justifiable. There are times when the target population is too small to warrant conventional advertising. It is hard to justify buying a 50,000 circulation base to reach 25 or 50 benefits managers in a particular market niche. In such instances a more targeted effort, such as a direct mail campaign, is preferable.

Direct Mail Communications

Direct mail is the media of choice when the target audience cannot be efficiently reached with conventional mass advertising. In many cases, mailing lists can be purchased which are subdivided by industry type, job titles, zip codes, and many other categories. If mailing lists are not available, a custom mailing list can be built. For a cost of $5 to $10 per name, telemarketing firms will call target companies and find out the names and titles of people who should receive information on a given subject. If time permits, this can be done by in-house staff.

There are times when direct mail is used even if mass advertising is more cost efficient. One key advantage of direct mail is its ability to deliver more information with more impact than a magazine page. A prospect might typically spend only ten seconds or so on any given page of a magazine, but might be willing to spend a great deal more time on an interesting, informative, engaging direct mail package. When your message requires more time to assimilate, direct mail can be the most effective vehicle.[6]

The contents of a direct mail package should be driven by the objective of the mailing. If the objective is to arouse curiosity and generate awareness, the package might contain attention-getting elements such as a wall poster or unique gift item that makes a point. If the objective is to explain the features and benefits, a clear, easy to read brochure and cover letter might be the best approach.

In designing the direct mail package, it is important to conform to the dimension and weight parameters set forth by the US postal service. A great deal of money can be wasted by using packages which are outside of the dimensions or a fraction of an ounce over the limits for certain price breaks. Additionally, if more than 200 pieces are being mailed at once, the sender can take advantage of bulk mail and presort discounts. It is a good idea to consult the customer service department of the local post office before finalizing the design of the direct mail package.

Whatever the objectives are, it is important to remember they should be expressed in terms of advancing the sale, not closing the sale. Some goods such as magazine subscriptions or audio tapes can close the sale with a single mailing, but this type of result would be highly unexpected in the case of Industrial Therapy products and services.

Every mailing should ask for an action step of some sort such as "Return the enclosed reply card," "Call us if you want to hear more," "Keep this rollodex card on file," or "Watch for our ad in this month's issue of (name of publication)." Always remember to keep it simple. Use no fewer than two pieces and no more than four pieces in the mailer. Avoid busy times like holidays. If the mailing is preceding a special event such as a trade show, it should be sent at least six to eight weeks ahead of the event.

Telephone Contact

Many times, prospective clients will not respond to advertising or direct mail contact. To reach these people it may be necessary to call them personally. While telephoning is primarily recommended for follow-up, it can also be the most effective way to get your message to someone. Some points to remember are:

- Always keep the conversation short.
- Ask if you are talking with the appropriate person. If not, get the name and title of the right person.
- Always suggest a next step. Ideally, this would be a meeting, but alternatively an informational packet can be sent or a date for a follow-up phone call can be set.
- If the prospect is not available, do not expect a call back simply because you have left your name and number.
- Keep trying. After enough messages, the prospect will feel obligated to respond and will be impressed with your persistance.

One of the key objectives of the selling process is to build a relationship over time. For this reason, the use of outside telemarketing services to contact potential clients is not a good idea. The person who will ultimately close the sale must start building a relationship with the prospect as early in the process as possible.

Public Relations and Press Releases

Public relations are a great way to get excellent coverage at no cost. The local paper may be 60 to 100 pages daily and 100 to 200 pages on Sunday. Magazines typically run 100 to 200 pages. Writers have to fill these publications with items of interest. They want topical stories that reward the reader with valuable information. The areas touched by Industrial Therapy are among the most newsworthy of topics; the rising cost of health care, America's penchant for litigation, the Americans with Disabilities Act, and the challenge of global competition.

Getting articles or information about the practice in print begins with the editor, who will indicate the appropriate columnist to call. Most newspapers have sections on business, jobs, health, fitness, and other areas where placements might be possible. Most magazines run custom articles where such information could be used. If the therapist or practice has something that will interest readers, a newspaper or magazine can provide a level of exposure that would otherwise cost a great deal if purchased in the form of paid advertising.

In addition, being covered by the media often carries more credibility than paid advertising. The reader is less likely to doubt what an impartial third-party has to say.

The disadvantages of this tool, however, are that there is no guarantee that the publication will provide the coverage and the practice or therapist will have no control over what is printed. Sometimes it is more newsworthy for a reporter to point out shortcomings or negative aspects of an issue than to focus on the good points. For this reason, it is important to be very careful as to what is said in interviews and the media.

Product and Service Brochures

One of the most important considerations when developing a brochure is what the brochure is intended to accomplish. The most common mistake in developing a brochure is to present everything there is to know about the practice, product, or service. The problems with such comprehensiveness are twofold. First, few people have the time or inclination to read such a voluminous piece, so it winds up in a stack of papers, a file, or in the wastebasket. Second, it is not a good idea to provide all of the information necessary for the buyer to make a decision. The risk is that the buyer will decide "no" before the sales person can make a presentation. A more effective strategy is to provide a small amount of information in one brochure which will make the buyer look forward to the next step in the selling process. Each step in the process should move the buyer one more easy and painless step forward.

Brochures can provide basic information that makes the next selling step more productive. Sending out an informational brochure in advance of a sales call covers basic information that might otherwise take up a lot of time at the beginning of the call. The name of the practice, the number of years in existence, key industrial customers, key principals or executives, and product lines are all items that an informational brochure can cover in advance of the sales call.

A brochure can also serve as a leave-behind piece that gives the prospective client more in-depth information to review after the sales presentation. This enables the presentation to focus on the big picture, leaving the details to be reviewed at the prospect's liesure.

Overall, brochures should concentrate on the key elements of persuasion, be straight forward, easy to read, and speak the prospect's language—no medical jargon. There should also be a lot of white space. A page that is cluttered with copy or visual elements tends to discourage reading.

Speeches and Presentations

As mentioned earlier, Industrial Therapy touches on a number of high profile topics in the news today, from health care to global competitiveness. Most public service and business roundtable clubs in any given metro area would undoubtedly be interested in what therapists have to say. By putting together a few speeches, one 15 minutes long and another 30 minutes long, the hardest part is done. Speaking engagements represent an efficient way to reach business people and promote the practice.

Newsletters

Compared to the $100+ cost of a personal sales call, newsletters are an economical way to make contacts. They are also an effective way to build credibility and begin building the relationship that must precede the sale. With desk top publishing, a professional looking newsletter is easily created and produced. There is also software available that is formatted especially for newsletters.

One way to gather material for a newsletter is to set up a file marked "Newsletter." When anyone in the office finds an interesting piece of information, they can put it in this file. With everyone in the office contributing, there should be more than enough information to fill the newsletter. Be aware, though, that as more and more businesses are using newsletters in their marketing efforts, they are becoming less unique. Newsletters need to be of high interest to keep from going unread or being quickly tossed. An alternative to a full blown newsletter is to send out quick-read bulletins with just one very interesting piece of information in each.

Health Fairs

Health fairs are growing in popularity as a way for health care providers to gain awareness and build relationships with industry and the public. They are usually publicized in the local media and are often sponsored by one or more participating organizations. Participation is simply a matter of keeping an eye out for health fairs, finding out who organizes them, and getting involved in them. In many instances it may be worthwhile to purchase booth space and demonstrate something useful to attendees like correct posture for lifting, or the correct way to sit in a chair. Health fairs are also good opportunities to meet other exhibitors and do some networking.

Logos

A company name and logo, and its placement on stationery, brochures, facility walls, and equipment is an important component of a practice's image in the marketplace. A great deal of thought should go into this verbal and visual identity that will appear so often and so prominently in association with the practice.

The organization's products and services will become known by the practice name. If the name says something about the strengths and unique qualities of the practice, so much the better. Using a person's name does not communicate an attribute or benefit, unless the name has been associated with positive values for a significant time in the marketplace. In addition, naming the practice after a person (i.e. the founder) may suggest to customers that they are not getting top attention unless that person is personally involved.

PERSONAL SELLING

Why it is Important

Personal selling is probably the most important issue discussed in this chapter. In some product categories, such as consumer products, personal selling is relatively unimportant. People prefer to buy the desired brand off the shelf or through the mail without sales assistance. However, in Industrial Therapy, the costs, benefits, and system wide ramifications are so significant that it is hard to imagine a sale being closed by means other than face-to-face personal selling. This does not discredit printed materials and other selling tools discussed in this chapter. Personal contact is essential in establishing the relationship necessary to consummate the sale.

The Fear Factor

Personal selling is regarded by many with fear and it is important to deal with this emotion from the beginning. Most therapists can remember working with patients during their first internship, and there was undoubtedly fear then, just as with any important first time experience. Repeated exposure, practice, and experience causes those fears to fade. The same is true with personal selling. Unlike therapy, if an error is made, no one is hurt. In fact, with personal selling, it is possible to make mistakes and still try again. When prospective customers see this kind of determination, their respect for the therapist and the practice will grow.

Selling Process Management

Of all aspects of marketing, the personal selling process is one of the most challenging, and like therapeutic processes, it follows an orderly progression.

The acquisition of a new customer must be managed by the therapist for a variety of reasons. First of all, only the therapist can see the end point, so only the therapist can effectively navigate to reach that destination where the solution (product or service) is matched with the customer's need or problem. For this discussion, the term "problem" is defined as the difference between what the customer has and what the customer wants.

It is important to emphasize that the therapist/ seller is in charge and is the only person who can envision the entire selling process. With proper management by the therapist, the prospective customer will not be left behind, but will be carried along through education, information, logic, proof, user testimonials, emotional reassurance, and a host of other resources.

Just as the overall selling process advances the prospective customer one step at a time toward contracting with the therapist, the personal selling event involves a series of small decisions and agreements that have to be reached with the prospective customer.

Personal selling can be illustrated as a six step process. These steps are:

1. Preparation
2. Opening
3. Exploration
4. Presentation
5. Clarification
6. Action

It is rare to achieve all of these steps in one meeting. Typically there will be several meetings spread out over many months (and sometimes years). As previously discussed, it is also important to use printed communication and other means of contact to assist and facilitate progress.

Preparation. Effective meetings begin with preparation. It is important to learn everything possible about the company before the first meeting and to stay on top of new information from then on.

Information gathering should start with basic industry trends to understand the environment in which Industrial Therapy products and services are to be introduced. The best resource for this basic information is the public library. The business section of the library has many periodicals relating to business and a Business Periodicals Index listing articles, by topic, that have been published in business magazines and journals. Many libraries have this and other indices on line, making searches easier and more efficient.

The daily newspaper often contains business reports of OSHA citations, injury frequencies, Workers' Compensation costs, and other related topics. Many city newspapers have indices of articles similar to the Business Periodicals Index and most libraries have the New York Times Index and the newspaper itself on microfilm.

Another tool for preparation is tracking. An Industrial Therapy Clinic might trace its clinic's Workers' Compensation claimants back to their place of work and use the workers' injuries as an opening. The therapist might call the company president and say, "We have seen four carpal tunnel patients who are employees of yours. Would you have time to talk about how you might prevent some of these injuries in the future?"

Also important in preparation is setting reasonable objectives for the meeting. As previously discussed, the sale will probably not be made in the first meeting or even by the second or third. Instead, the objective of each meeting should be to significantly build the relationship and advance the selling process.

It is important to visualize success before each meeting. Psychologists tell us that success is more easily attained if it is first visualized in our mind. Top athletes see themselves winning the race, executing the completed pass, or scoring the goal thousands of times before the actual event. When the event occurs, the mind has already been there and the body is ready. Therapists do the same thing when working with their patients, but need to carry that over to their personal selling. Visualization is best done in the quiet of a study or office. Visualizing solving the prospective customers' problems will help the entire selling process become more focused.

Opening.   After a thorough preparation, the therapist will be ready for the next step in personal selling, a face-to-face meeting with the prospective customer. In the first meeting, it is important for the therapist to confirm who each person is and to reiterate the purpose for the meeting.

Whenever people meet for the first time, tension is high. Think of some of the most important meetings in life; meeting a future spouse's parents for the first time, interviewing for acceptance into a professional school, sitting for an orals board, interviewing for a job. These are all tension-filled events. The first meeting with a prospective customer is no different. In fact, even therapists who are experienced in such meetings still feel this anxiety when first meeting with a prospective customer.

As therapist and prospective customer come together in the first sales call, task tension (the sense of urgency to take action) is low for the prospect. The prospect is relatively comfortable with the status quo or does not realize existing problems. They are curious to hear the message, but have little motivation to take action and are not willing to risk much. If task tension remains low, there will be no impetus to make decisions or take any action. At the same time, relationship tension (the interpersonal apprehension level) is high. Trust has not yet been established.

A good way to begin to build the trust of the prospective customer is to ask questions. It is also a way to raise the prospect's sensitivity to their problems and their interest in exploring ideas and solutions. For example, you might open by saying, "Would it be all right if I asked you a few questions?" Through this approach, relationship tension is reduced to a level of comfort and trust necessary for decision making and action. This question and answer sequence is one of the most important parts of the personal selling process.

While relationship tension is being reduced through questioning, task tension can be raised by drawing the prospect into the process of identifying problems and initiating small steps toward their solution. The prospect may be asked what their current injury rates are, and may agree to have this information for the next meeting. By identifying important areas of focus and assigning initial action steps, task tension begins to increase. At some point, relationship tension decreases and task tension increases to a point of alignment, culminating in the sale (Figure 27.1).

Exploration.   Exploration is the most important part of communication with a prospective customer; it is the art of asking questions. Exploration advances trust and allows for mutual discovery about needs and fulfillment. In the first meeting, during the question and answer exploration, prospects will make their first important decision which is sometimes referred to as the "affiliation decision." In making the affiliation decision, the prospect decides, "I like this person," "I feel good about what is happening," "I trust this person," "I can see myself going forward with this person." The affiliation decision happens with patients just as it happens with prospective customers.

Exploration sets the stage for the remaining steps in the selling process. If there are gaps in the information gathered, the solutions offered will be based on false premises and the results will not be successful. If the employer has spent one million dollars on sixty back injuries in the past year and most of the injuries were caused while lifting, a possible solution might be an education program, a back support program, and an audit assessment program. Other solutions might be a Job Placement Assessment program and a Job Analysis program. If the right questions are not asked, it will be impossible to know where to begin.

A common challenge is the process of deciding what information is most important and which is secondary. It may not be possible or practical to solve all of the problems immediately. It is important to avoid trying to deal with every issue. Four or five of the highest priority and most likely to be solved issues should be worked on first.

As information is gathered, it is important to stay focused on what the prospective client needs, and not on what the therapist can provide. That will come later. There is always a strong impulse to tell prospects about the practice's capabilities. This temptation must be resisted until the prospect is done telling their story through answers to the therapist's questions. Informa-

FIGURE 27.1   With questions and answer process, relationship tension diminishes and task tension can be elevated.

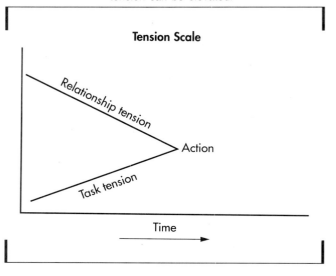

tion provided by the prospect can be categorized according to the kinds of therapy practice programs to which it pertains (Figure 27.2).

Questions and Answers. In addition to providing a forum for obtaining valuable information, questions asked by the therapist will be an important influence on the prospective customer's affiliation decision. There are two basic types of questions: fact questions and feeling questions. Box 27.3 lists examples of each type of question.

It is best to start off with the fact questions. They tend to be easier to answer and nonthreatening. These are questions like; How many?, What kind?, When?, and Where? Asking questions and being attentive to answers will help to build rapport and trust. The questions signal an interest in the prospect's business and show the therapist's base of knowledge. Listening attentively to the prospect's answers also communicates sincerity.

There should not be a menu of questions prepared ahead of time; just keep in mind the general approaches. The primary mission of the therapist is to listen. Not knowing what the next question will be compels the therapist to listen to the prospect's answer in order to determine the next question. This makes asking and listening a more natural process.

Once a comfortable relationship has been built with fact questions, it is then appropriate to begin asking questions such as, "If you could start with a clean sheet of paper, what would your program look like?"

Again, trust is very important. The prospect or customer will never know as much as the therapist about the solution or the pathway to find it. So, to a certain extent, they must make a leap of faith and trust that the therapist will come through for them.

The quality of a relationship is not a function of a duration of time, but what is done during that time. Interaction can either function as a trust builder or a diminisher of trust. Trust is not built based upon what is said, thought, or felt, but upon a person's actions. If a prospect is told they will receive a call and they do not, trust is diminished.

It is important to ask permission to take notes and to take those notes thoroughly. Many needs will be uncovered and the most tangible needs should be highlighted. This will help make the eventual presentation easier and more understandable. The prospect's company may have many needs, but it is important not to address them all at one time. The discussion and eventual presentation should be focused on one or two of the most important items with the highest impact and liklihood of the prospect's acceptance.

FIGURE 27.2 Information provided by the prospect is used to determine which therapy practice programs will be needed.

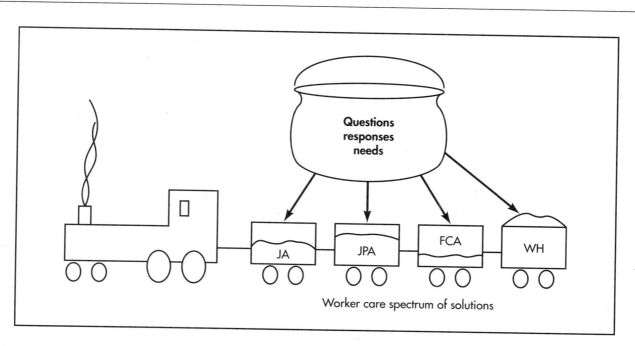

BOX 27.3

Twenty Good Questions

Fact questions:
　　How many employees?
　　　　Blue collar
　　　　White collar
　　Are you unionized?
　　　　Which unions?
　　Where are you located geographically?
　　Tell me about your products?
　　Tell me about your injury experience?
　　What kind of injuries?
　　　　Which departments?
　　Are you self insured?
　　Are you carrier insured?
　　What is your claims experience?
　　What is your cost experience?
　　Do you use a third-party administrator?
　　　　Which one?
　　What programs have you used in the past?
　　What has worked?
　　What hasn't?

Feeling questions:
　　What would you like to do?
　　Where would you like to start?
　　In your view, what constitutes a good program?

Presentation. A presentation may be made in the first meeting, but more than likely, it will be made in the second meeting as a response to issues raised in the first.

The purpose of a presentation is to match solutions to the prospective customer's needs. The presentation is where the product decision is made: is this the right product or service for the organization at this time? If the presentation is based on discussions from a previous meeting, it should ideally follow a format that incorporates the prospect's own words. When the prospect hears their own words or examples coming back to them, they can more easily associate with and accept the solution.

The Worker Care Spectrum can be an effective visual aid in a presentation. This schematic is comprehensive, yet very specific. Using the Worker Care Spectrum as a visual aid in a presentation helps to keep the focus on the primary components of the solution while putting everything in context. Viewing the entire spectrum also allows the therapist and prospective client to look at secondary solutions.

As discussed earlier, it is important to make services as tangible as possible. In the same manner, the presentation should make the solutions it presents seem tangible. The more substance perceived, the easier it is to make a purchase decision.

This chapter has also discussed how important it is for the therapist to visualize the end point. In addition, presentations are more effective if they help the prospect to visualize how the solution will look and feel in descriptive terms. This can be done through statements like, "Here is your situation now, and there is where you tell me you want to be . . . Is that right? . . . Here is what we will do to get you there . . . Can you see us doing this together? . . . I will be in the plant and will be accessible to each injured worker." Statements like this also help ensure that the presentation is staying on the right track. The strategy is to talk "solution," "mutual benefits," and in terms of "we," "us," and "together."

In addition to visualization, it is also important to keep the presentation simple and free of medical jargon. Range of motion and muscle grade strength means nothing on the shop floor. The Industrial Therapy prospect is almost always a non-medical person. The presentation must speak their language and the therapist must learn that language in order to communicate effectively and build trust.

Presentations should be developed into a written format that can serve as a formal proposal. As mentioned earlier, brochures and other written materials can be important tools in conveying basic principles and facilitating the selling process.

The presentation should end in a question and answer session with the focus on implementation. Questions, concerns, doubts, and fears may arise. These should be dealt with immediately in the next step.

Clarification. At the end of a presentation, the prospective customer may have fears such as, "I'll look bad if this doesn't work out." However, it is rare for the prospect to volunteer these concerns. The presenter must carefully identify these issues with questions such as, "Would it be all right if I asked you a few questions about that?" Questions like this help the prospect distinguish fears from real questions or confusion. Once these issues are clarified, the prospect and therapist are ready to take action.

Action. This is the step where arrangements are made for delivery of the product or service and fees are agreed upon. Cost should be the final decision the prospect faces. The reason price is left until the end is that it must first be determined whether or not the appropriate solution has been identified for the prospect. Price is not a determinant of that question.

If the solution is wrong, no price can make it right no matter how inexpensive. People buy things because they are right and fill a need, not because they are low priced.

SUMMARY

Each Industrial Therapist will have to choose the marketing program that works best for their practice. No matter how a marketing program is designed, chances for success will be increased by remembering that marketing starts with people and what they need. The therapist must also consider what the practice can provide in a competitively-sustainable fashion. With these things in mind, the therapist can move prospective customers toward proper solutions, using a combination of personal selling and written communications to achieve a mutually fulfilling outcome.

REFERENCES

1. Booz-Allen & Hamilton: *New Products Management for the 1980s*, New York, 1983, Booz-Allen & Hamilton.

2. Breen E, Blankenship AB: *Do-It-Yourself Marketing Research*, McGraw-Hill.

3. Brigham EF, Gapenski LC: *Intermediate Financial Management*, 1990, The Dryden Press.

4. Flamholtz EG, Diamond MA, Flamholtz DT: *Financial Accounting*, 1986, MacMillan Publishing.

5. Garrison RH: *Managerial Accounting, Concepts for Planning, Control, and Decision Making*, 1988, Business Publications.

6. Kotler P: *Marketing Management, Analysis, Planning, Implementation, and Control*, 1988, Prentice Hall.

7. Lee GG: *Adweek's Marketer's Guide to Media*, New York, 1990, A/S/M Communications.

8. McGraw-Hill Research: *Cost of a Business-to-Business Sales Call*, New York, 1987, McGraw-Hill.

9. Porter, ME: *Competitive Strategy, Techniques for Analyzing Industries and Competitors*, 1980, The Free Press.

10. *Advertising to Sales Ratios, 1990*, Evanston, Ill, 1990, Schonfeld and Associates.

11. Strategic Planning Institute: *What Approaches Succeed in Building a Strong Business?*, Cambridge, Mass, 1980.

Appendix III

Glenda L. Key

In the course of editing (and in some cases writing) the preceding 27 chapters on Industrial Therapy, it became evident that the multiplicity of therapeutic programs and procedures are undergoing a great deal of change. Pouring over the collective wisdom of so many experts in their respective fields, patterns become apparent and a picture of the future emerges. This picture may differ considerably from reader to reader, based on differences in background, field of expertise, regionality, and a host of other factors. Nevertheless, anyone involved in Industrial Therapy, whether an employer, payor, provider, or legal and regulatory player, should develop a working view of the future, so that investments of time and money can be targeted in directions that promise to be fruitful. It is to assist the process of anticipation and planning that this editor will attempt to distill some conclusions and make some predictions with regard to future trends in Industrial Therapy.

Industrial Therapy components, approaches, and reimbursement policies will be increasingly shaped by outcome studies that compare costs to long term bottom line impact.

As mentioned by nearly every contributing author, the evolution of Industrial Therapy is being driven primarily by the cost, productivity, and profit concerns of employers and insurers, concerns which have intensified under the heat of increasing global competition. Profits are the lifeblood of any commercial enterprise. In order to survive and prosper, employers and insurers must find ways to intelligently manage every factor that impacts their bottom line. Quantification is an inevitable requirement to objectively monitor and control operational variables. Outcome studies that provide statistical analyses of cause and effect will be in increasing demand. Industrial Therapy programs and procedures that can be validated by reliable outcome studies will gain increasing acceptance. Products, programs, or procedures with impact not measured in dollars and cents will decline.

A concern among many health care professionals is that over reliance on outcome studies may serve to limit Industrial Therapy to programs and procedures with easily measurable impact. But Therapists who believe strongly enough in more complex or innovative approaches will find ways to measure and correlate the factors necessary to support their approach. For example, studies on the impact of company funded employee fitness centers are successfully justifying costs on the basis of factors such as employee turnover and replacement costs, recruitment success, worker morale, and productivity.

The quantification of Industrial Therapy programs and procedures will become viewed less as infringements that restrict Therapists' latitude, and more as "tools" that amplify Therapists' capabilities.

Most fields of endeavor involve a combination of art and science. Industrial Therapy is no exception. The history of technological advancement in any field, however, indicates that practitioners tend to initially mistrust and resist the intrusion of new technology. The principle fear is that the advance might render a person's existing capabilities obsolete. The industrial age has generated fear in many workers, of being replaced by a machine. When new technology is on the horizon, people tend to argue that it is inappropriate, inaccurate, or a poor substitute for what it is replacing.

Yet when the new technology eventually gains acceptance, art does not disappear. It simply takes another form. The x-ray, CAT-scan and MRI did not obliterate the art of diagnosis. These advances merely enabled Physicians to practice their art on a higher plane, with more information, precision, and certainty of positive outcomes. Similarly, as therapeutic programs, procedures, and assessment protocols become more statistically or algorithmically driven, Therapists will simply apply their art on a higher plane, using new quantitative tools to amplify their capabilities to deliver successful outcomes with greater certainty.

As outcome studies target the most effective prevention and rehabilitation programs and procedures, consensus will broaden as to the best approaches, and Industrial Therapy components and procedures will become increasingly standardized.

There are currently many vendors and providers offering different approaches to Job Placement Assessment, Job Analysis, Functional Capacity Assessment,

Education and Training, Ergonomics, Work Conditioning, and Work Hardening. In marketing these products and services, vendors and providers must convince prospects that their approaches are the best, and that the points of difference offered by competitors are inferior. Since companies are driven by numbers and the bottom line, they will naturally gravitate toward those with the most reliable, statistically valid support for their approach. Accordingly, vendors will seek progressively greater statistical precision in tracking and analyzing their outcomes. As this process proceeds, the "best way" will become more tightly specified, and products, protocols, programs, and treatment procedures will become increasingly standardized.

> *As standardization progresses, equipment, programs, and procedures will become more easily "cookie cuttered," and national networks will spring up to mass produce, mass market, and nationally implement Industrial Therapy services, especially in the case of multi-site corporations.*

It is just a matter of time before the accumulating body of outcome studies begins to establish standards for performing Job Analysis, administering Job Placement Assessments and Functional Capacity Assessments, and equipping, staffing, and implementing Employee Fitness, Education and Training, Work Conditioning, Work Hardening, and other prevention and treatment programs. It is also just a matter of time before enterprising people propose to large corporations that implementation of these "best approaches" are established uniformly, at all corporate locations through geographically dispersed networks or alliances of Industrial Therapy providers.

Such networks may be initiated by manufacturers of therapy equipment in order to use the promise of corporate referrals as incentives for Industrial Therapists to buy their equipment. These relationships will evolve into mutually beneficial marketing partnerships.

Alternatively, networks may be formed by nationally-based prevention or rehabilitation consultants, or as subsidiaries of multi-site health care provider organizations.

Once networks are established, it will not be long before they begin offering their services to locally based firms, using their large corporate client list to establish credibility and help close the sale. For this reason, locally based, independent Industrial Therapy practices should watch this potential trend closely, and be on the lookout for opportunities to affiliate. Otherwise, they may be effectively locked out of the marketplace long term.

> *Standardization will enable nontherapist staff to increasingly assume functions that were once the exclusive realm of Therapists, just as paramedical and nursing staff have taken on an increasing number of functions that Physicians used to perform.*

As equipment, protocols, and processes become more standardized, the knowledge and experience required to make moment-to-moment judgments and decisions in some functions will be less necessary. For example, many Functional Capacity Assessments systems have developed standardized protocols that do not require administration by fully degreed Therapists. Analysis and reporting is performed through computerized algorithms. The advantages of standardization in this example are that the Industrial Therapy practice can offer a reduced price, or make a larger margin on assessments, while freeing experienced Therapists to focus on areas that require more expertise, and acquire higher fees.

> *The employer–employee relationship will become less adversarial as both sides realize the long term advantages of win–win outcomes that preserve the organization's competitive position—and hence the worker's job—in the global arena.*

Scarcely a week passes without an announcement of major layoffs at another large and formerly prosperous American corporation. This has fueled a great deal of concern among workers across the US, and they are increasingly willing to do whatever it takes to strengthen their employer's position in the global economy. As a result, corporations are obtaining heretofore unheard of wage and benefit concessions from their workers. At the same time, to strengthen commitment and productivity, employers are extending to employees greater "ownership" in decision making and rewards.

It is inevitable that this more cooperative relationship will permeate Industrial Therapy. Employers will increasingly recognize the advantages in morale and productivity of corporate-wide commitment and funding of employee fitness, safety education, ergonomics, and other prevention programs. When a worker becomes injured, return-to-work rehabilitation will increasingly be the preferred path over termination and replacement; both for long term cost and productivity considerations, and the positive signal it sends to the workforce regarding the company's commitment to its people.

Workers know that Workers' Compensation, litigation, and health care costs threaten their company's financial health and hence their job, therefore they will be more likely to reinforce a commitment to the company's prevention and rehabilitation programs.

Workers will also put pressure on injured peers if they try to exploit the system at the expense of the company's financial position.

| *Providers offering the convenience of delivering services at the employer's locations, will have a competitive advantage both in market preference and also in financial return on investment.*

As productivity continues to be the key to global competitiveness, employers will be increasingly sensitive to every hour an employee spends away from productive activity. Moreover, simulating actual job functions and working environment is gaining growing recognition as an important prerequisite to optimize prevention and rehabilitation. For both of these reasons, on-site Industrial Therapy services will become progressively more attractive to employers. Therapists who can deliver services on-site will gain a competitive advantage.

Equipment and materials that can be made mobile, such as Job Placement Assessment and Functional Capacity Assessment systems, will be brought to employers' locations. Employers providing on-site clinics, assessment stations, classrooms, fitness centers, and work simulation capabilities will be a competitive advantage for Industrial Therapy practices that can shed capital investment, overhead, and operating costs associated with providing services off-site.

| *Employers will comply with regulatory guidelines that benefit their long term bottom line, but will be forced by competitive necessity to circumvent those guidelines whose long term costs exceed the benefits.*

In some cases, regulations will cause employers to change in ways that actually benefit their long term bottom line. For example, certain OSHA safety and ergonomic regulations that effectively reduce injuries actually enhance the employer's profitability. In instances where this is true, firms that fully comply with such regulations will gain a long term competitive advantage over noncompliant firms.

In other cases, regulatory compliance costs will significantly exceed the offsetting benefits. One example might be the "reasonable accommodation" clause of the Americans with Disabilities Act (ADA). This clause compels employers to incur increased fixed and variable expenses to accommodate a disabled person without gaining a corresponding increases in productivity. Few would disagree with the laudable goal involved, and if every firm in the world complied with this regulation, the intended societal benefit would be realized with no adverse consequences.

But as often happens with regulations whose costs exceed bottom line benefits, certain firms will find ways to circumvent the requirements, as will foreign competitors who are not subject to similar laws. These noncompliant firms will gain competitive advantages over those that comply.

As a result, whether in connection with the ADA or other regulations, there may be as much demand for Industrial Therapy services to help companies tokenly comply with certain regulations as there may be for facilitating good faith compliance.

| *As the incidence of injuries is reduced, Industrial Therapists will evolve from providers of injury treatment to consultants and facilitators in employee wellness and productivity, with increasing focus on capability monitoring, case review, regulatory compliance, and bottom line outcomes.*

As outcome studies persuade more and more employers to fund and implement companywide employee fitness, education and training, safety, ergonomic, and other prevention measures, the incidence of injuries and the demand for rehabilitation services will inevitably subside. In the wake, however, will be a multiplicity of programs that require on-going supervision, monitoring, and adjustment in response to new outcome studies and technology. There will be growing demand for "audit assessments"—periodic functional assessments of workers on the job to ensure they are maintaining job requirement capabilities.

In addition, regulatory compliance will increasingly require Therapists' expertise in matters such as reviewing OSHA Logs, performing Workers' Compensation case review, and determining essential job functions for purposes of ADA compliance.

Firms that stay abreast of the best approaches to wellness, productivity, and regulatory compliance will gain competitive advantages over firms lagging behind in these spheres. And Industrial Therapists will be called upon to assume an ever-expanding role in managing companies' efforts in these fundamental areas.

In summary, it is important for everyone involved in Industrial Therapy to anticipate future trends as much as possible. But effective long range planning involves more than simply extrapolating trends and preparing for what might seem inevitable. It also involves envisioning the future, and then taking steps to bring that imagined future into being.

Perhaps the most important priority in every provider's imagined future is that the patient or client should always be given care based on the best long term outcome, not the least possible short term cost. And the most effective way this goal can be achieved is by generating reliable, reproducible outcome studies that provide the statistical proof and bottom line justification for programs and procedures. At the same time, the intensifying focus on outcomes, standardization, networks, and alliances should not be viewed as infringements on Therapist's traditional territory, but as tools that increase the Therapist's ability to successfully meet the needs of workers, employers, and insurers.

In addition, efforts must always be directed at achieving win-win outcomes for all concerned. No party to a process can maintain an unreasonable advantage for long. The fluidity of the marketplace has shortened the lifespan of unfair leverage. The best approach to the future, therefore, is to be open minded, receptive to change, committed to mutually beneficial goals, and dedicated to achieving increasingly higher levels of excellence.

INDEX